SCAI
Interventional Cardiology
Board Review Book

SCAI
Interventional Cardiology
Board Review Book

Edited by

Morton J. Kern, MD

University California Irvine
Orange, California

Associate Editors

Peter B. Berger, MD

Geisinger Center for Health Research
Danville, Pennsylvania

Peter C. Block, MD

Emory University Hospital
Atlanta, Georgia

Lloyd W. Klein, MD

Rush Medical College
Melrose Park, Illinois

Warren K. Laskey, MD

University of New Mexico Hospital
Albuquerque, New Mexico

Barry F. Uretsky, MD

University of Texas Medical Branch
Galveston, Texas

⊞. Lippincott Williams & Wilkins
a Wolters Kluwer business

Philadelphia · Baltimore · New York · London
Buenos Aires · Hong Kong · Sydney · Tokyo

Acquisitions Editor: Fran DeStefano
Developmental Editor: Rebeca Barroso
Production Editor: Dave Murphy
Manufacturing Manager: Kathleen Brown
Marketing Manager: Angela Panetta
Designer Coordinator: Doug Smock
Compositor: TechBooks
Printer: Edwards Brothers

Library of Congress Cataloging-in-Publication Data

SCAI interventional cardiology board review book / edited by Morton
    J. Kern ; associate editors, Peter B. Berger . . . [et al.].
      p. ; cm.
    Includes bibliographical references and index.
    ISBN-13: 978-0-7817-6197-0 (alk. paper)
    ISBN-10: 0-7817-6197-2 (alk. paper)
    1. Heart–Diseases–Treatment.   2. Heart–Surgery.   3. Angioplasty.
4. Cardiac catheterization.   I. Kern, Morton J.   II. Society of
Cardiac Angiography and Intervention.   III. Title: Interventional
cardiology board review book.
    [DNLM: 1. Cardiovascular Surgical Procedures–Examination
Questions. 2. Diagnostic Techniques, Cardiovascular–Examination
Questions.   WG 18.2 S278 2007]
RC683.8.S32 2007
616.1′20076–dc22   2006030567

Care has been taken to confirm the accuracy of the information presented and to describe generally accepted practices. However, the authors, editors, and publisher are not responsible for errors or omissions or for any consequences from application of the information in this book and make no warranty, expressed or implied, with respect to the currency, completeness, or accuracy of the contents of the publication. Application of this information in a particular situation remains the professional responsibility of the practitioner.

The authors, editors, and publisher have exerted every effort to ensure that drug selection and dosage set forth in this text are in accordance with current recommendations and practice at the time of publication. However, in view of ongoing research, changes in government regulations, and the constant flow of information relating to drug therapy and drug reactions, the reader is urged to check the package insert for each drug for any change in indications and dosage and for added warnings and precautions. This is particularly important when the recommended agent is a new or infrequently employed drug.

Some drugs and medical devices presented in this publication have Food and Drug Administration (FDA) clearance for limited use in restricted research settings. It is the responsibility of the health care provider to ascertain the FDA status of each drug or device planned for use in their clinical practice.

To purchase additional copies of this book, call our customer service department at (800) 638-3030 or fax orders to (301) 223-2320. International customers should call (301) 223-2300.

Visit Lippincott Williams & Wilkins on the Internet: http://LWW.com. Lippincott Williams & Wilkins customer service representatives are available from 8:30 am to 6 pm, EST.

10 9 8 7 6 5 4 3 2 1

Preface

Nowhere in medicine is there a more dynamic and rapidly changing body of knowledge and practice than in interventional cardiology. In 1999, the first ABIM Board Certification Examination for Interventional Cardiology was given. To prepare for this first board examination, the Society of Cardiac Angiography and Intervention (SCAI) teamed up with the American College of Cardiology. The review courses were initiated in August of that year and have been conducted every year after. Although this field has grown substantially and matured to a point, there is no single, collective work regarding the general material needed to review and help study for the Interventional Cardiology Board Examination.

The purpose of this book to provide a review of the general background information needed for the current and future practitioners of interventional cardiology. Well-known studies addressing current practice and guidelines are now incorporated into the field and comprise the bulk of material to be tested on any board certification examination. In view of the ever-expanding scope of interventional cardiology, we have attempted to cover the major topics as provided in the outline describing the ABIM certifying examination.

From basic to clinical science, the expert contributors have discussed and reviewed what are considered the most important aspects of the topics. Of course, much more could have been, or, perhaps, should have been, included in this first edition, and a question and answer section remains under development. We hope to improve on these shortfalls in the subsequent editions. Because of the need for continuing education of interventional cardiologists, the SCAI has always found it an enjoyable duty to take a leading role this area. We believe this book, in particular, exemplifies this role.

Acknowledgments

The coeditors and contributors for this book have been selected for their dedication and diligence in their fields. Many of the contributors are members of the SCAI Early Career Interventional Committee and reflect their competence and commitment in their contribution to the SCAI Review Book. It is the hope of the SCAI that all interventional cardiologists will benefit from this book and that the mission of the SCAI to provide interventional cardiology with high quality education for the advancement of patient care is accomplished.

The editor and coeditors wish to thank the contributors, the SCAI Board of Trustees and membership, and the publishers for their efforts in making this a helpful and rewarding review text. I include some of the thoughts of the coeditors, the SCAI president, and the chair of the Education Committee below.

On a personal note, I am ever indebted to my colleagues and friends in the SCAI and especially thank my coeditors who made this work possible. The SCAI plays a unique role in the life of a cardiologist. It had been apparent to me before but never more so after my sojourn out of university practice that the SCAI fills a vital need in a community cardiologist's life, and that it is as a stable resource for communication, education and professional support. I also thank my wife, Margaret, and daughter, Anna Rose, as we travel together to new personal and professional heights.

MORTON J. KERN, MD, FACC, FSCAI, FAHA
EDITOR IN CHIEF,
SCAI Interventional Board Review Book
SEPTEMBER 1, 2006

The curriculum for interventional cardiology has entered an exponential growth phase since the first SCAI Board Review course. The individual contributors to this volume deserve our utmost appreciation for it is they who strived to keep abreast of the "evidence" even as they were writing their chapters. It made our job that much easier.

WARREN K. LASKEY, MD, FACC, FSCAI
ASSOCIATE EDITOR,
SCAI Interventional Board Review Book

For my patients, who motivate me daily.
For my students, past and present, who challenge me constantly.

And for Barbara, who makes it all possible.

LLOYD W. KLEIN, MD FACC, FSCAI
ASSOCIATE EDITOR,
SCAI Interventional Board Review Book

The rapid pace of advances in interventional cardiology continues without pause. Even the "basics" of the subject require an update. This book fills that important need. I am honored to be part of the effort, particularly as it has provided me the opportunity to work with one of the long-time premier educators in invasive cardiology, Dr Morton Kern. I hope the reader finds the result as rewarding as I have in working on this project.

BARRY F. URETSKY, MD FACC, FSCAI
ASSOCIATE EDITOR,
SCAI Interventional Board Review Book

A major part of the SCAI mission statement focuses on education. In our field, this translates into an objective that reaches far beyond a simple didactic exercise; education in interventional cardiology is what we bring into the lab every day, and it yields solutions to cognitive and technical procedure problems, and, ultimately, to better outcomes. This book provides an important contribution to serving that mission.

TED FELDMAN, CHAIR
EDUCATION COMMITTEE,
BOARD OF TRUSTEES,
SOCIETY OF CARDIAC ANGIOGRAPHY
AND INTERVENTION

Like many who will read this, I acquired my training in percutaneous coronary intervention in an "on-the-job" fashion years before the first board examination in 1999. The field of interventional cardiology continues to change rapidly and those who passed that first board examination will soon face recertification. The SCAI is proud to offer this book to busy-practicing interventional cardiologists facing recertification and to those taking the examination for the first time. The society is committed to providing high-quality educational offerings to our profession and the *SCAI Interventional Board Review Book* is a prime example of that commitment.

GREGORY J. DEHMER, MD, FSCAI, FACC, FAHA, FACP
PRESIDENT,
SOCIETY FOR CARDIOVASCULAR ANGIOGRAPHY
AND INTERVENTIONS

Contributors

Joseph D. Babb, MD, FACC, FSCAI
Professor of Medicine
Department of Internal Medicine, Division of Cardiology
East Carolina University Brody School of Medicine
Director, Cardiac Catheterization Laboratories
Pitt County Memorial Hospital
Greenville, North Carolina

Thomas M. Bashore, MD, FACC, FSCAI
Professor of Medicine
Division of Cardiovascular Medicine
Duke University
Director, Cardiology Fellowship Training Program
Duke University Medical Center
Durham, North Carolina

Peter B. Berger, MD, FACC
Associate Chief Research Officer
Interventional Cardiologist
Geisinger Center for Health Research
Geisinger Health System
Danville, Pennsylvania

Peter C. Block, MD, FACC, FSCAI
Professor of Medicine/Cardiology
Director, Clinical Trials Office
Emory University Hospital
Emory School of Medicine
Atlanta, Georgia

Qi-Ling Cao, MD
Pediatric Cardiologist
Director of Echocardiographic Research Laboratory
University of Chicago
Chicago, Illinois

Charles J. Davidson, MD
Professor of Medicine
Department of Cardiology
Northwestern University
Chief, Cardiac Catheterization Laboratories
Northwestern Memorial Hospital
Chicago, Illinois

Larry S. Dean, MD, FSCAI, FACC
Professor of Medicine and Surgery
University of Washington School of Medicine
Director
UW Medicine Regional Heart Center
Seattle, Washington

John S. Douglas Jr., MD, FACC, FSCAI
Professor
Department of Medicine
Emory University School of Medicine
Director
Interventional Cardiology
Emory University Hospital
Atlanta, Georgia

James D. Flaherty, MD
Assistant Professor of Medicine
Interventional Cardiology
Northwestern University
Chicago, Illinois

Hussam N. Hamdalla, MD
Assistant Professor of Medicine
Division of Cardiovascular Medicine
University of Kentucky
Lexington, Kentucky

Robert A. Harrington, MD, FACC, FSCAI
Professor of Medicine
Department of Medicine
Duke University Medical Center
Director, Cardiovascular Clinical Trials
Duke Clinical Research Institute
Durham, North Carolina

Ziyad M. Hijazi, MD, MPH, FSCAI
George M. Eisenberg Professor
Department of Pediatrics and Medicine
Section of Pediatric Cardiology
University of Chicago
Chicago, Illinois

John McB. Hodgson, MD, FSCAI
Professor of Medicine
Chief, Academic Cardiology
St. Joseph's Hospital and Medical Center
Phoenix, Arizona

Ralf J. Holzer, MD, MSc
Assistant Director
Cardiac Catheterization & Interventional Therapy
The Heart Center, Columbus Children's Hospital
Assistant Professor of Pediatrics
Cardiology Division
The Ohio State University
Columbus, Ohio

Kenneth W. Kenyon, PharmD, BCPS

Clinical Instructor, University of Washington
    School of Pharmacy
Clinical Pharmacist, Cardiology
University of Washington Medical Center
Seattle, Washington

Morton J. Kern, MD, FSCAI, FAHA, FACC

Associate Chief Cardiology
Director Clinical Affairs
Department of Cardiology
University of California Irvine
Orange, California

Lloyd W. Klein, MD, FSCAI, FACC, FACP

Professor of Medicine
Rush Medical College
Chicago, Illinois

Arun Kuchela, MD, FRCPC, FACC

Assistant Professor of Medicine
Division of Cardiology
University of Washington
Seattle, Washington

Alexandra J. Lansky, MD, FACC, FSCAI

Associate Professor of Medicine
Director of Clinical Services,
    Center for Interventional Vascular Therapy
Columbia University Medical Center
Director of Angiographic Core Lab,
    Cardiovascular Research Foundation
New York, New York

Warren K. Laskey, MD, FSCAI

Professor
Department of Medicine
University of New Mexico School of Medicine
Chief
Division of Cardiology
University of New Mexico School of Medicine
Albuquerque, New Mexico

Michael J. Lim, MD, FACC

Assistant Professor of Medicine and
Director, Cardiac Catheterization Laboratory
Saint Louis University
St. Louis, Missouri

Michael J. Lipinski, MD

Medical College of Virginia Campus
Virginia Commonwealth University
Richmond, Virginia

Timothy A. Mixon, MD, FACC, FSCAI

Assistant Professor of Medicine,
    Texas A&M University System Health
Science Center
Interventional Cardiology, Scott & White Hospital
Temple, Texas

David J. Moliterno, MD, FACC

Chief, Division of Cardiovascular Medicine
Department of Internal Medicine
University of Kentucky
Medical Director
Gill Heart Institute
University of Kentucky Chandler Medical Center
Lexington, Kentucky

Douglass A Morrison, MD, PhD, FACC

Director, Cardiac Catheterization Laboratories, SAVAHCS
Professor of Medicine
University of Arizona
Tucson, Arizona

Kristen K. Patton, MD

Assistant Professor
University of Washington Medical Center
Division of Cardiology
Seattle, Washington

Karen S. Pieper, MD

Senior Statistician - DCRI
Statistical Manager - Clinical Trials Manuscripts
Duke Clinical Research Institute
Durham, North Carolina

Cody G. Pietras, BA

Cardiovascular Research Foundation
New York, New York

Michael Ragosta, MD, FSCAI

University Virgina Charlottesville
Charlottesville, Virgina

Bipin Ravindran, MD, MPH

Cardiology Fellow, Division of Cardiology
University of Washington
Seattle, Washington

Mark J. Ricciardi, MD

Associate Professor of Medicine
University of New Mexico School of Medicine
Director, Cardiac Catheterization Laboratories
    and Interventional Cardiology
University of New Mexico Health Sciences Center
Director, Interventional Cardiology
    and Cardiac Catheterization Labs
Albuquerque, New Mexico

Joel D. Robbins, MD
Interventional Cardiology Fellow
Northwestern University
Feinberg School of Medicine
Division of Cardiology
Chicago, Illinois

Campbell Rogers, MD
Associate Professor of Medicine
Harvard Medical School
Cambridge, Massachusetts

Timothy A. Sanborn, MD, FACC, FSCAI
Head, Division of Cardiology
Department of Medicine
Evanston Northwestern Healthcare
Professor of Medicine
Northwestern University
Feinberg School of Medicine
Evanston, Illinois

Daniel I Simon, MD
Chief
Division of Cardiovascular Medicine
Director
Heart & Vascular Institute
University Hospitals-Case Medical Center
Herman K. Hellerstein Professor of Medicine
Case Western Reserve University School
    of Medicine
Cleveland, Ohio

Leo Slavin, MD
Resident Physician, David Geffen School of Medicine at UCLA
Department of Medicine
UCLA Center for Health Sciences
Los Angeles, California

Jonathan M. Tobis, MD, FACC
Professor of Medicine
David Geffen School of Medicine at UCLA
Director of Interventional Cardiology Research
UCLA Medical Center
Los Angeles, California

Carl Tomasso, MD, FACC, FSCAI
Chicago, Illnois

Barry F. Uretsky, MD, FACC, FSCAI
Professor of Medicine
Chief Division of Cardiology
University of Texas Medical Branch
Galveston, Texas

George W. Vetrovec, MD, FACC
Chief, Cardiovascular Medicine
Virginia Commonwealth University
Richmond, Virginia

Frederick GP Welt, MS, MD
Director, Cardiac Catheterization Laboratory
St. Elizabeth's Medical Center
Boston, Massachusetts

Christopher J. White, MD, FACC, FSCAI
Chairman, Department of Cardiology
Ochsner Clinic Foundation
New Orleans, Louisiana

Contents

Basic Science

Peter B. Berger

CHAPTER 1

Arterial Disease—Atherosclerosis

Frederick GP Welt, Campbell Rogers, and Daniel I. Simon

Atherosclerosis

There is increasing understanding of the molecular and cellular pathophysiology of the vascular responses to injury, whether from the sustained effects of hyperlipidemia leading to atherosclerosis, or the sudden impact of placement of a stainless steel stent under high pressure leading to restenosis. A common thread that links these events is an inflammatory response to injury and it is increasingly appreciated that the inflammatory process not only initiates these lesions, but often dictates their clinical presentation. A fundamental knowledge of these processes is necessary to understand the natural history of the disease processes that affect the patients who present to the catheterization laboratory and, in addition, to understand the consequences of the therapies employed during coronary intervention. This chapter is therefore designed to describe the known pathophysiology of atherosclerosis, the conversion of stable atherosclerotic plaques to ones that cause acute coronary syndromes, the pathophysiology of restenosis emphasizing the differences between balloon- and stent-induced injury, and how vascular remodeling influence these processes.

Atherosclerosis: A Response to Injury

Atherosclerosis is a chronic inflammatory disease initiated and sustained by injury to the vascular wall (1). Largely through extensive epidemiologic studies, several injurious processes have been identified (Table 1–1). These include metabolic conditions such as sustained exposure to low density lipoprotein (LDL), hyperglycemia associated with diabetes, and hyperhomocysteinemia. However, other factors including physical (hypertensive changes in shear stress), environmental (tobacco smoke), and possibly infectious (Chlamydia Pneumoniae) processes have also been implicated. The common thread of injury to the vessel wall is an inflammatory response that involves a complex and still incompletely understood sequence of interactions between endothelial and smooth muscle cells, leukocytes, and platelets. These cells and their secreted growth factors and cytokines combine with lipid and components of the vessel wall to eventually form the mature atherosclerotic plaque. The central role of inflammation in the pathogenesis of atherosclerosis is evidenced by numerous epidemiologic studies that demonstrate a correlation between circulating markers of inflammation (e.g., fibrinogen, C-reactive protein [CRP], serum amyloid protein, myeloperoxidase) with subsequent risk of coronary events (2,3).

Atherosclerosis: Pathogenesis

There are several key biologic events involved in atherogenesis; extracellular lipid accumulation, leukocyte recruitment, foam cell formation, neointimal growth as a result of smooth muscle cell migration and proliferation and extracellular matrix deposition, and vessel remodeling (Fig. 1–1).

Extra- and Intra-Cellular Lipid Accumulation

The key event in the creation of the incipient atherosclerotic lesion is the accumulation of lipoproteins within the intima. These lipoproteins may subsequently be modified by processes such as oxidation, and glycation in the presence of aging and hyperglycemia. The modification of these lipoproteins helps to illicit a cascade of molecular and cellular events including stimulation of growth factor and cytokine production from endothelial and smooth muscle cells. These early events lead to recruitment of leukocytes and eventually to smooth muscle cell proliferation and migration, all of which act to form the mature atherosclerotic plaque. Of central importance is the understanding that hyperlipidemia is an inflammatory state. The interaction between inflammation and hyperlipidemia is evident in the presence of foam cells, the hallmark of the fatty streak, which is the initial lesion of atherosclerosis. The foam cell is a macrophage named for the abundance of lipid within the cell. Macrophages bind and internalize modified lipoprotein particles via a number of "scavenger receptors" including scavenger receptor-A family members, CD36, and macrosialin. Foam cells are able to further modify lipoproteins. In addition, lipoproteins can prove toxic to macrophages leading to necrotic debris and free cholesterol clefts and ester within the lesion. This necrotic debris, along with the expression of the tissue factor and other molecules, leads to a very pro-thrombotic environment within the plaque and is a serious threat to local blood flow in the setting of loss of integrity of the barrier between plaque and blood stream.

Table 1–1

Causes of Vascular Injury

Metabolic
- Hyperlipidemia
- Hyperglycemia
- Hyperhomocysteinemia

Physical
- Shear forces (hypertension)
- Laminar versus nonlaminar flow (i.e., bifurcations)

Environmental
- Tobacco Smoke

Infectious
- Chlamydia
- Herpes Simplex
- Cytomegalovirus

Leukocyte Recruitment

Leukocytes, especially macrophages, play pivotal roles in atherosclerosis through their release of critical cytokines and growth factors that influence not only atherogenesis, but also influence processes of plaque rupture and thrombosis. The process of leukocyte recruitment, attachment, and migration into the plaque is under the influence of a variety of molecules. As a response to injury, such as the accumulation of lipoproteins, endothelial cells express certain adhesion molecules such as e-selectin, which interact with ligands on the surface of circulating leukocytes to begin a process of loose association and rolling along the surface of the vessel (4). Subsequent tight binding mediated by the integrin class of adhesion molecules stops the leukocyte prior to the process of diapedesis. Although their pathologic role is uncertain, soluble forms of cell adhesion molecules (CAMs) can be found in plasma. Human studies have demonstrated that plasma levels of ICAM-1 and E-selectin correlate with clinical manifestations of coronary atherosclerosis (5).

Also central to recruitment of leukocytes to areas of vascular injury, chemokines are a group of chemoattractant cytokines produced by a variety of somatic cells including smooth muscle cells, endothelial cells, and leukocytes. One important chemokine of the C-C class, monocyte chemoattractant protein-1 (MCP-1), participates in the recruitment of monocytes in particular (6). Also critical is the C-X-C chemokine, interleukin-8 (IL-8), which participates in the recruitment of leukocytes to areas of vascular injury. IL-8 has been extensively documented in the recruitment of neutrophils (7), and more recent evidence suggests that the murine analogue of IL-8, KC also plays a critical role in the recruitment of monocytes to injured areas (8).

Several types of leukocytes can be identified within advanced human plaques that include macrophages and T-lymphocytes. However, the monocyte is thought to be the first leukocyte recruited to the incipient atheroma. As lesions mature, there tends to be excess accumulation of leukocytes at the "shoulder" regions of plaques where the eccentric plaque

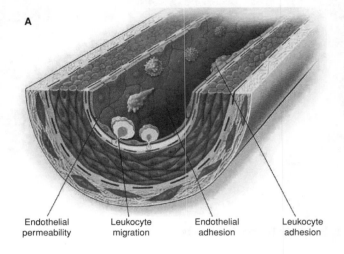

A

Endothelial permeability | Leukocyte migration | Endothelial adhesion | Leukocyte adhesion

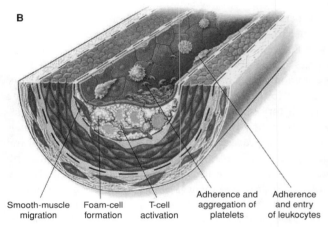

B

Smooth-muscle migration | Foam-cell formation | T-cell activation | Adherence and aggregation of platelets | Adherence and entry of leukocytes

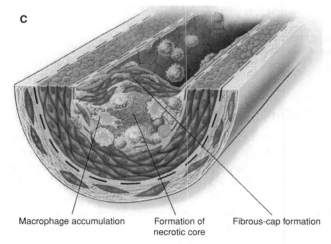

C

Macrophage accumulation | Formation of necrotic core | Fibrous-cap formation

Figure 1–1.

Stages of atherosclerotic plaque growth. **A:** Initial stage of atherosclerosis involves injury to the vessel wall with subsequent expression of inflammatory adhesion molecules, which leads to leukocyte recruitment. **B:** Intermediate lesions involve macrophages imbibing oxidized LDL leading to foam cell formation. There is continued leukocyte recruitment, formation of an early lipid core, and SMC proliferation and migration. **C:** The advanced or mature atherosclerotic plaque consists of a necrotic lipid core with foam cells, necrotic debris, and free cholesterol esters. In addition, there is a fibrous cap consisting of SMCs and extracellular matrix. (From: Ross R. *Atherosclerosis—An Inflammatory Disease. N Engl J Med.* 1999;340:115–126, with permission.)

merges with the more normal architecture of the vessel. This clustering is thought to make these "shoulder" regions more vulnerable to the consequences of atherosclerosis (9). In addition it has long been observed that atherosclerotic lesions develop preferentially at areas of bifurcations within the coronary tree. This likely is related to disturbances in flow patterns and resultant areas of flow separation and altered shear stress leading to preferential areas of upregulation of adhesion molecules and increased leukocyte recruitment.

Smooth Muscle Migration, Proliferation, and Extracellular Matrix Deposition

Smooth muscle cells and their products are responsible for giving structure to the mature atherosclerotic plaque which is, at first, little more than a collection of lipids and foam cells. Under the influence of growth factors and chemoattractants such as platelet derived growth factor and thrombin, smooth muscle cells migrate out from the media into the neointima where they begin to proliferate. In addition, SMC's produce extracellular matrix constituents including collagen, proteoglycans, elastin, fibrin(ogen), fibronectin, and vitronectin. These proteins often account for a substantial volume of the plaque and are important in determining the structural integrity of the fibrous cap. In some patients, an additional process of mineralization of the atherosclerotic plaque will occur with deposition of calcium and osteopontin. Although of uncertain biologic and prognostic significance, mineralization is of particular interest to the interventional cardiologist as it may influence technical aspects of the procedure.

Plaque Angiogenesis

A newly emerging area of interest to is the potential role of angiogenesis in plaque growth and in the pathogenesis of atherosclerotic complications (10). New vasculature, under the influence of angiogenic growth factors, may grow from the vaso vasorum within the adventitia into the plaque. These vessels may be disrupted and cause plaque hemorrhage independent of plaque rupture. In addition, analogous to tumor growth,

these vessels may stimulate plaque growth. There is experimental evidence demonstrating inhibition of plaque growth by angiogenic inhibitors in a mouse model of atherosclerosis (10).

The Mature Atherosclerotic Plaque

The mature atherosclerotic plaque is therefore composed of several components including a fibrous cap consisting of SMCs and extracellular matrix proteins overlying a necrotic lipid core consisting of free cholesterol esters, foam cells, other leukocytes such as T-cells, and necrotic debris of dead foam cells (Fig. 1–1). These plaques commonly are eccentric in nature and there is heterogeneity in terms of the thickness of the cap as well as distribution of leukocytes that tend to cluster in shoulder regions. Both of these features have potential import in terms of propensity of plaques to cause acute coronary syndromes.

Vascular Remodeling

While angiography remains the mainstay of diagnosis in coronary artery disease, its major limitation is that it provides information only on luminal encroachment of lesions, not in architecture of the vessel wall. Use of intravascular ultrasound has provided a much broader understanding of the nature of atherosclerosis by allowing systematic investigation of plaque architecture not only at sites of flow-obstructing lesions but throughout the vessel. Although the interventional cardiologist is most concerned with focal obstructive lesions in proximal portions of the vessel, it is important to realize that it is now recognized that atherosclerosis is almost always universally present throughout the coronary tree. The amount of impingement of the plaque on the lumen is controlled not only by the growth of plaque volume but also on vascular remodeling. Vascular remodeling involves restructuring of cellular or noncellular components of the wall, and can occur under a variety of stimuli (11). For example, under situations of hypertension, muscle mass of the vessel wall can increase in order to normalize wall stress. In atherosclerosis, remodeling may consist of compensatory enlargement of the vessel to preserve luminal area (Fig. 1–2). Central to the process of vascular

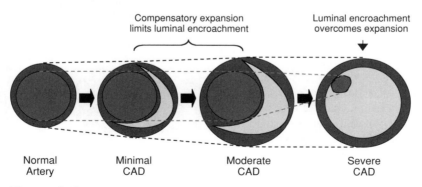

Figure 1–2.

Schematic of vascular remodeling. As the atherosclerotic lesions progresses, initial enlargement of the entire vessel allows preservation of luminal area. As atherosclerosis becomes severe, enlargement is overcome by progression of the atherosclerotic plaque and luminal area is compromised. (Adapted from: Glagov S., et al. *N Engl J Med.* 1987;316:1371–1375.)

remodeling are the matrix metalloproteinases (MMPs), a family of zinc dependent proteases which have been demonstrated to be upregulated in areas of vessel wall remodeling and are thought to play a central role also in plaque rupture (12).

Clinical Sequelae of Atherosclerosis

A convenient way of thinking about coronary artery disease is as a spectrum of syndromes from stable angina at one end associated with exertional angina and relatively benign outcomes to ST segment elevation MI at the other end associated with sudden complete thrombotic occlusion of an epicardial blood vessel and high rates of morbidity and mortality. The intermediate syndromes of unstable angina and non q-wave myocardial infarction exist between these two extremes. However, unstable angina, non q-wave MI and ST-segment elevation MI are collectively termed the acute coronary syndromes due to their similar pathophysiology and worse prognosis compared to stable angina. This is explained by the fact that complications from atherosclerosis can result from two related but distinct mechanisms: (a) simple luminal narrowing can lead to an imbalance between supply and demand for blood typically resulting in stable exertional angina, or (b) atheromatous plaques may rupture resulting in a thrombus of varying degrees of occlusion (13). Critical to the understanding of coronary disease is the knowledge that the propensity for thrombotic complications depends on a variety of vascular biologic factors, not the degree of stenosis.

Progressive Lumen Encroachment and Stable Angina

As atherosclerotic lesions grow in size and depending on the amount of compensatory vascular remodeling that occurs, they may gradually encroach upon the lumen of the vessel (Fig. 1–2). As a response to reduction in flow, there is vasodilation of the distal micro-circulation to increase in flow. This reduces coronary vascular reserve or the ability of the coronary circulation to increase blood flow in response to demand, which typically leads to exertional angina which is short in duration and relieved by rest. At what point luminal encroachment causes symptoms depends on many factors including the severity of the lesion, the demand of the distal cardiac bed, and the oxygen carrying capacity of the blood stream. However, in general, lesions begin to produce symptoms when they reach approximately 60% to 70% in diameter stenosis. Modern techniques of interrogating intra-coronary hemodynamics with flow and pressure wires have taught the interventional cardiologist that lesions with the same degree of angiographic stenosis may have very different hemodynamic consequences (14).

Plaque Rupture and Thrombosis and the Acute Coronary Syndromes

The historical view of the conversion of stable to acute coronary syndromes held that atherosclerotic lesions impinged upon the lumen of the vessel until some critical point was reached at

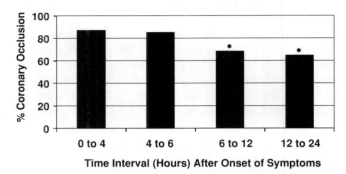

Prevalence of Total Coronary Occlusion

Figure 1–3.

Percent of vessels totally occluded in patients presenting after acute myocardial infarction as a function of time after onset of symptoms. (Adapted from: DeWood MA, et al. *N Engl J Med.* 1980;303:897–902, with permission.)

which either vasospasm or thrombosis in-situ developed to cause infarction. Considerable debate ensued as to whether thrombus found at autopsy was a premortem or postmortem phenomenon despite the fact that James Herrick had published his findings of thrombus as the predominant cause of sudden coronary obstruction in 1912 (15). The pivotal work was performed by DeWood, in his landmark 1980 paper (16), where he demonstrated angiographically that ST segment elevation was associated with occlusion of epicardial vessels (Fig. 1–3) and made the observation that thrombosis was present at the time of infarct. There is now considerable data to confirm this including autopsy studies (Fig. 1–4) as well as the use of angioscopy which has revealed the presence of visible thrombus associated with both unstable angina and acute myocardial infarction.

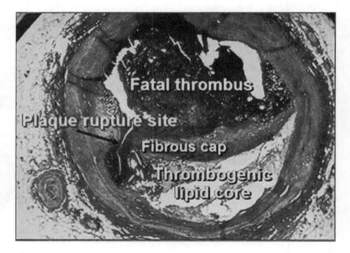

Figure 1–4.

Histologic example of a ruptured plaque with subsequent thrombosis leading to a fatal myocardial infarction. (From: Constantinides P. Plaque hemorrhages, their genesis and their role in supra-plaque thrombosis and atherogenesis. In: Glagov S, Newman WP III, Schaffer SA, eds. *Pathology of the Human Atherosclerotic Plaque.* New York: Springer-Verlag; 1990:393–411, with permission.)

Data from the early thrombolytic trials was instrumental in setting the stage for our modern understanding of acute coronary syndromes. As part of the design of these trials, patients presenting with acute MI underwent mandated angiography after randomization to either placebo or thrombolytic therapy. The angiograms revealed an unexpected finding, namely that the majority of lesions responsible for myocardial infarction were <50% in diameter stenosis (17). In addition, data from angiographic studies performed in patients before and after infarction show that mild and moderate stenoses may progress to cause myocardial infarction in a matter of weeks to months. In analysis of four serial angiographic studies, only ~15% of acute myocardial infarctions were found to arise from lesions with degrees of stenosis >60% on an antecedent angiogram (18) (Fig. 1–5). The implication of these data is that the vascular biologic state of the lesion is responsible for its propensity to cause an infarct, not the severity of stenosis. These data should not be misinterpreted to suggest that lesion severity is correlated with danger of infarction. Rather, noncritical lesions represent a larger population than critical lesions. In addition, as described earlier, compensatory enlargement of the vessel often accompanies atherosclerosis. Therefore, even mildly stenotic lesions may represent large plaques by volume. In summary, thrombosis, often on a noncritical stenosis, caused by lesion disruption causes the majority of myocardial infarctions.

The proximate event leading to thrombosis at a lesion is plaque rupture (or less commonly endothelial denudation) leading to exposure of blood to highly thrombotic subendothe-

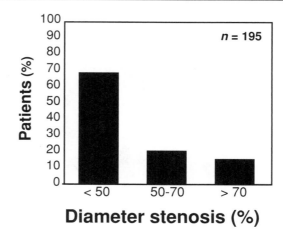

Figure 1–5.

Compiled data from 4 thrombolytic trials showing that the majority of underlying lesions responsible for acute myocardial infarction are less than 50% diameter stenosis. (From: Smith SC. *Circulation.* 1996;93:2205–2211, with permission.)

lial components of the plaque. Histologic studies have identified several features which appear to be associated with plaques more vulnerable to rupture. These include a thin fibrous cap, a large lipid core, and an abundance of inflammatory cells largely concentrated at the shoulder regions of the plaque (Fig. 1–6) (9). It is thought that inflammation is the key regulator of the structural integrity of the plaque.

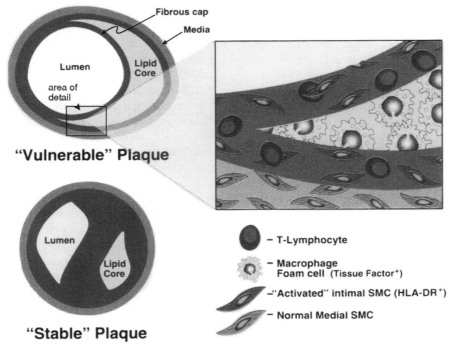

Figure 1–6.

Characteristics of stable vs. vulnerable plaques. Vulnerable plaques have thinner fibrous caps and larger, more inflammatory-cell-rich lipid cores. (From: Libby P. *Circulation.* 1995;91:2844–2850, with permission.)

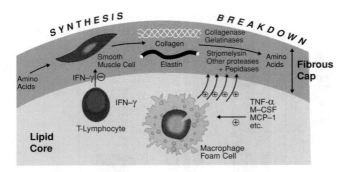

Figure 1–7.

Thickness of the fibrous cap is a balance between synthesis of extracellular matrix proteins by SMCs and the breakdown of these products by degradative enzymes. These processes are largely under the influence of inflammatory cells. (From: Libby P. *Circulation.* 1995;91:2844–2850, with permission.)

The structural integrity of the plaque is dependent on a balance between two components; smooth muscle cell mass and extracellular matrix content. In turn, smooth muscle cell mass is a balance between migration of cells from the media and subsequent proliferation in the neointima on the one hand, and cell death on the other. There is evidence to suggest that cytokines released from inflammatory cells control apoptosis, or programmed cell death (19). Extracellular matrix content is a balance between production from smooth muscle cells and degradation by a variety of proteases (Fig. 1–7). Production of extracellular matrix content is dependent on both the number of cells present and their activity. Activated T-cells in the plaque secrete interferon-γ (IFN-γ), an inhibitor of smooth muscle cell collagen synthesis. Inflammatory cells in atherosclerotic plaques also produce enzymes, such as matrix metalloproteinases and cathepsins, that are capable of degrading important constituents of the extracellular matrix (i.e., collagens, elastin) (9). Therefore, inflammatory cells can contribute to plaque weakening by decreasing smooth muscle cell mass, decreasing extracellular matrix content, and increasing extracellular matrix degradation.

How and why plaques rupture when they do is a subject of increasing study. It has long been observed that there is a circadian variation in presentation of myocardial infarction with a peak in the early morning hours (20). In addition, myocardial infarction rates are known to be effected by events that produce population wide stress as was observed after the Northridge earthquake in Southern California in 1994 (21). These observations have led researchers to suggest that cortisol and adrenaline levels may impact plaque rupture through there effects on systemic hemodynamic parameters. On a smaller scale, biomechanical studies utilizing finite element analysis indicate that rupture sites coincide with highest circumferential biomechanical forces. These are highest at the shoulder regions of plaques (22). Therefore, there is an interesting combination of both biochemical and biophysical characteristics that make rupture at the shoulder regions of plaques most likely. This is supported by histologic studies of coronary arteries of patients who died secondary to myocardial infarction.

While frank plaque rupture is the major antecedent cause of thrombotic complications of the acute coronary syndromes, other processes may also be responsible. Local superficial denudation of endothelial cells (perhaps secondary to apoptosis) may expose the internal elastic membrane representing an important thrombotic substrate. There is some evidence to suggest that these endothelial erosions occur more frequently in women and in diabetics. Mechanical injury during percutaneous coronary intervention is also another source of local plaque disruption which may lead to thrombotic complications.

The final pathway through which either plaque rupture or endothelial denudation lead to alterations in flow is through thrombosis. Exposure of blood to the lipid core is a potent stimulus for thrombus formation, largely on the basis of exposure to tissue factor associated with lipid-laden and necrotic macrophages. There is a balance between procoagulant-anticoagulant and fibrinolytic-antifibrinolytic factors in the blood stream which likely predetermines the consequence of any given plaque disruption. In the presence of an intact and robust fibrinolytic system, a mural thrombus might undergo rapid lysis, limiting its clinical consequences to unstable angina or non q-wave myocardial infarction. Similarly, patients on anti-platelet agents such as aspirin obviously are protected to some degree. In the presence of prothrombotic factors, such as elevated levels of fibrinogen or plasminogen activator inhibitor-1 (PAI-1), growth of a thrombus to occlusion may occur more frequently. Non-occlusive mural thrombus may be incorporated into the plaque during the process of healing, providing a mechanism for plaque growth.

There are numerous trials of anti-platelet therapy that corroborate the thrombotic paradigm of the acute coronary syndromes. Trials of lipid lowering therapy have similarly demonstrated an interesting corroboration of theories of plaque vulnerability. These trials have demonstrated marked reductions in subsequent coronary events associated with lipid lowering with essentially no change in lesion severity (18). As stated earlier, the hypothesis is that lipids within the plaque provide the critical initiating and sustaining inflammatory stimulus to plaque growth and rupture, and the beneficial actions of "statin" lipid-lowering agents may derive in part from the reduction of inflammation leading to stabilization of the fibrous cap and reduced thrombogenicity of the inner core. There is increasing evidence to support lipid lowering therapy as a vital adjunct to acute as well as chronic therapy for patients presenting with acute coronary syndromes.

A more complete understanding of the mechanisms of plaque rupture and the development of novel strategies to stabilize lesions represents a major goal of vascular biologists and clinical cardiologists. Complicating the clinical situation is the fact that many different lesions of varying vulnerable potential may coexist side by side in a vessel or throughout the coronary tree. Considerable interest exists in imaging techniques on both a macroscopic and molecular level to identify plaques most vulnerable to rupture in order to better prognosticate and direct therapy most effectively.

Restenosis

Gruntzig et al. ushered in the modern era of management of obstructive coronary artery disease with the introduction of coronary angioplasty. Yet, even in their first report on the subject (their 1,979 landmark publication "Non-operative dilatation of coronary-artery stenosis"), they found that 6 out of 32 patients undergoing successful initial angioplasty suffered restenosis, a rate of 19% (23). Large scale registries have since documented a restenosis rate closer to 33% (24). The clinical parameters that have been most closely associated with restenosis are final vessel diameter, lesion length, and presence of diabetes. Understanding of the pathophysiology of restenosis has evolved considerably over the last decade. Studies of human autopsy specimens revealed a fibrocellular response at sites of prior balloon angioplasty (25), whereas early animal studies revealed initial endothelial denudation, medial dissection, and platelet deposition as an immediate response to balloon injury, and described late restenosis as a consequence of smooth muscle cell (SMC) migration and proliferation as well as organized intraluminal thrombosis (26,27). Synthesizing the results of these studies and studies of wound healing, Forrester et al. proposed a paradigm for restenosis suggesting three phases in the process: (a) an inflammatory phase, (b) a granulation or cellular proliferation phase, and (c) a phase of remodeling involving extracellular matrix protein synthesis (28). As with atherogenesis, studies have revealed a critical role for inflammatory cells in the restenotic process. In addition, the thrombotic response to vascular injury imposed by coronary intervention appears to play a critical role in the initial recruitment of inflammatory cells. Coronary stenting, now performed in the majority of cases has a profound impact on the vascular biologic response to coronary intervention, particularly the impact on the inflammatory response and on vascular remodeling.

Neointimal Growth and Remodeling in Stent and Balloon Angioplasty Restenosis

Given the difficulty obtaining human restenotic tissue, our understanding of the pathophysiology is heavily dependent on imaging techniques such as intravascular ultrasound and animal models. Mintz et al. used intravascular ultrasound to determine the contributions of neointimal hyperplasia and negative remodeling after balloon angioplasty (29). They found that, although both negative remodeling (as measured by external elastic membrane area) and neointimal hyperplasia (as measured by plaque plus media cross sectional area) contributed to restenosis, negative remodeling contributed substantially more. In contrast, angiographic analysis of the first two large scale studies of coronary stents in humans (the STRESS [30] and BENESTENT [31] studies) revealed distinct differences between the pathophysiology of restenosis in balloon-injured and stented arteries. Arteries which received a stent experienced a much larger initial lumen gain, presumably due to the rigid scaffolding provided by the stent which prevents acute elastic recoil. At the 6-month follow-up, luminal area was greater and binary restenosis was less than balloon angio-

plastied arteries. However late loss (lumen immediately post minus lumen at follow-up) was actually greater in stented arteries. Therefore, stents cause greater neointimal growth, with their eventual benefit in restenosis attributable to their larger initial lumen gain and prevention of remodeling (Fig. 1–8). This was confirmed with a serial intravascular ultrasound study conducted by Hoffman and others (32).

Mechanisms of Leukocyte Recruitment and Infiltration

Expansion of a balloon or placement of a stent causes injury within the vessel wall including dissection, crush injury of SMCs, and de-endothelialization. Leukocyte recruitment and infiltration occur at these sites of injury where platelets and fibrin have been deposited. Within areas of injury, such as atherosclerotic and postangioplasty restenotic lesions, and in areas of ischemia-reperfusion injury, in vivo studies have shown that leukocytes and platelets are deposited together. For the inflammatory response after angioplasty, this interaction between platelets and leukocytes appears to be important (33,34).

This interaction has been explained by Diacovo et al. who have put forth a paradigm of leukocyte attachment to surface-adherent platelets followed by transmigration (35). As with atherosclerosis, the initial loose association of leukocytes is mediated through the selectin class of adhesion molecules (particularly by platelet P-selectin) (36) followed by their firm adhesion and trans-platelet migration, which are processes dependent on the integrin class of adhesion molecules (35). The β_2 integrin molecule Mac-1 (CD11b/CD18) is present on both neutrophils and monocytes and papers to be of central importance in leukocyte recruitment following vascular injury. In addition to promoting the accumulation of leukocytes at sites of vascular injury, the binding of platelets to neutrophils amplifies the inflammatory response by inducing neutrophil activation, upregulating cell adhesion molecule expression, and generating signals that promote integrin activation, and chemokine synthesis. These processes of activation may be mediated through the release of soluble CD40 ligand, a pro-inflammatory molecule stored most abundantly in platelets. Bolstering these data, both neutrophil-platelet and monocyte-platelet aggregates have been identified in the peripheral blood of patients with coronary artery disease and may be markers of disease activity and prognosis (37,38).

Evidence for a Role of Inflammation in Restenosis

Restenosis does not appear to be a case of accelerated atherosclerosis but rather a distinct temporal and pathophysiologic process. However, inflammation is an important common link between atherogenesis and restenosis. Observations in regards to restenosis have been hampered by the difficulty of obtaining human restenotic tissue. Farb et al. investigated stented arteries from pathologic samples of 116 stents from 87 patients >90 days postprocedure (39). They found a statistically significant association between extent of medial damage,

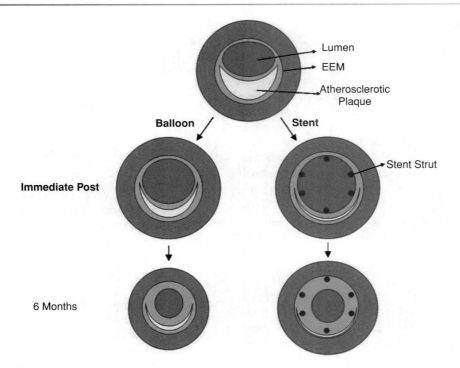

Figure 1–8.

Illustration of differences in mechanisms of restenosis between plain balloon angioplasty and stenting. In balloon angioplastied vessels, restenosis is caused by a combination of eointimal growth and negative remodeling. Stented arteries have lower rates of restenosis despite incurring greater neointimal growth due to their ability to achieve a larger initial lumen size, and the elimination of negative remodeling. (Adapted from: Welt FGP, Sobieszcczyk PS. Coronary artery stents: design and biologic considerations. *Cardiology.* 2003;9:9–14, with permission.)

inflammation, and restenosis. Also linking leukocytes and restenosis is data reported by Moreno et al. in which the authors present data from tissue retrieved from directional atherectomy at the time of angioplasty (40). They found a strong positive correlation between the number of macrophages present in the tissue at the time of angioplasty and subsequent risk of restenosis.

Systemic markers of inflammation following angioplasty have also provided insight into the mechanisms of restenosis. Neumann et al. investigated systemic inflammation utilizing a technique in which they collected blood samples both proximal to and just distal to the site of balloon dilatation in humans (41). Using flow cytometry to determine the expression of the neutrophil adhesion molecules L-selectin and CD11b, they found an upregulation of these markers of leukocyte activation after angioplasty measured as a gradient between distal and proximal specimens. Mickelson et al. were able to document upregulation of CD11b on both neutrophils and monocytes utilizing systemic venous specimens from patients undergoing angioplasty (42). They found that levels of CD11b had a positive correlation with adverse clinical events. Inoue et al. confirmed these data, demonstrating that elevated levels of neutrophil CD11b are predictive of future propensity for restenosis after balloon angioplasty (43) and stenting (44) (Fig. 1–9). Pietersma et al. showed that interleukin 1 production by stimulated monocytes isolated from blood pre-angioplasty

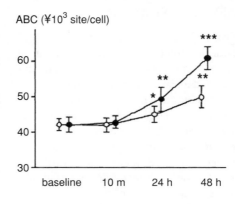

CD11b

ABC ($¥10^3$ site/cell)

-○- Patients without restenosis (n = 48)
-●- Patients with restenosis (n = 14)

Figure 1–9.

Serial changes in antibody-binding capacity (ABC) of CD11b after coronary stenting. Those patients with restenosis exhibit higher levels. *= $p < 0.05$, **= $p < 0.01$, ***= $p < 0.001$. (From: Inoue T, et al. *Circulation.* 2003;107:1757–1763, with permission.)

was correlated positively with late luminal loss while activation of granulocytes measured by CD66 levels was inversely correlated with late loss (45). Cipollone et al. demonstrated upregulated levels of MCP-1 following percutaneous intervention in humans and found that MCP-1 levels correlate with risk for restenosis (46). Gaspardone et al. showed a positive correlation between the nonspecific inflammatory marker C-reactive protein following stent placement and propensity for restenosis (47).

Animal models have been invaluable in elucidating basic cellular and molecular mechanisms of restenosis. In several experimental animal models, cell adhesion molecules critical for leukocyte recruitment have been found to be upregulated by an atherogenic diet (48–50), induction of diabetes (51), and increased shear stress (52). After balloon endothelial denudation in a rabbit model, vascular cell adhesion molecule-1, ICAM-1, and MHC class II antigens, all have been shown to be upregulated in a sustained fashion (53). A particularly potent inflammatory stimulus appears to be the implantation of a chronic indwelling endovascular stent leading to a brisk early inflammatory response with abundant surface adherent leukocytes of both monocyte and granulocyte lineage (54,55). Days and weeks later, macrophages invade the forming neointima and are observed clustering around stent struts often forming giant cells. Evidence of the importance of monocytes comes from studies utilizing blockade of early monocyte recruitment with antiinflammatory agents which result in reduced late neointimal thickening (54,56,57). In the stented rabbit iliac artery, a strong correlation exists between tissue monocyte number and neointimal area, suggesting a causal role for monocytes in restenosis (54). Activated macrophages may influence vascular repair through a variety of mechanisms including production of a variety of mediators, including members of the interleukin family, tumor necrosis factor, monocyte chemoattractant protein-1, and growth factors such as platelet derived growth factors, basic fibroblast growth factor, and heparin-binding epidermal growth factor (58).

Several studies have also shown infiltration of neutrophils within the arterial wall following vascular injury (59–61). As with macrophages, a concomitant reduction in neutrophil number and smooth muscle proliferation can be seen with administration of antiinflammatory agents resulting in less neointimal growth (55). The mechanisms by which neutrophils may affect vascular repair are not as fully understood as with monocytes/macrophages. While neutrophils are not typically thought to secrete growth factors, they can contribute to tissue injury through the release of reactive oxygen species and proteases (58). In addition, it has been reported that rabbit vascular smooth cells are stimulated to proliferate when co-cultured with neutrophils or neutrophil conditioned media (62). Neutrophils are also known to secrete cytokines including IL-1, TNF-alpha and IL-6 (63).

Differences Between Balloon and Stent Injury

Systematic investigation in both human and animal studies suggests important differences between vascular biologic responses to balloon- and stent-induced injury. Inoue et al. (64) used flow cytometry to measure CD11b (a member of the integrin family of adhesion molecules) expression on neutrophils following percutaneous coronary intervention and found substantially higher levels on neutrophils from patients undergoing stent implantation as compared to balloon angioplasty alone. This increased inflammatory response may help to explain the larger neointimal growth seen in stented arteries.

Animal studies have also demonstrated differences in response to vascular injury between balloon-angioplastied and stented arteries. Heparin, an archetypal modulator of vascular repair in animal models, has long been known to reduce neointimal growth following vascular injury (65,66). Heparin is equally effective at reducing neointimal hyperplasia following balloon injury or stent implantation (67,68). Studies have shown that heparin, the archetypal modulator of vascular repair following vascular injury, maximally inhibits neointimal hyperplasia in stented rabbit iliac arteries only when given in prolonged fashion (14 days) whereas maximal inhibition of balloon injured arteries requires only transient early heparin therapy (3 days) (68). An explanation of this difference is suggested by immunohistologic and molecular studies. Data demonstrate that there is a distinct pattern of leukocyte infiltration that distinguishes the superficial injury associated with simple balloon-induced de-endothelialization from the deep chronic injury associated with stent implantation. In a rabbit iliac artery model, balloon injury is associated with early and transient infiltration of neutrophils without monocyte accumulation, while stent implantation is associated with an early influx of neutrophils followed by sustained recruitment of monocytes over days to weeks. These differences are mirrored by molecular studies in which mRNA levels of the monocyte chemokine MCP-1 and the neutrophil chemokine IL-8 at sites of vascular injury were determined utilizing semi-quantitative reverse transcriptase polymerase chain reaction. In balloon injury, there is only transient (hours) expression of MCP-1 and IL-8. In contrast, in stented arteries, there was sustained expression of IL-8 and, more prominently, MCP-1 as late as 14 days (69).

An Integrated View of the Pathophysiology of Restenosis

When a balloon and stent are inflated at the site of a mature atherosclerotic plaque, a series of events are initiated (Fig. 1–10). The first is a predominant inflammatory phase. The initial consequences immediately following stent placement are de-endothelialization, crush of the plaque often with dissection into the tunica media and occasionally adventitia, and stretch of the entire artery. A layer of platelets and fibrin are deposited at the injured site. Activated platelets on the surface expressing adhesion molecules such as P-selectin and GP Ibα attach to circulating leukocytes via platelet receptors such as P-selectin glycoprotein ligand (PSGL-1) and begin a process of rolling along the injured surface. Leukocytes then bind tightly to the surface and stop rolling mediated through the leukocyte integrin (i.e., Mac-1) class of adhesion molecules

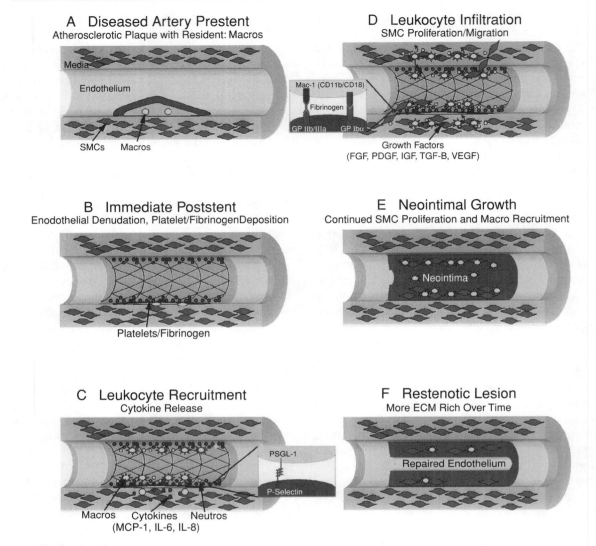

Figure 1–10.

Panel A illustrates a mature atherosclerotic plaque prior to intervention. Panel B illustrates the immediate result of stent placement with endothelial denudation and platelet/fibrinogen deposition. Panel C and D illustrate leukocyte recruitment, infiltration, and SMC proliferation and migration in the days following injury. Panel E demonstrates neointimal thickening in the weeks following injury with continued SMC proliferation and monocyte recruitment. Panel F illustrates the long-term (weeks to months) change from a predominantly cellular to a less cellular and more ECM-rich plaque. (From: Welt FGP, Rogers C. Inflammation and restenosis in the stent era. *Arterioscl Thromb Vasc Biol.* 2002;22:1769–1776, with permission.)

via direct attachment to platelet receptors such as GP 1bα and through cross linking with fibrinogen to the GP IIb/IIIa receptor. Migration of leukocytes across the platelet-fibrin layer and diapedesis into the tissue is driven by chemical gradients of cytokines released from smooth muscle cells and resident. Next is a granulation or cellular proliferation phase. Growth factors are subsequently released from platelets, leukocytes, and smooth muscle cells, which stimulate proliferation and migration of smooth muscle cells from the media into the neointima. The resultant neointima consists of smooth muscle cells, extracellular matrix, and macrophages recruited over a several week period of time. Over longer periods of time the artery enters a phase of remodeling involving extracellular matrix protein degradation and resynthesis. Accompanying this phase is a

shift to less cellular elements and greater production of extracellular matrix. In the balloon angioplastied artery, this leads to shrinkage of the entire artery and negative remodeling. In the stented artery, this phase has less impact due to the rigid scaffolding of the stent which prevents negative remodeling. In both balloon angioplastied and stented arteries, there is eventual re-endothelialization of at least part of the injured vessel surface.

Clinical Sequelae of Restenosis

Although inflammation is a common link between atherogenesis and restenosis, there are distinct differences between the two processes that manifest in clinical presentation. In terms of the temporal pattern, atherogenesis is a process that occurs over decades, while multiple studies have revealed that restenosis is a process which occurs predominantly during the first six months after angioplasty whether a stent is implanted or not. Restenotic lesions typically lack the complex architecture of mature atherosclerotic plaque consisting mainly of SMCs and extracellular matrix as well as numerous leukocytes. As such, the clinical sequelae of restenotic lesions are usually not plaque rupture and acute coronary syndrome, but more typically progressive exertional angina.

Implications for Antirestenotic Therapy

Antirestenotic therapy has largely focused on either direct antiproliferative strategies or antiinflammatory strategies. Interestingly, many of the proved and most promising therapies share both antiproliferative and antiinflammatory features. For example, sirolimus, which has shown remarkable efficacy against restenosis in a coated stent design (70), is an inhibitor of cell cycle progression, but also possesses important antiinflammatory properties as evidenced by its initial development as an antifungal agent and its current use as an immunomodulatory agent in the treatment of renal transplant rejection (71). Furthermore, in a porcine model of stent injury, sirolimus coated stents have been shown to downregulate vessel wall protein expression of the cytokines MCP-1 and IL-6 compared to bare metal stents (72). Also, the microtubule stabilizer paclitaxel, a promising therapy for restenosis, is known to interfere with SMC proliferation and migration through its effect on microtubules (71). However, some data suggest that paclitaxel effects leukocyte function, which has been said to be at least in part mediated through the interference with cytoskeletal interactions with the integrin class of adhesion molecules (73).

The data also suggest that there are important differences in the temporal and spatial pattern of inflammation between stent and balloon injury that must be taken into account when antirestenotic therapies are conceived. Specifically, the inflammatory response engendered by a stent is prolonged and contains more cells of the monocyte/macrophage lineage. Therefore, antiinflammatory therapies may likely need to be delivered over a prolonged period of time and be directed against macrophages in particular.

Conclusions

Over the past decades, the molecular and cellular pathophysiology of atherosclerosis and related arteriopathies has been extensively studied. A central role for inflammation has been confirmed as central to these processes. Important differences exist, however, between these processes likely as a result of the injury imposed against the artery which help to determine the clinical consequences of these processes. A more thorough knowledge of these processes has led to increasingly effective therapies for the treatment of atherosclerosis and the acute coronary syndromes as well as restenosis. However, there remains much to be determined regarding the molecular mechanisms of atherosclerosis, identification of plaques prone to rupture, and more effective and economic methods to treat restenosis.

REFERENCES

1. Ross R. The pathogenesis of atherosclerosis—an update. *N Engl J Med.* 1986;314:488–500.
2. Ridker PM, Rifai N, Rose L, et al. Comparison of C-reactive protein and low-density lipoprotein cholesterol levels in the prediction of first cardiovascular events. *N Engl J Med.* 2002;347:1557–1565.
3. Brennan ML, Penn MS, Van Lente F, et al. Prognostic value of myeloperoxidase in patients with chest pain. *N Engl J Med.* 2003;349:1595–1604.
4. Cybulsky MI, Gimbrone, Jr., MA. Endothelial expression of a mononuclear leukocyte adhesion molecule during atherogenesis. *Science.* 1995;251:788–791.
5. Ridker PM. Intercellular adhesion molecule (ICAM-1) and the risks of developing atherosclerotic disease. *Eur Heart J.* 1998;19:1119–1121.
6. Rollins BJ. Chemokines. *Blood.* 1997;90:909–928.
7. Webb LMC, Ehrengruber MU, Clark-Lewis I, et al. Binding to heparan sulfate or heparin enhances neutrophil responses to interleukin 8. *Proc Natl Acad Sci U S A.* 1993;90:7158–7162.
8. Huo Y, Weber C, Forlow SB, et al. The chemokine KC, but not monocyte chemoattractant protein-1, triggers monocyte arrest on early atherosclerotic endothelium. *J Clin Invest.* 2001;108:1307–1314.
9. Libby P. Molecular bases of the acute coronary syndromes. *Circulation.* 1995;91: 2844–2850.
10. Moulton KS. Plaque angiogenesis and atherosclerosis. *Curr Atheroscl Rep.* 2001;3:225–233.
11. Gibbons GH, Dzau VJ. The emerging concept of vascular remodeling. *N Engl J Med.* 1994;330:1431–1438.
12. Galis ZS, Khatri JJ. Matrix metalloproteinases in vascular remodeling and atherogenesis: the good, the bad, and the ugly. *Circ Res.* 2002;90:251–262.
13. Fuster V, Badimon L, Badimaon JJ, et al. The pathogenesis of coronary artery disease and the acute coronary syndromes. *N Engl J Med.* 1992;326:242–250.
14. Kern MJ. Coronary physiology revisited: practical insights from the cardiac catheterization laboratory. *Circulation.* 2000;101:1344–1351.
15. Herrick JB. Clinical features of sudden obstruction of the coronary arteries. *JAMA.* 1912;59:2015–2020.
16. DeWood MA, Spores J, Notske R, et al. Prevalence of total coronary occlusion during the early hours of transmural myocardial infarction. *N Engl J Med.* 1980;303:897–902.
17. Ambrose JA, Winters SL, Arora RR, et al. Coronary angiographic morphology in myocardial infarction: a link between the pathogenesis of unstable angina and myocardial infarction. *J Am Coll Cardiol.* 1985;6:1233–1238.
18. Smith SC, Jr. Risk-reduction therapy: the challenge to change. Presented at the 68th scientific sessions of the American Heart Association, November 13, 1995, Anaheim, California. *Circulation.* 1996;93:2205–2211.
19. Seshiah PN, Kereiakes DJ, Vasudevan SS, et al. Activated monocytes induce smooth muscle cell death: role of macrophage colony-stimulating factor and cell contact. *Circulation.* 2002;105:174–180.
20. Muller JE, Stone PH, Turi ZG, et al. Circadian variation in the frequency of onset of acute myocardial infarction. *N Engl J Med.* 1985;313:1315–1322.
21. Leor J, Kloner RA. The Northridge earthquake as a trigger for acute myocardial infarction. *Am J Cardiol.* 1996;77:1230–1232.
22. Lee RT, Schoen FJ, Loree HM, et al. Circumferential stress and matrix metalloproteinase 1 in human coronary atherosclerosis. Implications for plaque rupture. *Arterioscl Thromb Vasc Biol.* 1996;16:1070–1073.
23. Gruntzig AR, Senning A, Siegenthaler WE. Nonoperative dilatation of coronary-artery stenosis: percutaneous transluminal coronary angioplasty. *N Engl J Med.* 1979;301:61–68.

24. Bourassa MG, Wilson JW, Detre KM, et al. Long-term follow-up of coronary angioplasty: the 1977–1981 National Heart, Lung, and Blood Institute registry. *Eur Heart J.* 1989;10:36–41.

25. McBride W, Lange RA, Hillis LD. Restenosis after successful coronary angioplasty. Pathophysiology and prevention. *N Engl J Med.* 1988;318:1734–1737.

26. Faxon DA, Weber VJ, Haudenschild C, et al. Acute effects of transmural angioplasty in three experimental models of atherosclerosis. *Arterioscl.* 1982;2:125–133.

27. Faxon DP, Sanborn TA, Weber VJ, et al. Restenosis following transluminal angioplasty in experimental atherosclerosis. *Arterioscl.* 1984;4:189–195.

28. Forrester JS, Fishbein M, Helfant R, et al. A paradigm for restenosis based on cell biology: clues for the development of new preventive therapies. *J Am Coll Cardiol.* 1991;17:758–769.

29. Mintz GS, Popma JJ, Pichard AD, et al. Arterial remodeling after coronary angioplasty: a serial intravascular ultrasound study. *Circulation.* 1996;94: 35–43.

30. Fischman DL, Leon MB, Baim DS, et al. A randomized comparison of coronary artery-stent placement and balloon angioplasty in the treatment of coronary artery disease. *N Engl J Med.* 1994;331:496–501.

31. Serruys PW, de Jaegere P, Kiemeneij F, et al. A comparison of balloon-expandable-stent implantation with balloon angioplasty in patients with coronary artery disease. *N Engl J Med.* 1994;331:489–495.

32. Hoffmann R, Mintz GS, Dussaillant GR, et al. Patterns and mechanisms of in-stent restenosis. A serial intravascular ultrasound study. *Circulation.* 1996; 94:1247–1254.

33. Marcus AJ. Thrombosis and inflammation as multicellular processes: significance of cell-cell interactions. *Semin Hematol.* 1994;31:261–269.

34. Libby P, Simon DI. Inflammation and thrombosis: the clot thickens. *Circulation.* 2001;103:1718–1720.

35. Diacovo TG, Roth SJ, Buccola JM, et al. Neutrophil rolling, arrest, and transmigration across activated, surface-adherent platelets via sequential action of P-selectin and the beta 2-integrin CD11b/CD18. *Blood.* 1996; 88:146–157.

36. Yeo EL, Sheppard JA, Feuerstein IA. Role of P-selectin and leukocyte activation in polymorphonuclear cell adhesion to surface adherent activated platelets under physiologic shear conditions (an injury vessel wall model). *Blood.* 1994;83:2498–2507.

37. Ott I, Neumann FJ, Gawaz M, et al. Increased neutrophil-platelet adhesion in patients with unstable angina. *Circulation.* 1996;94:1239–1246.

38. Furman MI, Benoit SE, Barnard MR, et al. Increased platelet reactivity and circulating monocyte-platelet aggregates in patients with stable coronary artery disease. *J Am Coll Cardiol.* 1998;31:352–358.

39. Farb A, Weber DK, Kolodgie FD, et al. Morphological predictors of restenosis after coronary stenting in humans. *Circulation.* 2002;105:2974–2980.

40. Moreno PR, Bernardi VH, Lopez-Cuellar J, et al. Macrophage infiltration predicts restenosis after coronary intervention in patients with unstable angina. *Circulation.* 1996;94:3098–3102.

41. Neumann F-J, Ott I, Gawaz M, et al. Neutrophil and platelet activation at balloon-injured coronary artery plaque in patients undergoing angioplasty. *J Am Coll Cardiol.* 1996;27:819–824.

42. Mickelson JK, Lakkis NM, Villarreal-Levy G, et al. Leukocyte activation with platelet adhesion after coronary angioplasty: a mechanism for recurrent disease. *J Am Coll Cardiol.* 1996;28:345–353.

43. Inoue T, Sakai Y, Morooka S, et al. Expression of polymorphonuclear leukocyte adhesion molecules and its clinical significance in patients treated with percutaneous transluminal coronary angioplasty. *J Am Coll Cardiol.* 1996;28:1127–1133.

44. Inoue T, Uchida T, Yaguchi I, et al. Stent-induced expression and activation of the leukocyte integrin Mac-1 is associated with neointimal thickening and restenosis. *Circulation.* 2003;107:1757–1763.

45. Pietersma A, Kofflard M, de Wit LEA, et al. Late lumen loss after coronary angioplasty is associated with the activation status of circulating phagocytes before treatment. *Circulation.* 1995;91:1320–1325.

46. Cipollone F, Marini M, Fazia M, et al. Elevated circulating levels of monocyte chemoattractant protein-1 in patients with restenosis after coronary angioplasty. *Arterioscl Thromb Vasc Biol.* 2001;21:327–334.

47. Gaspardone A, Crea F, Versaci F, et al. Predictive value of C-reactive protein after successful coronary-artery stenting in patients with stable angina. *Am J Cardiol.* 1998;82:515–518.

48. Cybulsky MI, Gimbrone MAJ. Endothelial expression of a mononuclear leukocyte adhesion molecule during atherogenesis. *Science.* 1991;251: 788–791.

49. Li H, Cybulsky M, Gimbrone MA, Libby P. An atherogenic diet induces VCAM-1, a cytokine-regulatable mononuclear leukocyte adhesion molecule, in rabbit endothelium. *Arterioscl Thromb.* 1992;13:197–204.

50. Li H, Cybulsky MI, Gimbrone Jr. MA, Libby P. Inducible expression of vascular cell adhesion molecule-1 by vascular smooth muscle cells in vitro and within rabbit atheroma. *Am J Pathol.* 1993;143:1551–1559.

51. Richardson M, Hadcock SJ, DeReske M, et al. Increased expression in vivo of VCAM-1 and E-selectin by the aortic endothelium of normolipemic and hyperlipemic diabetic rabbits. *Arterioscl Thromb.* 1994;14:760–769.

52. Walpola PL, Gotlieb AI, Cybulsky MI, et al. Expression of ICAM-1 and VCAM-1 and monocyte adherence in arteries exposed to altered shear stress. *Arterioscl, Thromb Vasc Biol.* 1995;15:2–10.

53. Tanaka H, Sukhova GK, Swanson SJ, et al. Sustained activation of vascular cells and leukocytes in the rabbit aorta after balloon injury. *Circulation.* 1993;88:1788–1803.

54. Rogers C, Welt FGP, Karnovsky MJ, et al. Monocyte recruitment and neointimal hyperplasia in rabbits: Coupled inhibitory effects of heparin. *Arterioscl, Thromb Vasc Biol.* 1996;16:1312–1318.

55. Welt FGP, Edelman ER, Simon DI, et al. Neutrophil, not macrophage, infiltration precedes neointimal thickening in balloon-injured arteries. *Arterioscl, Thromb Vasc Biol.* 2000;20:2553–2558.

56. Rogers C, Edelman ER, Simon DI. A mAb to the beta2-leukocyte integrin Mac-1 (CD11b/CD18) reduces intimal thickening after angioplasty or stent implantation in rabbits. *Proc Natl Acad Sci U S A.* 1998;95:10134–10139.

57. Mori E, Komori K, Yamaoka T, et al. Essential role of monocyte chemoattractant protein-1 in development of restenotic changes (neointimal hyperplasia and constrictive remodeling) after balloon angioplasty in hypercholesterolemic rabbits. *Circulation.* 2002;105:2905–2910.

58. Libby P, Schwartz D, Brogi E, et al. A cascade model for restenosis. *Circulation.* 1992;86:III47–III52.

59. Jorgensen L, Grothe AG, Groves HM, et al. Sequence of cellular responses in rabbit aortas following one and two injuries with a balloon catheter. *Br J Exp Pathol.* 1988;69:473–486.

60. Richardson M, Hatton MW, Buchanan MR, et al. Wound healing in the media of the normolipemic rabbit carotid artery injured by air drying or by balloon catheter de-endothelialization. *Am J Pathol.* 1990;137:1453–1465.

61. Kockx MM, De Meyer GR, Jacob WA, et al. Triphasic sequence of neointimal formation in the cuffed carotid artery of the rabbit. *Arterioscler Thromb.* 1992;12:1447–1457.

62. Cole CW, Makhoul RG, McCann RL, et al. A neutrophil derived factor(s) stimulates [3H]thymidine incorporation by vascular smooth muscle cells in vitro. *Clin Invest Med.* 1988;11:62–67.

63. Lloyd AR, Oppenheim JJ. Poly's lament: the neglected role of the polymorphonuclear neutrophil in the afferent limb of the immune response. *Immunol Today.* 1992;13:169–172.

64. Inoue T, Sohma R, Miyazaki T, et al. Comparison of activation process of platelets and neutrophils after coronary stent implantation versus balloon angioplasty for stable angina pectoris. *Am J Cardiol.* 2000;86:1057–1062.

65. Clowes AW, Clowes MM. Kinetics of cellular proliferation after arterial injury: II. Inhibition of smooth muscle cell growth by heparin. *Lab Invest.* 1985;52:611–616.

66. Clowes AW, Clowes MM. Kinetics of cellular proliferation after arterial injury: IV. Heparin inhibits rat smooth muscle cell mitogenesis and migration. *Circ Res.* 1986;58:839–845.

67. Rogers C, Edelman ER. Controlled release of heparin reduces neointimal hyperplasia in stented rabbit arteries: Ramifications for local therapy. *J Intervent Cardiol.* 1992;5:195–202.

68. Edelman ER, Karnovsky MJ. Contrasting effects of the intermittent and continuous administration of heparin in experimental restenosis. *Circulation.* 1994;89:770–776.

69. Welt FG, Tso C, Edelman ER, et al. Leukocyte recruitment and expression of chemokines following different forms of vascular injury. *Vasc Med.* 2003;8:1–7.

70. Morice MC, Serruys PW, Sousa JE, et al. A randomized comparison of a sirolimus-eluting stent with a standard stent for coronary revascularization. *N Engl J Med.* 2002;346:1773–1780.

71. Oberhoff M, Herdeg C, Baumbach A, et al. Stent-based antirestenotic coatings (sirolimus/paclitaxel). *Catheter Cardiovasc Intervent.* 2002;55:404–408.

72. Suzuki TM, Kopia GP, Hayashi S-iM, et al. Stent-Based Delivery of Sirolimus Reduces Neointimal Formation in a Porcine Coronary Model. *Circulation.* 2001;104:1188–1193.

73. Zhou X, Li J, Kucik DF. The microtubule cytoskeleton participates in control of beta2 integrin avidity. *J Biol Chem.* 2001;276:44762–44769.

Fibrinolytic Therapy for Acute Myocardial Infarction

Timothy A. Mixon

With the advent of fibrinolytic therapy, the treatment of myocardial infarction changed from the management of complications to an active attempt to salvage myocardium. Not only was survival improved but also the study of this class of medications has refined the way that clinical investigation is carried out in the field of cardiovascular medicine.

Fibrinolytic medications are serine protease plasminogen activators. They work by facilitating the conversion of plasminogen to plasmin, which is an active enzyme involved in the degradation of fibrin to fibrin-degradation-products. Thus, the commonly used term *thrombolytics* is actually a misnomer, as these agents have no direct effect on thrombin, but rather the term *plasminogen activators* or *fibrinolytics* is more accurate. Of importance, fibrinolytic medications actually stimulate thrombin, and therefore have some inherent thrombogenic effects.

There are currently four FDA-approved fibrinolytic agents available that carry an indication for the treatment of acute myocardial infarction. (A fifth agent, anistreplase, a compound related to streptokinase, was previously approved but is no longer manufactured.) These include the first generation drug streptokinase, the second-generation agent alteplase, and the third generation compounds reteplase and tenecteplase. These agents will be reviewed individually and then important trials and concepts related to the administration of fibrinolytic therapy are reviewed.

Streptokinase

Streptokinase (SK) was the first fibrinolytic agent available and approved. Early interest in SK has led to it being one of the most studied compounds in cardiovascular medicine. SK is a single chain polypeptide derived from beta-hemolytic streptococci. Because the polypeptide forms a one-to-one complex with *both* circulating *and* thrombin-bound plasminogen, it is considered a fibrin "nonspecific" agent, which leads to excessive systemic depletion of not only plasminogen, but also fibrinogen, factor V, and factor VIII (Fig. 2–1). This depletion causes a system-wide "lytic" state associated with an increased risk of bleeding (although not intra-cerebral hemorrhage) and a lesser need for adjuvant anti-thrombotic therapy (e.g., heparin). SK is also an antigenic compound and is associated with formation of neutralizing antibodies, leading to the recommendation that it not be re-administered for fear of an important allergic reaction. These antibodies, once formed, are known to persist for more than 7 years. Although it has never been proven that re-administration years later would result in anaphylaxis, the general consensus is to avoid re-administration at any time (Table 2–1).

SK is associated with milder allergic reactions in up to 4% of the patients consisting of rash, fevers, chills, urticaria, and pyrexia. Anaphylactic shock is fortunately rare, occurring in <1% of the patients as shown in the ISIS-2 trial (1). These reactions prevent rapid or bolus administration. Hypotension (mean drop in the systolic blood pressure of 35 mm Hg) is common during administration; therefore, it is recommended that the drug be infused slowly. When minor allergic reactions or hypotension occurs, SK administration may be continued, but the infusion rate should be slowed; fluid boluses and dopamine may be necessary.

Because SK is a nonspecific agent, adjuvant heparin use is controversial and is not necessary in all cases. Current ACC/AHA guidelines recommend (class I indication) concomitant heparin with SK only in patients at "high risk of systemic emboli," such as those with atrial fibrillation, large anterior MI, those with a history of prior thromboembolic episodes, or with a known LV thrombus. For all others, heparin usage is considered a class IIb indication (2).

Data supporting the efficacy of SK include the GISSI trial, a placebo-controlled trial published in 1986, which was the first major fibrinolytic trial and the first to demonstrate a survival benefit with fibrinolytics. Mortality at 21 days was reduced from 13% to 10.7%, representing an 18% relative risk reduction. An important lesson learned from this study was the significantly greater benefit associated with very early drug administration (3). Subsequently the ISIS-2 trial again showed not only mortality benefit associated with SK usage, but also demonstrated the synergistic effects of adjuvant aspirin administration. Short-term mortality in the placebo arm was 13.2% with a 25% relative reduction seen in the treatment arms receiving either aspirin alone or SK alone, but a 45% relative

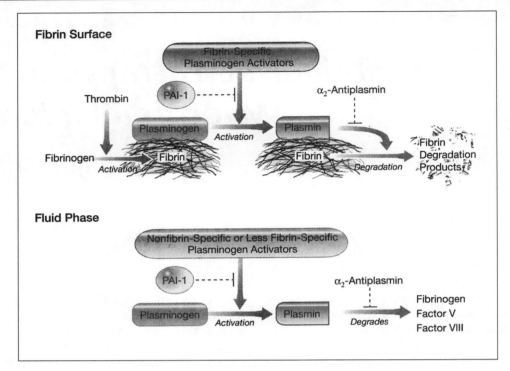

Figure 2–1.

Interaction of fibrin specific and nonfibrin specific plasminogen activators with plasminogen. Plasminogen is converted to plasmin due to the interaction with plasminogen activators. Fibrin specific plasminogen activators preferentially convert plasminogen that is on the fibrin surface, whereas fibrin nonspecific agents induce systemic plasminogen activation, which leads to widespread reduction in the plasma levels of fibrinogen, factor V, and factor VIII. PAI-1 (plasminogen activator inhibitor) and α2-antiplasmin are two of the main serine protease inhibitors. (From: Llevadot J, Giugliano RP, Antman EM. Bolus fibrinolytic therapy in acute myocardial infarction. *JAMA.* 2001;286:442–449, with permission.)

Table 2–1

Comparison of Currently Approved Fibrinolytic Agents in the United States

Feature	SK	t-PA	Reteplase	Tenecteplase
Fibrin-specific	−	++	+	++++
Half-life (minutes)	20	5	15	20
Antigencity	Y	N	N	N
90 minutes patency	60	84	83	85
90 minutes TIMI 3	32	54	60	66
Rate of ICH	0.34	0.69	0.76	0.69
Requires concomitant Heparin	+/−	Y	Y	Y
Weight adjusted dosing	N	Y	N	Y
Dose	1.5 mL units IV Over 60 minutes	15 mg IV/1–2 minutes 0.75 mg/kg IV/30 minutes (max 50 mg) 0.5 mg/kg IV/60 minutes (max 35 mg)	10 U IV bolus Repeat bolus in 30 minutes	One time weight-based bolus <60 kg = 30 mg 60–69 kg = 35 mg 70–79 kg = 40 mg 80–89 kg = 45 mg >90 kg = 50 mg
Bolus administration	N	N	Y (double bolus)	Y
Cost ($, US)	$613	$3609	$3016	$2917
Major Supportive Trials	GISSI 1 (3) ISIS II (1)	GUSTO I (5) (ASSENT III) (24)	GUSTO III (7) INJECT (8)	ASSENT III (24)

reduction in the group receiving both aspirin and SK (mortality 7.2%) (1).

Alteplase (t-PA)

Alteplase is a naturally occurring tissue plasminogen activator produced and secreted by mammalian endothelial cells, thus it is a component of the homeostatic coagulation cascade. It is produced by genetically inserting the human complimentary DNA sequence into a culture of hamster ovarian cells, which then secrete the enzyme that can be harvested, purified, and prepared. Alteplase was the first of the "fibrin-specific" agents, denoting an increased tendency for the enzyme to only attach to fibrin-bound plasminogen, thereby reducing systemic depletion of plasminogen and fibrinogen. Clinically some of its "fibrin-specificity" is reduced due to the large dose administered to promote rapid vessel patency. This agent achieves a higher and more rapid rate of vessel patency than SK, but is also associated with a higher rate of vessel re-occlusion and a higher rate of intracerebral hemorrhage. To reduce the likelihood of re-occlusion, aspirin and heparin (or another anti-thrombotic agent) are administered concomitantly. Also, it is more efficacious at dissolving an older, more mature clot than SK. Many dosing schemes were studied, but the most effective was the accelerated dosing schedule (4) (Table 2–1). Neutralizing antibodies are not formed after administration and, therefore, re-administration is possible. Hypotension during administration does not occur nor do allergic reactions.

Data supporting the efficacy of t-PA came from the large GUSTO-1 trial that randomized more than 41,000 patients to either SK or accelerated dose t-PA. Overall, short-term mortality was reduced from 7.3% to 6.3% with t-PA use, representing a 1% absolute and a 14% relative mortality reduction (p = 0.001) (5). A slight, but statistically significant increased rate of intra-cerebral hemorrhage was seen with t-PA (0.72% versus 0.52%, p = 0.03) with no clinically meaningful difference in other bleeding complications (5).

Reteplase

Reteplase is the first among the designed mutants of t-PA. It is produced by genetically engineered *E. coli* which produce a variant of t-PA containing 355 of the 527 amino acids of the mother compound. The engineered changes result in slightly less fibrin specificity but an increased plasma half-life of 13 to 16 minutes, which allows for bolus administration. The medication is administered as two 10-unit boluses (potency is expressed in units which are a reference standard specific to reteplase, and do not compare directly to other fibrinolytic agents) given 30 minutes apart, with no adjustment made for weight. Similar to other fibrin specific agents, aspirin and heparin are given as adjuncts to assist in preventing vessel re-occlusion. Initial pilot studies suggested superiority compared with t-PA (6); however, the large pivotal trial GUSTO-III compared accelerated dose t-PA with reteplase in 15,059 patients and found similar 30-day mortality rates (7.4% versus 7.2%) (7). Because of the expectation of the trial designers, the study

was undertaken as a superiority trial. Not only did reteplase fail to show superiority, but the study was underpowered to demonstrate statistical equivalency (although the primary and secondary endpoints appear similar at 30 days and one year). This illustrates the shortcomings of a valid, but limited surrogate endpoint (TIMI 3 flow rate) in predicting clinical outcomes and justifies large, adequately powered fibrinolytic trials that use outcomes such as mortality. Subsequently, the INJECT trial compared reteplase and SK in 6,010 patients. This study showed equivalent outcomes in terms of mortality and combined endpoints, and provided the impetus for its FDA approval for the indication of acute myocardial infarction (8).

Tenecteplase

Tenecteplase is a triple mutant variant of t-PA made by altering specific amino acids. The result is a highly fibrin specific agent (14 times more fibrin specific than t-PA) that causes significantly less fibrinogen and plasminogen degradation than less fibrin specific agents. This may be a biological explanation for a lower rate of hemorrhage seen clinically with tenecteplase. Tenecteplase also shows decreased plasma clearance and increased resistance to inactivation by plasminogen activator inhibitor-1 (PAI-1), a naturally occurring inhibitor to fibrinolytics. A prolonged half-life of 20 minutes allows for a single bolus, weight based administration, which is desirable to simplify therapy and reduce dosing errors that have been demonstrated in an appreciable percentage of patients receiving other agents requiring prolonged infusion. The pivotal ASSENT 2 trial randomized 16,949 patients to receive either accelerated dose t-PA or tenecteplase. At 30 days, equal rates of mortality, total strokes, and intra-cerebral hemorrhage were observed. There was a 20% lower rate of noncerebral bleeding and a slightly lower rate of transfusions in ASSENT 2; this formed the basis for its approval for clinical use (9).

Importance of Time to Treatment

As with any reperfusion strategy, the familiar adage "time is muscle" is true. The duration of symptoms before initiation of therapy has consistently been shown to be a major correlate of short and long-term mortality. Although studies have documented that mortality is highest in the first few hours, the possibility of mortality reduction is also highest at that time (Fig. 2–2) (10). It is estimated that fibrinolytic therapy administered within 90 minutes of symptom onset can result in a 50% myocardial salvage rate; in fact, in up to 40% of the patients treated very early, subsequent nuclear studies failed to show any evidence of infarction, suggesting the possibility of aborting permanent myonecrosis (11). Numerous studies have reported up to a 50% relative reduction in mortality in subsets of patients treated within the first 2 hours (1,3,12). The reasons for this impressive mortality benefit are multifactorial. One likely reason is that fibrinolytics are most effective hematologically if administered early because as the thrombotic occlusion ages, there is increased cross-linking of the

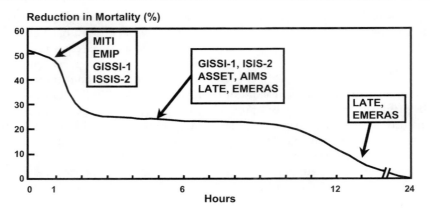

Reduction in Mortality (%)

Figure 2–2.

Two-step decline in mortality reduction with fibrinolytic therapy related to time of administration. Reduction in mortality benefit appears to occur in two step-wise declines. During the first "golden hour," relative mortality reduction is as much as 50%, after which it declines to an approximately 25% relative mortality reduction for 12 hours. After 12 hours, a further reduction in mortality benefit is seen, without consistent evidence of benefit at that time. AIMS, Anistreplase Intervention Mortality Study; ASSET, Anglo-Scandinavian Study of Early Thrombolysis; EMERAS, Estudios Multicentrico Estreptoquinasa Republicas de America del Sur; EMIP, European Myocardial Infarction Project; GISSI-1, Gruppo Italiano per lo Studio della Streptochinasif nell'Infarto Miocardico; ISIS-2, Second International Study of Infarct Survival; LATE, Late Assessment of Thrombolytic Efficacy; MITI, Myocardial Infarction and Triage Intervention Project. (From: Lincoff AM, Topol EJ. Illusion of reperfusion: does anyone achieve optimal reperfusion during acute myocardial infarction? *Circulation.* 1993;88:1361–1374, with permission.)

fibrin components rendering the clot more resistant to dissolution. Second, the possibility of myocardial salvage is present early but decreases rapidly after the first 2 hours (even if complete fibrinolysis is achieved and flow is adequately restored). There may be other mechanisms distinct from myocardial salvage by which therapy beyond 2 hours lowers mortality rates.

As depicted in Figure 2–2, there are two distinct time periods when the rate of mortality benefit drops, rather than a slow gradual decline. The first decline at 2 hours is related to factors discussed earlier: relative "thrombo-resistance" to lysis that develops as the clot matures, and permanent myonecrosis that has largely occurred by 2 hours (10). Subsequently, other mechanisms are thought to explain the continued modest reduction in mortality. One concept is that even late reperfusion may have beneficial effects on LV geometry, size, and shape (Fig. 2–3) (13). In addition, data suggest that regardless of the time administered, there is a reduction in late arrhythmia in patients who receive fibrinolytic therapy (14). Regardless of these interactions, it is imperative that the time to treatment be minimized, which can only be accomplished by continued education of patients as to the signs and symptoms of AMI, encouragement to seek medical treatment early, and by the adoption of protocols that minimize treatment delays.

Indications for Fibrinolytics

Current guidelines emphasize that all patients presenting with ST elevation myocardial infarction (STEMI) should be promptly evaluated for reperfusion therapy. Although the preponderance of evidence would favor primary percutaneous coronary intervention (PCI) by an experienced operator if a door-to-balloon time of <90 minutes can be achieved, the widespread availability of this procedure on a 24 hour-a-day basis is still a major issue. If primary PCI cannot be administered in a timely fashion, then consideration should be given to immediate administration of fibrinolytic medications.

Indications for fibrinolytic therapy include patients presenting within 12 hours of the onset of symptoms who show >0.1 mV ST elevation in at least two contiguous leads. Other indications include patients presenting with chest pain and a new or presumably new left bundle branch block (LBBB) or an ECG pattern of a true posterior myocardial infarction (MI) (Fig. 2–4). Patients presenting beyond 12 hours have little if any clinical benefit, although one trial did show some benefit. Therefore, it is prudent to use clinical judgment in this subset and consider fibrinolytic therapy if there is reason to believe viable tissue is still present. Specifically excluded from eligibility are patients presenting beyond 24 hours of symptom onset, and patients with ST depression only (unless indicative of a true posterior injury pattern) (2). The mortality benefit has been quantified in numerous trials, revealing up to 49 lives/1,000 patients treated if presenting with LBBB, 37 lives/1,000 treated if presenting with anterior MI, and a smaller, but still statistically significant 8 lives/1,000 treated among patients presenting with an inferior MI (15). The benefit is greatest among patients with an anterior MI, diabetes, and signs of significant myocardium

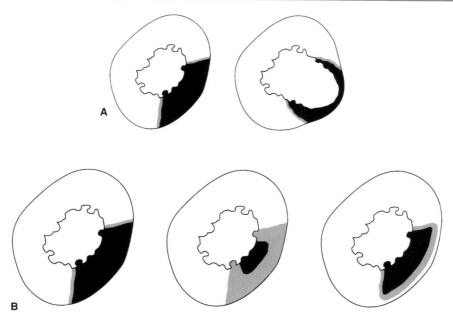

Figure 2–3.

Schemata of fibrinolytic therapy, infarct expansion, and left ventricular remodeling. **A:** The concept of infarct expansion is schematically shown with regional dilation and thinning after myocardial infarction. **B:** Three different situations are presented. The cross-section of no reperfusion (*left*) exhibits transmural necrosis, whereas the early perfusion schematic (*center*) shows sparing of the subepicardium and border zone. The potential benefit of late reperfusion may be preservation of the epicardial rim and a modest decrease in border zone necrosis, thus potentially inhibiting infarct zone expansion (*right*). (From: Topol EJ. Thrombolytic intervention. In: Topol EJ, ed. *Textbook of Interventional Cardiology.* 4th ed. Philadelphia: Saunders; 2003:91–118, with permission.)

at risk (low BP, high heart rate). Therapy is associated with a relatively greater benefit if given very early, with trials revealing a myocardial salvage rate up to 50% if given within the first 2 hours (11) (Fig. 2–5). Current national guidelines require a door-to-drug time (or more precisely, the time from first medical contact to drug administration) of no more than 30 minutes. This brief duration requires a cooperative effort

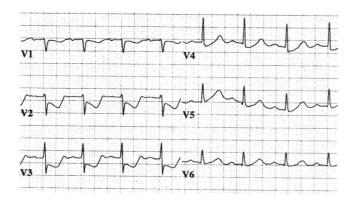

Figure 2–4.

ECG showing posterior injury current. Note down-sloping ST segment depression in leads V1-V3 with upright T waves. Posteriorly placed leads would reveal ST segment elevation, indicative of this posterior injury current. This pattern may be seen in isolation, or in association with an inferior injury pattern.

between all involved health care providers and strict protocols to guide EMS and emergency department triage personnel as well as physician management and decision-making once the patient arrives.

Contraindications

Absolute and relative contraindications exist, and are listed in Figure 2–6 (2). Hemorrhage and intra-cranial pathology represent the two greatest areas of risk with the agents. Models exist to allow the clinician to estimate the risk of intra-cerebral hemorrhage (ICH), which can then be weighed against the magnitude of expected benefit. Factors associated with an increased risk of ICH include increasing age, low body weight, the presence and degree of hypertension, and the use of any agent other than SK. Some models have also found higher rates of ICH among females, African-Americans, those with prior strokes, and those with excessive anticoagulation (e.g., INR <4) (2). Patients with contraindications to fibrinolytic therapy related to hemorrhage-risk are often still candidates for primary PCI and should be considered for rapid transfer to a facility with these capabilities.

Special Circumstances

Various clinical circumstances can complicate management decisions such as the decision to treat elderly patients or those

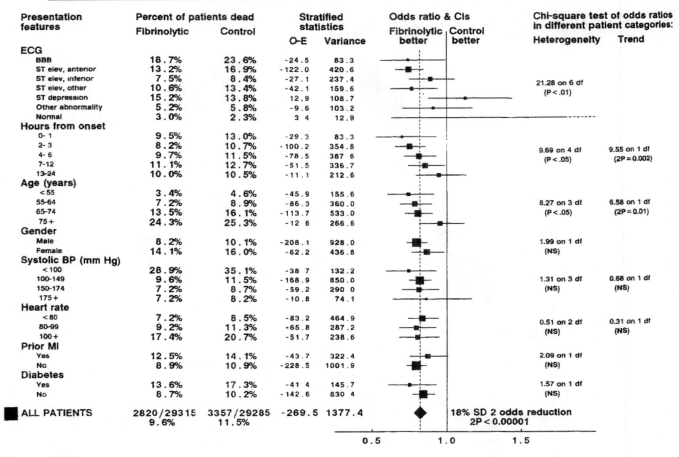

Presentation features	Percent of patients dead		Stratified statistics		Odds ratio & CIs	Chi-square test of odds ratios in different patient categories:	
	Fibrinolytic	Control	O-E	Variance	Fibrinolytic better / Control better	Heterogeneity	Trend
ECG							
BBB	18.7%	23.6%	-24.5	83.3			
ST elev, anterior	13.2%	16.9%	-122.0	420.6			
ST elev, inferior	7.5%	8.4%	-27.1	237.4		21.28 on 6 df	
ST elev, other	10.6%	13.4%	-42.1	159.6		(P < .01)	
ST depression	15.2%	13.8%	12.9	108.7			
Other abnormality	5.2%	5.8%	-9.6	103.2			
Normal	3.0%	2.3%	3 4	12.9			
Hours from onset							
0- 1	9.5%	13.0%	-29.3	83.3			
2- 3	8.2%	10.7%	-100.2	354.8		9.69 on 4 df	9.55 on 1 df
4- 6	9.7%	11.5%	-78.5	387 6		(P < .05)	(2P = 0.002)
7-12	11.1%	12.7%	-51.5	336.7			
13-24	10.0%	10.5%	-11.1	212.6			
Age (years)							
< 55	3.4%	4.6%	-45.9	155.6			
55-64	7.2%	8.9%	-86.3	360.0		8.27 on 3 df	6.58 on 1 df
65-74	13.5%	16.1%	-113.7	533.0		(P < .05)	(2P = 0.01)
75 +	24.3%	25.3%	-12 6	266.6			
Gender							
Male	8.2%	10.1%	-208.1	928.0		1.99 on 1 df	
Female	14.1%	16.0%	-62.2	436.8		(NS)	
Systolic BP (mm Hg)							
< 100	28.9%	35.1%	-38 7	132.2			
100-149	9.6%	11.5%	-168.9	850.0		1.31 on 3 df	0.68 on 1 df
150-174	7.2%	8.7%	-59.2	290 0		(NS)	(NS)
175 +	7.2%	8.2%	-10.8	74.1			
Heart rate							
< 80	7.2%	8.5%	-83.2	464.9		0.51 on 2 df	0.31 on 1 df
80-99	9.2%	11.3%	-65.8	287.2		(NS)	(NS)
100 +	17.4%	20.7%	-51.7	238.6			
Prior MI							
Yes	12.5%	14.1%	-43.7	322.4		2.09 on 1 df	
No	8.9%	10.9%	-228.5	1001.9		(NS)	
Diabetes							
Yes	13.6%	17.3%	-41 4	145.7		1.57 on 1 df	
No	8.7%	10.2%	-142.6	830 4		(NS)	
■ **ALL PATIENTS**	2820/29315 9.6%	3357/29285 11.5%	-269.5	1377.4	18% SD 2 odds reduction 2P < 0.00001		

0.5   1.0   1.5

Figure 2-5.

Mortality at 35 days stratified by various clinical parameters. Mortality differences during days 0 through 35 subdivided by presentation features in a collaborative overview of results from nine trials of fibrinolytic therapy. At center absolute mortality rates are shown for fibrinolytic and control groups for each clinical feature at presentation listed at left. The odds ratio of death in fibrinolytic group to that in control group is shown for each subdivision (*black square*) along with 95% confidence interval (*horizontal line*). The summary odds ratio at bottom corresponds to an 18% proportional reduction in 35-day mortality and is highly statistically significant. This translates to a reduction of 18 deaths per 1,000 patients treated with fibrinolytic agents. O-E indicates observed versus expected ratio; CIs, confidence intervals; ECG, electrocardiogram; BBB, bundle-branch block; ST elev, ST-segment elevation; df, degrees of freedom; BP, blood pressure; MI, myocardial infarction; SD, standard deviation. (Reprinted from: Fibrinolytic Therapy Trialsits' (FTT) Collaborative Group. *Lancet.* 1994;343:311–322, with permission.)

with a markedly elevated blood pressure. Fibrinolytic trials often excluded or discouraged enrollment of elderly patients, although in some studies patients older than 75 years of age have comprised up to 14% of the study patients. Retrospective trials have disagreed as to the benefit of fibrinolytic therapy in this cohort (16,17). However, it is important to emphasize that age is the single most important demographic risk factor for mortality. Frequently patients with the highest predicted short-term mortality are excluded from fibrinolytic therapy, although they stand to benefit the most (18). Data from the Fibrinolytic Therapy Trialists' (15) meta-analysis show that while the *relative* risk reduction of death is less among patients over 65 years of age compared with younger subgroups, the *absolute* reduction in mortality is greatest in those 65 to 74 years of age (Table 2–2) (19). Therefore, although primary PCI is an attractive alternative in elderly patients, if this is not available, fibrinolytic therapy should not be withheld strictly on the basis

of advanced age. Instead, the overall projected benefit should be weighed carefully against the overall projected risk.

Patients who present with a very high or very low systolic blood pressure also require special consideration. A prior history of hypertension, even if severe, is not of major concern. However, patients presenting with severe hypertension have an increased risk of ICH. The risk increases with an increasing baseline blood pressure (15). It is not known whether acute pharmacologic lowering of the blood pressure into a normal or acceptable range lowers the risk of ICH. Among these patients, consider primary PCI if available, but if not, carefully weigh all potential risk factors for bleeding and then treat accordingly.

Patients presenting with low blood pressure are a group at high risk for early mortality. Data are mixed regarding the efficacy of fibrinolytic therapy in this cohort (3,15,20). Experimental models suggest fibrinolytic therapy is less efficacious

Absolute Contraindications
1. Any prior ICH
2. Known structural intra-cerebral lesion (AVM, neoplasm)
3. Ischemic stroke within 3 months (unles swithin 3 hours)
4. Suspected aortic dissection
5. Active bleeding or bleeding diathesis (excluding menses)
6. Significant closed head or facial trauma

Relative Contraindications
1. History of long-standing, severe, poorly controlled hypertension
2. Severe uncontrolled hypertension on presentation (>180/110 mm Hg)
3. Traumatic or prolonged (>10 minutes) CPR
4. Major surgery within 3 weeks
5. Recent (<2 to 4 weeks) internal bleeding, or active peptic ulcer
6. Noncompressible vascular punctures
7. Pregnancy
8. Current use of anticoagulation (increasing risk with increasing INR)

Figure 2–6.

Contraindications to fibrinolytic therapy. (Adapted from: Antman EM, Anbe DT, Armstrong PW, et al. ACC/AHA guidelines for the management of patients with ST-elevation myocardial infarction—executive summary: a report of the American College of Cardiology/American Heart Association Task Force on Practice Guidelines (Writing Committee to revise the 1999 guidelines on the management of patients with acute myocardial Infarction). *J Am Coll Cardiol.* 2004;44:671–719, with permission.)

in this setting, perhaps related to poor perfusion and thus poor penetration of the drug into the intra-coronary thrombus. Data from the SHOCK trial (although lacking a control arm) may support the use of an intra-aortic balloon pump if fibrinolytics are administered. Nonetheless, data from that trial showed a superiority of primary PCI over fibrinolytic by reducing mortality at 6 months (21).

■ Limitations of Fibrinolytic Therapy

In addition to hemorrhagic risk and reduced efficacy with delayed administration, there are other limitations of fibrinolytic therapy that must be acknowledged. First, these drugs frequently do not completely restore normal coronary arterial flow. Early trials focused on arterial patency as it was appreci-

ated that an open artery correlated with improved outcomes. Fibrinolytic agents are known to produce TIMI 2 or TIMI 3 flow at 60 to 90 minutes in approximately 60% to 85% of the patients. However, it is now appreciated that TIMI 2 flow rates are not associated with statistically better outcomes than in patients who have TIMI 0 or TIMI 1 flow (22). Unfortunately, TIMI 3 flow is only achieved in 30% to 60% of patients at 90 minutes after fibrinolytic therapy. Second, among patients who achieve reperfusion, there is a 5% to 15% incidence of re-occlusion, a scenario associated with re-infarction and a poor clinical outcome. It appears that one important mechanism by which primary PCI is superior to fibrinolytic therapy is a reduction in re-infarctions. Finally, although fibrinolytic agents are more widely available as compared to primary PCI, there are many patients who are considered ineligible for fibrinolytic

Table 2–2

Revised Fibrinolytic Therapy Trialists' (FTT) Data Concerning Age, Relative and Absolute Benefit with Fibrinolytic Therapy (20)

Age Group (Years)	Control Group Mortality (%)	Treatment Group Mortality (%)	RRR (%)	ARR (%)
<55	5.4	3.8	29	1.6
55–64	10.7	8.1	24	2.6
65–74	19	15	21	4.0
>75	29.4	26	12	3.4

Despite less relative risk reduction in patients >65 years old, absolute risk reduction tends to be equal or slightly higher.

Table 2–3

Current Recommendations and Dosing for IV UFH in Association with Fibrinolytic Therapy

Class I:

1. Unfractionated heparin should be given intravenously to patients undergoing reperfusion therapy with alteplase, reteplase, or tenecteplase with dosing as follows: bolus of 60 U/kg (maximum 4,000 U) followed by an infusion of 12 U/kg/hour (maximum 1,000 U) initially adjusted to maintain activated partial thromboplastin time (aPTT) at 1.5 to 2.0 times control (approximately 50 to 70 seconds). *(Level of Evidence: C.)*
2. Unfractionated heparin should be given intravenously to patients treated with nonselective fibrinolytic agents (streptokinase, anistreplase, urokinase) who are at high risk for systemic emboli (large or anterior MI, atrial fibrillation (AF), previous embolus, or known LV thrombus). *(Level of Evidence: B.)*

Class IIb:

1. It may be reasonable to administer UFH intravenously to patients undergoing reperfusion therapy with streptokinase. *(Level of Evidence: B.)*

Class 1: Conditions for which there is evidence and/or general agreement that a given procedure or treatment is beneficial, useful, and effective.

Class IIb: Usefulness/efficacy is less well established by evidence/opinion.

Level of Evidence B: Data derived from a single randomized trial or nonrandomized studies.

Level of Evidence C: Only consensus opinion of experts, case studies, or standard-of-care.

Adapted from: Antman EM, Anbe DT, Armstrong PW, et al. ACC/AHA guidelines for the management of patients with ST-elevation myocardial infarction—executive summary: a report of the American College of Cardiology/American Heart Association Task Force on Practice Guidelines (Writing Committee to revise the 1999 guidelines on the management of patients with acute myocardial Infarction). *J Am Coll Cardiol.* 2004;44:671–719.

therapy. One meta-analysis of 50,000 patients presenting with AMI revealed that only 33% of patients were deemed eligible for fibrinolytic therapy and only about one half of the eligible patients received therapy (23). In addition to well-established contraindications to therapy, many patients are not treated because of late presentation, increased age, equivocal ECG findings, or other perceived medical contraindications. This emphasizes the need for physician education in regarding fibrinolytic therapy as well as the need for protocols to assist physicians in quantifying both the risk of complications and the predicted benefit so optimal and well-informed decisions can be made.

Adjuvant Therapies

Certain adjunctive medications have been shown to increase either the safety or efficacy of fibrinolytic therapy.

Aspirin

Aspirin was shown in the ISIS-2 trial to have synergistic effects when administered with SK, resulting in increased early arterial patency, which translated into a further reduction in mortality when compared to the SK-alone arm (1). The current recommended dose is 162 to 325 mg initially followed by oral administration of 75 to 162 mg daily (2).

Unfractionated Heparin

Unfractionated heparin (UFH) has been studied at various doses, with various routes of administration, and with multi-

ple different agents. Although UFH does not enhance thrombus dissolution, it has been shown to maximize sustained vessel patency. Studies have shown little additional benefit but increased bleeding complications when given along with SK. Therefore, it is given only in select circumstances in which there is a high risk of systemic embolism (atrial fibrillation, known LV thrombus, large anterior MI, prior thromboembolism). In contrast, IV UFH has a more important role when given concomitantly with the fibrin-specific agents. Efficacy is dependent on adequate dosing, requiring an aPTT level of 50 to 70 seconds. Current guidelines and dosing recommendations for IV UFH are summarized in Table 2–3 (2).

Low Molecular Weight Heparin

Recently the low molecular weight heparin enoxaparin has been studied as an adjunct to fibrinolytic therapy and a replacement for IV UFH. In the ASSENT 3 trial, there were three treatment arms, consisting of full dose tenecteplase with IV UFH (standard of care arm), full dose tenecteplase plus enoxaparin, and half dose tenecteplase with full dose abciximab and reduced dose IV UFH. Although there was no difference in the 30-day mortality between any arms, there was a lower rate of a pre-specified combined endpoint including death, re-infarction, or recurrent ischemia in the tenecteplase/enoxaparin arm and the arm containing abciximab, compared with the arm containing IV UFH. Specifically, re-infarction was lowest in those two groups, but unlike the abciximab group, bleeding was not increased in the enoxaparin arm (24).

Enoxaparin was also studied in the ExTRACT TIMI 25 trial, a 20,506 patient study using multiple different fibrinolytic agents chosen at the discretion of the clinician (25). The trial was designed to determine whether prolonged enoxaparin would be superior to IV UFH given at current recommended doses for 48 hours for maximizing sustained vessel patency. Previously, prolonged IV UFH had not been definitely shown to lower re-occlusion rates. The dose of enoxaparin utilized was a single 30 mg, nonweight based IV bolus, followed by 1 mg/kg subcutaneously every 12 hours that was not to exceed 100 mg, with the first SQ injection given within 15 minutes of the IV bolus. Important dose adjustments were made among patients >75 years of age, those with renal impairment, and patients who had previously received an IV bolus of UFH prior to entering the trial. The 30-day results showed a nonsignificant trend toward a reduction in total mortality in the enoxaparin arm, a statistically significant 33% relative reduction in re-infarction (4.5% versus 3.0%, p <0.001) in the enoxaparin arm, and lower rates of the softer endpoint of recurrent ischemia with enoxaparin. Bleeding tended slightly higher in the enoxaparin arm (2.1% versus 1.4% major bleeding rate). Taken together, these trials lend support to the use of enoxaparin as an adjunct to fibrinolytic therapy to promote sustained vessel patency and prevent re-occlusions (although it is not currently FDA approved for this indication).

Direct Thrombin Inhibitors

Direct thrombin inhibitors have also been studied as a substitute for IV UFH. The most studied agent is bivalirudin, which is currently approved and utilized during PCI for stable and unstable angina, but not STEMI or in conjunction with fibrinolytic therapy. Two trials have addressed the use of direct thrombin inhibitors with fibrinolytics, the GUSTO IIb and HERO 2 trials. GUSTO IIb, utilizing recombinant hirudin, showed no difference in mortality, but a modest reduction in re-infarction. This was achieved however, at the expense of increased "moderate" bleeds. Additionally, subgroup analysis suggested that the benefit was present when given along with SK, but not when given with the fibrin specific agent t-PA (the class of agent currently most commonly utilized in the United States) (26). The HERO 2 trial tested bivalirudin (previously called hirulog) against IV UFH in 17,000 patients who received SK. Again, an equivalent mortality with a reduction in re-infarction was seen, but this time with an increased rate of ICH and transfusion (27). Based on these findings, bivalirudin is not currently approved or recommended as an adjunct to fibrinolytic therapy.

Platelet Glycoprotein Receptor IIb/IIIa Antagonist

As fibrinolytic trials seem to hit a "ceiling" of myocardial salvage and mortality advantage, investigators speculated whether a combination of reduced dose fibrinolytics given with a platelet glycoprotein receptor IIb/IIIa antagonist could accelerate vessel patency and further improve survival. The rationale behind this was that fibrinolytics were inherently thrombogenic as they

did not directly lyse thrombin, and their action resulted in exposed thrombin that in turn activates platelets. Numerous pilot trials provided hope that this therapy would accomplish this goal, showing enhanced TIMI 3 flow rates. However, subsequent large-scale, multicenter randomized trials designed to examine the effect on mortality and safety endpoints failed to verify the expected benefit, and even created concerns about the safety of this approach. GUSTO V was the largest (n = 16,588) such trial, which utilized either full dose reteplase or half dose reteplase with full dose abciximab, with each arm also receiving IV UFH. Thirty day and one year mortality rates were equal while a reduction in the rate of nonfatal, recurrent MI was noted in the abciximab arm. The rate of ICH was not different between the two arms, but the rate of other bleeding was increased in the abciximab arm. Additionally, in patients >75 years of age, the rate of ICH was approximately doubled (2.1% versus 1.1%) in the abciximab arm. Conversely, the greatest benefit was seen in patients with an anterior MI; in fact among the subgroup of patients <75 years of age with an anterior MI, a reduction in the 30-day mortality rate was actually demonstrated, although this was not a durable finding at 1 year (28). The ASSENT 3 trial reported similar findings, with an abciximab arm showing no reduction in total mortality, an appreciable reduction in nonfatal re-infarction, but at the expense of increased bleeding complications. Again, patients >75 years of age seem to be at the greatest risk of being harmed by therapy (24).

As a result of these trials, the ACC/AHA guidelines assign a Class IIb indication to this combination of treatment, with consideration of this among patients <75 years of age with an anterior MI, or when an early (but not immediate) strategy of PCI is planned. The guidelines assign a Class III indication to this strategy among patients >75 years of age (2).

Clopidogrel

In another attempt to lower re-occlusion and re-infarction rates, two major trials using the platelet inhibitor clopidogrel have been reported. The larger Commit/CCS-2 Trial was performed in China, with only half of the patients receiving fibrinolytic therapy (predominantly urokinase), and a lower rate of subsequent angiography and revascularization than would occur in current western practices. Although it did show a small, statistically significant reduction in mortality in the clopidogrel arm, its applicability to western practice styles is limited (29). The CLARITY-TIMI 28 trial administered fibrinolytics, aspirin, and IV UFH to all patients who were then randomized to receive either clopidogrel or placebo. Although no further reduction in mortality was demonstrated, a reduction in the composite endpoint of death, re-infarction, or occluded infarct vessel at the time of angiography (performed at a median time of 3.5 days after infarction) was noted, primarily driven by a reduction in occluded vessels. No concerns of increased ICH or major bleeds were identified, with only a nonsignificant trend toward an increased number of minor bleeds in the clopidogrel treated group (30). In a prespecified subset population (the PCI-CLARITY trial) of patients who were sent for early angiography and PCI, a 41% relative risk reduction was seen in the combined endpoint of death, re-infarction, or stroke. Similar to other studies of clopidogrel, there was benefit derived both during the period before angiography, with additional benefit noted in the period between angiography and hospital discharge. While the numbers are too small for statistical significance, there was a roughly equal relative risk reduction among all three components of the endpoint (31). On the basis of this data, clopidogrel recently received FDA indication for use during STEMI.

Assessment and Treatment of Failed Fibrinolytics

Because fibrinolytics are not universally successful in restoring arterial patency, and because many patients are cared for at facilities without cardiac catheterization capabilities, there has been much interest in noninvasive methods to predict continued vessel occlusion. Three methods are commonly utilized in an effort to aid clinical decision-making.

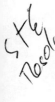

ST segment resolution is a useful tool to assess not only the presence of epicardial arterial flow, but also tissue level perfusion. Criteria have been proposed (at least 50% ST resolution at 90 minutes), but this finding suffers from imperfect sensitivity and specificity. Although this finding has a high positive predictive value of approximately 90% (i.e., >50% resolution predicts arterial patency well), failure to significantly resolve ST segment is not a particularly specific predictor of persistent occlusion, with a negative predictive value of only 50% (32). What is known is that patients with complete ST resolution seem to have the best prognosis, whereas those with ongoing ST elevation likely suffer either a persistently occluded artery or a patent epicardial artery with impaired tissue level perfusion. Among patients with TIMI 3 flow, those with persistent ST elevation have a noticeably poorer prognosis than those with ST resolution. Therefore, although ST resolution is an imperfect predictor of IRA patency, it does provide important prognostic information (32).

A second criterion proposed is resolution of chest pain. Although this is an intuitive clinical tool, in actual practice this can be a confusing variable to assess (varying types or severity of pain, evolving pain, intermittent pain), and, in fact, studies document that it is not sufficiently accurate to guide clinical decision-making. Even the circumstance of unchanged or worsened chest pain has been shown to be associated with infarct artery patency in 60% of cases (33).

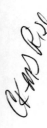

Finally, numerous attempts have been made to utilize cardiac biomarker data to predict arterial patency. Data are best in support of utilizing either CK-MB or myoglobin. Various reports have suggested that the rate of rise of the agents (as quantified by either absolute rise by 60 to 90 minutes or a ratio of the 60 to 90 minute value compared to the baseline value) may be used as "supportive evidence" of reperfusion. These data are probably best utilized in conjunction with other clinical clues, and schemes have been offered that combine these three variables in an attempt to distinguish vessel patency from persistent occlusion (34).

The presence of various ventricular arrhythmias is not thought to be a particularly sensitive or specific predictor of IRA patency.

Conclusion

Fibrinolytic therapy is a powerful tool to reduce mortality and morbidity associated with AMI. Its advantages include its widespread availability, the rapidity with which is can be administered, reasonable cost, and proven reduction in mortality. However, fibrinolytic therapy has well defined contraindications and a reasonably low, but serious incidence of side effects which renders many patients ineligible. Although there are still questions to be answered, large well-controlled, scientifically valid, prospective randomized trials have provided us valuable information on its anticipated benefits, and have significantly clarified the types and intensity of adjunctive therapies that should be administered. An adequate knowledge base concerning fibrinolytic therapy should assist the clinician in safely and effectively utilizing this vital therapy.

REFERENCES

1. Second International Study of Infarct Survival Collaborative Group. Randomized trial of intravenous streptokinase, oral aspirin, both, or neither among 17,187 cases of suspected acute myocardial infarction: ISIS-2. *Lancet.* 1988;2:349–360.
2. Antman EM, Anbe DT, Armstrong PW, et al. ACC/AHA guidelines for the management of patients with ST-elevation myocardial infarction—executive summary: a report of the American College of Cardiology/American Heart Association Task Force on Practice Guidelines (Writing Committee to revise the 1999 guidelines on the management of patients with acute myocardial Infarction). *J Am Coll Cardiol.* 2004;44:671–719.
3. Effectiveness of intravenous thrombolytic treatment in acute myocardial infarction. Gruppo Italiano per lo Studio della Streptochinasi nell'Infarto Miocardico (GISSI). *Lancet.* 1986;1:397–402.
4. Neuhaus KL, Feuerer W, Jeep-Tebbe S, et al. Improved thrombolysis with a modified dose regimen of recombinant tissue-type plasminogen activator. *J Am Coll Cardiol.* 1989;14:1566–1569.
5. The GUSTO investigators. An international randomized trial comparing four thrombolytic strategies for acute myocardial infarction. *N Engl J Med.* 1993;329:673–682.
6. Bode C, Smalling RW, Berg G, et al. Randomized comparison of coronary thrombolysis achieved with double-bolus reteplase (recombinant plasminogen activator) and front-loaded, accelerated alteplase (recombinant tissue plasminogen activator) in patients with acute myocardial infarction. The RAPID II Investigators. *Circulation.* 1996; 94:891–898.
7. The Global Use of Strategies to Open Occluded Coronary Arteries (GUSTO III) Investigators. A comparison of reteplase with alteplase for acute myocardial infarction. *N Engl J Med.* 1997;337:1118–1123.
8. International Joint Efficacy Comparison of Thrombolytics. Randomized, double-blind comparison of reteplase double-bolus administration with streptokinase in acute myocardial infarction (INJECT): trial to investigate equivalence. *Lancet.* 1995;346:329–336.
9. Assessment of the Safety and Efficacy of a New Thrombolytic Investigators. Single-bolus tenecteplase compared with front-loaded alteplase in acute myocardial infarction: the ASSENT-2 double-blind randomized trial. *Lancet.* 1999;354:716–722.
10. Lincoff AM, Topol EJ. Illusion of reperfusion: does anyone achieve optimal reperfusion during acute myocardial infarction? *Circulation.* 1993; 88:1361–1374.
11. Weaver WD, Cerqueira M, Hallstrom AP, et al. Prehospital-initiated vs hospital-initiated thrombolytic therapy. The Myocardial Infarction Triage and Intervention Trial. *JAMA.* 1993;270:1211–1216.

12. Boersma E, Maas AC, Deckers JW, et al. Early thrombolytic treatment in acute myocardial infarction: reappraisal of the golden hour. *Lancet.* 1996; 348:771–775.

13. Topol EJ, Califf RM, Vandormael M, et al. A randomized trial of late reperfusion therapy for acute myocardial infarction. Thrombolysis and Angioplasty in Myocardial Infarction-6 Study Group. *Circulation.* 1992;85: 2090–2099.

14. Sager PT, Perlmutter RA, Rosenfield LE, et al. Electrophysiological effects of thrombolytic therapy in patients with a transmural anterior myocardial infarction complicated by left ventricular aneurysm formation. *J Am Coll Cardiol.* 1988;12:19–24.

15. Fibrinolytic Therapy Trialists' (FTT) Collaborative Group. Indications for fibrinolytic therapy in suspected acute myocardial infarction: collaborative overview of early mortality and major morbidity from the all randomized trials of more than 1,000 patients. *Lancet.* 1994;343:311–322.

16. Thiemann DR, Coresh J, Schulman SP, et al. Lack of benefit for intravenous thrombolysis in patients with myocardial infarction who are older than 75 years. *Circulation.* 2000;101:2239–2246.

17. Berger AK, Radford MJ, Wang Y, et al. Thrombolytic therapy in older patients. *J Am Coll Cardiol.* 2000;36:366–374.

18. Cragg DR, Friedman HZ, Bonema JD, et al. Outcome of patients with acute myocardial infarction who are ineligible for thrombolytic therapy. *Ann Intern Med.* 1991;115:173–177.

19. Estess JM, Topol EJ. Fibrinolytic therapy for elderly patients with myocardial infarction. *Heart.* 2002;87:308–311.

20. Kennedy JW, Gensini GG, Timmis GC, et al. Acute myocardial infarction treated with intracoronary streptokinase: a report of the Society of Cardiac Angiography. *Am J Cardiol.* 1985;55:871–877.

21. Hochman JS, Sleeper LA, Webb JG, et al. Early revascularization in acute myocardial infarction complicated by cardiogenic shock. SHOCK Investigators. Should we emergently revascularize occluded coronaries for cardiogenic shock. *N Engl J Med.* 1999;341:625–634.

22. Anderson JL, Karagounis LA, Califf RM. Metaanalysis of five reported studies on the relation of early coronary patency grades with mortality and outcomes after acute myocardial infarction. *Am J Cardiol.* 1996;78:1–8.

23. Muller DW, Topol EJ. Selection of patients with acute myocardial infarction for thrombolytic therapy. *Ann Intern Med.* 1990;113:949–960.

24. Assessment of the Safety and Efficacy of a New Thrombolytic regimen (ASSENT)-3 Investigators. Efficacy and safety of tenecteplase in combination with enoxaparin, abciximab, or unfractionated heparin: the ASSENT-3 randomized trial in acute myocardial infarction. *Lancet.* 2001;358:605–613.

25. Antman EM, Morrow DA, McCabe CH, et al. ExTRACT-TIMI 25 Investigators. Enoxaparin versus unfractionated heparin with fibrinolysis for ST-elevation myocardial infarction. *N Eng J Med.* 2006;354:1477–1488.

26. The Global Use of Strategies to Open Occluded Coronary Arteries (GUSTO) IIb Investigators. A comparison of recombinant hirudin with heparin for the treatment of acute coronary syndromes. *N Eng J Med.* 1996;335:775–782.

27. White H; Hirulog and Early Reperfusion or Occlusion (HERO)-2 Trial Investigators. Thrombin-specific anticoagulation with bivalirudin versus heparin in patients receiving fibrinolytic therapy for acute myocardial infarction: The HERO-2 randomized trial. *Lancet.* 2001;358:1855–1863.

28. Topol EJ; GUSTO V Investigators. Reperfusion therapy for acute myocardial infarction with fibrinolytic therapy or combination reduced fibrinolytic therapy and platelet glycoprotein IIb/IIIa inhibition: the GUSTO V randomized trial. *Lancet.* 2001;357:1905–1914.

29. Chen ZM, Jiang LX, Chen YP, et al.; COMMIT (ClOpidogrel and Metoprolol in Myocardial Infarction Trial) collaborative group. Addition of clopidogrel to aspirin in 45,852 patients with acute myocardial infarction: randomized placebo-controlled trial. *Lancet.* 2005;366:1607–1621.

30. Sabatine MS, Cannon CP, Gibson CM, et al. ; CLARITY-TIMI 28 Investigators. Addition of clopidogrel to aspirin and fibrinolytic therapy for myocardial infarction with ST-segment elevation. *N Eng J Med.* 2005;352:1179–1189.

31. Sabatine MS, Cannon CP, Gibson CM, et al.; Clopidogrel as Adjunctive Reperfusion Therapy (CLARITY)-Thrombolysis in Myocardial Infarction (TIMI) 28 Investigators. Effect of clopidogrel pretreatment before percutaneous coronary intervention in patients with ST-elevation myocardial infarction treated with fibrinolytics, the PCI-CLARITY Study. *JAMA.* 2005; 294:1224–1232.

32. de Lemos JA, Braunwald E. ST segment resolution as a tool for assessing the efficacy of reperfusion therapy. *J Am Coll Cardiol.* 2001;38:1283–1294.

33. Califf RM, O'Neill W, Stack RS, et al. Failure of simple clinical measurements to predict perfusion status after intravenous thrombolysis. *Ann Intern Med.* 1988;108:658–662.

34. de Lemos JA, Morrow DA, Gibson CM, et al.; TIMI 14 Investigators. Thrombosis in Myocardial Infarction. Early noninvasive detection of failed epicardial reperfusion after fibrinolytic therapy. *Am J Cardiol.* 2001;88: 353–358.

CHAPTER 3

Medications Used in the Cardiac Catheterization Laboratory*

Morton J. Kern

Coronary Vasodilators

Nitroglycerin

Nitroglycerin is the most commonly used drug during coronary arteriography and ventriculography. Nitroglycerin dilates peripheral arteries, venous beds, and coronary arteries. Nitroglycerin is a very safe and short-acting drug. It can be given through the sublingual, IV, intracoronary, or intraventricular route. Sublingual (or oral spray) nitroglycerin (0.4 mg) is frequently given before coronary arteriography. Exceptions include patients in whom coronary spasm may be suspected and those with hypotension (<90 mm Hg systolic pressure). In patients with documented coronary spasm, sublingual or intracoronary nitroglycerin is given to eliminate coronary spasm. In patients with unstable angina, IV infusions of nitroglycerin of up to 250 micrograms/min with a systolic blood pressure of 90 mm Hg are permissible. In patients with elevated LV end-diastolic pressure in the catheterization laboratory from ischemia or from congestive heart failure, intraventricular or IV boluses of 200 micrograms of nitroglycerin will reduce LV end-diastolic pressure and are appropriate before and after ventriculography. Intracoronary micrograms nitroglycerin increases coronary blood flow without a marked reduction in pressure in doses of 50, 100, and 200 micrograms. In doses of more than 250 micrograms, hypotension without further increases in coronary blood flow may be evident. Care should be used to avoid hypotension when administering NTG to patients with known or suspected severe aortic stenosis, significant left main narrowing, or hypertrophic myopathy.

Calcium Channel Blockers

Calcium channel blockers dilate vascular smooth muscle and reduce heart muscle contractility, and some agents block AV nodal conduction. Calcium channel blockers are used to reduce peripheral vascular resistance, reduce blood pressure, block coronary spasm and increase coronary blood flow. Acute use in the cardiac catheterization is limited to treating arrhyth-

mias and "no-reflow" of coronary interventions or to treat radial artery spasm when performing transradial approach. Doses for calcium channel blockers are as follows:

1. Diltiazem: 30 to 60 mg po, 10 mg IV
2. Verapamil: 120 mg po, 2.5 to 5 mg IV (for coronary "no-reflow," intracoronary bolus Verapamil 200 μcg to be repeated 2 to 4 doses if needed).

Papaverine

Papaverine is a potent arterial vasodilator used in the investigation of coronary vasodilatory reserve. Intracoronary papaverine causes a marked increase in blood flow in the RCA in doses from 4 to 8 mg and in the LCA in doses from 8 to 12 mg. Doses exceeding these recommended levels do not appear to provide an increase over the maximal blood flow. Papaverine causes QT prolongation. Rare cases of papaverine-induced torsades de pointes have been reported, and antiarrhythmic preparations for this unusual event should be in place before administration of intracoronary papaverine.

Adenosine

Adenosine IV is used for breaking supraventricular tachycardia (SVT) and is the drug of choice for intracoronary induction of maximal hyperemia for coronary vasodilator reserve. For the RCA, intracoronary (IC) adenosine in 12 to 24 μg and for the LCA 24 to 40 mcg produces optimal results. Adenosine infusions, 140 mcg/kg/min IV, produce sustained hyperemia. Adenosine hyperemia lasts <60 seconds after drug administration is ended.

Acetylcholine

Acetylcholine dilates normal coronary arteries and constricts diseased vessels. In Japan, intracoronary doses of 20, 50, and 100 μg have been used to induce coronary spasm in patients. The drug is very short-acting and rapidly inactivated, making it suitable for catheterization laboratory use. Marked bradycardia, heart block, and vasospasm are common with acetylcholine. Temporary pacing is required during its administration. Continuous infusions of 0.02 to 2.2 mcg (10^{-8}, 10^{-7},

*Sections taken from: Kern MJ, ed. *The Cardiac Catheterization Handbook.* 4th ed. St. Louis, MO: Mosby-Yearbook; 2003, with permission.

10^{-6} M) have been used to identify normal endothelial function of coronary vessels (vasodilation not vasoconstriction).

Nitroprusside

For coronary "no-reflow," 25 to 100 μcg bolus can be used and repeated as needed.

Coronary Vasoconstrictor (for Provocation of Coronary Spasm Only)

Ergonovine

Ergonovine is used to provoke coronary vasospasm in patients with chest pain syndromes and normal or nearly normal coronary arteriograms. One commonly used dosing regimen is sequential dosing with 0.02, 0.18, and 0.2 mg intravenously at 3-minute intervals, obtaining ECGs at the end of each dose for a total dose of 0.4 mg. If the patient develops typical symptoms, an ECG is obtained and arteriograms performed immediately on both the left and right coronary arteries. Ergonovine-induced diffuse coronary vasoconstriction is a physiologic response. Ergonovine-induced focal coronary constriction (relieved with nitroglycerin) is a positive response for coronary spasm. These angiographic changes should be associated with electrocardiographic or symptomatic alterations. Ergonovine-induced coronary vasospasm or physiologic narrowing can be reversed immediately with intracoronary nitroglycerin.

Anticholinergics for Vagal Reactions

Atropine

Atropine is used to block vagally induced slowing of the heart rate and hypotension. Doses of 0.6 to 1.2 mg IV given immediately will reverse bradycardia and hypotension within 2 minutes. It is important to remember that in elderly patients and patients who are pacer dependent, heart rate may not slow during vagal episodes in which the only manifestation is that of low blood pressure. This low blood pressure can be alleviated by the administration of IV atropine and normal saline. In the rare patient in whom IV access is not immediately available, intraarterial atropine (in the aorta) can be administered. Vasoconstrictors are reserved for persistent hypotension after recovery of heart rate.

Antiarrhythmic Drugs

Lidocaine

Lidocaine is an antiarrhythmic drug used to block or reduce the number of ventricular extrasystoles. Lidocaine can be administered as a bolus of 50 to 100 mg intravenously before ventriculography if a stable and quiet catheter position within the left ventricle cannot be obtained. In patients in whom myocardial ischemia is developing during cardiac catheterization

or angioplasty, lidocaine for frequent ventricular ectopy is indicated. A bolus of 50 to 100 mg intravenously followed by 1 to 2 mg/min infusion is usually satisfactory.

Amiodarone

Amiodarone is indicated for recurrent ventricular fibrillation or recurrent hemodynamically unstable ventricular tachycardia nonresponsive to adequate doses of other antiarrhythmics or when alternative agents can't be tolerated.

The loading dose is 150 mg IV over 10 minutes (15 mg/min); then 360 mg IV over next 6 hours (1 mg/min), followed by 540 mg IV over next 18 hours (0.5 mg/min). After first 24 hours, continue with maintenance IV infusion of 720 mg/24 hours (0.5 mg/minute). In the cath lab, amiodarone has been associated with bradycardia, hypotension, arrhythmias, heart failure, heart block, sinus arrest, and edema.

Amiodarone may reduce hepatic or renal clearance of certain antiarrhythmics (especially flecainide, procainamide, and quinidine). Use of amiodarone with other antiarrhythmics (especially mexiletine, propafenone, quinidine, disopyramide, procainamide) may induce torsades de pointes. Use together cautiously with antihypertensives, beta blockers, calcium channel blockers, due to increased cardiac depressant effects and slowing of SA node and AV conduction.

Amiodarone may potentiate of anticoagulant response with the potential for serious or fatal bleeding. Decrease warfarin dosage 33% to 50% when amiodarone is initiated. Amiodarone is contraindicated in cardiogenic shock, second- or third-degree AV block, and severe SA node disease resulting in preexisting bradycardia unless a pacemaker is present.

Cardiac Agonists

Isoproterenol

Isoproterenol (Isuprel) is a pure beta agonist that increases heart rate and causes peripheral vasodilatation. It is indicated during cardiac arrest with refractory bradycardia. Isuprel has been used for provocation of cardiac stress (increased heart rate) in patients with valvular heart disease or hypertrophic cardiomyopathy. It is not used in the cardiac cath lab today.

Dopamine

Dopamine is a potent vasoconstrictor. In low doses it causes renal vasodilatation. In high doses it causes peripheral vasoconstriction, elevating the blood pressure and increasing myocardial contractility. Dopamine from 2 to 15 mcg/min will act to cause vasoconstriction, tachycardia, elevating the blood pressure for problems resulting in severe hypotension.

Dobutamine

Dobutamine is a potent inotropic agent with no peripheral vasoconstrictor effects. It increases cardiac contractility (inotropy) and is especially useful in patients with low cardiac

Table 3–1

Medications Used in the Cardiac Catheterization Laboratory*

Inotropics
Digitalis, 0.125 to 0.25 mg IV >4 hours apart
Dobutamine, 2 to 10 μg/kg/min IV drip
Dopamine, 2 to 10 μg/kg/min IV drip
Epinephrine, 1:10,000 IV
Isoproterenol, 1 mg/min IV drip

Antiarrhythmics, anticholinergics, beta blockers,
  calcium blockers
Adenosine, 5 to 12 mg IV bolus
Atropine, 0.6 to 1.2 mg IV
Bretylium, 100 to 300 mg IV bolus
Diltiazem, 10 mg IV
Esmolol, 4 to 24 mg/kg IV drip (beta blocker)
Lidocaine, 50 to 100 mg IV bolus; 2 to 4 mg/min IV drip
Procainamide, 50 to 100 mg IV
Propranolol, 1 mg bolus; 0.1 mg/kg in three divided doses
  (beta blocker)
Verapamil, 2 to 5 mg IV, may repeat dose to 10 mg (calcium
  channel blocker)

Analgesics, sedatives
Diazepam, 2 to 5 mg IV
Diphenhydramine, 25 to 50 mg IV
Meperidine, 12.5 to 50 mg IV
Morphine sulfate, 2.5 mg IV
Naloxone, 0.5 mg IV

Anticoagulants
Heparin 2,000 to 5,000 U IV; 1,000 U/hour IV drip; 40 to
  70 μ/kg for PCI

Vasodilators
Nitroglycerin 1/150 sublingual, 100 to 300 μg IC
Nitroprusside, 5 to 50 μg/kg/min IV

Vasoconstrictors
Aramine, 10 mg in 100 mL saline, 1 mL IV
Ergonovine, 0.4 mg IV in divided doses
Norepinephrine 1:10,000 IV, 1 mL doses IV

*The list is meant to be neither all inclusive nor exclusive of emergency life support techniques or standards.

Table 3–2

Table Applications of Physiologic Measurements in the Catheterization Laboratory

A. PCI Guideline Recommended Uses*
  1. Assessment of the effects of intermediate coronary stenoses (30%–70% luminal narrowing) in patients with anginal symptoms. Coronary pressure or doppler velocimetry may also be useful as an alternative to performing noninvasive functional testing (e.g., when the functional study is absent or ambiguous) to determine whether an intervention is warranted. (Class IIa, *Level of Evidence: B*)
  2. Assessing the success of PCI in restoring flow reserve and to predict the risk of restenosis. (Class IIb, *Level of Evidence: C*)
  3. Evaluating patients with anginal symptoms without an apparent angiographic culprit lesion. (Class IIb, *Level of Evidence: C*)
  4. Routine assessment of the severity of angiographic disease in patients with a positive, unequivocal noninvasive functional study is not recommended. (Class III, *Level of Evidence: C*)
B. Applications of FFR under Study**:
  1. Determination of one or more culprit stenoses (either serially or in separate vessels) in patients with multivessel disease.
  2. Evaluation of ostial or distal left main and ostial right lesions, especially when these regions cannot be well visualized by angiography.
  3. Guidance of treatment of serial stenoses in a coronary artery.
  4. Determination of significance of focal treatable region in vessel with diffuse coronary artery disease.
  5. Determination of prognosis after stent deployment.
  6. Assessment of stenosis in patients with previous (nonacute, >6 days) myocardial infarction.
  7. Assessment of lesions in patients with treated unstable angina pectoris.
  8. Assessment of the collateral circulation.
C. Applications of Coronary Doppler Flow under Study**
  1. Assessment of microcirculation
  2. Endothelial function testing
  3. Myocardial viability in acute myocardial infarction
D. Applications of Combined Coronary Pressure and Doppler Flow Velocity under Study**
  1. Assessment of intermediate stenosis
  2. Assessment of the microcirculation
  3. Identification of Lesion Compliance (change of pressure-velocity relationship)

*From: Smith SC Jr, et al. ACC/AHA/SCAI 2005 guideline update for percutaneous coronary intervention: a report of the American College of Cardiology/American Heart Association Task Force on Practice Guidelines (ACC/AHA/SCAI Writing Committee to Update the 2001. Guidelines for Percutaneous Coronary Intervention). American College of Cardiology Foundation and the American Heart Association, Inc., 2005. Available at: www.acc.org/clinical/guidelines/percutaneous/update/index.pdf.
**Not yet recommended by PCI Guidelines.

output or congestive heart failure. It may be used in conjunction with a potent vasodilator such as nitroprusside in those patients with markedly elevated filling pressures and poor cardiac output.

Epinephrine

Epinephrine (1:10,000) is a naturally occurring catecholamine that stimulates cardiac function. It is administered only during cardiac emergencies. This medicine will increase heart rate and blood pressure immediately, sometimes to very high levels. Epinephrine should be reserved for cases needing cardiac resuscitation or in which refractory hypotension is present and not responding to peripheral vasoconstrictors or in the treatment of anaphylactic reactions. Transthoracic administration of epinephrine through a long needle is no longer performed. IV or intraarterial administration of 1 mL of 1:10,000 dilution can increase systemic pressure transiently during hypotension to a safe level until IV vasopressors have been prepared. This dose of Epi has a duration of action between 5 and 10 minutes.

Arterial Vasodilator

Nitroprusside

Nitroprusside is a potent short-acting intravenous arterial vasodilator used in the treatment of aortic insufficiency, mitral regurgitation, hypertensive crisis, and congestive heart failure. Doses administered range from 10 to 100 μg/min and must be monitored by direct arterial pressure measurement. Table 3–1 lists medications used commonly during cardiac catheterization.

BIBLIOGRAPHY

Bech GJ, De Bruyne B, Bonnier HJRM, et al. Long-term follow-up after deferral of percutaneous transluminal coronary angioplasty of intermediate stenosis on the basis of coronary pressure measurement. *J Am Coll Cardiol*. 1998;31:841–847.

Bech GJ, Droste H, Pijls NH, et al. Value of fractional flow reserve in making decisions about bypass surgery for equivocal left main coronary artery disease. *Heart*. 2001;86:547–552.

Bech GJW, De Bruyne B, Pijls NHJ, et al. Fractional flow reserve to determine the appropriateness of angioplasty in moderate coronary stenosis: A randomized trial. *Circulation*. 2001;103:2928–2934.

Botman KJ, Pijls NHJ, Bech JW, et al. Percutaneous coronary intervention or bypass surgery in multivessel disease? A tailored approach based on coronary pressure measurement. *Catheter Cardiovasc Interv*. 2004;63:184–191.

Chamuleau SAJ, Meuwissen M, Koch KT, et al. Usefulness of fractional flow reserve for risk stratification of patients with multivessel coronary artery disease and an intermediate stenosis. *Am J Cardiol*. 2002;89:377–380.

De Bruyne B, Bartunek J, Sys SU, et al. Simultaneous coronary pressure and flow velocity measurements in humans: feasibility, reproducibility, and hemodynamic dependence of coronary flow velocity reserve, hyperemic flow versus pressure slope index, and fractional flow reserve. *Circulation*. 1996;94:1842–1849.

De Bruyne B, Hersbach F, Pijls NHJ, et al. Abnormal epicardial coronary resistance in patients with diffuse atherosclerosis but "normal" coronary angiography. *Circulation*. 2001;104:2401–2406.

De Bruyne B, Pijls NHJ, Heyndrickx GR, et al. Pressure-derived fractional flow reserve to assess serial epicardial stenoses: theoretical basis and animal validation. *Circulation*. 2000;101:1840–1847.

Di Segni E, Higano ST, Rihal CS, Holmes DR, Lennon R, Lerman A. Incremental doses of intracoronary adenosine for the assessment of coronary velocity reserve for clinical decision making. *Catheter Cardiovasc Interv*. 2001;54:34–40.

Gould KL, Kirkeeide RL, Buchi M. Coronary flow reserve as a physiologic measure of stenosis severity. *J Am Coll Cardiol*. 1990;15:459–474.

Jeremias A, Whitbourn RJ, Filardo SD, et al. Adequacy of intracoronary versus intravenous adenosine-induced maximal coronary hyperemia for fractional flow reserve measurements. *Am Heart J*. 2000;140:651–657.

Kern MJ, Donohue TJ, Aguirre FV, et al. Clinical outcome of deferring angioplasty in patients with normal translesional pressure-flow velocity measurements. *J Am Coll Cardiol*. 1995;25:178–187.

Kern MJ. Coronary physiology revisited: practical insights from the cardiac catheterization laboratory. *Circulation*. 2000;101:1344–1351.

Miller DD, Donohue TJ, Younis LT, et al. Correlation of pharmacologic 99mtc-sestamibi myocardial perfusion imaging with poststenotic coronary flow reserve in patients with angiographically intermediate coronary artery stenoses. *Circulation*. 1994;89:2150–2160.

Mintz GC, Popma JJ, Pichard AD, et al. Limitations of angiography in the assessment of plaque distribution in coronary artery disease: a systematic study of target lesion eccentricity in 1446 lesions. *Circulation*. 1996;93:924–931.

Pijls NH, De Bruyne B, Peels K, et al. Measurement of fractional flow reserve to assess the functional severity of coronary-artery stenoses. *N Engl J Med*. 1996;334:1703–1708.

Pijls NH, Van Gelder B, Van der Voort P, et al. Fractional flow reserve: a useful index to evaluate the influence of an epicardial coronary stenosis on myocardial blood flow. *Circulation*. 1995;92:3183–3193.

Pijls NHJ, De Bruyne B, Bech GJW, et al. Coronary Pressure Measurement to Assess the Hemodynamic Significance of Serial Stenoses Within One Coronary Artery: Validation in Humans. *Circulation*. 2000;102:2371–2377.

Pijls NHJ, Kern MJ, Yock PG, et al. Practice and potential pitfalls of coronary pressure measurement. *Catheter Cardiovasc Interv*. 2000;49:1–16.

Pijls NHJ, Klauss V, Siebert U, et al. Coronary pressure measurement after stenting predicts adverse events at follow-up. A multicenter registry. *Circulation*. 2002;105:2950–2954.

Pijls NHJ, van Som AM, Kirkeeide RL, et al. Experimental basis of determining maximum coronary, myocardial, and collateral blood flow by pressure measurements for assessing functional stenosis severity before and after percutaneous transluminal coronary angioplasty. *Circulation*. 1993;87:1354–1367.

Spaan JAE, Piek JJ, Hoffman JIE, et al. Physiological basis of clinically used coronary hemodynamic indices. *Circulation*. 2006;113:446–455.

Topol EJ, Nissen SE. Our preoccupation with coronary luminology. The dissociation between clinical and angiographic findings in ischemic heart disease. *Circulation*. 1995;92:2333–2342.

CHAPTER 4

Antiarrhythmic Drugs

Bipin Ravindran, Kenneth W. Kenyon, and Kristen K. Patton

General Principles of Antiarrhythmic Drug Pharmacology

Antiarrhythmic drugs are perhaps the most diverse and pharmacologically complex class of all cardiovascular agents. Many of these drugs are characterized by a relatively narrow therapeutic index, clinically significant inter-patient variability in metabolism, and considerable potential toxicity. Despite generalizing classification systems, such as the Sing-Vaughn Williams and the Sicilian Gambit, each of these agents is unique. Successful antiarrhythmic therapy entails appropriate selection of an agent for a presenting arrhythmia with concern for pharmacodynamic and pharmacokinetic properties. Failure to recognize these important properties of individual antiarrhythmic agents may lead to diminished efficacy, proarrhythmia, systemic toxicity and even death (1).

Pharmacodynamics

The pharmacodynamic effect of a given drug describes the relationship between the concentration of a drug and its effects at a specific site within the body. For antiarrhythmic drugs, this relationship refers to the way a drug affects specific ion channels and receptors throughout the myocardium, which ultimately affects the electrophysiologic properties of the myocardium (1,2). The ions of primary importance are sodium, potassium, and calcium. Although most antiarrhythmics are classified based upon their primary ion channel interaction, it is important to recognize that many, if not most, antiarrhythmic drugs have multiple electrophysiologic effects, and it is not easily discernable which effect imparts clinical efficacy. Furthermore, it is equally important to recognize that certain antiarrhythmic agents have active metabolites, and these metabolites may portend an innate electrophysiologic activity far different from the parent compound.

Pharmacokinetics

The principles of pharmacokinetics comprise the rate and extent of drug absorption, distribution to various organ systems, metabolic pathways, and elimination. Although these variables are important with regard to pharmacotherapy in general, they are particularly consequential because of the narrow therapeutic index of antiarrhythmic compounds and the inherent variability that exists with regard to these pharmacokinetic parameters in a given patient population.

Absorption

The bioavailability of a drug is the fraction of drug absorbed into the systemic circulation following administration. For drugs given intravenously, bioavailability is regarded as 100%, whereas drugs administered extravascularly are dependant upon a multitude of factors effecting absorption and presystemic clearance. This is of particular importance when transitioning from parenteral to oral administration (1). Factors influencing absorption may include, but are not limited to: gastric and bowel pH, bowel motility, food, concomitantly administered drugs, and tablet formulation (i.e., sustained release preparations) (1).

Distribution

Once absorption is complete, the extent to which a drug is distributed from the "central" compartment (e.g., heart, liver, and kidney) into the more "outward" compartments (e.g., adipose tissue, muscle, skin) is dependent upon the drug's volume of distribution (VD). This value represents the relationship between the drug dose and the resultant serum concentration. Antiarrhythmic agents with a relatively small VD may produce a clinical response sooner than those with a large VD which often require loading dose regimens. Amiodarone is an example of a drug with a long elimination phase and large VD; as such, onset of action with oral therapy is delayed as the drug distributes extensively into the tissue compartments and once a steady state is achieved, effects may persist for months upon discontinuation.

Many factors may influence how a drug is distributed, and protein-binding characteristics play an important role (2). Many antiarrhythmic agents are bases and bind extensively to alpha-1-acid glycoprotein; it is the unbound portion of a drug that interfaces with ion channels and receptors, producing an electrophysiologic effect (2,3). Factors that may alter protein binding, and thus the clinical effect of an antiarrhythmic drug, include the plasma concentration of the drug, serum pH, interactions with other highly protein bound drugs, and the concentration of the plasma protein itself, many of which are acute phase reactants (3).

Metabolism

The metabolism (biotransformation) of antiarrhythmic drugs is potentially the most important pharmacokinetic parameter clinicians should familiarize themselves with when prescribing these agents. All drugs entering the systemic circulation will either be metabolized before excretion or eliminated unchanged as the parent compound. Parameters that are of particular concern include the metabolic pathway, metabolite formation, and various other factors influencing metabolism.

Most antiarrhythmic drugs are metabolized (many to activate metabolites with distinct electrophysiologic properties) and eliminated by the liver; metabolism occurs primarily by the oxidative pathway via cytochrome P-450 isoenzymes (CYP). The two most important of these isoenzymes are CYP-2D6 and CYP-3A4 (1,2). An estimated 10% of the population is deficient in CYP-2D6 activity (classified as "slow metabolizers") and are subject to side effects of therapy due to accumulation of the parent compound. Slow metabolizers may require lower than expected doses to achieve the desired therapeutic effect. Even patients with functional expression of these isoenzymes are at risk if care is not taken in avoid drug interactions that inhibit isoenzyme activity and convert patients to slow metabolizer status (2,4). The enzyme N-acetyl transferase, which is responsible for the metabolism of procainamide, is another metabolic pathway influenced by genetic polymorphism. Approximately 50% to 65% of Caucasians and African-Americans are "slow" acetylators, whereas this phenotype is present in <20% of persons of Asian descent (5).

Drug metabolism and elimination occurring in the lumen of the intestine and liver prior to exposure to the systemic circulation is referred to as "first-pass" metabolism. The extent to which a drug undergoes first-pass metabolism will determine differences between parenteral and oral doses of a particular antiarrhythmic and in some cases render a drug inactive when administered orally (e.g., lidocaine, ibutilide) (2). Additional important factors influencing metabolism include a nonlinear (saturable) kinetic profile, coexisting diseases effecting biotransformation (i.e., decreased hepatic blood flow as a result of congestive heart failure), and drug-drug interactions.

Elimination

The major routes of drug elimination are hepatic and renal. Although most antiarrhythmic drugs undergo hepatic metabolism and elimination, drugs such as procainamide, flecainide and disopyramide are dependent upon both hepatic and renal elimination. Elimination half-life (i.e., time needed for 50% of the drug to be eliminated from the body) is an important consideration in prescribing antiarrhythmic agents. This parameter is of particular significance when assessing efficacy of therapy based upon time to steady-state plasma concentration (five half-lives) or when cross-titrating a patient from one antiarrhythmic drug to another in order to minimize the potential risk of proarrhythmia.

Class I Antiarrhythmic Agents

Class I antiarrhythmic agents possess "membrane-stabilizing" activity and exert antiarrhythmic potential primarily by blocking the sodium channel. The clinical use of many of these agents has diminished significantly over the past 10 to 15 years. This change is largely due to proarrhythmia, poor side-effect profiles, and alternative agents with enhanced efficacy.

The significant risk for proarrhythmia with these agents was demonstrated in the Cardiac Arrhythmia Suppression Trial (CAST) (6). This trial was designed to examine if suppression of premature ventricular complexes with the class IC antiarrhythmics encainide or flecainide would have a mortality benefit in patients with asymptomatic or mildly symptomatic ventricular arrhythmias post myocardial infarction. The result of this trial demonstrated that the rate of mortality with encainide and flecainide was 2 to 3 times greater than with placebo. Moricizine, another class IC agent, had similar results with regard to mortality in the CAST II trial (7). The proarrhythmic risk of class IC agents has often been extrapolated to include the class IA antiarrhythmic agents given because of their similar electrophysiologic and pharmacodynamic properties. However, the use of these agents to treat supraventricular tachycardias confers a low risk of proarrhythmia in patients with normal left ventricular anatomy and function (8).

Although not necessarily discussed in each individual section, or for each representative drug, it should be understood that all antiarrhythmic agents carry a risk for proarrhythmia and sudden cardiac death; the magnitude of this risk varies between individual agents. Pharmacokinetic and or pharmacodynamic interactions that lead to QT interval prolongation may enhance the risk for the development of polymorphic ventricular tachycardia, including torsades de pointes. (For additional information on drugs that may cause QT interval prolongation, please refer to www.torsades.org or www.qtdrugs.com.)

Class IA Antiarrhythmic Agents
Quinidine
Electrophysiologic and Pharmacodynamic Properties

Quinidine inhibits the rapid inward sodium current, resulting in an increased threshold for excitability and decreased automaticity. The cardiac action potential is prolonged as a result of potassium channel blocking properties, most notably inhibition of the rapidly activating component of the delayed rectifier current (I_{Kr}) (9). Quinidine's affinity for the sodium channel is greatest at faster rates, resulting in prolongation of the QRS interval. At slower rates, receptor occupancy is greater in the potassium channel, producing moderate prolongation of the QT interval (9,10). Quinidine produces modest alpha-adrenergic receptor blockade, which may result in hypotension and sinus tachycardia when administered intravenously or in large oral doses (9). Additionally, quinidine possesses moderate vagolytic activity and thus may enhance atrioventricular (AV) nodal conduction in patients with supraventricular tachyarrhythmias and as such should only be used in conjunction with AV nodal blocking agents in these patients (9,11).

Pharmacokinetics

Following oral administration, quinidine is rapidly absorbed and distributed with approximately 80% of the drug bound to plasma proteins including alpha-1-acid glycoprotein (9). Quinidine undergoes extensive hepatic metabolism via the oxidative pathway (CYP-3A4 isoenzyme substrate) to several metabolites, of which, the 3-hydroxyquinidine metabolite is the only one that confers relevant antiarrhythmic activity. Approximately 10% to 30% of the drug is eliminated by the kidneys unchanged; therefore dosage adjustments may be required with renal insufficiency. The elimination half-life of the drug is highly variable, ranging from 2 to 18 hours, with steady state being attained in the majority of patients within 24 hours (2,4).

Drug Interactions

Quinidine is responsible for a significant number of drug interactions. As a substrate of CYP-3A4, drugs that induce or inhibit this isoenzyme may significantly impact quinidine metabolism. Inhibition of metabolism is likely to occur with macrolide antibiotics (e.g., erythromycin), azole antifungals (e.g., ketoconazole), antiretroviral agents (e.g., nelfinavir), nondihydropyridine calcium channel antagonists (e.g., verapamil) and other inhibitors of the CYP-3A4 system, such as amiodarone. Inducers of the CYP-3A4 pathway (e.g., phenytoin, barbiturates, and rifampin) are likely to enhance metabolism of quinidine and potentially affect its efficacy (12). Quinidine is a very potent inhibitor of the CYP-2D6 pathway; as little as 50 mg of quinidine is sufficient to inhibit this isoenzyme. Extensive metabolizers are most susceptible to inhibition of CYP-2D6, as they effectively become slow-metabolizers, resulting in increased serum concentrations of drugs metabolized by this isoenzyme (e.g., metoprolol, propafenone, tricyclic antidepressants, and codeine) (12). Last, quinidine is an inhibitor of the efflux transporter protein, P-glycoprotein, and reduces the renal and nonrenal elimination of digoxin, which results in marked increases in the serum level. An empiric 50% dose reduction of digoxin is warranted at the onset of therapy (12).

Adverse Effects

Proarrhythmia, including torsades de pointes, is the most significant potential adverse effect associated with quinidine therapy. Often presenting as syncope or sudden cardiac death, torsades de pointes has been reported to occur with a frequency of 1.5% to 8% per patient-year of treatment, often occurring soon after treatment initiation (4,11). Gastrointestinal intolerance, primarily diarrhea, may occur in up to 50% of patients during quinidine therapy. Other potential adverse effects include tinnitus and headache (cinchonism); rarely thrombocytopenia

and systemic lupus erythematosus may occur. Quinidine may worsen neuromuscular blockade in patients with myasthenia gravis by impairing the synthesis or release of acetylcholine at the postsynaptic junction (10).

Clinical Indication and Utility

Quinidine is FDA approved for the conversion of symptomatic atrial fibrillation (AF), atrial flutter (AFL), and subsequent maintenance of sinus rhythm in patients at high-risk of symptomatic recurrence. Quinidine is also approved for the suppression of life-threatening ventricular arrhythmias. Clinically, quinidine is rarely utilized due to its adverse side effect profile.

Procainamide

Electrophysiologic and Pharmacodynamic Properties

Procainamide is a structural analog of the local anesthetic procaine and possesses electrophysiologic properties similar to quinidine. Unlike quinidine, procainamide lacks significant vagolytic activity and does not antagonize alpha-adrenergic receptors. The major metabolite of procainamide, N-acetyl procainamide (NAPA), does not inhibit the sodium current, but has equipotent activity at the potassium channel as the parent compound. Plasma concentrations of NAPA exceed those of procainamide and may result in increased refractoriness and QT-interval prolongation with long-term therapy (9). Hypotension may occur in patients treated with intravenous procainamide or in those with high serum levels as a result of the ganglionic blocking property of the drug.

Pharmacokinetics

Procainamide has nearly 100% bioavailability with a low-level of protein binding (~15%). Following oral administration, peak plasma levels are achieved within 2 hours and the drug is eliminated rapidly by both renal elimination and hepatic metabolism. The hepatic metabolism of procainamide is of clinical importance as conjugation to the metabolite NAPA occurs by N-acetyl transferase; an enzyme whose activity is determined by genetic polymorphism as described previously. In patients with the "slow" acetylator phenotype, serum concentrations of procainamide may exceed those of NAPA. This can account for interpatient variability with regard to electrophysiologic response to therapy as well as adverse effects. Dose reduction is warranted in patients with renal insufficiency, as both procainamide and NAPA are eliminated by active tubular secretion. The serum half-life of procainamide is 3 to 4 hours, and 6 to 10 hours for NAPA.

Drug Interactions

Procainamide does not undergo metabolism via the CYP450 isoenzyme pathway and has low-level protein binding, as such, drug interactions are limited to those that influence renal elimination. Inhibitors of cationic tubular secretion, such as cimetidine, ketoconazole and trimethoprim, may reduce renal clearance of procainamide. Monitoring of QT interval is warranted with concomitant therapy (13).

Adverse Effects

The side effect profile of procainamide limits its usefulness in long-term therapy. Approximately 40% of patients discontinue therapy within the first 6 months. Drug induced lupus syndrome may occur in up to 50% of patients with chronic therapy; early symptoms often present as rash and small-joint arthralgias and may progress to more severe symptoms including fever, malar erythematous rash, pleural and or pericardial effusions. Slow metabolizers of procainamide are at the greatest risk for developing the drug-induced lupus syndrome (10). Bone marrow aplasia and agranulocytosis occur in approximately 1 out every 500 patients treated with procainamide, which usually occurs in the first 12-weeks of therapy and proves fatal in up to 20% of these cases. Weekly monitoring of complete blood counts is warranted for the first 3 months of therapy and periodically thereafter.

Clinical Indication and Utility

Procainamide is FDA approved for the suppression and prevention of life-threatening ventricular arrhythmias (VA). Clinically the drug is utilized in both supraventricular and ventricular arrhythmias. Procainamide is useful in the acute management of patients with reentrant supraventricular tachycardia and atrial fibrillation or flutter associated with Wolff-Parkinson-White (WPW) syndrome (14). Additionally, procainamide may be utilized for treatment of wide-complex tachycardia and stable ventricular tachycardia in patients with preserved cardiac function and normal baseline QT interval.

Disopyramide

Electrophysiologic and Pharmacodynamic Properties

The electrophysiologic activity of disopyramide is similar to quinidine and procainamide with regard to sodium and potassium channel blockade; suppression of automaticity in the His-Purkinje system, and prolonging atrial and ventricular refractoriness. Disopyramide does not affect alpha- or beta-adrenergic receptors and rarely produces significant hemodynamic effects. The primary metabolite of disopyramide is mono-N-dealkyldisopyramide (MND) and while it confers minimal antiarrhythmic activity, it produces significant vagolytic activity, as its anticholinergic potency is 20 to 30 times the parent compound (9). As with quinidine, the vagolytic properties of disopyramide may enhance (AV) nodal conduction in patients with supraventricular tachyarrhythmias and should only be used in conjunction with AV nodal blocking agents in these patients.

Pharmacokinetics

Disopyramide is well absorbed with bioavailability >80%. It is bound to plasma proteins in a saturable, concentration-dependent manner; resulting in disproportionate increases in the fraction of unbound drug compared to the magnitude of the dosage increment (10). Disopyramide undergoes partial hepatic metabolism (via CYP-3A4) to minimally active metabolites. Approximately 50% of the drug is eliminated unchanged in the urine and 30% as metabolites, primarily MND. The dose of disopyramide should, therefore, be reduced in patients with underlying renal dysfunction. The half-life of disopyramide ranges from 4 to 10 hours.

Drug Interactions

As a substrate of the isoenzyme CYP-3A4, interactions involving disopyramide are similar to those seen with quinidine (e.g., macrolides, azole antifungals, and antiretrovirals). Additionally, consideration for pharmacodynamic interactions that may enhance the negative inotropic activity of disopyramide must be given (12).

Adverse Effects

The use of disopyramide is limited by the considerable, dose-dependent, anticholinergic effects it exerts, including exacerbation of glaucoma, constipation, urinary retention, dry mouth, blurred vision and gastric reflux. As a consequence of the negative inotropic effect of disopyramide, the development of new or worsened congestive heart failure is of significant concern.

Clinical Indication and Utility

Disopyramide is FDA approved for suppression and prevention of life-threatening VA. Clinically the drug has been utilized in a broad range of supraventricular and ventricular arrhythmias, however; the arrhythmogenic potential and significant anticholinergic side effects of the drug limit its clinical value. Of note, disopyramide has been shown to be effective at reducing mean outflow gradient and improving New York Heart Association functional class in patients with obstructive hypertrophic cardiomyopathy (15).

Class 1B Antiarrhythmic Agents

Lidocaine

Electrophysiologic and Pharmacodynamic Properties

Lidocaine blocks both open and inactivated cardiac sodium channels, and exhibits rapid recovery from blockade. Unlike other class I antiarrhythmics, lidocaine appears to act exclusively on the sodium channel with minimal effect on the QT interval. Lidocaine may decrease the action potential duration and the effective refractory period of Purkinje fibers and ventricular myocardium. Lidocaine has few electrophysiologic effects on normal conducting myocardium and best suppresses the electrical activity of depolarized myocardium. Therefore, it is particularly useful in ventricular arrhythmias associated with ischemia. There is little to no effect on atrial myocardium. In large doses, patients with left ventricular dysfunction my experience depressed myocardial contractility.

Pharmacokinetics

Lidocaine has a rapid distribution half-life from the central compartment, thus bolus dosing is recommended to achieve a therapeutic concentration in the plasma. Lidocaine undergoes hepatic metabolism, producing two distinct desethyl metabolites, both having less antiarrhythmic activity than the parent lidocaine. The half-life of the lidocaine is 1 to 2 hours in patients with normal heart and liver function, yet due to its high clearance rate, steady state is achieved in 8 to 10 hours for normal volunteers and 20 to 24 hours in those with heart failure or liver dysfunction. Clearance of lidocaine is reduced after 24 hours of administration due to competition for hepatic enzymes. Monitoring of lidocaine plasma levels is recommended to avoid the potential for serious toxicity.

Drug Interactions

Lidocaine is largely devoid of drug interactions; yet consideration for pharmacodynamic interactions with other antiarrhythmics should be considered.

Adverse Effects

Central nervous system toxicities are the most common side effect of lidocaine therapy, and may occur at therapeutic plasma concentrations. These side effects include tremor, nausea, paresthesia, and hearing disturbances. More deleterious effects include slurred speech, altered mentation, seizures and even coma, occurring more often in those with supratherapeutic plasma lidocaine levels. Monitoring of serum lidocaine level is recommended to avoid potential toxicity, especially in patients with hepatic dysfunction or heart failure.

Clinical Indication and Utility

Lidocaine is FDA approved for the acute management of life-threatening VA associated with myocardial infarction or during cardiac manipulative procedures, such as cardiac surgery and catheterization. Clinically, lidocaine remains useful for treatment of recurrent VA; however, it should not be considered a first-line agent (16). Amiodarone is used preferentially over lidocaine in the setting of ventricular arrhythmias and has been shown to confer a mortality benefit in resuscitated patients (17).

Mexiletine

Electrophysiologic and Pharmacodynamic Properties

Mexiletine is a conger of lidocaine and was developed to overcome the first-pass hepatic metabolism issues associated with oral lidocaine. As a conger, mexiletine has similar electrophysiologic properties (17). Both drugs block the rapid inward sodium current in Purkinje fibers and ventricular myocardium,

resulting in shortening of the action potential duration and the effective refractory period. Mexiletine is also use-dependent; there is greater sodium channel blockade at higher rates of excitation. Atrial myocardium is unaffected by mexiletine and there is no significant effect on left ventricular function.

Pharmacokinetics

Oral mexiletine has excellent bioavailability. Hepatic metabolism (via CYP-2D6) accounts for 85% to 90% of elimination, while 10% to 15% of the drug is excreted unchanged in the urine. The elimination half-life is 8 to 12 hours (18).

Drug Interactions

Inhibitors of the CYP-2D6 isoenzyme including amiodarone, quinidine, fluoxetine, and ritonavir are likely to increase serum concentrations of mexiletine (12).

Adverse Effects

Side effects during mexiletine therapy are relatively common and occur in a cumulative, dose-dependent manner. The most common side effects are due to central nervous system toxicity (e.g., tremor, dizziness, and dysphoria) followed by gastrointestinal intolerance (19).

Clinical Indication and Utility

Mexiletine is FDA approved for the treatment of life threatening VA. Clinical trials have not demonstrated its superiority over other class I antiarrhythmic agents. Mexiletine is often used in conjunction with other antiarrhythmics, such as amiodarone for the treatment of refractory ventricular arrhythmias (20). Mexiletine does not have a role in the treatment of supraventricular arrhythmias.

Class 1C Antiarrhythmic Agents

Flecainide

Electrophysiologic and Pharmacodynamic Properties

Flecainide blocks late-opening sodium channels, the delayed rectifier K^+ current (I_{Kr}) and blocks calcium channels. In atrial tissue, flecainide prolongs action potential duration at fast rates and conduction is slowed in the atria, AV node, His-Purkinje system and the ventricles. Sinus slowing and even profound bradycardia can be seen in patients with preexisting sinus node dysfunction. Flecainide prolongs the PR and QRS interval at normal heart rates; however, the QT interval is not prolonged because the drug has a limited affect on repolarization (21).

Pharmacokinetics

Flecainide has excellent bioavailability (>90%) with moderate protein binding (40%–60%). The drug is eliminated by hepatic metabolism (via CYP-2D6) to several metabolites, most of which confer no antiarrhythmic activity at plasma concentrations achieved during therapy, and undergoes extensive elimination by renal excretion (30% as unchanged drug). Because of the extensive renal elimination, genetic polymorphism of the CYP-2D6 isoenzyme does not result in accumulation of the parent drug. In patients with significant underlying renal dysfunction, dosage adjustments of flecainide are warranted to prevent alterations in the drugs pharmacokinetic profile (2,10). The elimination half-life of flecainide ranges from 8 to 14 hours in patients with normal renal function.

Drug Interactions

Similar to mexiletine, flecainide is a substrate of the CYP-2D6 isoenzyme and as such is subject to similar drug interactions previously described. Again, those at greatest risk from these drug interactions are the extensive-metabolizers who may require as much as a 50% reduction in flecainide dose. Flecainide may increase serum digoxin concentrations by 15%, prudent monitoring of digoxin levels is advised, but empiric dose reduction of digoxin is not warranted.

Adverse Effects

Flecainide is well tolerated in most patients; the most common compliant is dose-related blurred vision and dry eyes. The drug can also exacerbate congestive heart failure in patients with depressed left ventricular function.

Clinical Indication and Utility

Flecainide is FDA approved for the prevention of paroxysmal AF and supraventricular tachycardias (SVT) in patients without structural heart disease. Additionally, flecainide is FDA approved for the prevention of life-threatening VA.

Clinically, flecainide is mostly utilized in the suppression of supraventricular tachycardias including AF, AFL, and atrial tachycardia. In patients with AF or AFL, flecainide should be used with a concomitant AV nodal blocking agent to prevent 1:1 conduction of atrial flutter. In accessory pathway mediated tachycardia (e.g., WPW syndrome), the use of flecainide should be avoided due to the risk of inducing 1:1 conduction (22). As described previously, patients with known structural heart disease should not receive flecainide (6).

Propafenone

Electrophysiologic and Pharmacodynamic Properties

Propafenone is a racemate compound in which both enantiomers have equal activity at the sodium channels. The drug inhibits fast sodium channels, decreases membrane excitability, spontaneous automaticity, and triggered activity, thereby slowing conduction in the atria, AV node, and ventricles. The S-enantiomer of propafenone confers beta-adrenergic receptor blocking activity that results in sinus slowing particularly at high doses or with preexisting sinus node dysfunction (6).

The negative inotropic effect of the drug is well tolerated in patients with normal or only mildly depressed left ventricular systolic function. The drug should be avoided in patients with heart failure, because it can decrease cardiac output and increase left heart filling pressures (23).

Pharmacokinetics

Propafenone has low, dose-dependent bioavailability and has significant first-pass saturable hepatic metabolism that is mediated by the CYP-2D6 isoenzyme. In those patients not carrying the phenotype, propafenone will be rapidly and extensively metabolized to 5-hydroxypropafenone (via CYP-2D6) and to N-depropylpropafenone (via CYP-3A4, 1A2). For the 10% of the population who are lacking the CYP-2D6 isoenzyme, propafenone metabolism is slow and incomplete, and this has important implications in therapy.

Propafenone and the metabolite 5-hydroxypropafenone have equipotent activity at the sodium channel, however; propafenone has significantly more beta-adrenergic receptor antagonism than either metabolite. Because of the saturable metabolism of the drug, slow metabolizers will have five-times the serum concentration of propafenone at doses of <450 mg/day and at doses >450 mg/day only have twice the serum concentration of propafenone. At any dose, slow metabolizers are likely to experience more beta-adrenergic receptor antagonism and potentially therapeutic failure or increased adverse effects, as opposed to extensive metabolizers who may experience this only at higher doses. Metabolic pathway also determines the elimination half-life of propafenone. In the population lacking CYP-2D6 activity, the elimination half-life ranges from 10 to 32 hours, whereas in the extensive-metabolizers, the elimination half-life ranges from 2 to 10 hours (9,10).

Drug Interactions

Propafenone has the potential to be subject to numerous drug interactions as a substrate of CYP-2D6, -3A4, and -1A2. Clinically the most relevant is the CYP-2D6 isoenzyme since it is responsible for metabolizing propafenone to its most active metabolite, 5-hydroxypropafenone. Potential interactions related to this isoenzyme are similar to those described previously for flecainide and mexiletine. As was the case with those agents, the population at greatest risk of harm is those who express CYP-2D6 activity (extensive metabolizers). Propafenone also alters both renal and nonrenal clearance of digoxin and may result in serum digoxin concentrations of up to 80% greater than baseline. Empiric dosage reduction of 25% is warranted at initiation of therapy (12,13).

Adverse Effects

The most common side effect of chronic propafenone is a bitter, metallic taste that persists during the course of therapy. Other common side effects include gastrointestinal intolerance, dizziness, blurred vision and fatigue. Rare, but important side effects include risk for hepatotoxicity, lupus, blood dyscrasias and bronchospasm. Proarrhythmia develops in 5% of patients, with an increased risk seen in those with a reduced ejection fraction, and in those with prior episodes of ventricular tachycardia (24). Profound bradycardia can develop in patients with preexisting sinus node dysfunction.

Clinical Indication and Utility

Propafenone is FDA indicated when administered as an immediate-release tablet to prolong the time to recurrence of symptomatic, disabling SVT. Additionally, the immediate-release is also indicated to prolong the time to recurrence of SVT in patients without structural heart disease, and for the treatment of VA. The FDA-labeled indication for the extended-release tablet is to prolong the time to the first recurrence of symptomatic paroxysmal AF.

Clinically, propafenone is used to treat a variety of supraventricular tachyarrhythmias and the proarrhythmic risk is low in patients with structurally normal hearts (25). It is also effective reducing ventricular premature depolarizations.

Class II Agents

Beta-Blockers

Cardioselective beta-blockers, such as atenolol and metoprolol, block primarily $beta_1$ receptors, resulting in sinus rate slowing, decreased contractility, and slowing of AV nodal conduction. Nonselective beta-blockers interact with both $beta_1$ and $beta_2$ receptors, which are located in blood vessels and pulmonary bronchi. Both nonselective beta-blockers, and cardioselective beta-blockers at higher dosages, can exert $beta_2$ effects leading to bronchoconstriction.

Beta-blockers are ubiquitous in the management of cardiac arrhythmias, including acute and chronic management of SVT, and are considered the drug of first choice in controlling the ventricular response during episodes of atrial fibrillation and atrial flutter. They have been shown to reduce the incidence of sudden cardiac death mediated by ventricular tachyarrhythmias in patients with myocardial infarction (26), ischemic and non-ischemic heart failure (27,28), and congenital long QT syndrome (29).

Class III Antiarrhythmic Drugs Agents

Class III antiarrhythmic agents prolong action potential duration and the effective refractory period. Their primary mode of action is affected by blocking the delayed potassium rectifier channels that contribute to repolarization. The QRS interval and the QT interval may prolong on the surface ECG. There is considerable concern for proarrhythmia with these drugs due to the risk of torsades de pointes associated with QT interval prolongation.

Amiodarone

Electrophysiologic and Pharmacodynamic Properties

The electrophysiologic profile of amiodarone is unique compared to other class III antiarrhythmic agents due to its complex and ubiquitous receptor interactions. The principal mode of action of amiodarone is to prolong action potential duration and refractoriness via blockade of the delayed rectifier potassium current (I_{Kr}) and other potassium channels. However, amiodarone also has a multiplicity of effects including use dependent blockade of inactive sodium channels (class I effect), weak, noncompetitive alpha- and beta-adrenergic activity (class II effect) and reduction of calcium current by blockade of calcium channels (class IV effect) (2,4,9).

The primary metabolite of amiodarone is desethylamiodarone (DEA), which may be more potent than amiodarone with regard to sodium channel blockade and prolongation of refractoriness. The class II and IV effects result in slowing of the sinus node rate by 20% to 30% (30). Amiodarone is unlike other class III antiarrhythmics that have reverse-use dependency; the prolonged repolarization time persists at higher rates.

Electrophysiologic and hemodynamic differences are produced by amiodarone, dependent upon the route of administration. Amiodarone is insoluble in water and must be dispersed in a solvent (polysorbate-80) for intravenous (IV) administration (31). The solvent has been shown to decrease heart rate, depress AV node conduction, and increase refractoriness. Hypotension, which is not seen with oral therapy, can occur with IV administration and may be due to arterial dilation related to an anti-sympathetic effect or the solvent (32). The beta-adrenergic and calcium channel blockade properties of amiodarone may be more pronounced with the IV formulation of the drug (31). Left ventricular systolic function can be mildly and transiently depressed with IV amiodarone when rapidly infused, an effect not seen during oral therapy (33,34).

Pharmacokinetics

Amiodarone is a highly lipid soluble compound with variable bioavailability (mean 40%), presumably due to its slow and erratic absorption. Amiodarone undergoes extensive hepatic metabolism (CYP-3A4) to the desethyl metabolite (CYP-3A4, -2C8) with excretion into the bile. Renal elimination of the drug is negligible (<1%), and therefore dosage adjustments are not required even in severe renal dysfunction. Once metabolism has occurred, both amiodarone and DEA are distributed to all body tissues with highest concentrations found in the heart, adipose tissue, skin, liver and lungs. The cardiac tissue to plasma concentration ratio is >20:1, and the drug accumulates extensively into lipid tissue with a lipid to plasma concentration ratio >300:1. Amiodarone undergoes biphasic elimination with a 50% reduction in plasma concentration within 10 days of drug discontinuation. The elimination half-life of drug ranges from 26 to 107 days (mean 54 days) (35).

Drug Interactions

Amiodarone is a catalyst for a variety of drug interactions; it interferes with hepatic metabolism, and renal and nonrenal elimination of numerous drugs. Inhibition of hepatic metabolism is effected via the CYP-3A4, CYP2C9, and CYP2D6 isoenzyme pathways. Amiodarone also inhibits the P-glycoprotein transport protein. Drugs metabolized or eliminated by any of these pathways may require significant dose reduction during amiodarone therapy; empiric dose reductions of 50% are warranted with warfarin and digoxin. Additionally, concomitant use of other antiarrhythmics, tricyclic antidepressants, and certain antipsychotic agents may have a synergistic influence on the QT interval and should be avoided or used with caution to minimize the risk of torsades de pointes.

Adverse Effects

Amiodarone is very effective in treating both supraventricular and ventricular arrhythmias, but its widespread use is tempered by the adverse effects and toxicity associated with chronic therapy. Adverse effects early in therapy are limited and usually occur during oral loading (gastrointestinal intolerance) or with IV administration (hypotension, thrombophlebitis). Adverse effects during chronic therapy may be associated with the magnitude of the daily maintenance doses and the duration of therapy, owing to significant tissue accumulation (9). Common adverse reactions include pulmonary toxicity, hyper and hypothyroidism, hepatotoxicity, corneal microdeposits, peripheral neuropathy, and skin discoloration; the most morbid is pulmonary toxicity. Amiodarone induced pulmonary toxicity may affect as many as 15% of patients during long-term therapy and predisposing factors include advanced age, pre-existing restrictive lung disease, and maintenance doses >400 mg/day (36,37).

Manifestations of pulmonary toxicity include interstitial or alveolar pneumonitis, acute respiratory distress syndrome, and pulmonary fibrosis. Rarely, acute pulmonary toxicity may occur early in therapy but is usually limited patients with existing pulmonary disease and is most often seen in the critical care setting (37). The proarrhythmic risk of amiodarone is low compared to the other Class III agents. The incidence of amiodarone induced torsades de pointes is <1% (38).

Clinical Indication and Utility

Amiodarone is FDA approved for the treatment of life-threatening recurrent ventricular fibrillation and recurrent hemodynamically unstable ventricular tachycardia. Clinically, amiodarone is considered the most useful and widely effective of all antiarrhythmic agents due to its unique electrophysiologic and pharmacodynamic properties. Amiodarone is effective in suppressing and preventing the recurrence of a wide-array of supraventricular and ventricular tachyarrhythmias. Amiodarone used in patients with implantable cardioverter defibrillators can reduce the number of appropriate shocks for VA, as well as inappropriate shocks caused by SVT (39). Amiodarone is also the first line agent for sustained monomorphic ventricular tachycardia in patients with impaired left ventricular function.

Ibutilide

Electrophysiologic and Pharmacodynamic Properties

Ibutilide is a potent analogue of sotalol and effectively prolongs repolarization, action potential duration, and the effective refractory period in atrial and ventricular myocardium by blocking potassium rectifier currents and by activating a slow sodium inward current (40). This results in mild slowing of the sinus rate and prolongation of the QT interval. Left ventricular systolic function is unaffected (41).

Pharmacokinetics

Ibutilide undergoes extensive first-pass metabolism and therefore is only available for intravenous administration. Following a standard 10-minute infusion the half-life of ibutilide ranges from 2 to 12 hours. However, the drug has a large volume of distribution and rapid clearance from the central compartment, thus cardiac effects of the drug persist for <1 hour.

Drug Interactions

Drug interactions with ibutilide are limited to those agents that have the potential for additive effects with regard to prolongation of the QT interval.

Adverse Effects

Adverse effects of ibutilide are primarily limited to the risk of proarrhythmia and development of torsades de pointes, which may occur in up to 6% of the patients (9).

Most episodes of torsades de pointes are transient and self-limiting; however, sustained episodes requiring cardioversion occur in 1.7% to 2.4% (42). Ibutilide should not be given to patients who have hypokalemia, hypomagnesemia, or QT_c prolongation at baseline >440 ms. Intravenous administration of 1 to 2 grams of magnesium sulfate prior to or during ibutilide infusion may reduce the risk of torsades de pointes and increase cardioversion rates (43).

Clinical Indication and Utility

Ibutilide is FDA approved for the rapid conversion of recent onset atrial fibrillation or atrial flutter. Clinically, the drug is not utilized extensively due to the risk of torsades de pointes and should be used only in a telemetry monitored setting with personnel trained in cardiac resuscitation. The drug is also effective as pretreatment for atrial fibrillation or atrial flutter before electrical cardioversion (44).

Dofetilide

Electrophysiologic and Pharmacodynamic Properties

Dofetilide delays the rapid component of the delayed rectifier potassium current which acts to prolong repolarization. This effect is more prominent in the atria than in the ventricles. There is a linear dose dependent prolongation of the QT interval on the surface ECG.

Pharmacokinetics

Oral dofetilide has excellent absorption and 75% to 100% bioavailability (45). The drug is excreted almost equally by the kidneys and the liver (46). There are no significant left ventricular or hemodynamic effects associated with dofetilide.

Drug Interactions

Drugs that interfere with the CYP3A4 mediated metabolism of dofetilide should be avoided because they can lead to increased or toxic levels of dofetilide. These drugs include erythromycin, Ketoconazole, verapamil, and trimethoprim. Caution should be used if the patient has renal insufficiency, hepatic dysfunction, hypokalemia, or if the QTc is prolonged. The incidence of torsades de pointes is 3% (47).

Adverse Effects

The most serious potential adverse effect of Dofetilide is dose-dependant QT prolongation leading to torsades de pointes (3%) (47). Initiation of Dofetilide is therefore performed on an inpatient basis, with telemetry monitoring for a minimum of 3 days in a facility that can provide calculations of creatinine clearance, continuous electrocardiographic monitoring, and cardiac resuscitation. Dofetilide is available only to hospitals and prescribers who have received appropriate dosing and treatment initiation education. This drug should be avoided, or the dose adjusted in patients with renal dysfunction.

Clinical Indication and Utility

Dofetilide is used for the acute conversion of atrial fibrillation to sinus rhythm as well as for maintenance of sinus rhythm after reversion. The SAFIRE-D trial (48) assessed the efficacy of dofetilide in pharmacologic cardioversion of atrial fibrillation. At 500 mg there was conversion to sinus rhythm in 70% of patients by 24 hours and 91% by 36 hours. At 1 year, the probability of maintaining sinus rhythm was 58% with 500 mg BID versus 25% for placebo.

Sotalol

Electrophysiologic and Pharmacodynamic Properties

Sotalol exerts its effects via both potassium channel and nonspecific beta adrenergic receptor blockade. The available form of the drug contains both the *d*- and *l*-isomers which exhibit different electrophysiologic properties. Both isomers prolong repolarization by blockade of the rapid component of the delayed potassium rectifier (Ikr). However, the *l*-isomer is solely responsible for the beta-blocker activity. Sotalol shortens the sinus cycle period, lengthens the atrial and ventricular refractory periods, and lengthens the QT interval. The sinus rate is slowed by 25%. (49). The *l*-isomer has negative inotropic properties that can reduce left ventricular contractile force and increase filling pressure.

Pharmacokinetics

Sotalol is almost entirely excreted by the kidneys with an elimination half-life of 10 to 15 hours. This drug cannot be used in patients with renal failure, and renal insufficiency mandates reduced doses to avoid increased plasma levels (50).

Drug Interactions

The coadministration of drugs that prolong the QT interval, such as other antiarrhythmic medications and most antipsychotics, should be avoided. Hypokalemia and hypomagnesemia caused by diuretics can worsen QT prolongation caused by sotalol. Concomitant therapy with antihypertensives may lead to hypotension. Drugs that interact adversely with beta-blockers should be avoided.

Adverse Effects

Prolongation of the QT interval and subsequent development of torsades de pointes are the most concerning potential adverse effects of this drug. The majority of proarrhythmic events occur within the first 3 days of initiation. Initiation of Sotalol and dose increases should therefore be performed in an inpatient setting. Ventricular tachyarrhythmias occur in 4% of patients receiving the drug.

The drug should be avoided in patients with congenital or acquired long QT syndrome.

Clinical Indication and Utility

Sotalol is approved to treat patients for VA, as well as SVT. The SAFE-T study compared the efficacy of amiodarone to sotalol in converting atrial fibrillation to sinus rhythm (51). Both drugs had equal efficacy in spontaneous conversion and direct current cardioversion of AF. However, amiodarone proved superior in its ability to maintain sinus rhythm. Sotalol has also been shown to reduce the recurrence of ventricular tachycardia and ventricular fibrillation. It has been used in conjunction with implantable cardioverter defibrillators and reduces arrhythmia recurrence and defibrillator shocks (52).

Class IV Agents
Calcium Channel Blockers

Verapamil and diltiazem block slow calcium channels in the sinus and the AV nodes. These drugs decrease the slope of depolarization, slow conduction, and prolong the effective and functional refractory periods. The AV node actions exhibit use dependence, which results in more pronounced effects at higher heart rates. The dihydropyridines are a subclassification of calcium channel blockers that do not have clinically significant electrophysiologic properties. Both verapamil and diltiazem exert a negative inotropic effect, and caution should, therefore, be used in patients with left ventricular dysfunction or when combining with beta-blockers. Calcium channel blockers dilate coronary and peripheral arteries, and the resulting decrease in afterload may compensate for the negative inotropic effects. Verapamil and diltiazem are available in oral and intravenous forms for acute and chronic treatment of SVT (53,54). However, these drugs should be avoided in patients with Wolff-Parkinson-White syndrome because AV nodal blockade may lead to increased conduction of AF and AFL via the accessory pathway with resultant hemodynamic collapse.

Miscellaneous Antiarrhythmics

Adenosine

Adenosine is very effective for the acute conversion of SVT, particularly reentry tachycardias dependent on AV nodal conduction (55). Adenosine is rapidly removed from the circulation as it is transported into erythrocytes and vascular endothelial cells. The half-life is exceptionally short in duration, ranging for 1.5 to 10 seconds. The maximum effect of adenosine following a single bolus dose is seen within 30 seconds (9).

Adenosine is contraindicated in patients with sick sinus syndrome and second- or third-degree heart block in the absence of a functional pacemaker, as well as heart-transplant recipients due to the risk of prolonged asystole (55). Common side effects are often brief in nature and resolve rapidly; these include flushing, dyspnea and chest pressure. Adenosine should be used with caution in patients with underlying respiratory disease (e.g., asthma) due to the risk of bronchoconstriction. Methylxanthines, such as caffeine, theophylline and aminophylline, competitively antagonize the effects of adenosine, whereas dipyridamole increases the potency by blocking cellular uptake (9).

Digoxin

Digoxin decreases the atrial action potential duration and increases AV nodal refractoriness, making it useful in controlling ventricular response to supraventricular arrhythmias, such as atrial fibrillation (9). The role of digoxin in the management of atrial arrhythmias is that of a second- or third-line agent due to less than optimal rate control when compared to beta-adrenergic and calcium channel antagonists. Clinically, digoxin is primarily utilized for the management of rate control in response to atrial fibrillation in patients with systolic heart failure unable to tolerate the negative inotropic effects of beta-adrenergic and calcium channel antagonists (56,57). Digoxin is not extensively metabolized, has low-level protein binding (~25%) and is largely (>80%) excreted unchanged in the urine. The clearance of digoxin is strongly correlated to glomerular filtration rate and as such warrants dosage adjustment in patients with renal dysfunction. The half-life of digoxin is estimated at 36 hours in normal individuals. At therapeutic concentrations, digoxin is well tolerated and has minimal side effects. Digoxin has a narrow therapeutic index and periodic monitoring of serum levels is advised to avoid serious adverse effects, such as proarrhythmia, bradycardia, gastrointestinal intolerance, visual disturbances, and impaired cognitive function. Electrolyte abnormalities are likely to increase the risk of digoxin-induced arrhythmias (56). Digoxin is not a substrate of the CYP450 isoenzyme system, however, a number of drugs influence the renal and nonrenal clearance of digoxin requiring empiric dose reduction to prevent toxicity, most notably amiodarone (13).

Magnesium

Magnesium is a significant regulator of cardiac cell function and the electrical stability of the cardiac muscle (58). Magnesium may possess intrinsic antiarrhythmic properties by affecting atrial impulse conduction and effective refractory periods (43). Intravenous magnesium sulfate is recommended for the treatment of torsades de pointes with or without cardiac arrest.

REFERENCES

1. Kowey PR. Pharmacological effects of antiarrhythmic drugs. Review and update. *Arch Intern Med.* 1998;158:325–332.
2. Kowey PR, Marinchak RA, Rials SJ, Bharucha DB. Classification and pharmacology of antiarrhythmic drugs. *Am Heart J.* 2000;140:12–20.
3. Jurgens G, Graudal NA, Kampmann JP. Therapeutic drug monitoring of antiarrhythmic drugs. *Clin Pharmacokinet.* 2003;42:647–663.
4. Roden DM. Antiarrhythmic drugs: from mechanisms to clinical practice. *Heart.* 2000;84:339–346.
5. Evans P. N-acetyltransferase in pharmacogenetics of drug metabolism. In: Kalow W, eds. *International Encyclopedia of Pharmacology and Therapeutics.* Vol. 43. New York: Pergamon Press; 1992:95–178.
6. Akiyama T, Pawitan Y, Greenberg H, et al. Increased risk of death and cardiac arrest from encainide and flecainide in patients after non-Q-wave acute myocardial infarction in the Cardiac Arrhythmia Suppression Trial. CAST Investigators. *Am J Cardiol.* 1991;68:1551–1555.
7. The Cardiac Arrhythmia Suppression Trial II Investigators. Effect of the antiarrhythmic agent moricizine on survival after myocardial infarction. *N Engl J Med.* 1992;327:227–233.
8. Pritchett EL, Wilkinson WE. Effect of dofetilide on survival in patients with supraventricular arrhythmias. *Am Heart J.* 1999;138:994–997.
9. Roden, D., Antiarrhythmic Drugs. In: Hardman JG, Limbird LE, Gliman AG, eds. *Goodman and Gilman's the Pharmacologic Basis of Therapeutics.* New York: McGraw Hill; 2001:34:933–970.
10. Woosley RL, Indik JH. Antiarrhythmic Drugs. In: Fuster AR, O'Rourke V, Raisch DW, eds. *Hurst's the Heart.* New York: McGraw Hill; 2004:949–974.
11. Grace AA, Camm AJ. Quinidine. *N Engl J Med.* 1998;338:35–45.
12. Trujillo TC, Nolan PE. *Antiarrhythmic agents: Drug interactions of clinical significance. Drug Saf.* 2000;23:509–532.
13. Hansten PD, Horn JR. *The Top 100 Drug Interactions: A guide to Patient Management.* Freeland: H&H Publications; 2006.
14. Wellens HJ, Bar FW, Dassen WR, et al. Effect of drugs in the Wolff-Parkinson-White syndrome. Importance of initial length of effective refractory period of the accessory pathway. *Am J Cardiol.* 1980;46:665–669.

15. Sherrid MV, Barac I, McKenna WJ, et al. Multicenter study of the efficacy and safety of disopyramide in obstructive hypertrophic cardiomyopathy. *J Am Coll Cardiol*. 2005;45:1251–1258.

16. Marill KA, Greenberg GM, Kay D, Nelson BK. Analysis of the treatment of spontaneous sustained stable ventricular tachycardia. *Acad Emerg Med*. 1997;4:1122–1128.

17. Dorian P, Cass D, Schwartz B, et al. Amiodarone as compared with lidocaine for shock-resistant ventricular fibrillation. *N Engl J Med*. 2002;346:884–890.

18. Prescott LF, Pottage A, Clements JA. Absorption, distribution and elimination of mexiletine. *Postgrad Med J*. 1977;53:50–55.

19. Stein J, Podrid PJ, Lampert S, et al. Long-term mexiletine for ventricular arrhythmia. *Am Heart J*. 1984;107:1091–1098.

20. Yonezawa E, Matsumoto K, Ueno K, et al. Lack of interaction between amiodarone and mexiletine in cardiac arrhythmia patients. *J Clin Pharmacol*. 2002;42:342–346.

21. Pritchett EL, Wilkinson WE. Mortality in patients treated with flecainide and encainide for supraventricular arrhythmias. *Am J Cardiol*. 1991;67:976–980.

22. Aliot E, De Roy L, Capucci A, et al. Safety of a controlled-release flecainide acetate formulation in the prevention of paroxysmal atrial fibrillation in outpatients. *Ann Cardiol Angeiol (Paris)*. 2003;52:34–40.

23. Brodsky MA, Allen BJ, Abate D, Henry WL. Propafenone therapy for ventricular tachycardia in the setting of congestive heart failure. *Am Heart J*. 1985;110:794–799.

24. Buss J, et al. Malignant ventricular tachyarrhythmias in association with propafenone treatment. *Eur Heart J*. 1985;6:424–428.

25. Podrid PJ, Anderson JL. Safety and tolerability of long-term propafenone therapy for supraventricular tachyarrhythmias. The Propafenone Multicenter Study Group. *Am J Cardiol*. 1996;78:430–434.

26. Freemantle N, Cleland J, Young P, et al. Beta Blockade after myocardial infarction: systematic review and meta regression analysis. *BMJ*. 1999;318:1730–1737.

27. Effect of metoprolol CR/XL in chronic heart failure: Metoprolol CR/XL Randomised Intervention Trial in Congestive Heart Failure (MERIT-HF). *Lancet*. 1999;353:2001–2007.

28. Packer M, Bristow MR, Cohn, et al. The effect of carvedilol on morbidity and mortality in patients with chronic heart failure. U.S. Carvedilol Heart Failure Study Group. *N Engl J Med*. 1996;334:1349–1355.

29. Moss AJ, Zareba W, Hall WJ, et al. Effectiveness and limitations of beta-blocker therapy in congenital long-QT syndrome. *Circulation*. 2000;101:616–623.

30. Goldschlager N, Epstein AE, Naccarelli G, et al. Practical guidelines for clinicians who treat patients with amiodarone. Practice guidelines subcommittee, North American Society of Pacing and Electrophysiology. *Arch Intern Med*. 2000;160:1741–1748.

31. Kowey PR, Rials SJ, Filart RA. Intravenous amiodarone. *J Am Coll Cardiol*. 1997;29:1190–1198.

32. Scheinman MM, Levine JH, Cannom DA, et al. Dose-ranging study of intravenous amiodarone in patients with life-threatening ventricular tachyarrhythmias. The Intravenous Amiodarone Multicenter Investigators Group. *Circulation*. 1995;92:3264–3272.

33. Singh BN. Amiodarone: historical development and pharmacologic profile. *Am Heart J*. 1983;106:788–797.

34. Remme WJ, Kruyssen HA, Look MP, et al. Hemodynamic effects and tolerability of intravenous amiodarone in patients with impaired left ventricular function. *Am Heart J*. 1991;122:96–103.

35. Holt DW, Tucker GT, Jackson PR, et al. Amiodarone pharmacokinetics. *Am Heart J*. 1983;106:840–847.

36. Dusman RE, Stanton MS, Miles WM, et al. Clinical features of amiodarone-induced pulmonary toxicity. *Circulation*. 1990;82:51–59.

37. Donaldson L Fau–Grant IS, Naysmith MR, Thomas JS. Acute amiodarone-induced lung toxicity. In Print.

38. Hohnloser Sh Fau-Klingenheben T, Klingenheben T Fau–Singh BN, Singh BN. Amiodarone-associated proarrhythmic effects. A review with special reference to torsade de pointes tachycardia. In Print.

39. Connolly SJ, Dorian P, Roberts RS, et al. Comparison of beta-blockers, amiodarone plus beta-blockers, or sotalol for prevention of shocks from implantable cardioverter defibrillators: the OPTIC Study: a randomized trial. *JAMA*. 2006;295:165–171.

40. Murray KT. Ibutilide. *Circulation*. 1998;97:493–497.

41. Stambler BS, Beckman KJ, Kadish AH, et al. Acute hemodynamic effects of intravenous ibutilide in patients with or without reduced left ventricular function. *Am J Cardiol*. 1997;80:458–463.

42. Gowda RM, Khan IA, Punujollu G, et al. Use of ibutilide for cardioversion of recent-onset atrial fibrillation and flutter in elderly. *Am J Ther*. 2004;11:95–97.

43. Kalus Js Fau–Spencer AP, Tsikouris, et al. Impact of prophylactic i.v. magnesium on the efficacy of ibutilide for conversion of atrial fibrillation or flutter. In Print.

44. Oral H, Souza JJ, Michaud, et al. Facilitating transthoracic cardioversion of atrial fibrillation with ibutilide pretreatment. *N Engl J Med*. 1999;340:1849–1854.

45. Smith DA, Rasmussen HS, Stopher DA, et al. Pharmacokinetics and metabolism of dofetilide in mouse, rat, dog, and man. *Xenobiotica*. 1992;22:709–719.

46. Rasmussen HS, Allen MJ, Blackburn KJ, et al. Dofetilide, a novel class III antiarrhythmic agent. *J Cardiovasc Pharmacol*. 1992;20:S96–S105.

47. Norgaard BL, Wachtell K, Christensen PD, et al. Efficacy and safety of intravenously administered dofetilide in acute termination of atrial fibrillation and flutter: a multicenter, randomized, double-blind, placebo-controlled trial. Danish Dofetilide in Atrial Fibrillation and Flutter Study Group. *Am Heart J*. 1999;137:1062–1969.

48. Singh S, Zoble RG, Yellen L, et al. Efficacy and safety of oral dofetilide in converting to and maintaining sinus rhythm in patients with chronic atrial fibrillation or atrial flutter: the symptomatic atrial fibrillation investigative research on dofetilide (SAFIRE-D) study. *Circulation*. 2000;102:2385–2390.

49. Anderson JL, Prystowsky EN. Sotalol: an important new antiarrhythmic. *Am Heart J*. 1999;137:388–409.

50. Hohnloser SH, Woosley RL. Sotalol *N Engl J Med*. 1994;331:31–38.

51. Singh BN, et al. Amiodarone versus sotalol for atrial fibrillation. *N Engl J Med*. 2005;352:1861–1872.

52. Pacifico A, Hohnloser SH, Williams JH, et al. Prevention of implantable-defibrillator shocks by treatment with sotalol. d,l-Sotalol Implantable Cardioverter-Defibrillator Study Group. *N Engl J Med*. 1999;340:1855–1862.

53. Salerno DM, Dias VS, Kleiger, et al. Efficacy and safety of intravenous diltiazem for treatment of atrial fibrillation and atrial flutter. The Diltiazem-Atrial Fibrillation/Flutter Study Group. *Am J Cardiol*. 1989;63:1046–1051.

54. Steinberg JS, Katz RJ, Bren GB, et al. Efficacy of oral diltiazem to control ventricular response in chronic atrial fibrillation at rest and during exercise. *J Am Coll Cardiol*. 1987;9:405–411.

55. Delacretaz E. Clinical practice. Supraventricular tachycardia. *N Engl J Med*. 2006;354:1039–1051.

56. Gheorghiade M Fau–Adams KF Jr, Adams Kf JrFau–Colucci WS, Colucci WS. Digoxin in the management of cardiovascular disorders. *Circulation*. 2004;109:2959–2964.

57. Heist Ek Fau–Ruskin JN, Ruskin JN. Atrial fibrillation and congestive heart failure: risk factors, mechanisms, and treatment. *Circulation*. 2006;48:256–269.

58. Gums JG. Magnesium in cardiovascular and other disorders. *Am J Health Syst Pharm*. 2004;61:1569–1576.

Coronary Anatomy and Physiology

Warren K. Laskey

CHAPTER 5

Contrast Media

Warren K. Laskey and Carl Tomasso

■ Chemical Structure and Properties

Radiographic contrast media (CM), by virtue of containing iodine atoms that absorb x-rays in the diagnostic kV range (33 keV is the binding energy of electrons in the outer K shell of the iodine molecule) provide enchanced contrast between the blood-tissue interface. The basic structure of iodinated CM is a benzene ring with iodine atoms at the 2, 4, and 6 positions with substituted side chains at the 3 and 5 positions. Moieties at position 1 determine water solubility properties as well as the requirement for an accompanying cation when dissociated in solution. Figure 5–1 demonstrates this basic structure and Table 5–1 outlines pertinent physical properties of the commonly used CM. Agents that dissociate in solution are categorized as "ionic" CM while those that do not dissociate are categorized as "non-ionic" CM. Dissociation in solution contributes to the osmolality of the agent. Thus, CM are further categorized into high osmolal (HOCM), low osmolal (LOCM) and iso-osmolal (IOCM) (Table 5–1). A further categorization of CM is defined by the number of iodine atoms per particle in solution ("ratio"). Thus, a CM that dissociates in solution into two particles, and which possesses 3 iodine atoms per molecule, is defined as a "ratio 1.5" agent. CM ratio is an expression of the balance between the agent's imaging performance (directly related to the iodine concentration) and its adverse effects (directly related to osmolality).

Adverse Reactions Associated with CM

CM has one desirable feature—the enhancement of radiographic contrast—and numerous undesirable features. HOCM are associated with higher overall rates of adverse events when compared to non-ionic and ionic LOCM (Table 5–2) (1–4). However, rates of serious adverse events requiring treatment are generally <5% and a significant reduction in these rates with non-ionic LOCM is more likely to be seen in those patients identified as being at high risk (3–5).

Major Adverse Reactions

The major life-threatening reactions to CM are, fortunately, rare (2 to 10/100,000) and allergic in character. However, CM reactions are predominantly non-IgE- mediated and, therefore, are not truly anaphylactic. These "anaphylactoid" reactions cannot be easily screened for, or desensitized against. The clinical manifestations (angioedema, laryngospasm, shock) are due to liberation of histamine from mast cells and the actions of proinflammatory chemokines and cytokines triggered by hyperosmolar CM. Most severe reactions occur within minutes of CM administration although delayed presentations have been reported.

There is no cross reactivity with other iodine-containing foods or medications but individuals with allergic diatheses have a twofold higher risk of reactions compared to nonallergic individuals. Patients with documented prior reactions to CM have an even higher likelihood of recurrent reactions. Premedication with steroids (6) and H1 blockers (7) will significantly reduce the incidence and severity of these reactions in individuals at risk. Treatment of immediate systemic anaphylactoid reactions has been well-discussed elsewhere (8) and is summarized in Table 5–3.

Adverse Hemodynamic and Electrophysiologic Effects

The adverse cardiovascular effects of CM generally parallel their ratio (9) and include effects on myocardial contractility, oxidative metabolism, electrophysiologic properties, and intravascular volume. Adverse hemodynamic effects of CM are more pronounced with bolus injection and include rapid increases in intravascular volume, systemic arterial vasodilation, decreased systemic arterial pressure, and increased left ventricular filling pressure. All of the latter effects are most pronounced with calcium-binding formulations of ratio 1.5 CM. Adverse electrophysiologic effects include decreased sinus node automaticity, depressed AV nodal conduction, and decreased ventricular fibrillation threshold. The latter effects are more pronounced in diseased or ischemic hearts and, again, are most pronounced with calcium-binding formulations of ratio 1.5 CM.

The incidences of these adverse effects have decreased dramatically with the use of LOCM and, therefore, the latter are the preferred CM for hemodynamically unstable patients undergoing angiography (5,9).

Adverse Effects on Clotting

Controversy exists in the literature with respect to the effects of contrast media on coagulation and platelet function. Although all contrast media inhibit coagulation in vitro, the

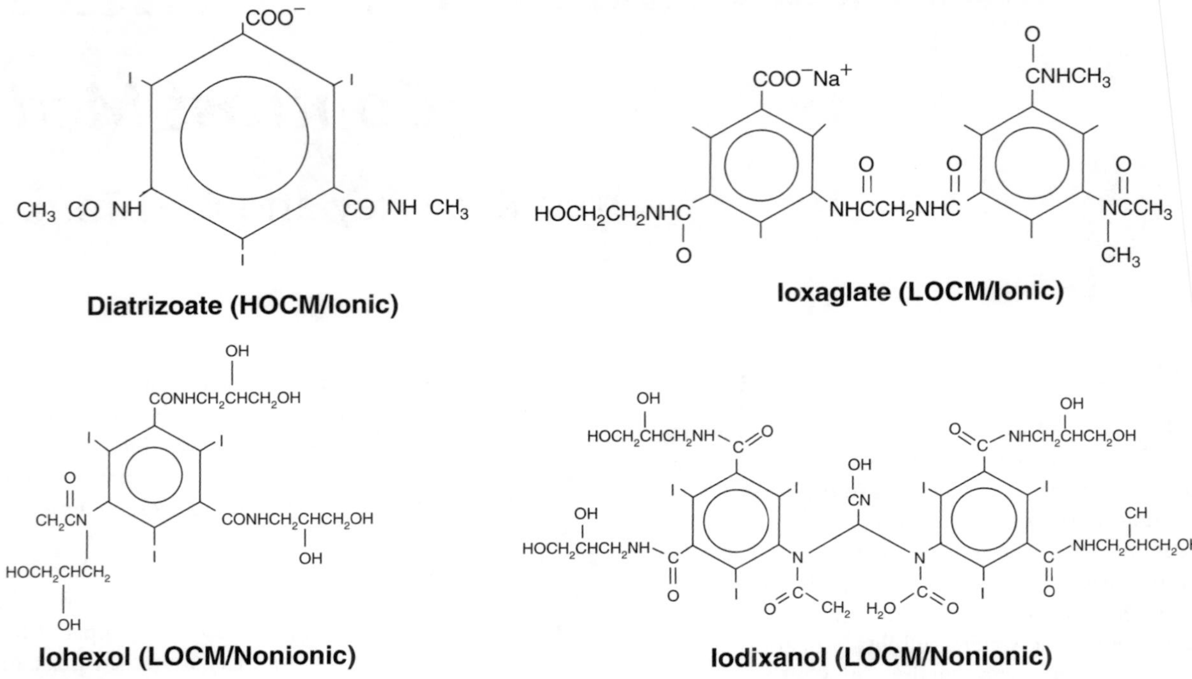

Diatrizoate (HOCM/Ionic)

Ioxaglate (LOCM/Ionic)

Iohexol (LOCM/Nonionic)

Iodixanol (LOCM/Nonionic)

Figure 5–1.

Molecular structure of representative contrast media.

anticoagulant effects of ionic HOCM are more potent than non-ionic LOCM (10). However, clinical studies to date have failed to identify an excess risk of thrombotic-related events in patients receiving non-ionic CM during angiographic procedures (11). The effects of CM on in vitro platelet function are complex and assay- and condition-dependent. Concerns surrounding an increased risk of thrombotic events during interventional procedures performed with non-ionic CM (12) have been allayed by two recent large-scale, double-blind, multicenter randomized controlled trials of an ionic LOCM compared to a non-ionic, iso-osmotic CM. In one study (13), no

increased risk of thrombotic events was seen with the use of a non-ionic iso-osmolal CM compared to an ionic LOCM (13) and another study reported a decreased risk of adverse events with the use of a non-ionic iso-osmolar CM (14) compared to an ionic LOCM.

Adverse Effects on Renal Function

Patients with renal insufficiency undergoing angiography represent a high risk group of patients not only as the result of depressed renal function per se but also as the result of multiple

Table 5–1

Chemical Composition and Physical Properties of Representative CM Used in Coronary Angiography

	Iodine (mg/mL)	Iodine Containing Molecule	Osmolality (mOsm/kg)	Viscosity (cP@37°C)	Na$^+$ (mEq/L)
Whole blood	0		290	4.0	140
Ionic, HOCM					
Renograffin-76	370	Diatrizoate	1940	8.4	190
Hypaque-76	370	Diatrizoate	2016	8.3	160
Non-ionic LOCM					
Isovue	370	Iopamidol	844	10.4	trace
Omnipaque	350	Iohexol	844	10.4	trace
Ionic LOCM					
Hexabrix	320	Ioxaglate	600	7.5	150
Non-ionic IOCM					
Visipaque	320	Iodixanol	290	11.4	trace

Table 5–2
Overall Adverse effects of CM

Reference	Ionic HOCM	Non-ionic LOCM
(1)	12.7%	3.1%
(3)	29%	9%
	(2.9% severe)	(0.8% severe)
(5a)		
• All reactions	194 per million	44 per million
• Severe reactions	37 per million	10.5 per million
• Death	3.9 per million	2.1 per million

Table 5–4
Pharmacologic Approaches to the Prevention of Contrast-Induced Nephropathy Based on Hypothesized Pathogenetic Mechanisms

"Vascular" hypothesis	Calcium channel blockers Dopamine Atrial natriuetic peptide Fenoldopam Prostaglandin E1
"Humoral" hypothesis	Endothelin receptor antagonist Theophylline
"Cytotoxic" hypothesis	N-acetylcysteine

comorbidities (15). As renal insufficiency is a powerful risk factor for the development of contrast-associated nephropathy (CAN), the mitigation of the adverse effects of CM on renal function are of clinical relevance. CAN is generally defined as either a 25% rise over the baseline creatinine or an absolute rise of 0.5 mg%. CAN is the third leading cause of renal failure in hospitalized patients and accounts for 10% of all cases of in-hospital oliguric renal failure. The time course of CAN is such that there is a deterioration of renal function within 24 to 72 hours after contrast administration which, in the majority of patients, returns to baseline over 7 to 10 days. However, as many as 5% of these patients may require dialysis. The overall risk of CAN in patients undergoing cardiovascular angiography (with coronary intervention) is ~ 3% (16) while the overall risk of CAN in patients with preexistent renal insufficiency is ~22% (16). CAN has been shown to be an independent risk factor for both in-hospital and long-term adverse outcomes (16).

The precise pathogenesis of CAN is as yet unknown although several not-mutually exclusive schools of thought have developed (Table 5–4). Importantly, a common substrate for most experimental models of CAN is dehydration/hypovolemia and figures prominently in the prophylaxis for CAN. Preexisting renal insufficiency, treated diabetes, degree of hydration, age, amount of contrast injected, hypotension, and repeated exposure to CM over a short time period have served as traditional risk factors for CAN. Diabetes mellitus appears to be a risk factor only in association with evident renal disease although as more sophisticated measures of both the diabetic state and preclinical renal disease evolve, the incidence of CAN in diabetic patients may likely increase. A number of studies have developed risk prediction algorithms for the development of CAN and support the validity of the previously mentioned "traditional" risk factors (17).

Numerous randomized clinical trials targeting hypothetical pathogenetic mechanisms (Table 5–4) of CAN have failed to convincingly identify an effective treatment. However, the fundamental importance of "meaningful hydration" cannot be over-emphasized and remains a mainstay of treatment of these patients (18–20). The use of N-acetylcysteine (NAC), in addition to hydration, prior to angiography in patients with renal insufficiency has been demonstrated to reduce the risk of CAN (21). While there is debate surrounding the magnitude, and consistency, of treatment effect (22), given its lack of toxicity and low cost NAC should be strongly considered in patients with renal insufficiency scheduled for angiography. Discontinuation of concomitant nephrotoxic or nephrotoxic potentiator medications (ACE-I, diuretics, NSAID, antibiotics) prior to the procedure is further recommended in individuals at risk. De novo institution of such agents in the immediate post-CM

Table 5–3
Treatment of Systemic Anaphylactoid Reactions to CM

Urticaria	Bronchospasm	Angioedema	Hypotension/Shock
• No specific Rx • Diphenhydramine	• Supplemental O_2 • Epinephrine 0.3 cc of 1:1,000 Sub-Q every 15 minutes or • 5–10 mcg/min bolus followed by 1–4 mcg/min infusion • Diphenhydramine 50 mg IV • Hydrocortisone 200–400 mg IV	• Call anesthesiologist • Assess airway • Supplemental O_2 • Epinephrine (as for bronchospasm) • Diphenhydramine 50 mg IV	• Epinephrine 10 mcg/min bolus IV to desired BP followed by • 1–4 mcg/min infusion • 0.9% normal saline • O_2 by mask or intubation • Diphenhydramine 50–100 mg IV

Adapted from: Goss JE, Chambers CE, Heupler FA, et al. Systemic anaphylactoid reactions to iodinated contrast media during cardiac catherization procedures. Guidelines for prevention, diagnosis, and treatment. *Cath Cardiovasc Diagn.* 1995;34:99–104, with permission.

exposure period (24–72 hours) in patients at risk for CAN is clearly ill-advised.

The type of CM used has a significant effect on the risk of CAN in high risk subjects. Randomized trials have demonstrated a significant reduction in the risk of CAN with the use of non-ionic LOCM compared to ionic HOCM (23,24). The treatment effect is most notable in patients at highest risk-those with diabetes and renal insufficiency (23). In this regard, a striking reduction in the risk of CAN was observed in a recent study of diabetic patients with renal insufficiency randomized to iodixanol, an iso-osmolal non-ionic agent, compared to iohexol, a low osmolal non-ionic agent (25).

Adverse Events in Diabetic Patients Treated with Metformin and Receiving CM

Metformin, a biguanide oral hypoglycemic agent, has been (rarely) associated with the development of lactic acidosis in diabetic patients with renal insufficiency. Although the manufacturer provides guidelines in the product brochure for such patients scheduled for angiography, these guidelines present limitations to current standards of care. Given the rarity of the development of lactic acidosis in patients receiving metformin, a revised set of guidelines has been proposed (26) and is summarized in Table 5–5. It should be emphasized that renal

---

Table 5–5
Guidelines for Management of Metformin-Treated Patients Undergoing Angiography

Elective cases
Normal renal function
Discontinue metformin (preferably 2 days prior, but
  not mandatory)
Proceed with angiography
Hydrate patient appropriately
Resume metformin *after* establishing normal renal function
Abnormal renal function
Consult with referring physician
Consider rescheduling study

Urgent/emergent cases
Normal renal function
Proceed as in elective case
Abnormal or unknown renal function
Discontinue metformin
Proceed with angiography as per guidelines for patients
  with renal insufficiency
Appropriate hydration
Minimum volume of low/iso-osmolal CM
Adjunctive therapy
Monitor renal function postprocedure
Resume metformin, if indicated, after re-establishing
  baseline renal function

---

function should be assessed in all diabetic patients receiving metformin prior to angiography.

Minor Adverse Effects

Minor reactions include symptoms such as nausea (sometimes intense), flushing, itching, urticaria and severe local discomfort (particularly with selective injections into peripheral vessels). These reactions generally occur within minutes of CM administration although delayed (>24 hours) reactions have been reported as well (27,28). LOCM have essentially eliminated the risk of these minor events (1,2).

Cost-Effectiveness and Risk Stratification Issues

LOCM were initially slow to be accepted due to cost concerns and inadequate data on appropriate use. However, the improved side effect profile and patient tolerance of LOCM relative to HOCM increasingly favored the former and LOCM have currently become the CM of choice in most cath labs (29). Formal cost-effectiveness analyses of the universal use of LOCM for diagnostic coronary angiography have failed to identify a significant advantage to this practice (4). A more acceptable approach from the standpoint of resource allocation employs a strategy of risk stratification, that is, reserving use of LOCM for those patients at highest risk of CM-associated adverse events, (4,5).

Although it has been established in a number of studies that the use of LOCM mitigates the risk of CAN in patients with chronic renal insufficiency, the persistently elevated risk of CAN despite LOCM use has led to investigations of differences in this risk among LOCM. Several studies have suggested such an interaction by demonstrating reduced rates of CAN in high risk patients undergoing angiography with the use of an iso-osmolar agent compared to a LOCM agent (25,30). Improved cost-effectiveness of such a strategy was demonstrated in a recent report from the NEPHRIC investigators (31).

Recommendations Regarding the Use of LOCM for Coronary Angiography
Class I Indication

- Use of (non-ionic) LOCM or IOCM in setting of prior contrast hypersensitivity to HOCM or LOCM, respectively—Level of evidence: C
- Use of (non-ionic) LOCM (compared to HOCM) or IOCM (compared to LOCM) in setting of renal insufficiency (w or w/o diabetes)—Level of evidence: A

Class IIa Indication

- Use of LOCM or IOCM in patients at "high risk" for acute complications of angiographic procedures—Level of evidence: A
- Use of IOCM in patients at risk of acute complications of interventional procedures—Level of evidence: A

REFERENCES

1. Katayama H, Yamaguchi K, Kozuka T, et al. Adverse reactions to ionic and nonionic contrast media. *Radiology.* 1990;175:621–628.
2. Bettmann MA, Heeren T, Greenfield A, et al. Adverse events with radiographic contrast agents: Results of the SCVIR Contrast Agent Registry. *Radiology.* 1997;203:611–520.
3. Barrett BJ, Parfrey PS, Vavasour HM, et al. A comparison of non-ionic, low osmolality radiocontrast agents with ionic, high-osmolality agents during cardiac catheterization. *N Engl J Med.* 1992;326:431–436.
4. Steinberg EP, Moore RD, Powe NR, et al. Safety and cost-effectiveness of high osmolality as compared with low osmolality contrast material in patients undergoing cardiac angiography. *N Engl J Med.* 1992;326:425–430.
5. Matthai WH Jr, Kussmaul WG, Krol J, et al. A comparison of low-with high-osmolality contrast agents in cardiac angiography. Identification of criteria for selective use. *Circulation.* 1994;89:291–301.
5a. Lasser EC, Lyon SG, Berry CC. Reports on contrast media reactions: analysis of data from reports to the US Food and Drug Administration. *Radiology.* 1997;203:605–610.
6. Lasser EC, Berry CC, Talner LB, et al. Pretreatment with corticosteroids to alleviate reactions to intravenous contrast material. *N Engl J Med.* 1987;317:845–849.
7. Thomsen HR. Guidelines for contrast media from the European Society of Urogenital Radiology. *Am J Roentgenol.* 2003;181:1463–1471.
8. Goss JE, Chambers CE, Heupler FA, et al. Systemic anaphylactoid reactions to iodinated contrast media during cardiac catheterization procedures. Guidelines for prevention, diagnosis and treatment. *Cathet Cardiovasc Diagn.* 1995;34:99–104.
9. Hirshfeld JW. Radiographic contrast agents. In: Marcus ML, ed. *Cardiac Imaging: A Companion to Braunwald's Heart Disease.* Philadelphia, PA: WB Saunders, 1996:1209–1215.
10. Corot C, Perrin JM, Belleville J, et al. Effect of iodinated contrast media on blood clotting. *Invest Radiol.* 1989;24;390–393.
11. Davidson CJ, Mark DB, Pieper KS, et al. Thrombotic and cardiovascular complications related to nonionic contrast media during cardiac catheterization: Analysis of 8,517 patients. *Am J Cardiol.* 1990;65:1481–1484.
12. Grines CL, Schreiber TL, Savas V, et al. A randomized trial of low osmolar ionic versus nonionic contrast media in patients with myocardial infarction or unstable angina undergoing percutaneous transluminal coronary angioplasty. *J Am Coll Cardiol.* 1996;27:1381–1386.
13. Bertrand ME, Esplugas E, Piessens J, et al. Influence of a nonionic, iso-osmolar contrast medium (iodixanol) versus an ionic, low-osmolar contrast medium (ioxaglate) on major adverse cardiac events in patients undergoing percutaneous transluminal coronary angioplasty: a multicenter, randomized, double-blind study. Visipaque in Percutaneous Transluminal Coronary Angioplasty. *Circulation.* 2000;101:131–136.
14. Davidson CJ, Laskey WK, Hermiller JB, et al. Randomized trial of contrast media utilization in high-risk PTCA: The COURT trial. *Circulation.* 2000;101: 2172–2177.
15. Culleton BF, Larson MG, Wilson PWF, et al. Cardiovascular disease and mortality in a community-based cohort with mild renal insufficiency. *Kidney Int.* 1999;56:2214–2219.
16. Rihal CS, Textor SC, Grill DE, et al. Incidence and prognostic importance of acute renal failure after percutaneous coronary intervention. *Circulation.* 2002; 105:2259–2264.
17. Mehran R, Aymong ED, Nikolsky E, et al. A simple risk score for prediction of contrast-induced nephropathy after percutaneous coronary intervention: development and validation. *J Am Coll Cardiol.* 2004;44:1393–1399.
18. Solomon R, Werner C, Mann D, et al. Effects of saline, mannitol, and furosemide to prevent acute decreases in renal function induced by radiocontrast agents. *N Engl J Med.* 1994;331:1416–1420.
19. Stevens MA, McCullough PA, Tobin KJ, et al. A prospective randomized trial of prevention measures in patients at high risk for contrast nephropathy: results of the P.R.I.N.C.E. Study. Prevention of Radiocontrast Induced Nephropathy Clinical Evaluation. *J Am Coll Cardiol.* 1999;33:403–411.
20. Mueller C, Buerkle G, Buettner HJ, et al. Prevention of contrast media-associated nephropathy: randomized comparison of 2 hydration regimens in 1620 patients undergoing coronary angioplasty. *Arch Intern Med.* 2002; 162:329–336.
21. Tepel M, Van der Giet M, Schwarzfeld C, et al. Prevention of radiographic contrast agent induced reductions in renal function by acetylcysteine. *N Engl J Med.* 2000;342:180–184.
22. Birck R, Krzossok S, Markowetz F, et al. Acetylcysteine for prevention of contrast nephropathy: a meta-analysis. *Lancet.* 2003;362:598–603.
23. Rudnick MR, Goldfarb S, Wexler L, et al. Nephrotoxicity of ionic and nonionic contrast media in 1196 patients: a randomized trial. The Iohexol Cooperative Study. *Kidney Int.* 1995;47:254–261.
24. Barrett BJ, Carlisle EJ. Meta-analyis of the relative toxicity of high- and low-osmolality iodinated contrast media. *Radiology* 1993;188:171–178.
25. Aspelin P, Aubry P, Fransson SG, et al. Nephrotoxic effects in high-risk patients undergoing angiography. *N Engl J Med.* 2003;348:491–499.
26. Heupler FA Jr., for members of the Laboratory Performance Standards Committee of the Society for Cardiac Angiography and Interventions. Guidelines for performing angiography in patients taking metformin. *Cathet Cardiovasc Diagn.* 1998;43:121–123.
27. Webb JA, Stacul F, Thomsen HS, et al. Late adverse reactions to intravascular iodinated contrast media. *Eur Radiol.* 2003;13:181–184.
28. Sutton AG, Finn P, Grech ED, et al. Early and late reactions after the use of iopamidol 340, ioxaglate 320 and iodixanol 320 in cardiac catheterization. *Am Heart J.* 2001;141:677–683.
29. Johnson LW, Krone R and the Registry Committee of the Society for Cardiac Angiography and Interventions. Cardiac catheterization 1991: a report of the Registry of the Society for Cardiac Angiography and Interventions. *Cathet Cardiovasc Diagn.* 1993;28:219–220.
30. Chalmers N, Jackson RW. Comparison of iodixanol and iohexol in renal impairment. *Br J Radiol.* 1999;72:701–703.
31. Aspelin P, Aubry P, Fransson S-G, et al. Cost-effectiveness of iodixanol in patients at high risk of contrast-induced nephropathy. *Amer Heart J.* 2005;149:298–303.

CHAPTER 6

Coronary Anatomy and Lesion Characteristics for the Interventional Cardiologist

Michael J. Lipinski and George W. Vetrovec

High-quality coronary angiography is essential for optimal percutaneous coronary intervention (PCI). Angiographic parameters effecting PCI outcome include vessel tortuosity, calcification, and associated side branches as well as the severity, composition, and characteristics of the target lesion. Thus, anticipated PCI markedly enhances the requirements for high-quality coronary angiography.

Essentials of High-Quality Coronary Angiography

Optimal angiography requires adequate contrast delivery to avoid streaming, which can blur vessel and lesion borders leading to overestimation of lesion severity. The coronary catheter must be properly positioned and with a sufficiently large lumen to allow adequate contrast injection for the given patient and anatomical circumstances. Thus, a 4F catheter in the setting of aortic insufficiency, extreme left ventricular hypertrophy, or a large dominant left system may be inadequate to provide sufficient dye to optimally assess lesion severity. It is also important to "reflux" the coronary ostium to avoid overestimating ostial lesions and to identify the borders of the ostium and the aorta, should stenting be necessary. Culprit vessel angiography should include orthogonal views to identify lesion severity, characteristics, and local branches. Identifying small branches at the site of a lesion may significantly enhance guide wire passage while reducing the risk of small branch dissection and/or perforation.

Identification of collateral vessels is also important particularly for assessing total occlusions. Longer injections allow visualization of retrograde collateral filling, enhancing identification of the length of the obstruction and course of the distal vessel. Specific matched left and right views can be helpful. For example, lateral right and left injections can identify the length of a mid RCA occlusion. Similarly, matched AP cranial views can identify the characteristics of a mid LAD occlusion. In addition to contrast injections, careful visualization of the skipped area for calcification can help identify the course of an occluded artery.

Following a coronary intervention, it is important to repeat the preprocedure orthogonal views to identify vessel, lesion, and, in particular, stent edge dissection; inadequate stent deployment; or downstream reduced flow, or obstruction. Identification of such findings, discussed later, can limit the risk of late ischemic events.

Optimal Coronary Views

Table 6–1 illustrates optimal native coronary views defined by vessel segment. Utilizing a limited number of basic standard angiographic views supplemented by targeted special views allows one to get optimal angiography with limited contrast administration (Fig. 6–1). However, in complex anatomy, adjunctive views are frequently helpful to best visualize specific vessel or lesion characteristics. Sequential, small variations in angulation can help identify overlapping branches, bifurcation points, or other complex anatomy.

Bypass graft anatomy poses an additional challenge. First, identifying the graft ostium in a perpendicular view to the aortic takeoff is important for stenting an ostial lesion. Dye tests are often required to obtain the best view. Although the graft body is easily visualized, orthogonal views are important to identify eccentricity of vein graft lesions.

Assessing graft insertion site and distal native vessel disease generally involves the same segmental views used for native coronary angiography. However, the angle of graft insertion into the segments may require adjustment of the angulation to obtain a perpendicular view of the insertion site (Table 6–2). Examples include an AP caudal view for the insertion site of the RCA vein graft into the proximal posterior descending. Likewise the LIMA-LAD insertion is best identified in a lateral projection (Fig. 6–2).

Identifying the presence, extent, and complexity of proximal subclavian artery stenosis is important in evaluating LIMA-LAD steal as a possible cause of ischemia. Pressure

Table 6–1

Optimal Coronary Angiographic Views

Vessel	Segment	Routine View	Adjunctive View
LM	Ostial/Body	LAO Caudal RAO Caudal	AP Caudal RAO Cranial
	Distal/Bifurcation	LAO Caudal RAO Caudal	LAO Cranial
LAD	Ostial	LAO Caudal	AP/RAO Caudal
	Body	LAO/RAO Cranial	AP Cranial
	Distal	RAO	RAO Caudal
CIRC	Ostium	LAO Caudal	AP Caudal
	Body	RAO Caudal/LAO	AP Caudal
	Distal	RAO Caudal AP Caudal	LAO Cranial
RCA	Ostial/Prox	LAO Cranial	AP Caudal Steep LAO
	Mid Vessel	Shallow RAO	Lateral LAO Caudal
	Distal Bifurcation	LAO Cranial	AP Cranial
	Posterior Descending	Shallow RAO	AP Cranial
	Posterior Lateral Branches	Shallow RAO	AP Caudal Lateral-Cranial

damping on catheter entry into the subclavian artery warrants careful vessel assessment. Subclavian angiography should include reflux into the aorta to assess the ostium and proximal vessel. An RAO cranial view can "straighten" the subclavian artery to best identify a lesion and if present the relation to the LIMA and vertebral arteries.

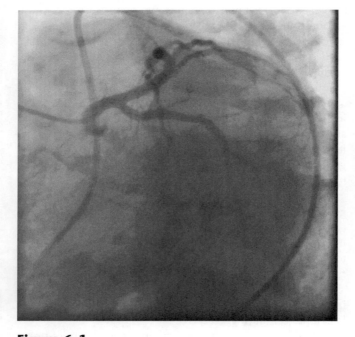

Figure 6–1.
LAO caudal projection demonstrating excellent display of the distal LM and proximal LAD and circumflex vessels.

Angiographic Characteristics and Classifications of Lesions

Although controversy exists whether 50% or 75% diameter stenosis criteria should define significant angiographic coronary artery disease, animal and human studies demonstrate that ischemia typically occurs with a diameter stenosis of greater than 70%. The CASS criteria for defining significant angiographic coronary artery disease was diameter stenosis $\geq$50% in the left main coronary artery or diameter stenosis $\geq$70% in any other major epicardial coronary artery or major branch.

Lesion morphology is likewise important to identify lesion calcification, ulcerated plaques, and thrombus (Fig. 6–3).

Table 6–2

Optimal Coronary Angiographic Views: Bypass Graft Insertion Site

Segment	Routine*	Adjunctive
Lad/Diag	AP Cranial	Lateral
Circ	LAO	AP Caudal RAO Cranial
RCA	LAO Caudal	Lateral RAO Caudal
PDA/PLB (Bifurcation)	AP Cranial	Lateral
PDA/PLB (Mid vessels)	LAO Cranial	RAO Caudal

*Similar views for same area of native vessel.

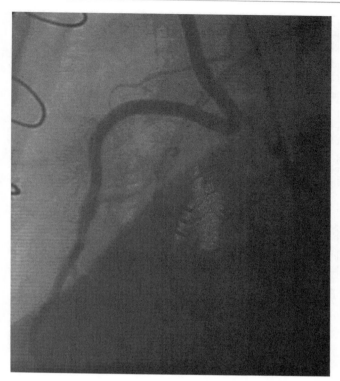

Figure 6–2.
Lateral view of LIMA insertion site with a diagonal graft anastomosis to LIMA also visualized.

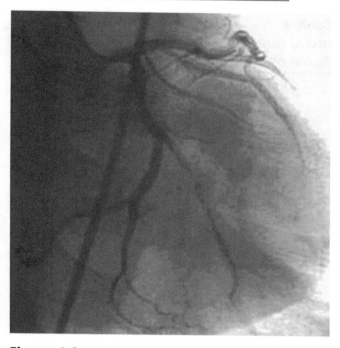

Figure 6–3.
A series of round, hazy filling defects consistent with thrombus seen in a partially thrombosed recent stent placed in the mid-circumflex marginal.

Angiographic characteristics of coronary lesions have been classified (Table 6–3) to estimate PCI procedural risk and outcome. Type A are simple lesions, Type B are moderately complex lesions divided into B1 (lesions with only one B characteristic), and B2 (lesions with ≥2 or more B characteristics), and C are high-risk lesions. An early analysis of balloon angioplasty results by Ellis et al. (1) identified a 92% success and 2%

complication rate for Type A lesions, with sequentially declining outcomes as lesion severity increased with only a 61% success and a 21% complication rate for Type C lesions. Likewise, in a study by Krone et al., PCI for Type A lesions had a success rate of 98%, B1 97.7%, B2 95.7%, and C 89.9% (2). An analysis by Kastrati et al. of PCI outcomes in the stent era demonstrated that the restenosis rate correlated with increasing lesion complexity (21.7% restenosis for Type A lesions to 32.6% for Type C lesions) (3). Likewise, the 1-year event-free survival

Table 6–3
ACC/AHA Lesion Classification

Low-Risk Lesion	Moderate-Risk Lesion	High-Risk Lesion
(Type A)	(Type B)	(Type C)
Discrete (Length <10 mm)	Tubular (Length 10–20 mm)	Diffuse (Length >20 mm)
Concentric	Eccentric	Excessive tortuosity of proximal segment
Readily accessible	Moderate tortuosity of proximal segment	Extremely angulated segment >90°
Nonangulated segment (<45°)	Moderately angulated segment (>45°, <90°)	Total occlusion >3-months old and/or bridging collaterals
Smooth contour	Irregular contour	Inability to protect major side branches
Little or no calcification	Moderate or heavy calcification	Degenerate vein grafts with friable lesions
Less than totally occlusive	Total occlusion <3-months old	
Not ostial in location	Ostial location	
No major side branch involvement	Bifurcation lesions requiring of double guidewires	
Absence of thrombus	Some thrombus present	

Table modified from the ACC/AHA Guidelines for Percutaneous Coronary Intervention. Type B1 lesions have one characteristic of Type B lesions, whereas Type B2 lesions have two or more of the Type B lesion characteristics.

Table 6–4

Distal Blood Flow/Collateral Classification Based on TIMI Classification Scheme

	TIMI Grade	Contrast Flow
0	(No perfusion)	Antegrade flow to lesion: no flow beyond occlusion
1	(Penetration with minimal perfusion)	Contrast passes beyond lesion but does not opacify distal vessel during cine run
2	(Partial perfusion)	Contrast passes obstruction and fills distal vessel; however, rate of filling and/or washout slower than vessel segments outside lesion
3	(Complete perfusion)	Contrast passes freely into distal at same visual rate as unaffected adjacent vessels

Table 6–5

NHLBI Classification System for Coronary Dissection

	Dissection
A	Small radiolucent area within the lumen of the vessel
B	Linear, nonpersisting extravasations of contrast
C	Extraluminal, persisting extravasations of contrast
D	Spiral-shaped filling defect
E	Persistent lumen defect with delayed antegrade flow
F	Filling effect accompanied by total coronary occlusion

Length (in mm)

Measure end-to-end for Type B through F dissections

Staining

Persistence of contrast within the dissection after washout of contrast from the remaining portion of the vessel

was 85.2% for Type A lesions, 79.4% for Type B1, 75.9% for Type B2, and 75.2% for Type C lesions. A 2004 report from the Mayo Clinic on 5,064 PCI patients again demonstrated that lesion risk correlated with the rate of in-hospital major adverse cardiovascular events (MACE) (4). Patients undergoing PCI for Type A lesions had a 1.2% event rate, increasing to 4.9% for Type C lesions. Therefore, although improvements in PCI have led to better outcomes, lesion complexity determined by the ACC/AHA lesion classification continues to serve as a predictor of outcome.

Another predictor of clinical outcome following PCI is coronary blood flow distal to the lesion postrevascularization. Several complementary grading systems have been established to define residual coronary flow and myocardial perfusion. The traditional TIMI criteria are based on operator visual assessment of flow (Table 6–4). To improve the predictability of the visual TIMI flow score, a corrected TIMI frame count was developed to denote the number of frames required for contrast to travel from the coronary ostium across a target lesion to a distal landmark. Last, TIMI myocardial perfusion grade (TMP) was established to angiographically evaluate tissue perfusion based on myocardial blush. Thus, in decreasing severity, grade 0 is minimal or no myocardial dye stain or blush, grade 1 is dye staining that persists to the next injection, grade 2 is dye that washes out slowly such that the dye staining is strongly persistent at the end of the injection, and grade 3 is normal dye washout being mildly persistent at the end of the injection. Several studies (5) using the TIMI flow grade, TIMI perfusion grade (6), and TIMI frame count (7,8) have demonstrated that improved coronary flow and myocardial perfusion following revascularization, whether by PCI or thrombolytic therapy, resulted in improved survival and decreased clinically adverse events.

Last, as noted earlier, postangiographic assessment includes identifying vessel or stent edge dissection as well as rare vessel perforation. The extent of coronary dissection has been classified as shown in Table 6–5.

Anomalous Coronary Arteries

Coronary anomalies have been shown in several angiographic studies to have an occurrence rate of 0.6% to 1.55%. Of 126,595 patients undergoing coronary angiography at the Cleveland Clinic (9), 1.3% had a coronary anomaly of which 13% were coronary artery fistulae. Most (81%) were considered benign. However, coronary anomalies can cause symptoms such as angina pectoris, myocardial infarction, syncope, cardiac arrhythmias, heart failure, and sudden death. Pathologic coronary anomalies may result in symptoms or death secondary to inadequate myocardial perfusion due to unusual angling of the anomalous coronary artery (left main arising from the right coronary sinus and coursing between the aorta and pulmonary artery) or perfusion of the myocardium with inadequately oxygenated blood (anomalous coronary artery arising from the pulmonary artery). Examples of benign and pathologic coronary artery anomalies are listed in Table 6–6. The most common anomaly is separate ostia for the LAD and circumflex arteries, followed by an anomalous circumflex arising from the right sinus. Angiographic identification of the LAD passing between the great vessels has been described by Serota et al. (10) as a superior "dot" visualized just beyond the left coronary sinus and above the aortic valve during an RAO left ventriculogram produced by sharp angulation of the LAD as it turns to enter its usual course in the anterior interventricular groove.

Summary

The acute and late outcomes for coronary intervention have improved dramatically over the last 25 years. Optimal angiographic assessment of coronary anatomy pre- and

Table 6–6

Benign and Pathologic Coronary Anomalies

Benign Coronary Anomalies	Pathologic Coronary Anomalies
LAD and LCX with separate origins in the left sinus of Valsalva	Ectopic coronary artery arising from the pulmonary artery
Ectopic origin of circumflex artery from the right sinus of Valsalva	Ectopic coronary artery arising from the opposite coronary sinus
Ectopic origin of a coronary artery from the posterior sinus of Valsalva	Large coronary artery fistulae
Coronary artery origin from the ascending aorta	
Small coronary fistula	

post-PCI has contributed to this success. Given the ever-increasing complexity of coronary intervention, the need for optimal angiography will persist.

REFERENCES

1. Ellis SG, Vandormael MG, Cowley MJ, et al. Coronary morphologic and clinical determinants of procedural outcome with angioplasty for multivessel coronary disease. Implications for patient selection. Multivessel Angioplasty Prognosis Study Group. *Circulation.* 1990;82:1193–1202.

2. Krone RJ, Kimmel SE, Laskey WK, et al. Evaluation of the Society for Coronary Angiography and Interventions' lesion classification system in 14,133 patients with percutaneous coronary interventions in the current stent era. *Catheter Cardiovasc Interv.* 2002;55:1–7.

3. Kastrati A, Schomig A, Elezi S, et al. Prognostic value of the modified American College of Cardiology/American Heart Association stenosis morphology classification for long-term angiographic and clinical outcome after coronary stent placement. *Circulation.* 1999;100:1285–1290.

4. Singh M, Rihal CS, Lennon RJ, et al. Comparison of Mayo Clinic risk score and American College of Cardiology/American Heart Association lesion classification in the prediction of adverse cardiovascular outcome follow-ing percutaneous coronary interventions. *J Am Coll Cardiol.* 2004;44:357–361.

5. Gibson CM, Cannon CP, Murphy SA, et al. Relationship of the TIMI myocardial perfusion grades, flow grades, frame count, and percutaneous coronary intervention to long-term outcomes after thrombolytic administration in acute myocardial infarction. *Circulation.* 2002;105:1909–1913.

6. Gibson CM, Cannon CP, Murphy SA, et al. Relationship of TIMI myocardial perfusion grade to mortality after administration of thrombolytic drugs. *Circulation.* 2000;101:125–130.

7. Gibson CM, Murphy SA, Rizzo MJ, et al. Relationship between TIMI frame count and clinical outcomes after thrombolytic administration. Thrombolysis in Myocardial Infarction (TIMI) Study Group. *Circulation.* 1999;99:1945–1950.

8. Hamada S, Nishiue T, Nakamura S, et al. TIMI frame count immediately after primary coronary angioplasty as a predictor of functional recovery in patients with TIMI 3 reperfused acute myocardial infarction. *J Am Coll Cardiol.* 2001;38:666–671.

9. Yamanaka O, Hobbs RE. Coronary artery anomalies in 126,595 patients undergoing coronary arteriography. *Cathet Cardiovasc Diagn.* 1990;21:28–40.

10. Serota H, Barth CW III, Seuc CA, et. al. Rapid identification of the course of anomalous coronary arteries in adults: The "dot and eye" method. *Am J Cardiol.* 1990;65:898.

CHAPTER 7

Coronary Physiology for the Interventional Cardiologist: Theory and Practice of Using Coronary Pressure and Flow Measurements in the Cath Lab*

Morton J. Kern

Coronary angiography remains the standard for the diagnosis of epicardial coronary disease. However, precise quantification of stenosis severity is limited by the inability to provide accurate two- or three-dimensional resolution on coronary "luminograms." The limitations of coronary angiography have been well documented by comparisons to intravascular ultrasound and ischemic stress testing. Direct measurement of coronary blood flow velocity and distal perfusion pressures allow the interventional cardiologist to have a complete assessment of both coronary anatomy and physiology (1,2). The weakness of the luminograms and the rationale for using coronary physiology can be seen by examination of Figure 7–1. A pathologic specimen of a coronary artery shows a normal lumen with the plaque underlying this normal lumen. Atherosclerosis is indeed present despite an angiographic presence of this location of a normal artery. In the middle segment, the plaque has ruptured. The cap of plaque can be seen at the upper right. The shoulder is split and hematoma formed beneath the cap. The lumen at this location would appear angiographically as mildly narrowed with no evidence of significant obstruction. On the far right specimen, the lumen has been compromised to a significant degree surrounded by hematoma and the ruptured plaque. Contrast entered and mixed with blood behind the plaque gives a hazy and indistinct appearance to this portion of the luminograms. Thus, the true lumen may not appear severely narrowed despite the fact the physiologic response is abnormal. The corresponding angiograms show a hazy and indistinct lesion segment in two orthogonal views. The complex nature of the many plaques can be identified by ultrasound (Fig. 1–8, *right lower panel*). A serpiginous border

with many crevices and cracks fill in with contrast resulting in an angiographic appearance of nonphysiologic significance. In many circumstances, there is a failure to identify the critical lesion. In addition, a single view of an eccentric lesion may show only one diameter narrowed and may give a false impression of the flow limiting nature of the stenosis. For these reasons, coronary physiologic measurements can address and at times solve the dilemma faced by angiographer where no objective evidence is at hand.

Measuring coronary blood flow and pressure provides unique information that complements the angiographic evaluation and in most cases facilitates decision-making regarding appropriateness of therapy (1,2).

Fundamentals of Coronary Blood Flow

Because the extraction of oxygen in the coronary circulation is almost maximal even under "resting" conditions, coronary blood flow is intricately matched to myocardial oxygen demand. For the most part, the large epicardial conduit arteries offer little resistance to coronary blood flow, and arteriolar vasomotion can increase blood flow to the normal heart more than threefold (3–5). However, in the presence of a hemodynamically significant epicardial stenosis, the capacity of the arterioles to vasodilate becomes limited, and under conditions of increased oxygen demand, may lead to a mismatch between oxygen delivery and demand resulting in ischemia and often angina. Other conditions, including left ventricular hypertrophy and diabetes, may also impair coronary microvascular vascular regulation producing ischemia in the absence of epicardial coronary obstructions. Coronary artery disease (i.e., atherosclerosis) is a diffuse process throughout the coronary

---

*Some sections reproduced from: Kern, MJ. Curriculum in international cardiology: coronary pressure and flow measurements in the cardiac catherization laboratory. *CCI.* 2001;54:378–400.

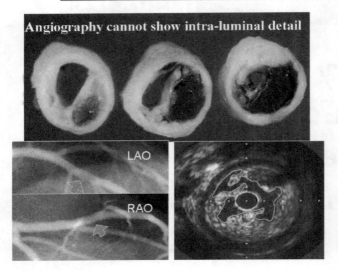

Figure 7–1.
Limitations of angiography and the rationale for use of coronary physiology. *Top panel* shows artery cross sections proximal and at a distal ruptured plaque. The corresponding angiogram **(lower left)** demonstrates a hazy appearance without lumen narrowing. The IVUS image **(lower right)** shows the reason why angiography fails. Detail of plaque rupture is below the resolution of the angiogram.

arterial tree as illustrated in Figure 7–2, where an epicardial lesion can be easily seen (*large circle*). This stenosis obstructs flow by a mechanical narrowing in the lumen resulting in loss of distal pressure and flow. Note that arterial branches proximal to this stenosis, which have no obstruction, may divert flow before the significant lesion. Coronary flow measured proximal to the stenosis will not give an accurate reflection of the physiology of stenosis itself. Moreover, from a clinical point of view, a stenosis of this type may be flow limiting but not clinically active, whereas less obstructive lesions elsewhere may become activated and thrombotic at some future date resulting in acute coronary syndromes.

In addition, the function of the microcirculation is a major contributor to the ability of coronary flow to increase in response to myocardial demand. A normal coronary epicardial conduit may be associated with reduced maximal flow due to microvascular impairment at the precapillary arterial level. This means that a normal coronary reserve (maximal/basal flow) represents the response of two components, the epicardial artery and microvasculature. If either of the two systems is abnormal, an abnormal coronary flow reserve is the result. For this reason, coronary flow reserve is not a specific measurement for lesion assessment. In contrast, measurement of translesional pressure is specific only for the epicardial narrowing and especially useful to identify lesion significance for those of intermediate severity.

The relationship between pressure and flow is illustrated in Figure 7–3. The frame from an angiogram of a significant stenosis is shown with blood traversing the angiogram (*left to right* in Fig. 7–3). This stenosis produces resistance to flow with pressure loss distal to the stenosis due to the complex interaction of rheologic coefficients. Viscous friction is generated by the intrinsic narrowing. Further pressure loss occurs

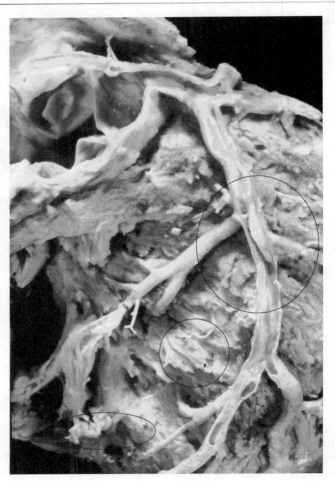

Figure 7–2.
Pathologic specimen of a coronary artery. The *large circle* is epicardial narrowing. The *small circle* points to microvascular region. The *oval* indicates region of potential collateralization.

due to separation and reestablishment of laminar flow in the post-stenotic turbulent region. These components of the geometry are different for different stenosis configurations and, thus, vessels with a similar percent diameter narrowing may have two very different physiologic responses. This response is illustrated in Figure 7–4 in which the pressure flow curves of two patients, A and B, are shown in the lower left panel. The pressure and flow responses can be measured in the cardiac cath lab using sensor guidewire techniques. Doppler flow velocity measurements are shown in the lower right panel. However, because of the complexity of using Doppler flow, the hemodynamic significance of a stenosis is better assessed by pressure measurements.

Coronary Doppler Flow Velocity

Coronary Doppler flow velocity is the speed of red blood cells flowing past an ultrasound emitting and receiving crystal. Velocity can be measured by the Doppler phase shift in frequency:

$$\text{Velocity (cm/sec)} = (\text{freq 1} - \text{freq } \emptyset)^*(\text{constant})/$$
$$(2^*\text{freq } \emptyset)^* \text{Cos } \Phi \qquad (7.1)$$

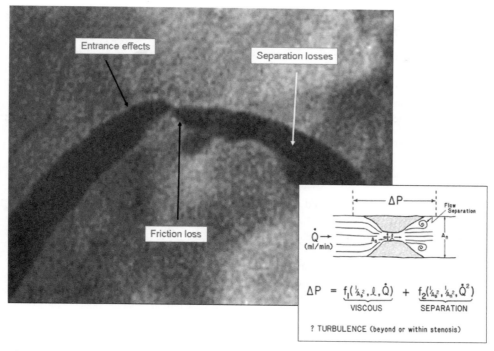

Figure 7–3.

Pressure loss across a stenosis is derived from two sources: frictional losses along the entrance and inertial losses of flow separation. Frictional losses are linearly related to flow, Q (law of Poiseuille) and inertial and exit losses increase with the square of the flow (law of Bernoulli). The pressure gradient (delta P) thus is delta P = f_1*Q + f_2*Q^2. The loss coefficients f_1 and f_2 are a function of both geometry and rheologic properties of blood (viscosity and density). This formula results in a quadratic relationship, where the curvilinear shape is derived from nonlinear stenosis exit losses. When no stenosis is present, the second term is zero and the curve becomes a straight line (with a positive slope that depends on the diameter of the vessel, law of Poiseuille). A_s = area of the stenosis; L = length; A_n = area of the normal segment.

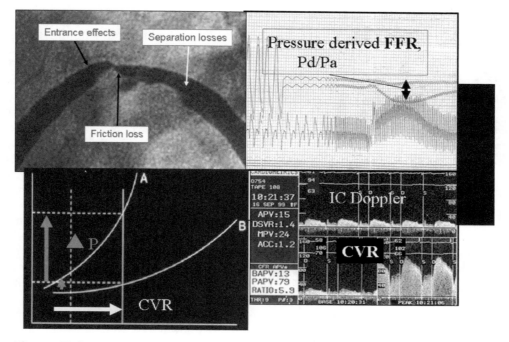

Figure 7–4.

Angiogram used to determine flow across a stenosis **(upper left)**; aortic and coronary pressure tracings during hyperemia **(upper right)**. FFR is fractional flow reserve. Pressure-flow relationships in two patients with 60% angiographic stenoses **(lower left)**. Abscissa is coronary flow (CVR) and ordinate is delta P, pressure. Coronary Doppler flow signals across a stenosis **(lower right)**.

Where:

Velocity = velocity of coronary blood flow
Freq Ø = transmitting frequency of the Doppler crystal
Freq 1 = returning frequency to the Doppler crystal
Constant = speed of sound in blood
Cos Φ = angle of incidence at the crystal

Volumetric flow in the epicardial artery can be obtained by multiplying the flow velocity above by the vessel cross-sectional area (cm^2) measured by online quantitative imaging techniques, yielding a value in cm^3/sec.

Coronary Doppler flow velocity can be measured using a 0.014-inch Doppler angioplasty guidewire. Velocity signals are generated by the reflected sounds from the moving red cells. A spectral velocity signal is then produced for the operator to examine, and measurements at baseline and hyperemia are created to produce coronary flow velocity reserve (CFR) measurements (Figure 7–5). The continuous trend of velocity (*lower panel*) is interrupted by the artifact of intracoronary adeno-

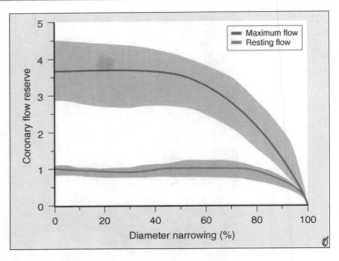

Figure 7–6.

Coronary flow reserve expressed as ratio of maximum to resting flow plotted as a function of percent diameter narrowing. With progressive narrowing, resting flow does not change. Maximum potential increase in flow and coronary flow reserve begins to be impaired at approximately 50% diameter narrowing (*dash line*). The shaded area represents the limits of variability of data about the mean. (Adapted from: Gould KL, Lipscomb K, Hamilton GW. Physiologic basis for assessing critical coronary stenosis: instantaneous flow response and regional distribution during coronary hyperemia as measures of coronary flow reserve. *Am J Cardiol.* 1974;33:87–94.)

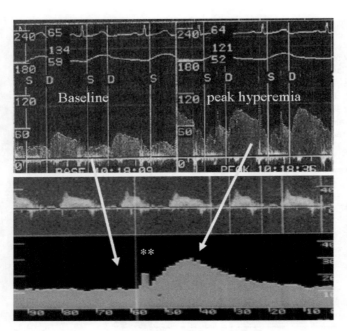

Figure 7–5.

Coronary Doppler flow velocity signals used for the measurement of coronary flow velocity reserve in the cardiac cath lab. The *top panel* is divided into the baseline **(left)** and the peak hyperemic velocity **(right)** signals. Phasic flow velocity tracing is demarcated by systolic (S) and diastolic (D) markers, corresponding to the electrocardiogram and aortic pressure at top of panels. Diastolic flow predominates over systolic flow. Flow velocity scale is from 0 to 240 cm per second. Continuous trend plot of average peak velocity showing the baseline and time course of peak hyperemia (*bottom panel*). The intracoronary bolus adenosine injection can be seen by the square wave signal preceding the rapid increase in average peak velocity. The phasic peak hyperemic velocity signal was captured and displayed in the *upper right panel*. The trend plot scale is from 0 to 60 cm per second with a time base of 0 to 90 seconds (*bottom panel*). In this example, baseline flow is 13 cm per second and peak hyperemic flow is 30 cm per second for a coronary flow reserve of 2.3.

sine injection to stimulate hyperemia. The peak hyperemic response occurs over the next 30 seconds. The peak to basal flow velocity ratio is the CFR. CFR is equivalent to the volumetric coronary flow reserve, assuming the vessel cross-sectional area remains constant over the measuring period.

CFR decreases when a stenosis exceeds a critical threshold (Fig. 7–6). At a diameter narrowing of approximately 60%, coronary flow reserve begins to diminish. Resting flow diminishes when the stenosis is 90% or greater. However, the variability of CFR responses is large as evidenced by the white-gray band around each line of flow (6–8).

The clinical limitation of coronary flow reserve is the requirement of interpret the CFR as a result of the two-component system (Fig. 7–7). When both the conduit and microvasculature are normal, coronary flow reserve is normal (*top panel*, Fig. 7–7). When an epicardial stenosis is present, coronary flow reserve is diminished. Likewise, when microvascular disease is present in the absence of stenosis, coronary flow reserve can also be diminished. Thus, the limitation of differentiating microvasculature from epicardial coronary obstruction becomes difficult if not impossible. An attempt has been made to resolve this dilemma by employing the concept of relative coronary flow reserve (Fig. 7–8) whereby the ratio of coronary flow reserve in a target vessel to the coronary flow reserve in an unobstructed reference vessel is made by producing relative coronary flow reserve with the assumption that the microvascular bed is the same. Unfortunately, a large variability around the coronary flow reserve measurements both for the target and reference vessel make the two ratios unreliable. This value is no longer used for lesion assessment (9.10).

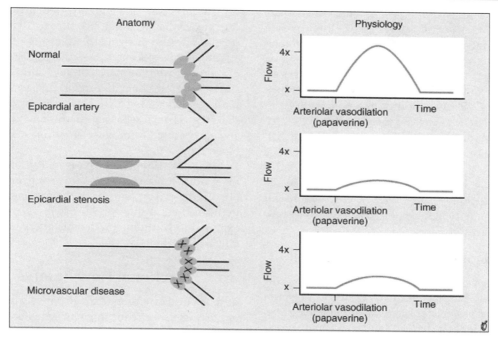

Figure 7–7.

Limitations of CFR. A normal epicardial and microvascular bed results in a normal CFR (**right side**, top panel). If either a stenosis or microvascular disease is present then CFR is reduced (middle and lower panels. (From: Wilson R, CCI 1998.)

Coronary Flow Reserve

There are two indices that suggest an epicardial stenosis is significant: (i) post-stenotic absolute coronary flow reserve (CVR) <2.0 and (ii) relative coronary flow reserve (rCVR) <0.8. CVR is subject to variations in conditions that may alter resting flow and limit maximal hyperemic flow (5,6). Tachycardia increases basal flow; CVR is reduced by 10% for each 15 beats heart rate (7). Increasing mean arterial pressure reduces maximal vasodilatation reducing hyperemia with less alteration in basal flow. CVR may be reduced in patients with essential hypertension and normal coronary arteries and in patients with aortic stenosis and normal coronary arteries (5).

In patients referred for coronary arteriography with chest pain syndromes, CVR has been measured at 2.7 ± 0.6, suggesting a degree of patient variability or microvascular disease beyond the resolution of the coronary angiogram. In patients with obstructive coronary disease in other arteries or in patients with orthotropic heart transplantation, CVR ranges from 2.5 ± 0.95 and 3.1 ± 0.9, respectively (10). CVR >2.0 has a strong correlation with nonischemic nuclear stress imaging (1). CVR values <2.0 occur in approximately 12% of patients referred for catheterization for chest pain with normal arteries, which suggests the less frequent incidence of isolated microvascular disease (10).

Age and basal flow affect CVR (12). ($CVR_{corr} = 2.85*$ $CVR_{measured}* 10^x$, where $X = 0.48$ log (BAPV) $+ 0.0025*$ age $- 1.16$). Use of the corrected CVR standardizes for variations in basal average peak velocity and patient age and may discriminate between intrinsic and extra cardiac factors impairing CVR (8).

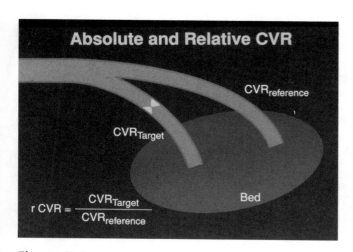

Figure 7–8.

Diagram of absolute and relative coronary reserve calculations. The target coronary reserve CVR_{target} and $CVR_{reference}$ vessel in the unobstructed artery both supply a bed with common microvascular responses. Relative coronary flow reserve or CVR is the ratio of CVR_{target} to $CVR_{reference}$.

Relative Coronary Flow Velocity Reserve

Because of a two-component system (epicardial and microvascular), there is some uncertainty in accepting an abnormal CVR as the sole indicator of lesion significance. To measure lesion severity independent of the microvascular influence, a relative CVR (rCVR), defined as the ratio of maximal flow in the coronary with stenosis (Q^S) to flow in a normal coronary without stenosis (Q^N), has been suggested (3,4). For patient studies, rCVR is the ratio of CVR_{target} to CVR in an angiographically normal reference vessel, ($rCVR = (Q^s/Q_{base})/(Q^N/Q_{base}) = (CVR_{target}/CVR_{reference})$ (9). Basal flow in the two vessels is assumed to be similar and thus, rCVR mathematically resembles Gould's derivation. rCVR cannot be used in patients with three-vessel coronary disease who have no suitable reference vessel. rCVR relies on the assumption that the microvascular circulatory response is uniformly distributed among the myocardial beds; therefore, rCVR is of no value in patients with myocardial infarction, left ventricular regional dysfunction, or patients in whom the microcirculatory responses are heterogeneous. This may explain why the normal range for rCVR in patients is so large at 0.65 to 1.0 (9,10).

Pharmacologic Hyperemic Stimuli

CFR and stenosis severity should always be assessed using measurements obtained during maximal hyperemia. The most widely used maximal vasodilator agents are dipyridamole, papaverine, and adenosine. The hyperosmolar ionic and low osmolar, nonionic contrast media do not produce maximal hyperemia. Nitrates increase volumetric flow, but because these agents also dilate epicardial conductance vessels, the increase in coronary flow velocity is less than with adenosine or papaverine. Intracoronary nitroglycerin (100 to 200 μcg) should be given before flow velocity measurements to paralyze vasomotion and minimize any flow-mediated vasodilation.

Intracoronary papaverine increases coronary blood flow velocity four to six times over resting values in patients with normal coronary arteries. Papaverine (8 to 12 mg) produces a response equal to that of an IV infusion of dipyridamole in a dose of 0.56 to 0.84 mg/kg of body weight, but can occasionally cause QT prolongation and ventricular tachycardia or fibrillation.

Both IC and IV adenosine have short half-lives. The total duration of the hyperemic response of IC adenosine is only 25% that of papaverine or dipyridamole. Adenosine is benign in the appropriate dosages (20 to 30 μcg in the right coronary artery or 40 to 60 μcg in the left coronary artery or infused intravenously at 140 μcg/kg/min). A rare patient may be hypersensitive to standard doses of adenosine in the right coronary artery with transient heart block lasting <10 seconds. Because bolus IC adenosine does not increase the vessel cross-sectional area, coronary flow velocity reserve can be used as a surrogate for coronary volumetric flow reserve.

The vasodilatory effects of adenosine are primarily on the microcirculation, with little effect on the epicardial conduit arteries. Both intracoronary and intravenous adenosine infusions produce maximal hyperemia in humans.

Pressure-Derived Fractional Flow Reserve

Myocardial perfusion is closely linked to myocardial ischemia and is directly dependent on the coronary "driving" pressure associated with three major coronary vascular resistances (epi-cardial, arteriolar, and intramyocardial capillary resistance). The myocardial perfusion pressure (aortic pressure–left ventricular pressure or right atrial pressure) is reduced when an epicardial stenosis causes pressure loss distal to the stenosis in proportion to the flow rate. If the myocardial bed resistances are stimulated to maximal hyperemia and remain constant, then the post-stenotic hyperemic coronary artery pressure represents the maximal achievable perfusion available in that vessel and can be used to produce an estimate of normal coronary blood flow.

Using coronary pressure measured at constant and minimal myocardial resistances (i.e., maximal hyperemia), Pijls et al. (11,12) derived an estimate of the percentage of normal (i.e., in the theoretical absence of the stenosis) coronary blood flow expected to go through a stenotic artery called the fractional flow reserve (FFR).

Fractional Flow Reserve

As a practical extension of the previously mentioned concept, one can assess the reduction in maximal flow due to a stenosis in an indirect way by a pressure measurement distal to a stenosis under hyperemic conditions. The pressure-derived myocardial FFR was originally defined as the ratio of distal pressure to aortic pressure during maximal hyperemia, assuming that venous pressure can be regarded as zero.

$$\text{FFR} = \frac{Q_s}{Q_n} = \frac{(P_d - P_v) \cdot R_{m,n}}{(P_a - P_v) \cdot R_{m,s}} \approx \frac{P_d}{P_a} \qquad (7.2)$$

where Q_s is flow in the stenotic artery, Q_n is flow in the theoretic normal artery, and P_d, P_a, and P_v represent the pressure in the distal artery, aorta, and right atrium (vein, v), respectively. Note that this relationship is only true under the assumption that microvascular resistance in the dilated myocardial vascular bed distal to a normal ($R_{m,n}$) and to a diseased ($R_{m,s}$) artery is fixed, minimal, and the same.

A cut-off value of 0.75 was derived based on clinical studies where the FFR was compared to a number of noninvasive indices of reversible ischemia. This simply means that at an aortic pressure of 100 mm Hg, a pressure of 75 mm Hg or higher distal of the stenosis during hyperemia, is regarded as sufficient to guarantee adequate blood supply of the coronary microcirculation during maximal flow. The applicability of the FFR for decision-making in diagnosis and treatment evaluation has been established in a number of clinical trials.

The FFR reflects antegrade and collateral myocardial perfusion rather than merely trans-stenotic pressure loss (i.e., a stenosis pressure gradient). Because it is calculated only at peak hyperemia, the FFR is further differentiated from CVR by being largely independent of basal flow, driving pressure, heart rate, systemic blood pressure, or status of the microcirculation (13). The FFR, but not the resting pressure or hyperemic pressure gradient, is strongly related to provocable myocardial ischemia (FFR <0.75) established by rigorous comparisons to different clinical stress testing modalities in patients with stable angina.

An example of translesional pressure measurements (Fig. 7–9) shows the guiding catheter pressure (aortic pressure) is

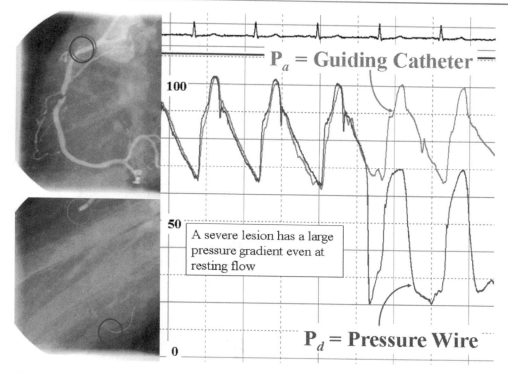

Figure 7–9.

Angiogram of significant RCA lesion (*left panels*) and corresponding pressures in aorta and coronary pressure wire before crossing lesion **(left side)** and after crossing lesion **(right side)**. A severe lesion has a large pressure gradient even at rest. (Courtesy of Dr. B. De Bruyne.)

matched against the guidewire sensor pressure before crossing the stenosis. The wire is then advanced beyond the stenosis to acquire distal coronary artery pressure (P_d). A severe lesion at rest has a large pressure gradient even under basal conditions. However, not all stenoses have significant angiographic narrowing nor do they produce significant gradients at rest. For

example, examine Figure 7–10 in which the proximal left anterior descending stenosis is only mildly narrowed. Pressure will be measured proximal to the lesion, across the lesion, and again distal to the lesion at rest and during hyperemia with IC or IV adenosine (Fig. 7–11). The aortic pressure (P_A) measured by the guide catheter is matched against coronary pressure (P_D). Intracoronary adenosine is given. For illustration purposes,

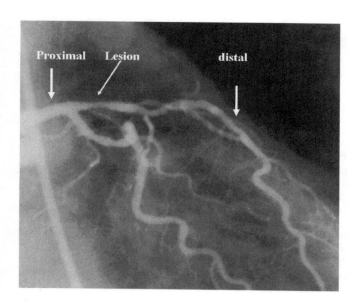

Figure 7–10.

Angiogram of intermediate LAD lesion showing locations of pressure measurements.

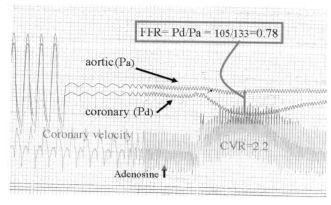

Figure 7–11.

Pressure-derived fractional flow reserve (FFR) is the ratio of distal coronary pressure, (Pd), divided by aortic pressure, (Pa), at maximal hyperemia. In this example, a coronary flow velocity tracing is also provided, which demonstrates that the maximal decline Pd occurs at peak velocity after IC adenosine. FFR = 0.78 while coronary vasodilatory reserve (CVR = CFR) = 2.2, both values above the ischemic threshold. (Courtesy of Dr. B. De Bruyne.)

the coronary flow velocity tracing is also provided beneath the pressure tracings. Within 15 seconds after the administration of adenosine, peak hyperemia is achieved, increasing coronary flow to a maximum of 2.2 times baseline level. The distal coronary pressure decreases along the pressure flow curve to its nadir during peak flow. The ratio of distal coronary pressure to proximal aortic pressure at maximal hyperemia in this example is 105/133, resulting in a calculated fraction flow reserve of 0.78. The FFR represents the percentage of normal flow that would occur through this artery. The normal FFR is 1.

How a Flow Ratio Is Derived from Pressure Measurements

The derivation of fractional flow reserve is presented in Figure 7–12. It is known that normal coronary artery pressure is the same as aortic pressure and is distributed equally along the entire length of a coronary vessel. The resistance to flow is equal to pressure divided by flow. Flow, therefore, is equal to pressure divided by resistance. If one would like the ratio of flow in the target vessel with the stenosis, Qs, to flow in the same vessel in of theoretic normal vessel, Qn, without the stenosis, then the ratio can be computed as shown in Figure 7–12. Because the resistance bed is assumed to be minimal and fixed during hyperemia and it is identical for both the theoretic and target arteries, the resistance term, R, can be canceled leaving the ratio of coronary flow (Qs/Qn) equal to ratio of pressures (Pd/Pa) obtained at maximal hyperemia, a ratio called FFR.

FFR has advantages over coronary flow reserve. As shown in Figure 7–13, coronary flow reserve is altered by changing hemodynamics or shifting the line of maximal hyperemia. FFR on the other hand is not influenced by basal flow and is only the ratio of the measured hyperemic maximal flow to the theoretic maximal hyperemic flow. Thus, hemodynamics, changing heart rate, blood pressure, or contractility do not affect FFR, whereas alterations of these variables are expected to change coronary flow reserve and, thus, complicate the measurement over time and under different clinical circumstances. The reproducibility of FFR and coronary flow reserves can be shown

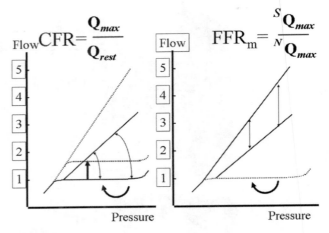

$$CFR = \frac{Q_{max}}{Q_{rest}} \qquad FFR_m = \frac{{}^S Q_{max}}{{}^N Q_{max}}$$

Figure 7–13.

Comparison of features of CFR and FFR. CFR is affected both by changing baseline hemodynamic influences as well as those factors altering the line of maximal hyperemia. FFR is the ratio of hyperemic responses between measured and maximal theoretical and is unaffected by baseline flow status.

in Figure 7–14. Changes in heart rate, blood pressure, and contractility did not significantly affect the FFR in contrast to the CFR (13).

To summarize, coronary flow reserve is the ratio of maximal flow to resting flow in the target vessel measured by Doppler. Relative coronary flow reserve is the ratio of coronary flow reserve in the target vessel to the reference vessel, and fractional flow reserve is the ratio of pressure measured in the distal target artery to aortic pressure at maximal hyperemia. A comparison of the characteristics of the coronary flow reserve, rCVR, and

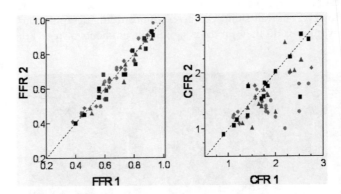

Figure 7–14.

Reproducibility of fractional flow reserve by serial measurements in a multicenter study of 325 patients in whom FFR was measured twice within a 10-minute interval **(left)**. (From: G. Jan Willem Bech, Bernard De Bruyne, Nico H. J. Pijls, et al. Fractional flow reserve to determine the appropriateness of angioplasty in moderate coronary stenosis: A randomized trial. *Circulation*. Jun 2001;103:2928–2934.) Changing heart rate, blood pressure, and contractility with pacing (△) nitroprusside (▼) and dobutamine (●). Despite variations in heart rate of 40%, blood pressure of 35%, and contractility of 50%, FFR was unaffected by these changes **(right)**. (From: De Bruyne B, Bartunek J, Sys SU, et al. Simultaneous coronary pressure and flow velocity measurements in humans: feasibility, reproducibility, and hemodynamic dependence of coronary flow velocity reserve, hyperemic flow versus pressure slope index, and fractional flow reserve. *Circulation*. 1996;94:1842–1849.)

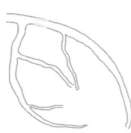

Normal artery pressure, Pa, is the same along the length of the vessel

Resistance=P/Q

Flow, Q=P/R

Qs/Qn = (Pd/Rs)

Pa/Rn

If Rs=Rn, then

Qs/Qn = Pd/Pa

FFR= Qs/Qn = Pd/Pa,

Measured during maximal hyperemia

NHJ Pijls et al. Circulation 1993

Figure 7–12.

Derivation of FFR (see text).

Table 7–1

Comparison of Absolute and Relative CFR and FFR

	Hemodynamic Independence	Independent of Microcirculation Abnormalities	Unequivocal Normal Values	Use in Multivessel CAD	Use for Collateral Measurements
CVR	−	−	Range >2.0	+	+
rCVR	+	+	Range >0.8	−	−
FFR	+	+	1.0	+	+

+, useful; −, not useful.
Reprinted from: Kern MJ. Coronary physiology revisited: Practical insights from the cardiac catheterization laboratory. *Circulation.* 2000;101:1344–1351, with permission.

FFR are displayed in Table 7–1. Hemodynamic independence is attributable to rCVR and FFR. Microvascular independence is also present for FFR and rCVR. Normal values of 1 are present for rCVR and FFR. For CFR, normal values are associated with nonischemic stress testing with CFR >2.0 associated with negative testing. Assessment of lesions in patients with multivessel disease can be made with CFR and FFR, but not relative coronary flow reserve (no reference vessel). Assessment of collateral flow can be obtained using both Doppler flow velocities as well as by distal pressure measurements.

Clinical Associations of FFR and CFR

The physiologic criteria associated with the best clinical outcomes for CFR, rCVR, and FFR are shown in Table 7–2. Studies presenting correlations of physiologic measurements with ischemia stress testing modalities is provided in Table 7–3. A substantial number of studies have reproduced similar endpoints. For coronary flow reserve, the detection of myocardial ischemia using a coronary flow reserve was a value of <2.0. For safely deferring PCI, a CFR >2.0 has excellent outcomes. For a physiologic endpoint regarding balloon angioplasty, CFR >2.5 with an angiographic percent diameter stenosis <35% is associated with a low 2-year restenosis rate. The CFR methodology is no longer used in clinical practice as it is considered obsolete in the era of coronary stenting.

For rCVR, ischemia detection had only a few studies with a wide range of normal values, ranging from 0.65 to 0.80 values make this variable not clinically suitable.

For FFR, nonischemic threshold values are >0.75 to 0.80. As a gray zone, values above 0.80 are associated with negative perfusion stress ischemia and excellent long-term outcomes. An FFR endpoint after angioplasty of >0.90 is associated with stent-like restenosis rates. An FFR endpoint of stenting >0.94 is associated with low major adverse cardiac event rates (6%) over a 2-year period. The higher the FFR after the stenting, the fewer the MACE rates.

The use of FFR to defer or perform coronary intervention for intermediate lesions is associated with good clinical outcomes. PCI performed on intermediate lesions with normal FFR has more events than those that are medically treated. Bech et al. (14) examined the results of FFR on three groups of patients undergoing percutaneous clinical intervention. The first group of patients that had intermediate lesions with normal FFR was treated medically; a 2-year event-free survival rate was 89%. The second group of patients with intermediate lesions with normal FFR underwent PCI anyway. Their 2-year event-free survival rate was approximately 83% (Fig. 7–15). The third group of patients with intermediate lesions had FFR <0.75 and underwent PCI as usually practiced. Their event-free survival rate at the end of 2 years was 78%, a typical value for patients having coronary interventions. From these outcome

Table 7–2

Catheter-based Anatomic and Physiologic Criteria Associated with Clinical Outcomes

Application	IVUS	CVR	rCVR	FFR
Ischemia detection	<3 to 4 mm^2	<2.0	<.08	<0.75
Deferred angioplasty	>4 mm^2	>2.0	—	>0.75
Endpoint of angioplasty	—	>2.0 to 2.5 with <35% DS	—	>0.90
Endpoint of stenting	>9 mm^2 >80% ref area, full apposition	—	—	>0.94

Modified from: Kern MJ. Coronary physiology revisited: Practical insights from the cardiac catheterization laboratory. *Circulation.* 2000;101:1344, with permission.

Table 7–3
Physiologic Measurements and Noninvasive Stress Test Results

Index	Reference	Ref #	N	Ischemic Test	BCV Accuracy	%
FFR	Pijls	16	60	X-ECG	0.74	97
	DeBruyne	20	60	X-ECG/SPECT	0.66	87
	Pijls	18	45	X-ECG/SPECT/pacing/DSE	0.75	93
	Bartunek	79	37	DSE	0.67	90
	Abe	80	46	SPECT	0.75	91
	Chamuleau*	45	127	SPECT	0.74	77
	Caymaz	81	40	SPECT	0.75	95
	Fearon	82	10	SPECT	0.75	95
	DeBruyne#	57	57	SPECT	0.78	85
	Jimenez-Navarro	83	21	DSE	0.75	90
	Meuwissen	23	151	SPECT	0.74	75
	Usui#	84	167	SPECT	0.75	79
	Yanagisawa	85	165	SPECT	0.75	76
CFR	Joye	86	30	SPECT	2.0	94
	Miller	87	33	SPECT	2.0	89
	Deychack	88	17	SPECT	1.8	96
	Tron	89	62	SPECT	2.0	84
	Donohue	90	50	SPECT	2.0	88
	Heller	91	55	SPECT	1.7	92
	Schulman	92	35	X-ECG	2.0	86
	Danzi	93	30	DSE	2.0	87
	Verberne	94	37	SPECT	1.9	85
	Piek	95	225	X-ECG	2.1	76
	Abe	80	46	SPECT	2.0	92
	Chamuleau*	45	127	SPECT	1.7	76
	Duffy	96	28	DSE	2.0	88
	El-Shafei	14	48	SPECT	1.9	77
	Meuwissen	23	151	SPECT	1.7	75
	Voudris	97	48	SPECT	1.7	75
rCFR	Verberne	94	37	SPECT	0.65	85
	Chamuleau*	45	127	SPECT	0.60	78
	Duffy	96	28	DSE	0.75	81
	El-Shafei	14	48	SPECT	0.75	75
	Voudris	97	48	SPECT	0.64	92
H-SRv	Meuwissen	23	151	SPECT	0.80	87

From: Kern MJ. Coronary physiology revisited: Practical insights from the cardiac catheterization laboratory. *Circulation.* 2000;101:1344–1351, with permission. N, number; BVC, best cut-off value (defined as the value with the highest sum of sensitivity and specificity); SPECT, single photon emission tomography; DSE, dobutamine stress echocardiography; X-ECG, exercise ECG; *, multivessel disease, #, myocardial infarction.

data, performing PCI on FFR normal lesions did not improve the patient's late outcome. In fact, this approach increased the adverse event rates related to the procedure as compared to those continuing medical therapy.

Fractional flow reserve after stenting does not indicate whether the stent is successfully implanted and fully apposed to the vessel wall. This issue is an anatomic diagnosis requiring an anatomic tool like IVUS. However, although FFR does not indicate if the stent is apposed to the wall, it does provide long-term prognostic data. Pijls et al. (15) examined outcomes in 750 patients with corresponding FFR measurements after stenting. The adverse event rates at 6 and 12 months were correlated to decreasing FFR (Fig. 7–16). Of the 206 patients with FFR of 0.96 to 1.0 after stenting, the adverse event rate

was 5%. The adverse event rate increased as FFR decreased. For the patients with an FFR of 0.86 to 0.90, the event rate was 16%; for the 44 patients who had an FFR of 0.76 to 0.80, the event rate was higher at 30%. These data likely indicate that the patients with lowest residual FFR after stenting still have residual plaque elsewhere in the artery and, thus, are prone to more complications and major adverse events after stenting.

Diffuse and Focal Coronary Artery Disease

FFR can also differentiate diffuse coronary artery disease from focal narrowings (16). A patient with a proximal left anterior

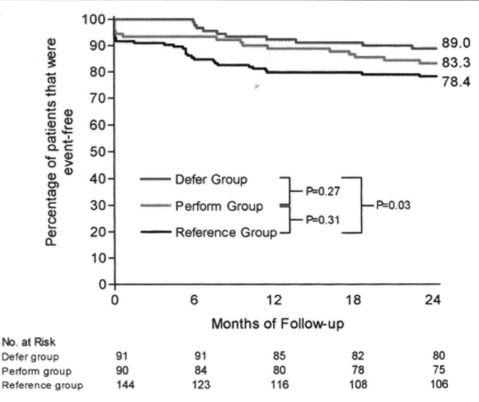

No. at Risk					
Defer group	91	91	85	82	80
Perform group	90	84	80	78	75
Reference group	144	123	116	108	106

Figure 7–15.

Fractional flow reserved guided angioplasty results. (From: Bech GJW, De Bruyne B, Pijls NHJ, et al. Fractional flow reserve to determine the appropriateness of angioplasty in moderate coronary stenosis: A randomized trial. *Circulation.* 2001;103:2928–2934, with permission.)

descending stenosis undergoing coronary artery stenting would be one example of how FFR can be used (Fig. 7–17). After stent placement, FFR immediately distal to the stent demon-

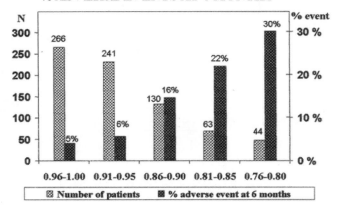

Figure 7–16.

Clinical outcome of stenting and relationship to FFR. A strong inverse correlation was present between FFR after stenting and event rate at 6-month follow-up. Distribution of percentage residual stenosis in the five FFR categories with very similar minimal luminal diameter (MLD) in the five FFR categories **(middle)**. (Reproduced from: Pijls NHJ, Klauss V, Siebert U, et al. Coronary pressure measurement after stenting predicts adverse events at follow-up. A multicenter registry. *Circulation.* 2002;105:2950–2954, with permission.)

strates a satisfactory value of 0.95 (Fig. 7–18), whereas more distally, FFR was 0.41. The reason for this marked disparity between locations is the presence of diffuse disease, which can be verified by pressure pullback (Fig. 7–19). As shown, the most distal pressure gradient is to the summed resistance of the diffuse accumulation of atherosclerotic material throughout the length of vessel. There is no focal or regional location where pressure is suddenly lost. Mechanical therapy by PCI for this vessel would be unsuitable and continued medical therapy can be recommended. De Bruyne et al. (17) compared FFR in patient arteries that were angiographically normal to those with unobstructed arteries in patients who had significant disease in another artery (Fig. 7–20). Those patients with atherosclerotic arteries had a wide range of FFR values from 0.70 up to 1.0, whereas patients with complete normal arteries and no evidence of atherosclerosis all had FFR greater than 0.92. The low FFR in some patients with diffusely diseased arteries may explain why many of these patients have persistent chest discomfort or positive ischemic testing despite having no epicardial lesions that can be treated by PCI.

Coronary Physiology for Acute Myocardial Infarction

In patients having acute myocardial infarction, coronary physiology cannot be utilized because of the dynamic condition in

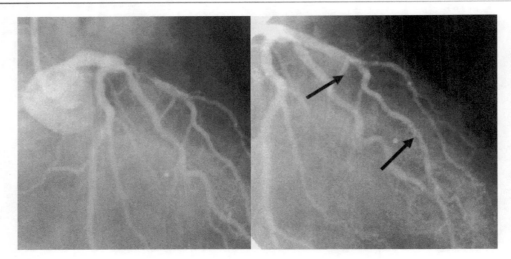

Figure 7–17.
Angiographically severe left anterior descending coronary stenosis with diffusely narrowed distal vessel (*left panel*). Resting P_d to P_a ratio, FFR of <0.4.

which changes of the vessel, the active coronary lesion, and the myocardial bed are occurring simultaneously. Measurements on the first day of the event may not necessarily reflect those findings on day 5 or 6. However, in patients having had a myocardial infarction and are studied more than 6 days after the event, the use of FFR can identify those patients with positive or negative SPECT Sestamibi myocardial perfusion scanning. De Bruyne et al. (17) examined 57 patients after myocardial infarction. The study occurred from 6 days to 3 months after the myocardial infarction. The investigators found an 85%

concordance with FFR and SPECT scanning (Fig. 7–21). For investigators wishing to examine acute myocardial infarction physiology, the use of coronary flow velocity in the acute setting has been studied by Kawamoto et al. (18) (Fig. 7–22). The phasic patterns of coronary flow velocity indicated that a marked diastolic deceleration time and systolic flow reversal were associated with nonviable myocardium as compared to the patients with a normal phasic flow velocity (gradual diastolic deceleration and antegrade systolic flow) who had evidence of myocardial viability.

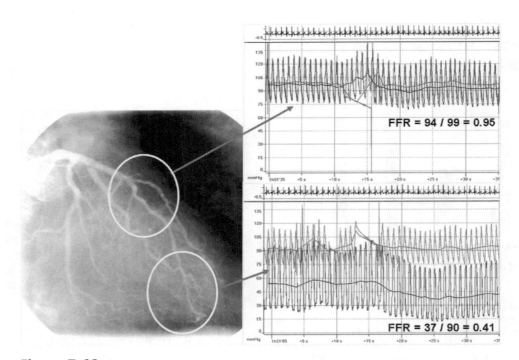

Figure 7–18.
Left anterior descending coronary artery after stenting. Measurements of FFR distal to the stent are 0.95 and in the distal LAD is 0.41 (*right panel*).

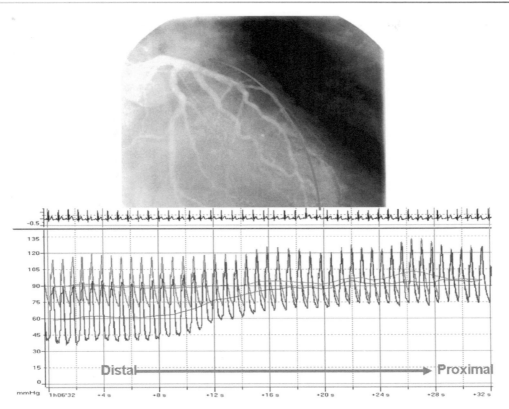

Figure 7–19.

Continuous hyperemic pressure pullback from the distal to proximal regions demonstrates a gradual pressure recovery consistent with diffuse coronary artery disease as the explanation for persistently abnormal distal FFR. (Courtesy of Dr. B. De Bruyne.)

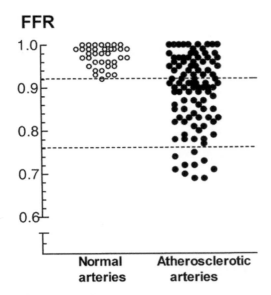

Figure 7–20.

Graphs of individual values of FFR in normal arteries and in atherosclerotic coronary arteries without focal stenosis on arteriogram. The *upper dotted line* indicates the lowest value of FFR in normal coronary arteries. The *lower dotted line* indicates the 0.75 threshold level. (Reproduced from: De Bruyne B, Hersbach F, Pijls NHJ, et al. Abnormal epicardial coronary resistance in patients with diffuse atherosclerosis but "normal" coronary angiography. *Circulation.* 2001;104:2401–2406, with permission.)

Differentiation of IVUS versus Physiology

Intravascular ultrasound imaging measures vessel dimension, the extent of the plaque segment, characteristics of the plaque segment, full apposition of the stenting, and complications of the percutaneous coronary intervention, such as thrombus or dissection. FFR, on the other hand, measures only myocardial flow at the epicardial level and determines whether the physiologic significance of the lesion is optimal. If the most relevant measurement at the current time is whether the physiologic characteristics of the lesion are ischemia producing or not, FFR provides the ability to optimize the opportunities for necessary complete coronary revascularization.

Collateral Circulation

One of the greatest areas of new information provided by the sensor guidewire techniques has been the appreciation of collateral function and physiology (19–21). The collateral circulation can be described by intracoronary pressure and flow relationships. Ipsilateral collateral flow and contralateral arterial responses have been described in numerous studies using both pressure and flow to provide new information regarding mechanisms, function, and the clinical significance of collateral flow in patients, as well as provide new insights into coronary artery disease. For example, Seiler et al. (19) examined

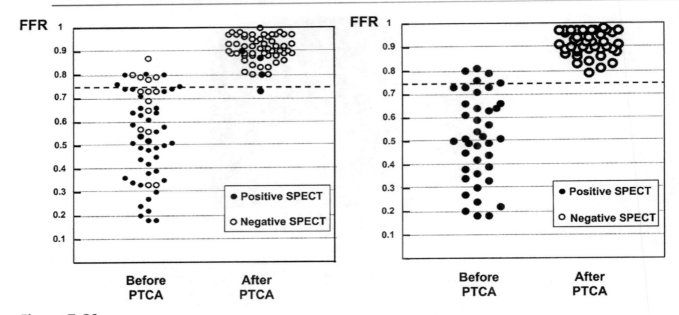

Figure 7–21.

Values of FFR before and after PCI according to results of Sestamibi SPECT myocardial perfusion imaging in patient population as a whole **(top)** and in patients with truly positive and truly negative SPECT imaging **(bottom)**. (From: De Bruyne B, Pijls NHJ, Bartunek J, et al. Fractional flow reserve in patients with prior myocardial infarction. *Circulation.* 2001;104:157–162, with permission.)

coronary pressure and flow in 51 patients with coronary artery stenosis treated by PTCA. Simultaneous measurements were used to calculate collateral flow indices using velocity or pressure. Both CFI$_v$ and CFI$_p$ were compared with conventional methods for collateral assessment using ST segment elevation greater than 1 mm on IC or surface electrocardiogram during coronary occlusion with balloon angioplasty. In 11 patients without ECG signs of ischemia during coronary occlusion, relative collateral flow amounted to 46% (0.46) as determined by pressure flow indices. Patients with insufficient collaterals, (n = 40), had relative coronary flow values of 18% (0.18). Using a CFI of 0.30, sufficient and insufficient collaterals could be diagnosed with 100% sensitivity and 93% specificity by IC Doppler, and 75% sensitivity and 92% specificity by IC pressure measurements. Intracoronary flow velocity or pressure measurements during routine coronary occlusion represent an accurate and at least quantitative method for assessing the collateral coronary artery circulation in man.

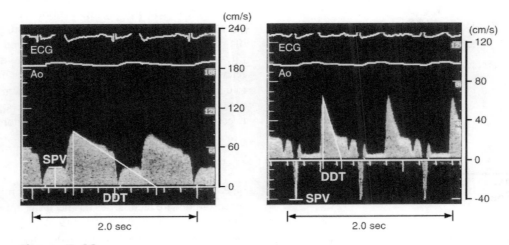

Figure 7–22.

Phasic flow velocity signals in patients with acute myocardial infarction demonstrating diastolic deceleration time (DDT) and systolic flow reversal (SPV). Rapid DDT and the presence of SPV are associated with poor myocardial functional recovery after infarction. (From: Kawamoto T, Yoshida K, Akasaka T, Hozumi T, Takagi T, Kaji S, Ueda Y. Can coronary blood flow velocity pattern after primary percutaneous transluminal coronary angiography predict recovery of regional left ventricular function in patients with acute myocardial infarction? *Circulation.* 1999;100:339–345, with permission.)

Key Points for FFR and CFR

1. Anatomy does not equal physiology. Intermediate lesion may or may not be flow limiting.

2. Stenoses produce resistance-limiting flow distally limiting distal hyperemic flow.

3. Adenosine intravenously at a dosage of 140 mcg/kg/minute or intracoronary 20/30 for the right coronary artery and 40 to 60 mcg for the left coronary artery stimulates maximal hyperemia that produces minimal resistance of the microvascular bed.

4. Coronary flow reserve measures both conduits (i.e., the stenosis and the microvascular bed flow). Normal or nonischemic values for CFR are those greater than 2.0.

5. Relative coronary flow reserve normalizes for abnormal microvascular flow, nonischemic values greater than 0.65 to 0.80.

6. Stenosis resistance produces energy loss that results in distal pressure loss.

7. FFR, that is, pressure distal to pressure proximal during hypermedia, is independent of microvascular flow and is specific for stenosis resistance, nonischemic values of greater than 0.75.

8. FFR does not identify lesions which benefit from treatment but does not address adequacy of stent implantation. This is an anatomic diagnosis.

REFERENCES

1. Kern MJ. Coronary physiology revisited: Practical insights from the cardiac catheterization laboratory. *Circulation.* 2000;101:1344–1351.

2. Topol EJ, Nissen SE. Our preoccupation with coronary luminology. The dissociation between clinical and angiographic findings in ischemic heart disease. *Circulation.* 1995;92:2333–2342.

3. Gould KL, Lipscomb K, Hamilton GW. Physiologic basis for assessing critical coronary stenosis: instantaneous flow response and regional distribution during coronary hyperemia as measures of coronary flow reserve. *Am J Cardiol.* 1974;33:87–94.

4. Gould KL, Kirkeeide RL, Buchi M. Coronary flow reserve as a physiologic measure of stenosis severity. *J Am Coll Cardiol.* 1990;15:459–474.

5. Baumgart D, Haude M, Liu F, et al. Current concepts of coronary flow reserve for clinical decision making during cardiac catheterization. *Am Heart J.* 1998;136:136–149.

6. Kern MJ, Bach RG, Mechem C, et al. Variations in normal coronary vasodilatory reserve stratified by artery, gender, heart transplantation and coronary artery disease. *J Am Coll Cardiol.* 1996;28:1154–1160.

7. McGinn AL, White CW, Wilson RF. Interstudy variability of coronary flow reserve: influence of heart rate, arterial pressure, and ventricular preload. *Circulation.* 1990;81:1319–1330.

8. Wieneke H, Haude M, Ge J, et al. Corrected coronary flow velocity reserve: a new concept for assessing coronary perfusion. *J Am Coll Cardiol.* 2000;35:1713–1720.

9. Baumgart D, Haude M, Goerge G, et al. Improved assessment of coronary stenosis severity using the relative flow velocity reserve. *Circulation.* 1998;98:40–46.

10. Kern MJ, Puri S, Bach RG, et al. Abnormal coronary flow velocity reserve after coronary artery stenting in patients: role of relative coronary reserve to assess potential mechanisms. *Circulation.* 1999;100:2491–2498.

11. Pijls NH, Van Gelder B, Van der Voort P, et al. Fractional flow reserve: a useful index to evaluate the influence of an epicardial coronary stenosis on myocardial blood flow. *Circulation.* 1995;92:3183–3193.

12. Pijls NH, De Bruyne B, Peels K, et al. Measurement of fractional flow reserve to assess the functional severity of coronary-artery stenoses. *N Engl J Med.* 1996;334:1703–1708.

13. De Bruyne B, Bartunek J, Sys SU, et al. Simultaneous coronary pressure and flow velocity measurements in humans: feasibility, reproducibility, and hemodynamic dependence of coronary flow velocity reserve, hyperemic flow versus pressure slope index, and fractional flow reserve. *Circulation.* 1996;94:1842–1849.

14. Bech GJW, De Bruyne B, Pijls NHJ, et al. Fractional flow reserve to determine the appropriateness of angioplasty in moderate coronary stenosis: a randomized trial. *Circulation.* 2001;103:2928–2934.

15. Pijls NHJ, Klauss V, Siebert U, et al. Coronary pressure measurement after stenting predicts adverse events at follow-up. A multicenter registry. *Circulation.* 2002;105:2950–2954.

16. Kern MJ. Focus for the new millennium: diffuse coronary artery disease and physiologic measurements of severity. *Am Coll Cardiol Curr J Rev.* 2000:13–19.

17. De Bruyne B, Pijls NHJ, Bartunek J, et al. Fractional flow reserve in patients with prior myocardial infarction. *Circulation.* 2001;104:157–162.

18. Kawamoto T, Yoshida K, Akasaka T, et al. Can coronary blood flow velocity pattern after primary percutaneous transluminal coronary angioplasty predict recovery of regional left ventricular function in patients with acute myocardial infarction? *Circulation.* 1999;100:339–345.

19. Seiler C, Fleisch M, Billinger M, et al. Simultaneous intracoronary velocity- and pressure-derived assessment of adenosine-induced collateral hemodynamics in patients with one- to two-vessel coronary artery disease. *J Am Coll Cardiol.* 1999;34:1985–1994.

20. Pijls NHJ, Bech GJW, elGamal MIH, et al. Quantification of recruitable coronary collateral blood flow in conscious humans and its potential to predict future ischemic events. *J Am Coll Cardiol.* 1995;25:1522–1528.

21. Piek JJ, van Liebergen RAM, Koch KT, et al. Clinical, angiographic and hemodynamic predictors of recruitable collateral flow assessed during balloon angioplasty coronary occlusion. *J Am Coll Cardiol.* 1997;29:275–282.

CHAPTER 8

Cardiac Hemodynamics for the Interventional Cardiologist

Morton J. Kern

Cardiac hemodynamics are important to the interventional cardiologist in the performance of basic and complex cardiac and noncardiac interventions. An understanding of the clinical problems and related hemodynamic presentations will assist the interventionalist in determining the best treatment options for resuscitation and survival.

There are two major hemodynamic problems that present during coronary interventions: hypotension and hypertension. Table 8–1 lists the most common causes of hypotension during coronary percutaneous interventions, which include volume loss, anaphylaxis, cardiac tamponade, arrhythmia, new valvular lesions, and shock, either hypovolemic and/or cardiogenic. Artifactual causes of hypotension due to errors in pressure measurement should be considered.

Hypertension is uncommon during coronary interventions, but may be due to labile hypertension previously untreated or related to medication delay or hypertension due to overzealous vasopressor support, a recognizable condition that is easily treated.

Other common diagnostic dilemmas that present for both coronary and noncardiac interventions are listed in Table 8–2. These include coronary hemodynamic lesion assessment, hypertrophic obstructive cardiomyopathy, mitral valve disease, mitral stenosis, diastolic cardiac dysfunction, constrictive and restrictive pathophysiology, intracardiac shunting, low gradient aortic stenosis, and prosthetic valve dysfunction. The hemodynamics of each of these conditions are pertinent to the intervention performed for both the diagnostic results and recognition of complications.

Hypotension during Coronary Intervention

Simultaneous measurement of femoral artery and left ventricular pressure provides information for the diagnosis of the majority of the typical cause of hypotension in the cath lab. Figure 8–1 shows simultaneous aortic and left ventricular pressure using high fidelity catheters (from 0 to 200 mm Hg scale). Within several minutes of this recording, after ventriculography is performed, hypotension is identified. The operator was observing left ventricular pressure at the time aortic pressure had fallen significantly. Note that left ventricular end diastolic pressure (Fig. 8–2) is not elevated. There is no left ventricular outflow tract obstruction manifested by a gradient between the aortic and left ventricular pressure. The correct diagnosis is an anaphylactic reaction with vasodepressor response, and the treatment for this episode of hypotension is immediate volume replacement and epinephrine for presumed anaphylactic reaction. Figure 8–3 shows the rapid change of pressure from normal to hypotensive in the setting of contrast administration demonstrating the immediate nature of this anaphylactoid reaction rather than another cause of hypotension.

In the setting of coronary interventions, the possibility of arterial perforation should be considered. Hypotension following arterial manipulation should raise the suspicion of pericardial tamponade as a cause of systemic hypotension. Examine the arterial and right atrial pressure tracings obtained during a rotablator atherectomy of the right coronary artery (Fig. 8–4) in a 53-year-old man. Note the distinct cyclical nature of the arterial pulse wave corresponding to respiration (0 to 200 mm Hg scale). The femoral artery pressure ranges from 180/120 to 120/90 mm Hg, and then on subsequent inspiration, a loss of arterial pressure transmission can be identified on the right side of tracing (Figure 8–4b) showing group beating with marked pulsus paradoxus. On further examination of the right atrial and arterial pressure simultaneously (Fig. 8–4a), it can be seen that the right atrial pressure is markedly elevated with a mean of approximately 35 mm Hg and loss of the phasic pressure waveforms. The right atrial pressure changes markedly over the inspiratory cycle with the tachypneic effort of the patient. A blunted pressure waveform and equalization of diastolic pressure across the heart (Fig. 8–5) shown by the pulmonary artery and right ventricular pressures (0 to 100 mm Hg pressure scale) emphasize the loss of phasic components and elevated diastolic pressures. The mean pulmonary capillary wedge pressure is equal to right atrial pressure of approximately 38 mm Hg. Because of these hemodynamics and the high suspicion of cardiac tamponade, echocardiography was performed demonstrating significant fluid accumulation. Pericardiocentesis was then performed. Simultaneous right

Table 8–1

Common Hemodynamic Problems in Coronary Interventions

1. Hypotension:
   a. Volume loss
   b. Anaphylaxis
   c. Tamponade
   d. Arrhythmia
   e. New valvular lesion
   f. Shock
   g. Pressure miscalibration
2. Hypertension

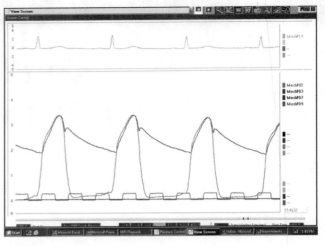

Figure 8–1.

Left ventricular and aortic pressure measured with high fidelity catheter 0 to 200 mm Hg scale.

atrial and pericardial pressures were measured before and after pericardiocentesis (Figs. 8–6 and 8–7). Pericardiocentesis reduced the right atrial pressure from 40 to 20 mm Hg and the pericardial pressure fell to approximately 40 mm Hg. The arterial pressure waveform normalized. Hypotension was eliminated and phasic waveforms of the right heart pressure tracings could be again demonstrated (Fig. 8–8).

Intraventricular Pressure Gradients

The measurement of left ventricular–aortic pressure to gauge supravalvular, valvular, or subvalvular pressure gradients commonly employs a pigtail catheter and femoral artery pressure measured from the sidearm of the femoral artery sheath. The two measurements are critical to the accurate determination of valvular or intraventricular obstruction. Close attention to the waveforms is needed for accurate diagnosis. Simultaneous left ventricular and femoral artery pressure can demonstrate this relationship (Fig. 8–9, 0 to 200 mm Hg scale). In panel A of Figure 8–9, aortic stenosis is shown with a 60 mm Hg

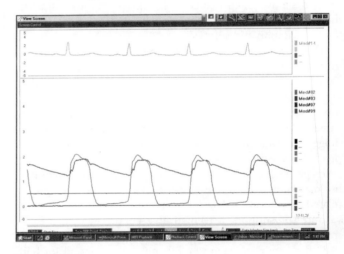

Figure 8–2.

Left ventricular and aortic pressure measured with high fidelity catheter 0 to 200 mm Hg scale. Immediately after contrast injection.

Table 8–2

Common Diagnostic Hemodynamics Problems in Coronary and Noncardiac/ Noncoronary interventions

1. Valvular Heart Disease
   a. Aortic stenosis/insufficiency
   b. Mitral stenosis/insufficiency
   c. Tricuspid/pulmonary stenosis/insufficiency
   d. Prosthetic valve dysfunction
2. Hypertrophic Cardiomyopathy
3. Coronary Hemodynamic Lesion Assessment
4. Congestive Heart Failure
   a. Diastolic dysfunction
   b. Constrictive pericardial disease
   c. Restrictive cardiomyopathy
5. Pulmonary Hypertension

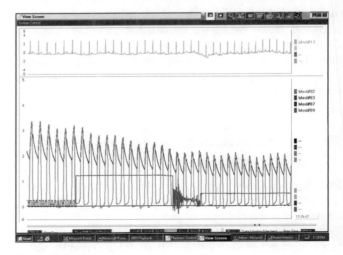

Figure 8–3.

Continuous recording of left ventricular and aortic pressure after contrast administration.

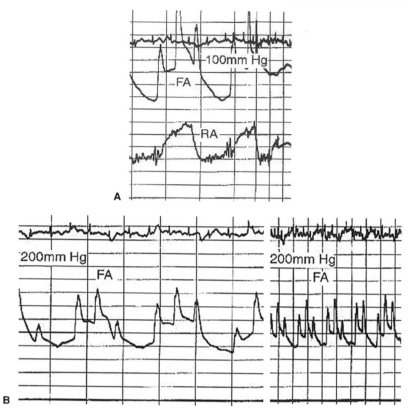

Figure 8–4.

A: Aortic and right pressure on 0 to 100 mm Hg scale. FA, femoral artery; RA, right atrial pressure. **B:** 0–200 mm Hg scale, 25 mm/sec paper speed, (right pane shows 10 mm/sec recording speed).

peak-to-peak LV-Ao pressure difference. In panel B, this left ventricular–aortic pressure gradient is markedly diminished. Is this an indication of severe aortic stenosis? On closer examination of panel B, it can be noted there is no change in the aortic pressure or diastolic pressure, but there is marked re-duction in left ventricular systolic pressure with an abnormal left ventricular diastolic pressure waveform. The highest left ventricular diastolic pressure occurs at the earliest point in the diastolic as opposed to a normal left ventricular diastolic pressure configuration with the earliest diastolic pressure being the lowest or nadir. This left ventricular diastolic pressure wave-form continues to decline across diastole, a finding that has been reported to occur in patients with marked left ventricular

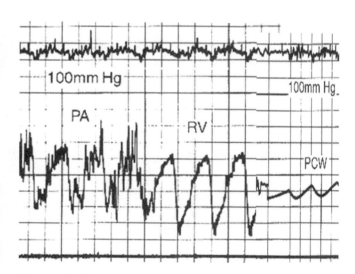

Figure 8–5.
Pulmonary artery (PA), right ventricular pressure (RV) on 0 to 100 mm Hg scale. PCW, pulmonary capillary wedge pressure.

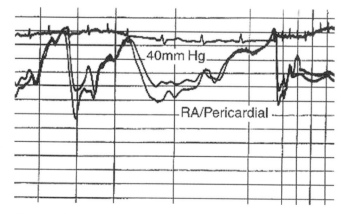

Figure 8–6.
Right atrial and pericardial pressures before pericardiocentesis on 0 to 40 mm Hg scale.

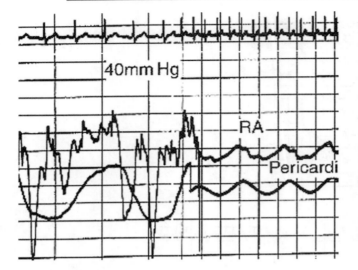

Figure 8–7.

Right atrial and pericardial pressures after pericardiocentesis on 0 to 40 mm Hg scale.

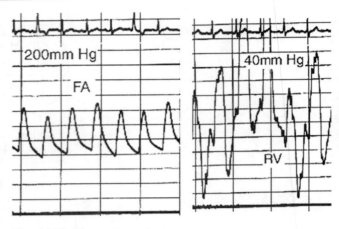

Figure 8–8.

Femoral artery and right ventricular pressure. FA, femoral artery; RV, right ventricular pressure on 0 to 200 mm Hg scale and 0 to 40 mm Hg scale, respectively.

diastolic dysfunction. It is also the result of a measurement artifact with one or more side holes of the catheter shaft being across the aortic valve with the remaining two side holes underneath the aortic valve. This artifact of catheter placement is easily detected by slight repositioning of the catheter and reacquisition of the pressure tracings (Fig. 8–9).

Another example of changing left ventricular–aortic pressure gradient appearing and disappearing is seen in Figure 8–10. The marked left ventricular–aortic gradient following a premature ventricular beat is associated with reduction of arterial pulse pressure on the following beat. In addition, the arterial waveform demonstrates an early systolic peak (a spike) with a delay in relaxation and dome-like configuration of arterial pressure waveform. Given these findings of the post-PVC pulse pressure and left ventricular–aortic gradient, the diagnosis of obstructive cardiomyopathy is evident. The reduction in pulse pressure in the post-PVC beat with the largest left ventricular–aortic gradient is known as the Brockenbrough-Braunwald-Morrow sign, hallmark of hypertrophic obstructive cardiomyopathy. In distinction to the hemodynamics of aortic

stenosis, the pulse pressure is not diminished or even increased in the post-PVC beat with an obstructive valvular lesion. Note that in this individual (as compared to Figure 8–9, Panel B), the diastolic pressure waveform is elevated both in early diastole and late diastole and increases across the diastolic. This individual with hypertrophic obstructive cardiomyopathy then undergoes a therapeutic procedure (Fig. 8–11) eliminating the gradient between the left ventricle and aorta (left side of Fig. 8–11). The spike and dome-like configuration of the aortic pressure wave is somewhat reduced and the left ventricular diastolic function is unchanged. This hemodynamic result follows treatment with transluminal alcohol septal ablation for hypertrophic cardiomyopathy (TASH). TASH resulted in a complete abolition of the LVOT gradient without induction of electrical heart block. First-degree block or bundle branch block commonly occurs in some individuals during TASH.

Mitral Valve Hemodynamics

Mitral valve disease requires the simultaneous assessment of left atrial and left ventricular pressures. In majority of cases, a

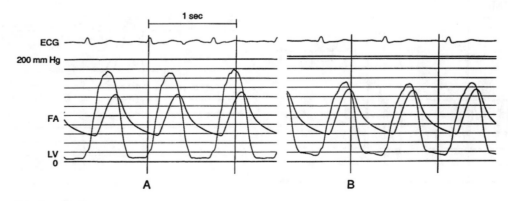

Figure 8–9.

Left ventricular and aortic pressure in patients with aortic stenosis on 0 to 200 mm Hg scale. **A:** before maneuver. **B:** after maneuver.

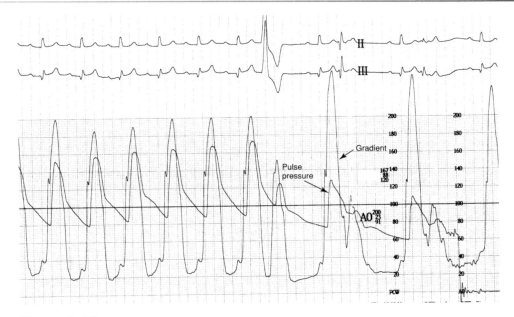

Figure 8–10.

Left ventricular and aortic pressure on 0 to 200 mm Hg scale. PP, pulse pressure. This is an example of Hypertrophic Obstructive Cardiomyopathy.

pulmonary capillary wedge pressure is used to represent the left atrial pressure. A normal pulmonary capillary wedge and left ventricular pressure tracing are shown in Figure 8–12. The pulmonary capillary wedge pressure tracing is delayed in time (100 to 140 msec) due to the transient through the lungs before the pressure is acquired in the catheter and transmitted

to the transducer. A small A wave (A′) can be seen following the A wave of the left ventricle (*first large arrow*) and the V wave is identified thereafter with its peak occurring at or after downsloping of the left ventricular pressure (*second large arrow*). In many clinical settings, these pressure waveforms are often damped or obscured using a pulmonary capillary

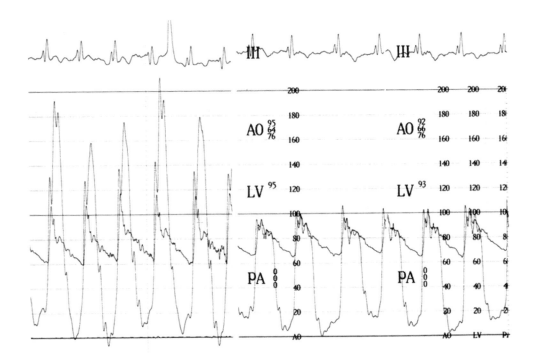

Figure 8–11.

Left ventricular and aortic pressure before (*left panel*) and after Alcohol septal ablation for hypertrophic cardiomyopathy (TASH) (*right panel*), 0 to 200 mm Hg scale.

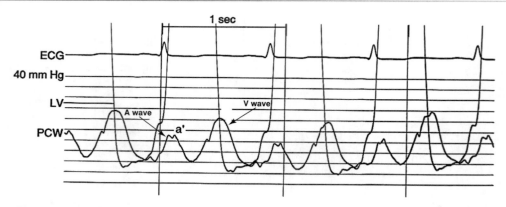

Figure 8–12.

Normal pulmonary capillary wedge pressure (PCW) and left ventricular pressure on 0 to 40 mm Hg scale.

wedge catheter. Overcoming the poor-quality tracing presents a technical challenge due to both artifact and compliance of the pulmonary circuit. A comparison of pulmonary capillary wedge and direct left atrial pressure measurements in a patient with mitral stenosis is shown on Figure 8–13. A marked V wave of the left atrium can be seen easily in the left atrial pressure waveform but not appreciated as well in the pulmonary capillary wedge pressure tracing (*left panel*). A mean pressure data acquired with both catheters is similar, differing only by 1 mm Hg (*right side of panel*). The mitral valve area is only slightly greater with direct left atrial pressure measurement (1.7 versus 1.9 cm^2). In some cases, the pulmonary capillary wedge pressure may not be useful to determine mitral valve gradients. For example, a 49-year-old woman with a diastolic murmur of mitral stenosis undergoes cardiac catheterization, the pulmonary capillary wedge and left ventricular pressures are simultaneously recorded on Figure 8–14. The pulmonary capillary wedge pressure is damped without good phasic pressure waveforms. This tracing makes it nearly impossible to assess a true mitral gradient. The direct left atrial pressure

measurement via trans-septal technique as compared to PCW is shown on Figure 8–15 and demonstrates that although the mean pressure tracings are identical, the phasic waveforms are distinctly different. The pulmonary capillary wedge pressure cannot be used to assess the mitral gradient in this individual. The left atrial pressure is matched against left ventricular pressure on Figure 8–16. It is quite easy to appreciate the mitral gradient with prominent A and large V waves. Note the position of the V wave occurring at or inside the down stroke of the left ventricular pressure, an indicator that this waveform is left atrial rather than pulmonary capillary wedge pressure. A mitral balloon valvuloplasty was performed using the In-oue technique (Fig. 8–17). The pulmonary capillary wedge pressure and left ventricular pressures were again remeasured (Fig 8–18). Given the poor quality of the initial pulmonary capillary wedge pressure, it is difficult for the operator to accept the residual gradient shown by the PCW. Although this mitral gradient is small, the operator might be tempted to proceed further with a larger valvuloplasty balloon. Fortunately, direct left atrial pressure was measured and matched against

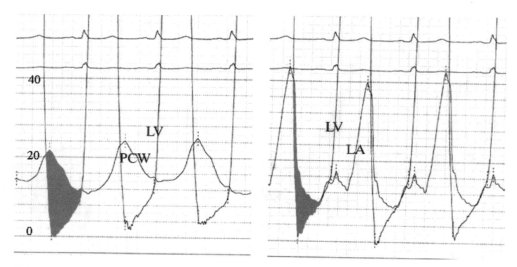

Figure 8–13.

Pulmonary capillary wedge pressure and left atrial pressure measured against left ventricular pressure. *Left-sided panel* is pulmonary capillary wedge pressure. *Right-sided panel* is left atrial pressure. Courtesy of Ted Feldman, MD.

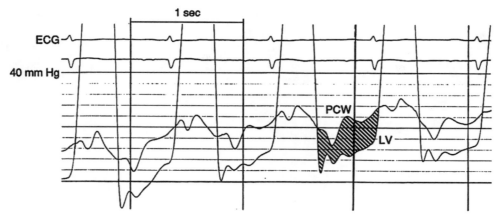

Figure 8–14.

Pulmonary capillary wedge and left ventricular pressure in patient with mitral stenosis, 0 to 40 mm Hg scale.

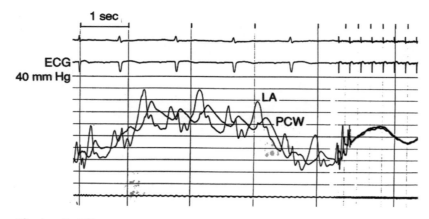

Figure 8–15.

Left atrial and pulmonary capillary wedge pressure, 0 to 40 mm Hg scale.

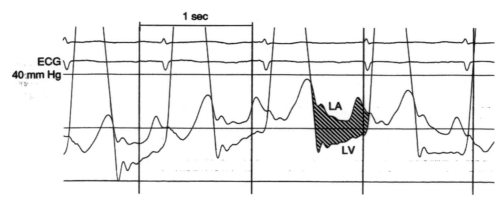

Figure 8–16.

Left atrial and left ventricular pressure, 0 to 40 mm Hg scale.

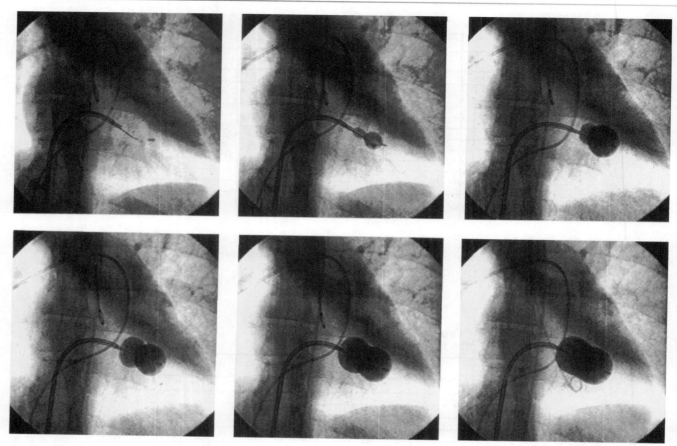

Figure 8–17.

Cineangiographic frames of the Inoue mitral balloon valvuloplasty procedure.

left ventricular pressure for the determination of the true mitral gradient (Fig. 8–19). Direct left atrial pressure corresponds to left ventricular diastolic pressure and no mitral gradient is evident. The V wave is small. The A wave is absent with the A wave matching the left ventricle in this tracing. The mitral valvuloplasty procedure is successful and completed at this point.

In other patients undergoing mitral balloon valvuloplasty, examination of the postprocedure left atrial pressure may re-

veal another endpoint has occurred. Hemodynamic tracings obtained after 28 mm Hg Inoue valvuloplasty balloon to treat a mitral valve stenosis with an echo score of 10 is shown on Figures 8–20 and 8–21. Simultaneous left atrial and ventricular pressures demonstrate a large V wave. The large V wave is twice the mean left atrial pressure and characterizes severe mitral regurgitation. The peak of the V wave occurs at the down stroke of the left ventricular pressure and corresponds closely to left ventricular diastolic pressure across the entire diastolic. There

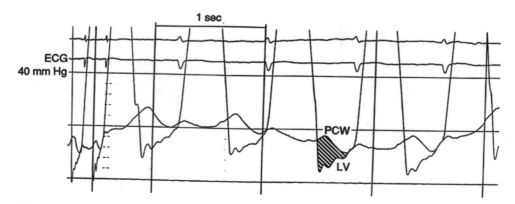

Figure 8–18.

Pulmonary capillary wedge and left ventricular pressures after mitral balloon valvuloplasty, 0 to 40 mm Hg scale.

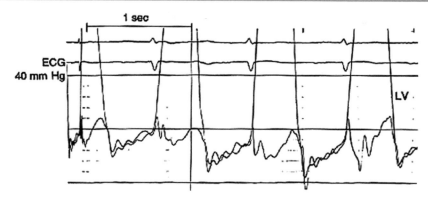

Figure 8–19.

Left atrial and left ventricular pressure on 0 to 40 mm Hg scale, postvalvuloplasty.

is no obstructive component to mitral flow consistent with severe mitral regurgitation. Other causes of large or prominent V waves are ventricular septal defects, pulmonary-aortic window, high systemic flow, or low compliant atrial conditions.

Another patient undergoing hemodynamic assessment for mitral stenosis has measurements of left atrial and left ventricular pressure obtained (Fig. 8–22, *left panel*). A usual late diastolic gradient is evident between the left atrium and left ventricular pressure. This later-appearing gradient can be eliminated by slight movement of the catheter on withdrawal from its position (Fig. 8–22, *right panel*). The positional demonstration of the late gradient within the atrium occurring only at the A wave is not characteristic mitral stenosis, but rather left atrial appendage hemodynamics and may be used to identify the correct positioning in the left atrial appendage for occluding device placement should such a procedure become routine. Demonstration of left atrial appendage hemodynamics is un-

usual and uncommon, but should not be mistaken for mitral stenosis.

Diastolic Cardiac Dysfunction

A 49-year-old woman comes to the emergency room with congestive heart failure and a small heart. The patient responds initially to diuretics. An echocardiogram reveals normal systolic function with a question of diastolic dysfunction. Left and right heart hemodynamics are obtained (Fig. 8–23). The simultaneous left and right ventricular pressure tracings show an abrupt cessation of early diastolic pressure (dip) with a plateau and matching the LV/RV diastolic pressure waveforms. These hemodynamic data are consistent with constrictive cardiac physiology. The most important differentiating factor between constrictive and restrictive cardiac physiology is the dynamic respiratory variation of left and right ventricular

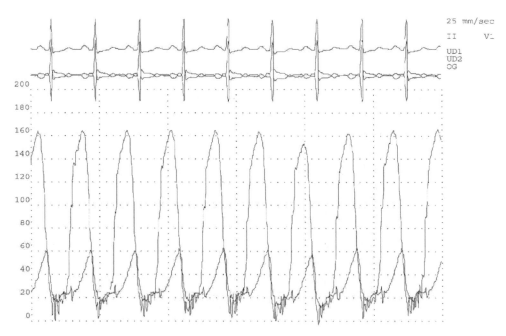

Figure 8–20.

Left atrial and left ventricular pressures on 0 to 40 mm Hg scale.

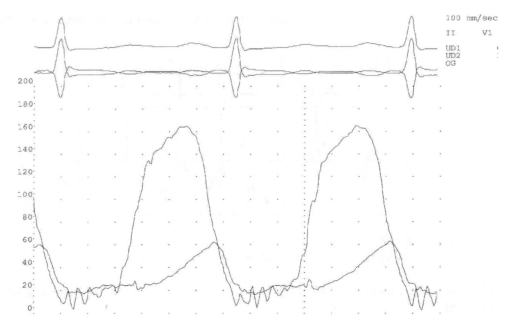

Figure 8–21.

Left ventricular and left atrial pressure on 0 to 200 mm Hg scale at 100 mm paper speed.

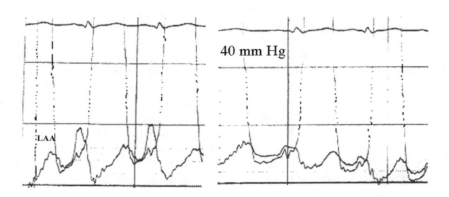

Figure 8–22.

Left atrial and left ventricular pressure. Left panel shows left atrial appendage (LAA) and right panel shows left atrial pressure against left ventricular pressure on 0 to 40 mm Hg scale.

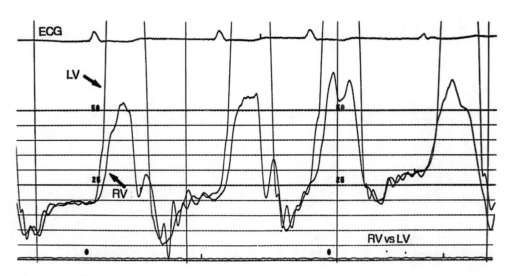

Figure 8–23.

Simultaneous LV and RV pressures on 0 to 40 mm Hg scale.

Table 8–3

Comparison of Traditional and Dynamic Respiratory Criteria for Diagnostic Constrictive Pericarditis

	Criteria	Sensitivity	Specificity	PPV	NPV
Traditional:	LVEDP versus RVEDP <5	60	38	4	57
	RVEDP versus RVSP >1/3	93	38	52	89
	PASP <55	93	24	47	25
	Right ventricular free wall >7 mm	93	57	61	92
	Respiratory: Change of right atrial pressure <3 mm Hg	93	48	58	92
Dynamic Respiratory Factors:	Pulmonary capillary wedge versus LV >5 mm Hg	93	81	78	94
	LV/RV interdependence	100	95	94	100

systolic pressures, also known as ventricular interdependence. In a study by Hurrel et al. from the Mayo Clinic in 1996, left and right ventricular systolic pressure discordance over the first beats of the respiratory cycle is highly consistent with constrictive pericardial physiology, whereas left and right ventricular systolic pressure concordance is associated with restrictive cardiomyopathy. The hemodynamic criteria of constrictive physiology are provided in Table 8–3. The most sensitive and specific findings of constrictive pericardial disease are the relationships between the pulmonary capillary wedge and left and right ventricular systolic pressures over a respiratory cycle. Examples of these criteria are shown in Figure 8–24. In restrictive cardiomyopathy during respiration, both right and left systolic ventricular pressures fall and rise over each inspiratory phase. This pressure pattern is different than that in constrictive physiology (Fig. 8–24, *right side*) in which left ventricular pressure increases and right ventricular systolic pressure decreases during inspiration. This pattern differentiates the two major etiologies of constrictive cardiac physiology.

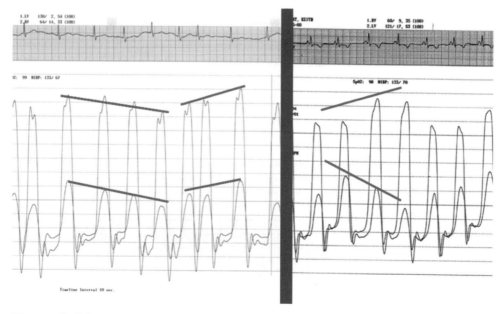

Figure 8–24.

Simultaneous right and left ventricular pressures during respiration demonstrating restrictive (concordant) and constrictive (discordant respiratory variations of systolic pressures) physiologic responses, *left and right panels,* respectively.

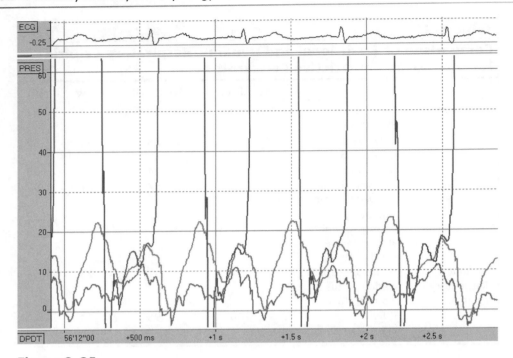

Figure 8–25.

Simultaneous left ventricular and left atrial and right atrial pressures, 0 to 40 mm Hg scale, before Valsalva maneuver.

Atrial Hemodynamics

A 59-year-old man has a transient ischemic attack. No obvious cardiac source of emboli was identified. However, on echocardiographic contrast bubble study during Valsalva maneuvers, agitated saline bubbles were evident in the left atrium. Hemodynamic data was obtained. Simultaneous left atrial and right atrial pressures were measured during the Valsalva maneuver (Figs. 8–25 to 8–29). The right atrial pressure is nearly always lower than the left atrial pressure at rest with an A and V wave beneath those of the left atrium (Fig. 8–25). At the beginning of the Valsalva maneuver, the right and left atrial pressure tracings both rise and are shown changing over the strain phase and plateau phase (Figs. 8–26 to 8–28). During the early strain phase, the left and right atrial pressures match each other (Figure 8–28) and at the lateral strain phase before release the right atrial pressure exceeds the left atrial pressure. At this time, intra-atrial blood can be shunted from the right side to the left side through patent foramen ovale, which in some individuals may result in a TIA or stroke. On release of the Valsalva maneuver (Fig. 8–29, *right sided panel*), the left atrial pressure rises normally above that of right atrial pressure, thus closing any patent foramen ovale that may exist. Other reasons why right atrial pressure may exceed left atrial pressure should be considered. For example, a 79-year-old woman is admitted to the Intensive Care Unit with an acute myocardial infarction, persistent hypoxia despite 100% FI O_2. The left and right atrial pressures were made on pullback from the left to right atrium in this

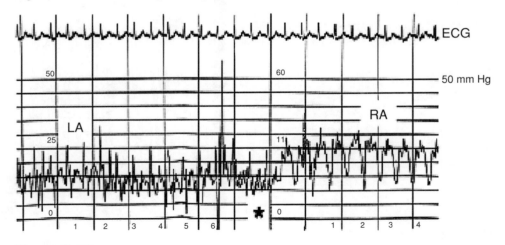

Figure 8–26.

Simultaneous left atrial and right atrial pressures, 0 to 40 mm Hg scale in patient following inferior myocardial infarction and hypotension.

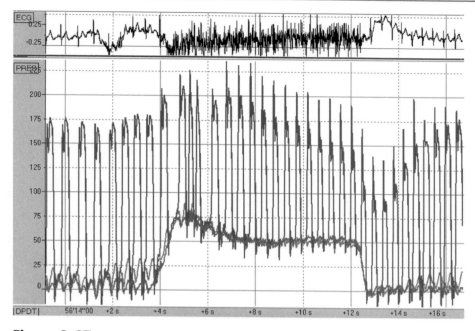

Figure 8–27.
Simultaneous left ventricular, left atrial, and right atrial pressures, 0 to 40 mm Hg scale, during Valsalva maneuver.

patient (Fig. 8–29). Why is the left atrial pressure lower than the right atrial pressure? Although the complete hemodynamic picture of cardiogenic shock was not presented, an acute right ventricular infarction with a patent foramen ovale explained the persistently elevated right atrial pressure with shunting of deoxygenated blood from right to the left side resulting in persistent hypoxia. An attempt to close the patent foramen ovale was made with a Rashkind balloon (Fig. 8–30), and was only partially successful. Today, the interventional cardiologist has several patent foramen ovale closure devices available (Fig. 8–31).

In summary, the most common hemodynamic problems during coronary intervention include hypotension due to volume loss, anaphylaxis, tamponade, arrhythmia, new valvular lesions, hypovolumic, or cardiogenic shock or pressure miscalibration due to artifact. Hypertension due to labile vascular

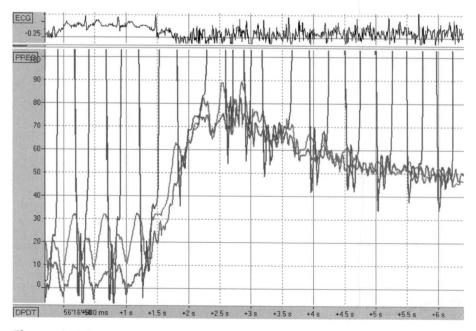

Figure 8–28.
Simultaneous left ventricular, left atrial, and right atrial pressures, 0 to 40 mm Hg scale, during peak Valsalva maneuver.

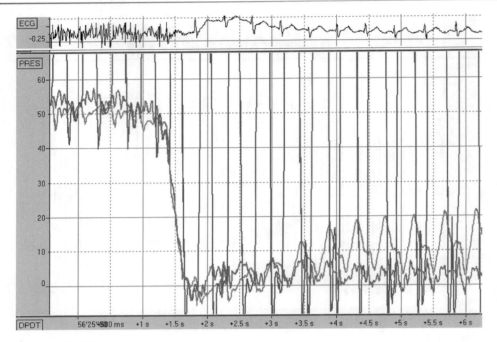

Figure 8–29.
Simultaneous left ventricular, left atrial and right atrial pressures, 0 to 40 mm Hg scale, during release of the Valsalva maneuver.

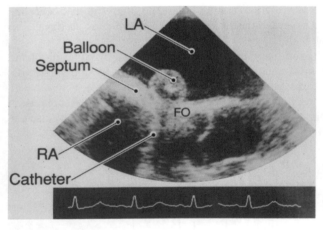

Figure 8–30.
Rashkind balloon across patent foramen ovale.

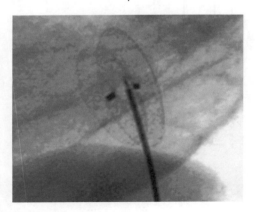

Figure 8–31.
Demonstration of patent foramen ovale Amplatzer occluder.

resistance intrinsic to the individual or to the medication misadministration should be considered. Other common diagnostic dilemmas in which hemodynamic data may assist in solving the problems, principally for noncardiac interventions include hypertrophic obstructive cardiomyopathy, mitral stenosis, diastolic cardiac dysfunction with constrictive or restrictive physiology, intracardiac shunting, low-gradient aortic stenosis, and prosthetic valve malfunction. Examination of the hemodynamic tracings in these individuals during the critical period will assist the interventional cardiologist in making a correct diagnosis and instituting potentially lifesaving therapy.

BIBLIOGRAPHY

Kern MJ. *Hemodynamic Rounds.* New York: Wiley Liss; 1994.

Kern MJ. *The Cardiac Catheterization Handbook,* 4th ed. St. Louis: Mosby; 2003.

Baim DS, Grossman W, eds. *Grossman's Cardiac Catheterization, Angiography and Intervention,* 6th ed. Baltimore: Lippincott Williams & Wilkins; 2000.

Pepine CJ, Hill JA, Lambert CR. Diagnostic and Therapeutic Cardiac Catheterization, 3rd ed. Baltimore: Williams & Wilkins; 1998.

Assey ME, Zile MR, Usher BW, et al. Effect of catheter positioning on the variability of measured gradient in aortic stenosis. *Catheter Cardiovasc Diagn.* 1993;30:287–292.

Gorlin R, Gorlin G. Hydraulic formula for calculation of area of stenotic mitral valve, other cardiac valves and central circulatory shunts. *Am Heart J.* 1951;41:1–29.

Cohen MV, Gorlin R. Modified orifice equation for the calculation of mitral valve area. *Am Heart J.* 1972;84:839–840.

Folland ED, Parisi AF, Carbone C. Is peripheral arterial pressure a satisfactory substitute for ascending aortic pressure when measuring aortic valve gradients? *J Am Coll Cardiol.* 1984;4:1207–1212.

Hakki AH. A simplified valve formula for the calculation of stenotic cardiac valve areas. *Circulation.* 1981;63:1050–1055.

Imaging

Warren K. Laskey

CHAPTER 9

Fundamentals of X-ray Imaging and Radiation Safety

Thomas M. Bashore

Every invasive cardiologist should have a working knowledge of how x-rays are produced and of how these x-rays eventually result in visual images of the heart and its structures during angiography. By understanding some of the fundamental principles behind the workings of the x-ray system, the ways in which the patient, the staff, and the cardiologist are exposed to ionizing radiation becomes more evident, and, thus, ways to protect oneself and others from radiation exposure becomes clearer. The following is meant to be a brief, schematic look at these issues for the purposes of board review.

The Basic X-ray Imaging System

Figures 9–1A to 9–1C outline the basic x-ray systems still in use today. Figure 9–1A describes an older traditional x-ray system that produces cine film utilizing a generator, x-ray tube, and traditional image intensifier (I.I.). Images from the I.I. are directly fed to a video camera for fluoroscopic viewing on an analog monitor or a partially silvered mirror splitter may be inserted during cineangiography to divert some of x-rays (up to 80%) to a 35-mm cine camera. These images are then processed onto cine film for later review on a cine projector. Figure 9–1B outlines the typical digital x-ray system commonly in use today. The system is similar to the traditional system except the mirror splitter, the cinefilm capture, and the resultant processing components are eliminated; the analog video signal that results is digitized by an analog-to-digital converter, undergoes computer processing, and then is made available for viewing on computer monitors. Figure 9–1C reveals a newer flat panel system wherein the image intensifier and the video pickup are replaced by the flat panel acquisition system. Digitization of the video signal occurs on the flat panel, and a digital signal is sent directly to a computer for processing then to the monitor in this configuration.

To understand how an x-ray system works, follow the flow of energy of a typical digital cardiac catheterization system (Fig. 9–2). Energy begins in the generator where electrons are sent to the x-ray tube where they are converted to x-rays. The x-rays emerge from the x-ray tube and diverge immediately. They travel through the table and patient where most are absorbed or scattered. A few make it to the I.I. where they strike an input phosphor, where they converted to a number of light photons, that subsequently strike a photocathode layer. Here the light photons are converted back to electrons, and the electrons are accelerated toward the output phosphor of the I.I. The image is minified and also intensified a thousand-fold. The image at the output phosphor can be visually seen at this point (the energy is light again). The light then passes through the image distributor where it strikes the face of a video camera (usually a CCD chip). Here the light is converted back to electrons in the form of an analog video signal. This signal is digitized in the A/D converter, processed by a variety of computer algorithms, and sent to a computer monitor for viewing.

The Formation of the X-ray Beam

Figure 9–3 summarizes the general concept of what happens between the generator and the x-ray tube. The x-ray tube is a vacuum tube with a cathode coil (or coils) facing a spinning anode. Electrons are sent to the cathode from the generator, and the cathode becomes white hot (about 3,000°F). At this temperature, the electrons virtually boil off (thermionic emission). The generator also sets up a voltage potential across the x-ray tube. The electrons from the cathode are encouraged to jump from the cathode to the anode by this voltage potential. A cup with a local voltage potential helps focus the electrons toward the anode. The maximal (peak) voltage across the x-ray tube is referred to as the kVp of the system, and the number of electrons that jump from the cathode to the anode is called the mA of the system. Most of the electrons that jump from the cathode to the anode simply produce heat, but some result in striking the anode and producing x-rays. To control the heat generated, the anode rotates rapidly (3,500 to 10,000 rpm) and circulating oil around the x-ray tube helps cool it.

X-rays are produced when electrons strike the tungsten anode. The face of the anode is steeply angulated (8° to 15°), so that the x-rays emerge from as much a point source as possible (the x-ray beam focal point). If a large patient is on the table, a second coil may be brought into play. Because lower frequency x-rays are not clinically useful and only contribute to noise, many of them are absorbed in the output of the x-ray

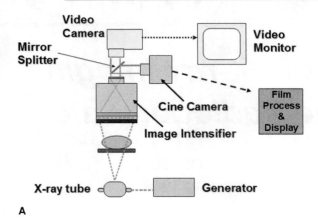

A

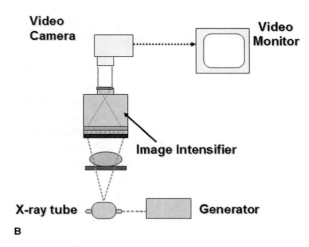

B

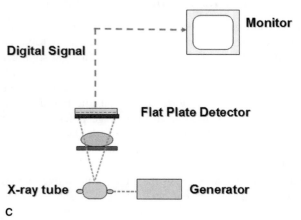

C

Figure 9-1.

Panel A schematically represents the classic x-ray system in the cardiac catheterization laboratory with cinefilm capability. **Panel B** represents the major components in the all-digital x-ray system using the traditional image intensifier and video pickup. **Panel C** displays the newer flat panel x-ray system. See text for details.

tube by copper and aluminum filters. Collimation also helps shape the x-ray beam as it emerges and reduces scatter.

Figures 9–4A and 9–4B outline how the electrons are converted to x-rays in the tungsten. Most x-rays are produced when electrons from the cathode pass near the tungsten nucleus, causing the electrons to slow down (brake). As the

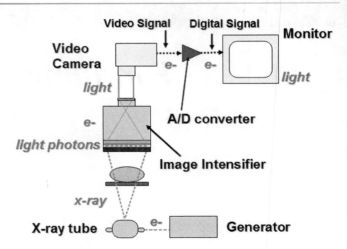

Figure 9-2.

The flow of energy through the digital x-ray system. Electrons from the generator are converted to x-rays in the x-ray tube. These x-rays traverse the patient and a few reach the image intensifier. Here they release light photons that are converted back to electrons and accelerated to the output phosphor of the image intensifier. The video camera converts the light image into a video signal that is digitized and displayed on the computer monitor.

electron loses energy, an x-ray is emitted (the braking or Bremsstrahlung x-ray). An alternative, and less important, method may occur when the traveling electron knocks out an inner shell tungsten electron. When the inner shell electron is replaced by an outer shell electron, energy is released in the form of a characteristic x-ray.

The X-ray Spectrum and Iodinated Contrast

Figure 9–5 represents the x-ray spectrum that emerges from the x-ray tube. The highest energy in the spectrum correlates

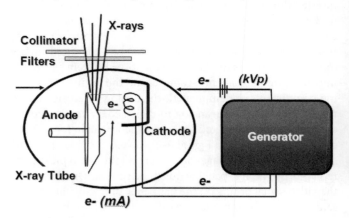

Figure 9-3.

The generator and the x-ray tube. The generator sets up a voltage potential across the x-ray tube and also sends electrons to the cathode within the tube. The maximal voltage across the tube is called the kVp. Electrons sent to the cathode "boil off" and jump to the spinning anode. The number that takes the leap correlates with the mA of the system, and it corresponds to the total number of x-rays produced. Collimators shape the beam and filters absorb low frequency x-rays. See text for further details.

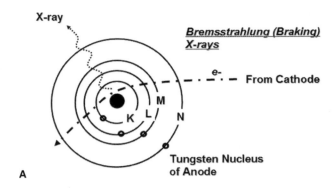

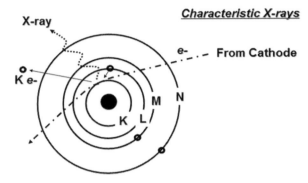

Figure 9–4.
Panel A outlines the generation of the majority of the x-rays of clinical value via the Bremsstrahlung (braking) method. Energy from the traveling electron is lost as it slows down (brakes). **Panel B** outlines how characteristic x-rays are formed. Here x-rays are produced when the traveling electron knocks out an inner shell electron, and it is subsequently replaced by an outer shell electron. The loss of energy produces the characteristic x-rays.

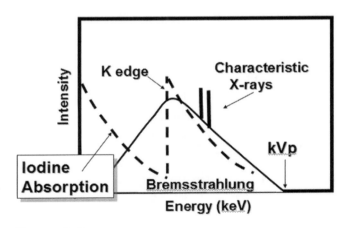

Figure 9–5.
The emitted x-ray spectrum and the iodine absorption curve. The spectrum of x-rays produced by the braking method (Bremsstrahlung) and the characteristic x-rays are represented in this schematic. Note the maximal energy is the kVp of the x-ray tube. The superimposed iodine absorption curve points out that progressively less of the x-rays emitted are absorbed as the x-ray energy increases, until suddenly most are absorbed. This point is the energy of the K electron of the iodine (K edge).

with the highest energy potential across the x-ray tube (the kVp). Most of the x-rays are produced by the Bremsstrahlung method, and their intensity versus energy (keV) is shown. Iodine is a particularly good absorber of the x-rays in this energy range, and that is why it is used as a contrast agent. The iodine absorption spectrum is shown superimposed on the x-ray spectrum (1). Note that as the energy increases, the iodine absorbs fewer and fewer of the x-rays until suddenly there is marked absorption. This is the energy of the K shell electron of the iodine and is referred to as the K edge. Progressively increasing the x-ray energy again results in progressively less absorption past this K edge. As noted, much of the energy spectrum produced by the x-ray tube is absorbed by iodine.

X-ray exposure is defined by the following equation:

$$\text{Exposure} = \text{mA} \times \text{kVp} \times \text{pulse width} \qquad (9.1)$$

What then happens when the kVp is increased? When this occurs, there are more high energy x-rays produced with many of them penetrating through any iodine column (Fig. 9–6A). The result is a washed out, gray image with little contrast between the angiogram and background. For this reason, the kVp should not be too great, and most systems limit it. What happens when the mA is increased? When this occurs, there is a significant increase in the radiation exposure, but radiographic imaging contrast is preserved (Fig. 9–6B). In very large patients, it may be difficult to generate enough mA, though,

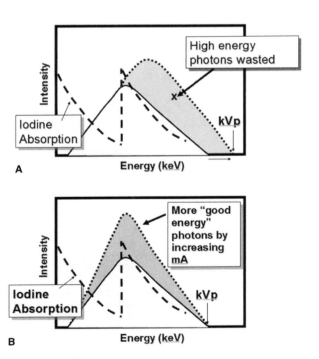

Figure 9–6.
Panel A: The effect of increasing the kVp. As the kVp is increased, the x-rays "penetrate" the iodine column, more radiation occurs, and the image contrast is lost. **Panel B:** The effect of increasing the mA. If the kVp is not increased, then contrast is preserved, though more radiation occurs as the mA rises.

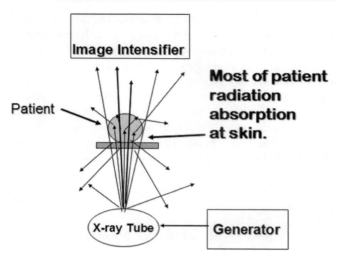

Figure 9–7.

The patient and x-ray scatter. The patient lies in the x-ray path to the image intensifier. Most of the absorption of the x-rays emitted is in the skin, with radiation scatter greatest at the skin level.

and the second cathode in the x-ray tube is brought into play to increase the number of eventual x-rays. If the pulse width is too long, then blurring of the image may occur.

From the X-ray Tube to the Image Intensifier: The Inverse Square Law

Figure 9–7 outlines the course of the x-rays as they leave the x-ray tube and travel toward the I.I. through the table and patient. Most of the x-rays never make it to the I.I., but are absorbed, attenuated, and scattered by the patient and table. To the operator, most of the exposure occurs from the scatter from the entry side of the patient. When the x-ray tube is closest to the operator, the amount of radiation exposure to the operator is the greatest (Fig. 9–8). Thus, in a cranial LAO view, with the x-ray tube on the same side of the table as the

operator, six times more operator exposure occurs than in a caudal RAO, where the x-ray tube is on the opposite side of the table (2).

Radiation exposure decreases by the inverse square law:

$$Radiation\ exposure = 1/distance^2 \qquad (9.2)$$

Thus, the greater the distance the operator can be from the radiation source and patient, the less the exposure. The same issue applies to the patient, i.e. the closer the patient is to the x-ray source, the greater the exposure. Indeed, the patient is the major absorber of the x-ray, with most of the impact of the ionizing radiation occurring in the patient's skin. X-rays also scatter from within the patient to both the operator and the patient's internal organs.

An estimate of how much radiation absorption has occurred at the skin has been devised and is available on many recent x-ray systems. Figure 9–9 demonstrates how this method derives the "interventional reference point." From an ionization chamber placed at the output of the x-ray tube, an estimate of the radiation dose, the dose-area product (DAP), can be derived. Using an average distance between the patient to the x-ray tube of 15 cm and the inverse square law, the radiation dose at the skin level can be mathematically derived. There is some uncertainty as to how well these derived data actually correlate with the measured peak skin dose (3), but the value has correlated with total effective dose to the patient (4). During a diagnostic cardiac catheterization study, the reported values vary widely, but an average DAP for a diagnostic cath is about 60 Gy-cm^2; the average dose during an interventional study is about 90 Gy-cm^2 (5–7).

The Image Intensifier, Image Distributor, and Exposure Control

Figure 9–10 is a schematic of the key features of the classic I.I. On the face of the I.I., a grid helps screen out any scattered

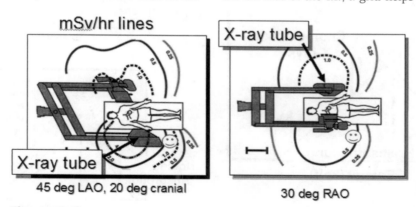

Figure 9–8.

The relationship between the x-ray source and the operator. The amount of radiation to the operator is dependent upon the relationship of the operator to the scatter from the patient and from the x-ray source. In the *left panel*, the x-ray tube is close to the operator and one might receive 6 times the radiation dose as from the setup in the right panel, where the x-ray tube is on the opposite side of the table. (From: Balter S. Stray radiation in the cardiac catheterisation laboratory. *Radiat Prot Dosimetry.* 2001;94:183–188, with permission.)

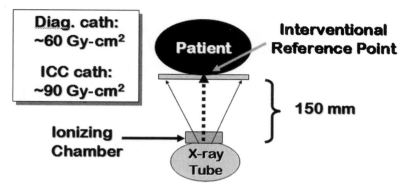

Figure 9–9.

The interventional reference point. An estimate of skin exposure can be made by measuring the amount x-rays produced (by an ionizing chamber (the dose-area product) at the output of the x-ray tube) and assuming the patient is 15 cm (150 mm) away. The average dose-area product for a diagnostic cath is about 60 Gy-cm^2 and about 90 Gy-cm^2 for an interventional procedure. (From: Balter S. A new tool for benchmarking cardiovascular fluoroscopes. *Radiat Prot Dosimetry.* 2001;94:161–166, with permission.)

x-rays. Once through the grid that screens out x-rays entering at an angle, the x-rays interact with a cesium iodide crystal, causing it to scintillate, producing around 1,600 light photons for each x-ray that strikes it. These light photons then travel forward toward a photocathode layer that has an efficiency of about 10% to 15% where the light photons result in the final production of about 200 electrons for each of the original x-rays (8). The electrons are accelerated through the I.I. due to the large voltage potential placed across the I.I. These electrons strike the smaller output phosphor creating an image about 1,000 times brighter on the input phosphor. The light then emerges from the output phosphor, with an image that can be visualized by the naked eye. This light is then sent through a series of lenses in the image distributor to the video camera or CCD. Within the image distributor is a prism or partially silvered mirror that directs some of the light to a photodetector that feeds back the exposure to the generator via the exposure control system (Fig. 9–11). The output from the generator is then altered to satisfy the exposure control equation. (Exposure = mA × kVp × PW).

While continuous emission of the x-rays has traditionally been used during fluoroscopy and pulsing of the x-ray beam used during cineangiography, newer systems now pulse the fluoroscopic beam as well. Pulsing the fluoroscopic beam reduces total x-ray exposure, and most studies in adults are now done at a fluoroscopic rate of 7.5 to 15 frames/sec, with cineangiography rates of 15 frames/sec. At higher heart rates, framing rates need to be increased to prevent inadequate sampling (aliasing); so many pediatric laboratories still sometimes use 30–60 frames/sec imaging rates.

Regardless of the pulsing rate, each exposure must still satisfy the exposure equation. The exposure control prism usually samples about 60% of the output phosphor phosphor (8). As one pans over the bones rather than the lungs, for instance,

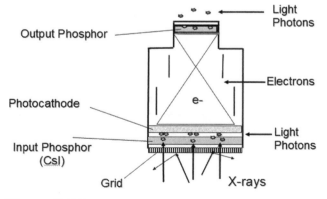

Figure 9–10.

The traditional image intensifier. As x-rays approach the image intensifier, scattered x-rays are screened out by use of a grid. Useable x-rays then strike a cesium iodide crystal that scintillates, producing light photons. These then strike a photocathode that converts them into electrons that are subsequently accelerated through the image intensifier to the output phosphor. Here an x-ray image is formed and can be viewed with the naked eye.

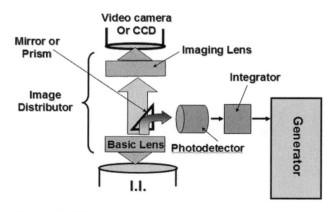

Figure 9–11.

The image distributor and automatic exposure control. A portion of the light sent from the output phosphor to the video camera is intercepted by a partially silvered mirror or prism that deflects this to a photodetector that feeds back to the generator as to whether there has been appropriate exposure for that frame.

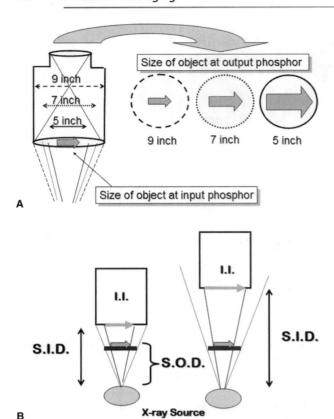

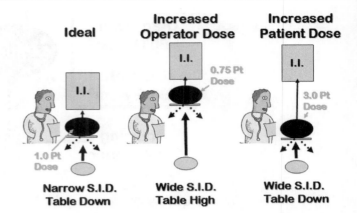

Figure 9–13.

Effect of table height and S.I.D. on operator and patient, radiation exposure. The various relationships between the S.I.D., the patient, and the operator are shown. The *left panel* shows an ideal situation. If the S.I.D. is too high and the patient is elevated, *middle panel*, more x-rays are needed to image (as noted in Fig. 9–12) and the dose to the operator is increased even though the dose to the patient is less (due to the inverse square law). In the *right panel,* the S.I.D. is high, but the patient is close to the x-ray tube. Because the overall dose is increased due to the wide S.I.D., the patient gets an excessive radiation dose from being close to the x-ray source.

Figure 9–12.

Panel A: Magnification within the image intensifier. When the entire face of the I.I. is used to acquire the image, it appears smaller than when less of the face of the I.I. is used. The difference between using the entire surface (9-inch diameter) is shown contrasted with only using 7-inch or 5-inch diameters. Because the exposure equation must still be met, yet less x-rays are being acquired from the I.I. surface, it takes more x-rays to obtain magnified views. **Panel B:** Magnification due to increasing the source-to-image distance (S.I.D.). The x-ray source is shown in relationship to the image intensifier (I.I.)—the S.I.D. and to the patient or object, the S.O.D. As the S.I.D. is increased there is more magnification due to the divergence of x-rays. There is also a loss of x-rays for the same reason. More x-rays are thus required in order to meet the exposure equation as the S.I.D. is increased.

more exposure is required due to the increased density of bone. Similarly in obese patients and using angulated views, more exposure is required to satisfy the exposure equation. To preserve image contrast and to prevent blurring, the kVp or the pulse width cannot be increased too much, so a lot of the increased dose needed is achieved by increasing the mA (and overall radiation dose).

Another factor that increases the x-ray dose is magnification. Figure 9–12A shows how magnification is electronically accomplished in the I.I. When the entire face of the I.I. is used to acquire an image on the input phosphor (9-inch diameter mode, for example), then the image at the output phosphor appears much smaller than when only either 7-inch diameter mode or the 5-inch diameter mode is used. Said another way, the less of the face of the I.I. used to create the image, the larger the image appears on the output phosphor. However, because less of the face of the I.I. is used, and the exposure equation

must still be satisfied, the x-ray dose must necessarily increase proportionately. A final factor that results in magnification is an increase in the source-to-image (S.I.D.) (Fig. 9–12B). Because of the diversion of x-rays, the more narrow the S.I.D. the more x-rays are captured and the image appears smaller compared to when the S.I.D. is wide. Therefore, it is important to keep the I.I. as close to the patient as possible. Recall, though, that the closer the patient is to the x-ray source, the more radiation exposure to the patient via the inverse square law. Figure 9–13 outlines the various relationships between the patient, the operator, the x-ray source, and the I.I. If the S.I.D. is high and the patient is elevated, then there is excessive exposure to the operator. If the S.I.D. is too high and the patient is close to the x-ray tube, then there is excessive exposure to the patient.

Cinefilm

With the advent of digital imaging systems, Cinefilm is uncommonly used nowadays in most cardiac catheterization laboratories. Cinefilm is a composite material made of a polyester film base coated with an emulsion layer that contains silver halide crystals suspended in a gelatin. The base layer is coated on both sides with emulsion, and when the film is exposed to light, a latent image forms. This latent image is enhanced in processing that includes development (conversion of latent image to a visible image) and fixing (removal of undeveloped silver halide crystals and making the image permanent) followed by washing and drying. The resultant image is projected using a Cinefilm projector that typically shows each image twice in sequence to simulate 60 frames/sec, because the original film is usually acquired at 30 frames/sec and flicker would be otherwise noted.

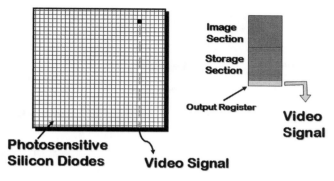

Figure 9–14.
The charge coupled device (CCD). As light strikes each of the squares of the CCD (photosites), a charge occurs proportional to the intensity of the light. These charges are collected in potential wells or "buckets" and shifted row by row from an image section to the storage section. Here they are read out a line at a time as a video signal that contains where the photosite was located and shows the intensity of the charge.

The Video Chain

Once the image is passed through the image distributor, it strikes the face of either a video camera or, now more commonly, a charge-coupled device (CCD) (Figs. 9–14 and 9–15). This device has rows of photo-sensitive silicon squares called photosites (about 300,000 to 500,000 per chip) (8). When light strikes each photosite, a charge occurs. The brighter the light, the more the charge that occurs. These charges are col-

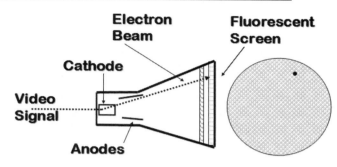

Figure 9–15.
The traditional CRT. The traditional CRT reverses the process from the CCD chip. The CRT has rows of phosphor dots that glow when struck by electrons. The incoming video signal provides the location and intensity that each dot needs to be struck to correspond to the image that was acquired.

lected in potential wells or charge "buckets." Electrons in this image section are then shifted in parallel, one row at a time, to the storage section. From the storage section, the charges from each photosite are read out horizontally, creating a video signal that contains information as to where each photosite is located on the face of the CCD and the charge at each of these sites.

In an analog system, this video signal is sent to a cathode ray tube (CRT) (Fig. 9–16) where the process is reversed. Rather than a row of silicon-sensitive squares, the CRT has rows of phosphor dots that glow when struck by electrons accelerated

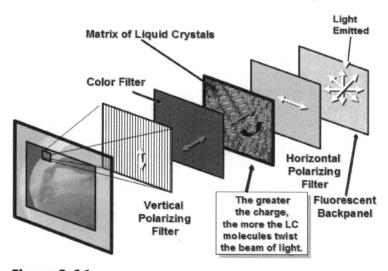

Figure 9–16.
The LCD monitor. The flat LCD monitor is made up of a series of panels. A matrix of thin-film transistors (TFTs) is located on polarizing and color filters. Each pixol has its own transistors. Light vibrating in all directions is produced by the fluorescent back panel. This light passes through a horizontal polarizing panel. These light waves then travel through the liquid crystal panel, where the liquid crystals twist the light in proportion to the amount of voltage applied by the incoming video signal. The greater the signal intensity, the more the light is twisted. This twisted light is now sent through a color filter then to another polarizing panel that only allows mostly vertical light to pass. If the light was not twisted by the LCD panel, it will not pass through this polarizing panel, and the pixel will appear black. If it was twisted to 90° (maximally), the pixel will appear white. Any twisting between 0° and 90° results in various shades of gray. In this manner the image is formed on the monitor.

through the tube. The incoming video signal provides the location and intensity that each dot needs to be struck to provide the image. Because flicker is generally perceived whenever <50 frames/sec is observed by the human eye, the rows of phosphor dots are divided into A-rows alternating with B-rows. By scanning only the A-rows then scanning only the B-rows, each frame is scanned twice and the apparent framing rate is doubled as far as the human brain is concerned. Scanning of fields in this manner is referred to as interlaced scanning. Because there is always some overlap in the process, the image is downgraded somewhat, however.

If the video signal is first converted to digital data by use of an analog-to-digital converter, the data can be displayed on a computer monitor where the screen is divided into a series of pixels (picture elements) and the brightness of each pixel defined by a grayscale value. The pixel array is 512 × 512 or 1024 × 1024 for most systems. The actual display matrix is somewhat less than this, but the concept is what is important. The computer display of the images is not limited by the acquisition rate as computer monitors can read each line in order (sequential or progressive scanning), with the whole frame being read much faster than the human eye can detect flicker. Most scanning rates are in the range of 60 to 100 times/sec (Herz). The great advantage of such progressive scanning is that it has higher resolution and allows for the use of lower acquisition rates, thus helping to reduce radiation exposure.

The growing alternative to heavy CRT monitors is the liquid crystal display (LCD) panel. The LCD panel is actually a series of panels sandwiched together (Fig. 9–16). An active-matrix structure is used. A matrix of thin-film transistors (TFTs) is added to polarizing and color filters. Each pixel has its own dedicated transistors. The back panel provides fluorescent light that spreads out in waves that vibrate in all directions. The next panel is a polarizing filter that lets only the light waves that are more or less horizontal through. The light then passes to a panel with a matrix of liquid crystal twisted nematic (TN) cells. When voltage is applied to each cell, the long rod-shaped liquid crystal molecules react by forming a spiral. The horizontally polarized light entering the cell is twisted along the spiral path. If the cell is fully charged, the light is rotated a full 90°. If no charge, the light passes through. If partially charged, the light is rotated between 0° and 90°. The light then passes through color filters, then to a second polarizing filter that only allows light that is vibrating vertically to pass through. Light that was not twisted at all is now blocked by this second polarizing panel, and the pixel on the monitor appears black. Light that was twisted a full 90° now passes through this second polarizing panel, and the pixel on the monitor appears white. Light that was partially twisted appears as various shades of gray. In this manner the complex final image appears on the monitor screen.

Image Storage

Digital imaging allows for high-resolution image data to be filtered and made available for immediate reading. Once in a digital format, the data are then written to disk using the DICOM (Digital Communication in Medicine) format that provides

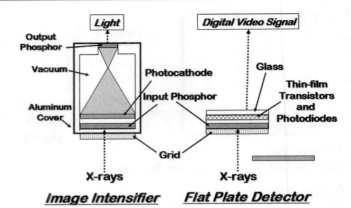

Figure 9–17.
The traditional versus flat panel imaging system. The traditional I.I. is contrasted with the flat panel system. The flat panels in current use still have a grid over the surface and a cesium iodide crystal that scintillates and converts the light photons to electrons. Rather than accelerating these electrons to an output phosphor, though, the electrons strike individual photodiodes that represent each pixel. The data are thus converted on the flat panel to a digitized video signal that represents each pixel and the intensity of the charge at each pixel. There is no aluminum cover over the flat panel to alternate x-rays, reducing the dose needed by 5–10%.

for standardization across the various cardiac catheterization laboratories. The digital data are also available for viewing across internal and external network connections and can be stored in a variety of archival media devices. As the cost of digital storage has dramatically dropped and the availability of large storage media in the terabyte range has become a reality, the expense involved with the all digital imaging system has dropped, and it has increasingly become the norm.

A Brief Primer on Flat Panel X-ray Systems

Figure 9–17 schematically compares a newer flat panel system with that of a traditional image intensifier system. Compared to the traditional digital x-ray system, many of the steps involved in producing an x-ray image are consolidated or eliminated in the flat panel system. Certain similarities between the two systems still exist, and are schematically shown in the figure. For example, there is a grid in front of the flat panel to reduce exposure to scattered x-rays, and the x-rays still strike a cesium iodide crystal that scintillates and releases light photons. The next layer consists of glass coated with a thin layer of millions of silicon transistors (thin-film transistor array or TFTs) similar to that described in the LCD panel earlier. Each of these TFTs is attached to a light-absorbing photodiode making up an individual pixel (Fig. 9–18). The light photons from the cesium iodide strike the photodiode, producing electrons. The TFTs are essentially switches, and the matrix on the flat panel is normally scanned one line at a time from the top to the bottom. The output from the system is A/D converted right on the flat panel, so that a digital signal is sent directly from the flat panel to the monitor system. Magnification involves selection of only

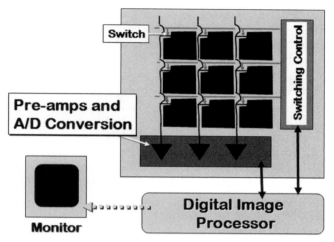

Figure 9–18.

TFT chip array. The array of TFT chips on the flat panel is shown here. Each transistor corresponds to a pixel on the monitor much as the CCD chip or LCD panel. See text for details.

the more central pixels prior to display, and in theory does not increase dosage as much as in the traditional I.I. The final image is also square rather than the round image from the standard I.I., and there is no distortion or brightness nonuniformity to deal with. The DQE (detective quantum efficiency), a measure of noise, signal loss, sensitivity, and resolution, is much higher for flat panel systems than those based on the standard I.I. with its CCD video acquisition (9). The main radiation dosage savings, though, is the elimination of the attenuation created by the aluminum covering material that is normally around the image intensifier. Biplane flat panel systems are also now becoming available.

Radiation Safety Issues and Terms

There are several recent reviews of radiation safety specifically for cardiac catheterization laboratories (2,10–15). The National Council on Radiation Protection and Measurement (NCRP) is responsible for providing guidelines for the public and medical workers. The traditional use of the ALARA (As Low As Reasonably Achievable) concept still holds, as theoretically no dose of ionizing radiation is without harm.

Much of the confusion in the radiologic literature relates to the interchangeable use of various terms to describe radiation, radiation absorption, and radiation exposure. The basic unit of radiation ionization is defined as the Roentgen (R). It is the amount of ionization that a defined mass of air undergoes when bombarded by x-rays or gamma rays. The amount of energy actually absorbed by material is the radiation absorbed dose (rad). The amount of energy absorbed by differing materials varies according to the type of radiation and the atomic number of the material. Radiation protection units are simply rads times some quality factor that is dependent on the type of radiation, and these units are called rems. In cardiology the quality

factor is 1.0 for either x-rays or gamma rays, so rems and rads are equal.

The units for rads are now expressed in Gray units (Gy) and for rems in Seiverts (Sv). One Sv equals 100 rem or 1 rem equals 10 mSv. For consistency, we will express radiation terms in mSv, because this has now become the recommended norm.

The Biologic Effects Resulting from X-ray Exposure

Radiation may be classified as directly or indirectly ionizing (16). *Direct ionization* means the radiation has enough energy to disrupt the atomic structure of the material it strikes, producing chemical and biologic changes. X-rays (and gamma rays) are *indirectly ionizing*, meaning that when they are absorbed, they produce a variety of fast-moving particles that can ionize other atoms of the absorber, breaking vital chemical bonds. The biologic effects of x-rays results principally from damage to DNA. For x-ray radiation, this damage is primarily due to the production of free radicals (a free radical is an atom or molecule with an unpaired orbital electron in the outer shell), and most of this is from the hydroxyl radical. When cells are irradiated, the DNA may suffer a single-strand break or a double-strand break. Single-strand breaks are readily healed and the cell normally is not killed. The repair may be incorrect and a mutation may occur. Double-strand breaks are less common, but more serious, and result in cell death as well as mutations and carcinogenesis.

For most organs, the loss of a few cells is unimportant until a threshold dose is reached. Effects such as this are called *deterministic*, and this kind of injury is dose dependent. Examples of this type of injury include skin erythema, skin desquamation, cataracts, bone marrow suppression, gonadal injury, sterility, fibrosis, and organ atrophy. If irradiation to the cell keeps it viable, but modified, it may become cancerous. This latter type injury is called *stochastic* (a word generally meaning "random"). Stochastic effects have no threshold (a single x-ray can cause it), but the probability of occurrence increases as the dose increases.

Each of the body's organs has a variable susceptibility to radiation injury. In general, the more biologically active an organ, the more susceptible it is to radiation. The International Commission on Radiation Units and Measurement has suggested a tissue weighting factor for the various organs, and this generally corresponds to the organ susceptibility to the effects of ionizing radiation. Table 9–1 outlines the tissue weighting factors for different tissues based on this report (17). Note that the sum of all the weighting factors is unity.

We live on a planet where radiation has been a fact of life since the beginning. In fact, most of the background radiation (18) we receive comes from the earth (radon = 55% of total background dose). Natural radiation accounts for about 82% of the radiation we receive, and man-made radiation for 18%. Though the numbers vary widely depending on location, altitude, etc., the average background radiation per year received in the United States is about 3.6 mSv (18). Compare this with

Table 9–1

Tissue Weighting Factors.

Tissue or Organ	Tissue Weighting Factor
Gonads	0.20
Bone marrow	0.12
Colon	0.12
Lung	0.12
Stomach	0.12
Breast	0.05
Bladder	0.05
Thyroid	0.05
Liver	0.05
Esophagus	0.05
Skin	0.01
Bone surface	0.01
All other tissues not listed	0.05

From: National Council on Radiation Protection and Measurement. Recommendations for Limits on Exposure to Ionizing Radiation. Report 116. Bethesda, MD, 1993, with permission.
These Factors Approximate the Susceptibility of Various Tissues to Stochastic Effects from Ionizing Radiation. The Number Represents the Risk Being Induced in the Organ When Singly Irradiated Compared to the Total Risk if the Same Radiation Dose is Received by the Whole Body.

a patient's exposure from a routine chest x-ray being around 0.02 to 0.04 mSv.

Table 9–2 outlines the current recommendations for maximal occupational radiation dose limits (17,19). Note that the total recommended maximal dose for an invasive cardiologist is 50 mSv (5 rem) per year, and the total accumulative dose is the age × 10 mSv (age × total rems). The cancer risk has variously been estimated for the general population at about 20% or greater. The cumulative additional risk for cancer in

Table 9–2

Recommended Dose Limits from the NCRP

Background radiation	3.6 mSv (0.36 rem)
Chest x-ray	0.02–0.04 mSv
Annual Dose Limits	
Stochastic Effects	
Cumulative	10 mSv x age (rem x age)
Annual	50 mSv (5 rems)
Deterministic Effects (Annual)	
Eye	150 mSv/year (15 rem)
Skin	500 mSv/year (50 rem)
Embryo or fetus	0.5 mSv/month (0.05 rem)

From: Hall EJ. Radiation Protection. In: Hall EJ, ed. *Radiobiology for the Radiologist*. Philadelphia: Lippincott Williams & Wilkins, 2000:234–248; International Commission on Radiation Units and Measurements. Recommendations. Report 60. New York: Pergamon Press, 1991; National Council on Radiation Protection and Measurement. Recommendations for Limits on Exposure to Ionizing Radiation. Report 116. Bethesda, MD, 1993, with permission.

those exposed to occupational radiation is about 0.004% × mSv (or 0.04% × rem) (10). If a busy interventionalist receives 25 mSv/year and practices for 20 years, his total dose would be about 500 mSv (50 rem). The added risk would thus be 500 × 0.004% or 2%. The additional radiation exposure received would thus increase the cancer risk from baseline 20% to 22%.

During an average interventional cardiac catheterization, the physician operator receives about 0.04 mSv (about that of a chest x-ray). In a year, the average interventionalist receives from 2 to 60 mSv per year (20). Nurses in the room receive around 8 to 16 mSv per year, and the technologists about 2 mSv per year (21).

Radiation exposure to the fetus is particularly an issue during the first trimester (22). The principle effects on the developing embryo or fetus are growth retardation, death, congenital malformations, and functional impairment, such as mental retardation. Microcephaly has also been linked, as has childhood malignancies, especially leukemia. A pregnant worker may make a conscious decision to work in the cardiac catheterization laboratory, however, without fear of repercussions. The United Nations Scientific Committee on the Effects of Atomic Radiation (UNSCEAR) suggests that the risk of a fetal congenital malformation or a malignancy is about 0.0002% per mSv (0.002% per rem) exposure (10). Based on the Japanese survivors of the atomic bomb (arguably not the analogous situation, because this was an enormous dose over a brief period), the fetal sensitivity appears greatest between 8 and 15 weeks. The pregnant woman should wear a dosimeter under the outer lead as well as on the thyroid collar, and there should be no more than 5 mSv (0.5 rem) total exposure and no more than 0.5 mSv (0.005 rem) per month (10). A dose of 100 mSv (10 rem) during the most sensitive period (10 days to 26 weeks) is often regarded as the cutoff point for considering a therapeutic abortion (22). Legal precedent has been established that the pregnant worker may remain in the laboratory if she chooses, but that she should receive counseling from the radiation safety officer regarding her decision.

Measuring the Dose of Radiation Exposure

Radiation exposure nowadays is usually measured with either a TLD (thermoluminescent dosimeter) badge or an OSL (optically simulated luminescent) badge. The TLD badge has a LiF crystal that absorbs x-rays. When heated, it releases light photons in proportion to the amount of x-ray absorbed. The OSL badge is similar, but the substrate is aluminum oxide doped with carbon, and it releases light in proportion to the amount of x-ray absorbed when struck with a laser. The badges have differing filters to mimic attenuation for different parts of the body. The results are usually reported for shallow, lens or deep dose exposure. It is recommended that radiation badges be worn on both the thyroid collar and beneath the lead apron at the waist.

Table 9–3
Minimizing Radiation Exposure to the Patient
Proper collimation.
Use of filters at the output of the x-ray tube.
Keep the kVp as high as possible to maintain good image contrast.
Use the minimal number of views.
Keep the I.I. as close to the patient as possible.
Keep the S.I.D. as narrow as possible.
Use the lowest framing rate possible.
Use pulsed fluoroscopy.
Keep the number of magnified views to a minimum.
Use direct shielding of gonadal organs.

Table 9–4
Minimizing Occupational Exposure
Time
Keep the time per frame to a minimum.
Keep the number of shots to a minimum.
Don't ignore fluoroscopic time.
Distance
Remember the inverse square law.
Stay as far away from the x-ray source as possible.
Barriers
Use all available shielding, barriers, and eyewear.
Pay attention to relationship of patient, the x-ray source, the S.I.D., and you.
Use all the efforts to minimize exposure outlined for the patient in Table 9-3.

Patient Exposure to Ionizing Radiation

Patients may receive a considerable amount of radiation from x-ray studies in the cardiac catheterization laboratory. From continuous fluoroscopy alone, the patient may receive about 20 mSv/minute. That is anywhere from 100 to 200 chest x-rays per minute. Pulsing the fluoroscopic dose can reduce radiation exposure; for example, reducing the fluoroscopic framing rate to 7.5 frames/sec can reduce the overall dose by about half (23,24). Because the patient's skin absorbs most of the direct impact from the x-ray in the cardiac catheterization laboratory, the majority of reported injuries to patients relate to excessive skin dosages (25). In general, skin epilation can be expected after about 2,000 mSv (200 rem), erythema after about 6,000 mSv (600 rem), and necrosis after about 15,000 mSv (1,500 rem). In one study, this corresponded to 0.7, 2, and 6 hours of continuous fluoro time, respectively (25).

Minimizing Radiation Exposure

Table 9–3 outlines ways to minimize radiation exposure to the patient. These include proper beam shaping with collimation, the use of copper and aluminum filters at the output of the x-ray tube, using the fewest magnified views, keeping the S.I.D. as narrow as possible, keeping the kVp as high as good image contrast will allow in order to keep the mA as low as possible, using the minimal number of exposures, using pulsed fluoroscopy, and using the lowest practical framing rates. Direct shielding of sensitive areas helps protect the gonads from direct exposure (although it does not protect someone from internally scattered radiation).

Table 9–4 outlines similar issues for the occupational worker. All of the ways to reduce exposure to the patient also apply to the operator. The three basic tenets for minimizing occupational exposure are:

1. Time
2. Distance
3. Barriers

Keep the studies as short as possible. While a minute of fluoroscopy time may only result in 1/10 the dose of 1 minute of cineangiography, most of the radiation exposure in the laboratory is due to fluoroscopy. In fact the operator typically receives about six times more dose from fluoroscopy than cine (26). Remember the inverse square law and stay as far from the x-ray source as possible. Note the relationship of the patient, the S.I.D., and you to keep your exposure to a minimum (Fig. 9–13). Use barriers such as shields, lead aprons, thyroid collars, and eye protective glasses— all are very effective in reducing your exposure, but they are of little value unless properly used.

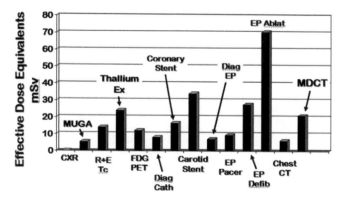

Figure 9–19.

Comparative radiation dosages from various cardiovascular studies that produce ionizing radiation. (From: Hall EJ. Radiation Protection. In: Hall EJ, ed. *Radiobiology for the Radiologist*. Philadelphia: Lippincott Williams & Wilkins, 2000:234–248; Duke Medical Center, Duke Radiation Safety Committee. Radiation risk determinations. Available at: www.safety.duke.edu/radsafety/consents; Hunold P, Vogt FM, Schmermund A, et al. Radiation exposure during cardiac CT: effective doses at multi-detector row CT and electron-beam CT. *Radiology*. 2003;226:145–152, with permission.)

Summary

Many cardiologists have minimal knowledge of the relative radiation risks for various cardiovascular tests (13,27). A working knowledge of how x-ray images are derived in the cardiac catheterization is important in order to take full advantage of the technology and for troubleshooting. Equipped with such knowledge, ways of reducing the risk of ionizing radiation to the patient, to the operator, and to the staff becomes more intuitive. The dangers from radiation have taken on a larger profile recently with the advent of multi-slice computerized tomography for cardiology. As an addendum, Figure 9–19 is provided as a guide to contrast the patient radiation exposure in the cardiac catheterization laboratory with various other cardiovascular imaging studies that employ ionizing radiation (16,28,29).

REFERENCES

1. Balter S. Managing radiation in the fluoroscopic environment. In: Philips Medical Systems. The Netherlands: Best, 1995:1–15.

2. Balter S. Radiation safety in the cardiac catheterization laboratory: operational radiation safety. *Catheter Cardiovasc Interv.* 1999;47:347–353.

3. Fletcher DW, Miller DL, Balter S, et al. Comparison of four techniques to estimate radiation dose to skin during angiographic and interventional radiology procedures. *J Vasc Interv Radiol.* 2002;13:391–397.

4. Bacher K, Bogaert E, Lapere R, et al. Patient-specific dose and radiation risk estimation in pediatric cardiac catheterization. *Circ.* 2005;111:83–89.

5. Betsou S, Efstathopoulos EP, Katritsis D, et al. Patient radiation doses during cardiac catheterization procedures. *Br J Radiol.* 1998;71:634–639.

6. Lobotessi H, Karoussou A, Neofotistou V, et al. Effective dose to a patient undergoing coronary angiography. *Radiat Prot Dosimetry.* 2001;94:173–176.

7. van de Putte S, Verhaegen F, Taeymans Y, et al. Correlation of patient skin doses in cardiac interventional radiology with dose-area product. *Br J Radiol.* 2000;73:504–513.

8. Blume H. The imaging chain. In: Nickoloff EL, Strauss KJ, eds. *RSNA Categorical Course in Diagnostic Radiolgy Physics: Cardiac Catheterization Imaging.* Oak Brook, IL: RSNA, 1998:83–103.

9. Holmes DR, Jr., Laskey WK, Wondrow MA, et al. Flat-panel detectors in the cardiac catheterization laboratory: revolution or evolution-what are the issues? *Catheter Cardiovasc Interv.* 2004;63:324–330.

10. Limacher MC, Douglas PS, Germano G, et al. ACC expert consensus document. Radiation safety in the practice of cardiology. *J Am Coll Cardiol.* 1998;31:892–913.

11. Balter S. An overview of radiation safety regulatory recommendations and requirements. *Catheter Cardiovasc Interv.* 1999;47:469–474.

12. Balter S. Radiation safety in the cardiac catheterization laboratory: basic principles. *Catheter Cardiovasc Interv.* 1999;47:229–236.

13. Hirshfeld JW, Jr., Balter S, Brinker JA, et al. ACCF/AHA/HRS/SCAI clinical competence statement on physician knowledge to optimize patient safety and image quality in fluoroscopically guided invasive cardiovascular procedures: a report of the American College of Cardiology Foundation/American Heart Association/American College of Physicians Task Force on Clinical Competence and Training. *Circ.* 2005;111:511–532.

14. Bashore TM. Fundamentals of X-ray imaging and radiation safety. *Catheter Cardiovasc Interv.* 2001;54:126–135.

15. Bashore TM. Radiation safety in the cardiac catheterization laboratory. *Am Heart J.* 2004;147:375–378.

16. Hall EJ. Radiation Protection. In: Hall EJ, ed. *Radiobiology for the Radiologist.* Philadelphia: Lippincott Williams & Wilkins, 2000:234–248.

17. International Commission on Radiation Units and Measurements. Recommendations. Report 60. New York: Pergamon Press, 1991.

18. National Council on Radiation Protection and Measurement. Exposure of the Population in the United States to Ionizing Radiation. Report 93. Bethesda, MD, 1987.

19. National Council on Radiation Protection and Measurement. Recommendations for Limits on Exposure to Ionizing Radiation. Report 116. Bethesda, MD, 1993.

20. Zorzetto M, Bernardi G, Morocutti G, et al. Radiation exposure to patients and operators during diagnostic catheterization and coronary angioplasty. *Cathet Cardiovasc Diagn.* 1997;40:348–351.

21. Renaud L. A 5-y follow-up of the radiation exposure to in-room personnel during cardiac catheterization. *Health Phys.* 1992;62:10–15.

22. Hall EJ. Effects of radiation on the embryo and fetus. In: Hall EJ, ed. *Radiobiology for the Radiologist.* Philadelphia: Lippincott Williams & Wilkins, 2000:178–192.

23. Holmes DR, Jr., Wondrow MA, Gray JE, et al. Effect of pulsed progressive fluoroscopy on reduction of radiation dose in the cardiac catheterization laboratory. *J Am Coll Cardiol.* 1990;15:159–162.

24. Aufrichtig R, Xue P, Thomas CW, et al. Perceptual comparison of pulsed and continuous fluoroscopy. *Med Phys.* 1994;21:245–256.

25. Wagner LK, Eifel P, Geise R. Effects of ionizing radiation. *J Vasc Interv Radiol.* 1995;6:988–989.

26. Pitney MR, Allan RM, Giles RW, et al. Modifying fluoroscopic views reduces operator radiation exposure during coronary angioplasty. *J Am Coll Cardiol.* 1994;24:1660–1663.

27. Correia MJ, Hellies A, Andreassi MG, et al. Lack of radiological awareness among physicians working in a tertiary-care cardiological centre. *Int J Cardiol.* 2005;103:307–311.

28. Duke Medical Center, Duke Radiation Safety Committee. Radiation risk determinations. Available at: www.safety.duke.edu/radsafety/consents.

29. Hunold P, Vogt FM, Schmermund A, et al. Radiation exposure during cardiac CT: effective doses at multi-detector row CT and electron-beam CT. *Radiology.* 2003;226:145–152.

30. Balter S. Stray radiation in the cardiac catheterisation laboratory. *Radiat Prot Dosimetry.* 2001;94:183–188.

31. Balter S. A new tool for benchmarking cardiovascular fluoroscopes. *Radiat Prot Dosimetry.* 2001;94:161–166.

CHAPTER 10

Intravascular Ultrasound

John McB. Hodgson

Intravascular ultrasound allows direct visualization of coronary anatomy during diagnostic and interventional catheterization (1–6). Unlike angiography, which depicts a silhouette of the coronary lumen, intravascular ultrasound displays a tomographic, cross-sectional perspective. This facilitates direct measurements of the lumen dimensions, including the minimum and maximum diameter and cross-sectional area (7). By employing a timed pullback, length measures may be obtained (8). Ultrasound-derived measurements are more accurate than angiographic dimensions (9,10). In addition to luminal measurements, the ability of coronary ultrasound to image the soft tissues within the arterial wall enables characterization of atheroma size, plaque distribution, and lesion composition (11–13). Accordingly, ultrasound can detect the presence or absence of structural abnormalities of the vessel wall after mechanical interventions, including dissections, tissue flaps, intramural hematomas, perforations, and irregular surface features (14–17). Since intracoronary ultrasound was first performed in 1988, it has been instrumental to our understanding of coronary anatomy and pathophysiology and allowed detailed evaluation of interventional procedures.

Intravascular Ultrasound Devices

Intracoronary ultrasound equipment requires two components; a catheter incorporating a miniaturized transducer and a console containing the necessary electronics to reconstruct an ultrasound image. Catheters typically range in size from 2.9F to 3.5F, a corresponding diameter of 0.96 to 1.17 mm. Two technical approaches to transducer design have emerged: mechanically rotated imaging devices and a multi-element electronic array device. The mechanically rotated design requires an imaging sheath; the electronic design is inserted directly into the artery. Most systems use a monorail design to facilitate rapid catheter exchange.

Artifacts and Limitations

Mechanical transducers may exhibit variations in rotational speed arising from mechanical drag on the catheter driveshaft, creating nonuniform rotational distortion (NURD) and producing visible distortion. NURD is most evident when the driveshaft is bent into a small radius of curvature by a tortuous vessel and is recognized as circumferential "stretching" of a portion of the image with "compression" of the contralateral vessel wall. An additional artifact, transducer ring-down, appears in virtually all medical ultrasound devices. This artifact arises from acoustic oscillations in the piezoelectric transducer material, resulting in high-amplitude signals that obscure near-field imaging. In mechanical systems, this artifact may be merged with the imaging sheath artifact. In electronic array catheters, this artifact may be largely removed by mask subtraction. All intravascular imaging systems are vulnerable to geometric distortion produced by oblique imaging. Thus, when the ultrasound beam interrogates a plane not orthogonal to the vessel walls, an artery with a circular lumen appears elliptical in shape. Some transducer designs position the guide wire external to the transducer, thereby introducing an obligatory "wire artifact." In general, higher frequency transducers have a lower penetration depth; in practice this is not usually an issue for coronary imaging, but may become evident if peripheral arterial imaging is attempted. Alternative catheters with reduced frequency are used for large-vessel peripheral imaging and for intracardiac examination.

Safety of Coronary Ultrasound

Although intravascular ultrasound requires intracoronary instrumentation, initial studies conducted during diagnostic catheterization demonstrated few serious untoward effects (18–20). The imaging transducer can transiently occlude the coronary when advanced into a tight stenosis or a small distal vessel, but patients generally do not experience chest pain if the catheter is promptly withdrawn. Preinstrumentation nitroglycerine is advised to prevent spasm. In interventional practice, operators have safely used coronary ultrasound after most types of procedures, including balloon angioplasty and stent deployment. Despite the relative safety of coronary ultrasound, any intracoronary instrumentation carries the potential risk of intimal injury or acute vessel dissection. Although many centers use intravascular ultrasound during diagnostic catheterization, most laboratories limit credentialing for intravascular imaging procedures to personnel with interventional training. In the unlikely event of intimal disruption, this safety measure ensures that the necessary personnel and equipment are immediately available to initiate appropriate interventional corrective action.

Quantitative Luminal Measurements

Diagnostic and interventional practitioners routinely use luminal measurements to evaluate the severity of stenoses, determine the size of the "normal" reference segment, and assess gain in lumen size achieved by revascularization. Comparisons of vessel dimensions by angiography and intravascular ultrasound generally reveal a limited correlation, particularly for vessels with an eccentric luminal shape (21), presumably owing to the inability of angiography to accurately portray the complex, irregular cross-sectional profiles of atherosclerotic vessels. Poor correlations have been found between angiographic and intravascular ultrasound evaluation after balloon angioplasty due to the complex dissections that occur (22). In general, angiography overestimates lumen dimensions compared to intravascular ultrasound, even after symmetric stent implantation (23). By performing a timed or calibrated pullback through the vessel, a third dimension of information can be collected (length) allowing the calculation of the lumen, vessel, and plaque volume (24). This information has been instrumental in evaluating the mechanism of different interventional techniques, the pathology of restenosis, and the effect of drug therapy aimed at treating atherosclerosis.

Angiographically Unrecognized Disease

Intravascular ultrasound commonly detects atherosclerotic abnormalities at angiographically normal coronary sites (25–28). The long-term implications of these findings remain uncertain. However, Little et al. (28) have demonstrated that plaques with minimal to moderate angiographic narrowing are the most likely to rupture and cause acute coronary syndromes. Accordingly, the presence of angiographically occult coronary disease may have important prognostic significance. Studies are currently under way to determine the predictive value of intravascular ultrasound in determining the prognosis in patients with coronary disease. Several studies have shown that plaque burden or lumen size in the left main coronary may be an indicator of the behavior of the coronary vasculature and that left main disease seen on IVUS predicts adverse cardiac events (29,30).

Using volumetric intracoronary ultrasound, minor changes in plaque and lumen volume can be reliably detected. By comparing baseline and repeat studies, the effects of drug therapy on atheroma can be assessed (31–33). Due to the precise measures, such methodology allows pharmaceutical studies to be completed using far fewer patients than necessary if only clinical endpoints are collected (34,35).

The impact of calcium on lesion response to intervention is one of the most important contributions of intravascular ultrasound imaging. Calcium is frequent in target lesions (75%), but poorly detected by angiography (sensitivity only 40%) (36,37).

Lesions of Uncertain Severity: Left Main Lesions

Despite thorough radiographic examination with multiple projections, angiographers commonly encounter lesions that elude accurate characterization. Coronary atherosclerosis can be associated with vessel remodeling and dilatation, thus the angiographic appearance of the vessel may be normal despite significant accumulation of plaque. Lesions of uncertain severity often include ostial lesions and moderate stenoses (angiographic severity ranging from 40% to 70%) in patients whose symptomatic status is difficult to evaluate. For these ambiguous lesions, ultrasound provides tomographic measurements, enabling quantification of the stenosis independent of the radiographic projection (21,38). Bifurcation lesions are particularly difficult to assess by angiography because overlapping side branches often obscures the lesion (39). Intravascular lesion cross-sectional areas have shown a statistically significant, however, weak correlation with noninvasive stress imaging studies and other measures of stenosis severity (40–44). In general, lumen areas less that 3 to 4 mm^2 correlate with a positive stress study. In most situations, functional measures, such as fractional flow reserve, are better suited for assessing the prognostic significance of intermediate lesions.

As the severity of left main disease is of critical importance for properly determining patient treatment, intravascular imaging of this vessel deserves special mention. The normal diameter of the left main has been characterized by IVUS. Using a definition of the mean minus 2 standard deviations, the lower limit of normal left main luminal area is 7.5 mm^2 (45). With respect to functionally significant lesions, comparison with fractional flow reserve has revealed that the best cut points for predicting an FFR <0.75 is an IVUS left main diameter of <2.8 mm or area <5.9 mm^2 (46). Several studies have documented the negative impact of left main disease discovered by intravascular ultrasound on patient prognosis (29,30,47–50). In one study of 122 consecutive patients who had left main imaging and were treated medically, lesions in the left main with lumen diameters less than 3 mm clearly predicted a higher incidence of subsequent cardiac events (30).

Cardiac Allograft Disease

Identification of atherosclerotic lesions in cardiac allograft recipients represents a particularly challenging task (26,51). These patients may have diffuse vessel involvement that for reasons already enumerated conceals the atherosclerosis from angiography. Many large transplant centers now routinely perform intravascular ultrasound as an annual catheterization in all cardiac transplant recipients. Studies have revealed two pathways to transplant-associated atherosclerosis, with some patients receiving atherosclerotic plaques from the donor heart, whereas others develop immune-mediated vasculopathy (51,52).

Intravascular Ultrasound and Restenosis

The relatively poor correlation between angiographic and ultrasonic dimensions after PCI raises the issue of whether poor long-term results represent recurrence of disease or an inadequate initial procedure (53). Several multicenter clinical trials have shown that certain findings on ultrasound, such as minimal lumen area and plaque burden, can predict restenosis after intervention. The GUIDE trial evaluated the predictive value of intravascular imaging after balloon angioplasty. A residual plaque burden in the lesion of >65% or a minimal lumen area of <2 mm^2 was associated with a higher rate of restenosis (54). A careful longitudinal study of balloon angioplasty and directional atherectomy documented that the primary mechanism of restenosis was vessel contraction (negative remodeling) (SURE Trial) (55). Although stent placement abolishes this negative remodeling, it stimulates intimal hyperplasia inside the stent (56). The major predictor of in-stent restenosis has repeatedly been shown to be the final minimal stent area. Areas over 8 to 10 mm^2 are generally associated with target lesion revascularization rates of 10% or less (57–60). Although inadequate minimal stent area is the predominant factor associated with in-stent restenosis lesions, nearly 5% of cases are found to have significant mechanical implantation abnormalities (61). Many experts recommend that all cases of in-stent restenosis be interrogated by intravascular ultrasound to define the mechanism and guide therapy.

Intracoronary brachytherapy is an effective treatment for in-stent restenosis, resulting in significant retardation of neointimal hyperplasia formation. Although intravascular imaging was helpful in developing the brachytherapy delivery systems and dosing strategies, it is not generally felt to be necessary for the guidance of commercial brachytherapy delivery systems (62,63).

Balloon Angioplasty

Early intravascular studies determined the mechanism of balloon angioplasty (15,64–66). The primary mechanism of lumen enlargement is overstretching of the adventitia with axial plaque redistribution away from the lesion center. Specific predictors of restenosis following balloon PTCA include residual plaque area and minimal lumen area (54,67–69). After intravascular imaging confirmed marked occult atheroma in the "reference" segments surrounding target lesions, several investigators explored the use of oversized balloons to enhance balloon angioplasty (70–76). This "provisional-stent" strategy resulted in excellent angiographic and clinical outcomes (77). Approximately 50% of lesions could be effectively treated in this way, with the other 50% requiring stenting to achieve optimal results. Although this strategy was once proposed as a way to avoid costly stents, it has not been widely used.

New variations of balloon angioplasty, including the cutting balloon and variable diameter balloon, have also been investigated by intravascular ultrasound (78–81).

Atherectomy

Directional (65,82–84) and rotational atherectomy (85) have been extensively evaluated by intravascular ultrasound. Both clearly remove plaque; however, directional atherectomy also results in adventitial expansion. Stent expansion is impaired in regions of calcification; however, asymmetric expansion is rarely a clinical problem (86). A number of studies using IVUS-guided directional coronary atherectomy have shown excellent clinical outcomes compared to balloon angioplasty (87–89) or

stenting (90,91). Regardless, since the widespread acceptance of stenting, directional atherectomy is a rarely used technique in most laboratories.

Coronary Stent Deployment

Intravascular ultrasound has significantly influenced our understanding of the mechanism underlying stent deployment and is now widely used in guiding clinical procedures. A small observational study documented that angiographically guided stent deployment using first generation stents and low-pressure techniques resulted in an average residual stenosis of 51% (comparison of minimum stent diameter with reference segment diameter) (92). Subsequently, this same center used IVUS criteria and high-pressure balloon postdilation to optimize stent implantation (93). This study reported a subacute thrombosis rate of only 0.3% with antiplatelet agents alone and forever altered the technique of stent implantation, allowing elimination of coumadin from the poststent regimen.

Since that study, the mechanism of deployment, and subsequently criteria for optimal ultrasound-guided bare metal stent deployment, have been extensively explored (94–99). To minimize restenosis, most authorities recommend that operators attempt to achieve a minimum stent lumen cross-sectional area of over 8 mm^2 when vessel size will allow (57–60). High pressure and upsized balloons are sometimes necessary to achieve these results.

Calcium in the lesion is an important limitation to appropriate stent expansion, even after high-pressure balloon dilation (86,100–102). Pretreatment with rotational atherectomy improves stent results in these calcified lesions (103,104).

Many studies have defined predictors of restenosis following stenting. The plaque burden, plaque composition, and minimal lumen area are the most important predictors of late outcome (105–116). Most trials of angiographic versus intravascular ultrasound guidance for optimizing stent deployment have suggested a benefit for IVUS guidance (117–123). The results of the CRUISE (Can Routine Intravascular Ultrasound Impact Stent Expansion) subset of the STARS (Stent Anti-Thrombotic Regimen Study) showed that IVUS guidance significantly reduced lesion revascularization rates from 15.3% (angiographic guidance) to 8.5% (IVUS guidance) (119). The AVID study also showed a clear benefit for IVUS-guided stenting with first generation stents in several important subgroups (small vessels, vein grafts) (120). OPTICUS, however, was a neutral study (122). In this randomized European study, no long-term angiographic or clinical advantage was seen for IVUS, although the acute angiographic results were slightly better in the IVUS group. It is generally accepted that angiographic appearance can be deceiving, and IVUS can be very useful in determining suboptimal expansion and quantifying the additional gain achieved by higher pressure or larger diameter repeat balloon expansion. Additional studies have documented benefit for ultrasound guidance in small vessels (124) and long lesions (125,126) as well as high-risk bifurcation and left main lesions (127,128). The finding that many "small" vessels are actually not small but severely diseased has justified oversized stenting in these positively remodeled vessels (129).

Table 10–1

IVUS Versus Angiographically Guided PCI Trials

Year	Study	Study Design	Primary Results	Take Home Points
1995	Colombo (93)	Single-center registry. 359 patients. IVUS after angiographically adequate stent implantation.	30% of stents placed had optimal expansion after angiographic guidance (CSA >60% of reference). After, IVUS guidance increased to 96%. Six-month SAT 1.4% on antiplatelet therapy only.	IVUS guidance resulted in a 26% increase in minimal stent area (MSA). Study led to now routine process of high pressure stent implant without postprocedure coumadin.
1997	Albiero (117)	Case control (two sites) 346 patients. IVUS versus angiographically guided stent.	Early after stent implant, restenosis is less with IVUS guidance (9.2% IVUS versus 28.3% angio, p = 0.04) No difference at late follow-up (22.7% versus 23.7%).	Acute results of stent implantation can be optimized with IVUS.
1997	Stone (70) CLOUT	Multicenter registry 102 patients. IVUS-guided PTCA after angiographically adequate result.	IVUS-measured EEM diameter in reference vessel used to define oversized balloon diameter. Increased balloon size in 73% of lesions. No increase in dissections after use of IVUS-determined oversized balloon.	Due to positive remodeling, oversized balloons (B:A ratio 1:3) may safely be used for PTCA. IVUS is needed to assess degree of remodeling (not apparent angiographically).
1998	de Jaegere (118) (MUSIC)	Multicenter registry 161 patients. IVUS-guidance of stent implantation.	Stents implanted using IVUS-guided criteria associated with a 6-month TVR rate of 4.5% and angiographic restenosis rate of 9.7%. Antiplatelet agents only with optimal IVUS result. No acute Q-wave MI, one CABG, 1.3% SAT.	Tested hypothesis that criteria-driven IVUS-guidance could improve restenosis after stenting. Compared to contemporary stent studies had lowest reported TVR rate.
1998	Schiele (121) (RESIST)	Randomized multicenter trial. 155 patients. IVUS versus angiographically guided stent.	80% achieved IVUS criteria. Stent CSA in IVUS group 20% larger. Restenosis at 6 months (22.5% IVUS versus 28.8% angio p = 0.25). Lumen area by IVUS only predictor of restenosis.	IVUS group had larger 6-month MSA. Study was underpowered for restenosis endpoint.
1999	Schroeder (73)	Single-center registry 252 consecutive patients. IVUS-guided PTCA.	PTCA with balloon sized 1:1 with lesion EEM resulted in a low MACE rate (14%) and low angiographic restenosis rate (19%). Only 2% received stents.	Aggressive PTCA strategy based on vessel remodeling. Many dissections were left untreated and were not associated with adverse events.
1999	Abizaid (74)	Single-center registry 284 consecutive patients. IVUS guided provisional stenting.	PTCA with balloon sized 1:1 with lesion EEM. Stents placed for inadequate results. 47% of procedures successful with balloon only. Overall 1-year TLR 12% (IVUS-guided PTCA lesions: 8%, stented lesions: 16%.)	Aggressive PTCA strategy with more liberal use of stents for dissections than in the Schroeder study. Clinical results after IVUS-guided balloon only are excellent.
2000	Frey (71) SIPS	Randomized single-center trial. 291 consecutive patients. IVUS-guided versus angiographically guided PCI.	Stent use encouraged only for inadequate PTCA result and was similar in two groups: (47.7% versus 49.0%). 6-month restenosis: 29% IVUS versus 35% angio p = 0.42. 2-year TLR: 17% versus 29%, p = 0.02.	Clinical outcome at 2 years improved by routine IVUS guidance of PCI. IVUS strategy was cost effective (75).
2000	Fitzgerald (119) CRUISE	Case control (multicenter) 525 patients. IVUS versus angiographically guided stent.	Acute MSA: 7.78 mm^2 IVUS versus 7.06 mm^2 angio, p <0.001. 9-month TLR: 8.5% IVUS versus 15.5 angio, p <0.05.	Clinical outcomes at 9 months improved by routine IVUS guidance of Palmaz-Schatz stent implantation.

(Continued)

Table 10–1

(Continued)

Year	Study	Study Design	Primary Results	Take Home Points
2000	Russo (120) AVID	Randomized multicenter trial. 759 patients. IVUS versus angiographically guided stent.	Acute MSA: 7.54 mm^2 IVUS versus 6.94 mm^2 angio, p <0.01. 12-month TLR significantly better in IVUS-guided graft or smaller vessel (<3.25) lesions.	Final report not yet publicized. TLR reported as 4.9% IVUS versus 10.8% angio in protocol-compliant patients.
2001	Mudra (122) OPTICUS	Randomized multicenter trial. 550 patients. IVUS versus angiographically guided stent.	6-month restenosis: 24.5% IVUS versus 28.8% angio, p = 0.68. 12-month MACE: Relative risk 1.07, p = 0.71. 12-month TLR: Relative risk 1.04, p = 0.87.	Only neutral randomized trial. Acute gain greater in IVUS group (2.07 mm^2 versus 1.93 mm^2, p <0.001).
2003	Oemrawsingh (125) TULIP	Randomized single-center trial. 144 patients. IVUS versus angiographically guided stents.	Stenosis >20-mm long. 6-month restenosis: 23% IVUS versus 45% angio, p = 0.008. 12-month TLR: 10% versus 23%, p = 0.018).	Clinical outcome improved with IVUS guidance of long lesion stenting.
2003	Schiele (76) BEST	Randomized multicenter trial. 254 patients. IVUS-guided PTCA versus angiographically guided stent.	Noninferiority design. 44% of IVUS "PTCA" group received stents. 6-month restenosis: 16.8% IVUS versus 18.1% stent, noninferior.	IVUS-guided PTCA with provisional stenting not inferior to routine angiographically guided stent implantation.

Definitive evidence to support routine IVUS guidance of *all* stent procedures is lacking (123), although positive studies in varied subgroups suggest that IVUS can be of benefit in many stent procedures (Table 10–1).

In-stent restenosis is primarily due to intimal hyperplasia. Treatment of in-stent restenosis with various balloon and other devices can be effectively monitored by IVUS (130–132). The most important predictor of subsequent restenosis is the final minimal stent area. Maximizing the minimal stent area is of paramount importance regardless of the technique used. Subacute stent thrombosis is a rare but serious complication of stent placement. IVUS has usually demonstrated abnormalities in cases of thrombosis. These are often not appreciated by routine angiography (133,134). Due to the low incidence of thrombosis, studies after high pressure stent implantation have not demonstrated a benefit for IVUS guidance on subsequent subacute thrombosis rates (135). Data from core laboratories with careful clinical follow-up have allowed investigation of particular IVUS findings. Minor stent malapposition (136) or small edge tears (17) have not adversely affected patient outcome after stenting, and may be left untreated.

In everyday practice, the most important measurements to be obtained from IVUS include the reference lumen diameter, the poststent lumen area, and the lesion length. The reference lumen diameter is used to determine the appropriate stent diameter, the lesion length (measured from a timed pullback), the stent length, and the stent lumen area the adequacy of expansion and apposition (Fig. 10–1). Operators should also be familiar with the relationship between diameter and area for the devices used in coronary intervention (Table 10–2). Use of the package inserts listing expected balloon (or stent) diameters at given pressures should be discouraged. Direct measurement by IVUS will detect the actual degree of expansion. Determinants of expansion at any given pressure are dependent on the compliance of the vessel, not just the balloon material (137).

Drug-eluting Stents

Drug-eluting stents have replaced bare metal stents for the treatment of many lesions. The development of drug-eluting stents was extensively monitored by intravascular ultrasound (138–142). The predominant mechanism of improved patient outcome is marked suppression of neointimal hyperplasia. Most early studies testing drug-eluting stents have involved intravascular imaging; however, randomized studies comparing ultrasound-guided and angiographic-guided drug-eluting stent placement are lacking. Due to the near-complete suppression of neointimal hyperplasia, the optimal minimal stent area to prevent target lesion revascularization is less for drug-eluting stents than for bare metal stents (143). Restenosis following drug-eluding stent placement, although infrequent, is generally due to continued intimal hyperplasia (144–146). The site of restenosis is also most often associated with the stented portion having the smallest postdeployment minimal stent area (147).

Intravascular ultrasound is of continued utility in the drug eluting stent era. Proper sizing, full lesion coverage, and proper expansion are best accomplished with IVUS. It is important to remember that the drug-eluting stents are virtually identical to the bare metal stent with respect to their mechanical

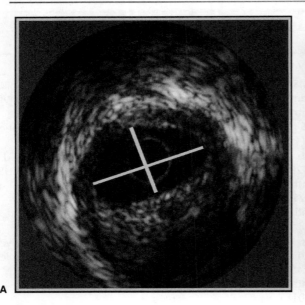
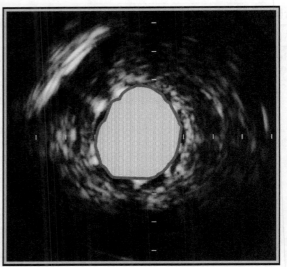

A   **B**

Figure 10–1.

Most useful measurements during PCI. **A:** Device size selection: reference lumen diameter. **B:** Result optimization: lesion (stent) lumen cross-sectional area.

properties. Thus, the issues of proper sizing, impact of calcium or lesion morphology on expansion, and proper placement are not different with these new devices. The lessons learned from years of IVUS use in bare metal stents continue to apply to drug-eluting stents.

Vulnerable Plaque

Due to the ability of IVUS to characterize vessel wall composition, new insights are now possible regarding vulnerable plaque and clinical syndromes (12–14,148–160). Studies using IVUS have documented diffuse multifocal abnormalities in patients presenting with unstable syndromes (14,156,158). New processing techniques for IVUS that incorporate phase information in addition to amplitude show promise for further characterizing plaque content and potentially identifying vulnerable plaque (161,162). Additional studies will be required

to define the optimal management of patients identified by IVUS to have vulnerable plaque.

Summary

IVUS adds significantly to day-to-day decision making in the catheterization laboratory. Optimal techniques for stent placement have been developed using IVUS. Drug-eluting stents are predicted to expand the number and complexity of lesions treated percutaneously in the catheterization laboratory. IVUS is particularly useful in small vessels, complicated anatomy, and long lesions. Therefore, active interventionalists should have a good working knowledge of IVUS and how it can be used to optimize PCI.

REFERENCES

1. Hodgson JM, Graham SP, Savakus AD, et al. Clinical percutaneous imaging of coronary anatomy using an over the wire ultrasound catheter system. *Int J Card Imaging*. 1989;4:187–193.
2. Bom N, Lancée CT, VanEgmond FC. An ultrasonic intracardiac scanner. *Ultrasonics*. 1972;10:72–76.
3. Nissen SE, Grimes CL, Gurley JC, et al. Application of a new phased-array ultrasound imaging catheter in the assessment of vascular dimensions: in vivo comparison to cine angiography. *Circulation*. 1990;81:660–666.
4. Yock PG, Starksen N. Clinical applications of intravascular ultrasound imaging. *Am J Card Imaging*. 1991;12:54–59.
5. Di Mario C, Gorge G, Peters R, et al. Clinical application and image interpretation in intracoronary ultrasound. Study group on intracoronary imaging of the working group of coronary circulation and of the subgroup on intravascular ultrasound of the working group of echocardiography of the European Society of Cardiology. *Eur Heart J*. 1998;19:207–229.
6. Oesterle SN, Limpijankit T, Yeung AC, et al. Ultrasound logic: the value of intracoronary ultrasound imaging for the interventionist. *Cathet Cardiovasc Intervent*. 1999;47:475–490.

Table 10–2	
Target Lumen Areas Based on Vessel Diameter or Chosen Balloon (Stent) Size	
Lumen Diameter (Balloon Size) (mm)	**Expected Lumen CSA (mm^2)**
2.00	3.14
2.25	3.98
2.50	4.90
2.75	5.94
3.00	7.07
3.25	8.30
3.50	9.62
3.75	11.00
4.00	12.57

7. Mintz GS, Nissen SE, Anderson WD, et al. ACC clinical expert consensus document on standards for the acquisition, measurement and reporting of intravascular ultrasound studies: a report of the American College of Cardiology Task Force on Clinical Expert Consensus Documents. *J Am Coll Cardiol.* 2001;37:1478–1492.

8. Prati F, Di Mario C, Gil R, et al. Usefulness of on-line three-dimensional reconstruction of intracoronary ultrasound for guidance of stent deployment. *Am J Cardiol.* 1996;77:455–461.

9. Ziada KM, Kapadia SR, Tuzcu EM, et al. The current status of intravascular ultrasound imaging. *Current Problems in Cardiology.* 1999;24.

10. Gil R, von Birgelen C, Prati F, et al. Usefulness of three-dimensional reconstruction for interpretation and quantitative analysis of intracoronary ultrasound during stent deployment. *Am J Cardiol.* 1996;77:761–764.

11. Schoenhagen P, Tuzcu EM, Stillman AE, et al. Non-invasive assessment of plaque morphology and remodeling in mildly stenotic coronary segments: comparison of 16 slice computed tomography and intravascular ultrasound. *Coronary Artery Disease.* 2003;14:459–462.

12. Hodgson JM, Reddy KG, Suneja R, et al. Intracoronary ultrasound imaging: correlation of plaque morphology with angiography, clinical syndrome and procedural results in patients undergoing coronary angioplasty. *J Am Coll Cardiol.* 1993;21:35–44.

13. Rasheed Q, Dhawale P, Anderson J, et al. Intracoronary ultrasound defined plaque composition: Computer-aided plaque characterization and correlation with histologic samples obtained during directional coronary atherectomy. *Am Heart J.* 1995;129:631–637.

14. Rioufol G, Finet G, Ginon I, et al. Multiple atherosclerotic plaque rupture in acute coronary syndrome: a three-vessel intravascular ultrasound study. *Circulation.* 2002;106:804–808.

15. Potkin BN, Keren G, Mintz GS, et al. Arterial responses to balloon coronary angioplasty: an intravascular ultrasound study. *J Am Coll Cardiol.* 1992;20:942–951.

16. Fitzgerald PJ, Ports TA, Yock PG. Contribution of localized calcium deposits to dissection after angioplasty. *Circulation.* 1992;86:64–70.

17. Sheris SJ, Canos MR, Weissman NJ. Natural history of intravascular ultrasound-detected edge dissections from coronary stent placement. *Am Heart J.* 2000;139:59–63.

18. Hausmann D, Erbel R, Alibelli-Chemarin M-J, et al. The safety of intracoronary ultrasound. A multicenter survey of 2207 examinations. *Circulation.* 1995;91:623–630.

19. Batkoff BW, Linker DT. Safety of intracoronary ultrasound: data from a Multicenter European Registry. *Cathet Cardiovasc Diagn.* 1996;38:238–241.

20. Pinto FJ, St. Goar FG, Gao S-Z, et al. Immediate and one-year safety of intracoronary ultrasonic imaging. Evaluation with serial quantitative angiography. *Circulation.* 1993;88:1709–1714.

21. Nissen SE, Gurley JC, Grines CL, et al. Intravascular ultrasound assessment of lumen size and wall morphology in normal subjects and patients with coronary artery disease. *Circulation.* 1991;84:1087–1099.

22. Nakamura S, Mahon DJ, Maheswaran B, et al. An explanation for discrepancy between angiographic and intravascular ultrasound measurements after percutaneous transluminal coronary angioplasty. *J Am Coll Cardiol.* 1995;25:633–639.

23. Blasini R, Neumann FJ, Schmitt C, et al. Comparison of angiography and intravascular ultrasound for the assessment of lumen size after coronary stent placement; impact of dilation pressures. *Cathet Cardiovasc Diagn.* 1997;42:113–119.

24. Dhawale PJ, Wilson DL, Hodgson JMcB. Volumetric intracoronary ultrasound: methods and validation. *Cathet Cardiovasc Diagn.* 1994;33:296–307.

25. White CJ, Ramee SR, Collins Tj, et al. Ambiguous coronary angiography: clinical utility of intravascular ultrasound. *Cathet Cardiovasc Diagn.* 1992;26:200–203.

26. St. Goar FG, Pinto FJ, Alderman EL, et al. Detection of coronary atherosclerosis in young adult hearts using intravascular ultrasound. *Circulation.* 1992;86:756–763.

27. Mintz GS, Painter JA, Pichard AD, et al. Atherosclerosis in angiography "normal" coronary artery reference segments: an intravascular ultra-sound study with clinical correlations. *J Am Coll Cardiol.* 1995;25:1479–1485.

28. Little WC, Constantinescu M, Applegate RJ, et al. Can coronary angiography predict the site of a subsequent myocardial infarction in patients with mild to moderate coronary artery disease? *Circulation.* 1988;78:1157–1166.

29. Riccardi MH, Meyers S, Choi K, et al. Angiographically silent left main disease detected by intravascular ultrasound: a marker for future adverse cardiac events. *Am Heart J.* 2003;146:507–512.

30. Abizaid AS, Mintz GS, Abizaid A, et al. One-year follow-up after intravascular ultrasound assessment of moderate left main coronary artery disease in patients with ambiguous angiograms. *J Am Coll Cardiol.* 1999;34:707–715.

31. Nissen SE, Tsunoda T, Tuzcu EM, et al. Effect of recombinant ApoA-1 Milano on coronary atherosclerosis in patients with acute coronary syndromes. *JAMA.* 2003;290:2292–2300.

32. Nissen SE, Tuzcu EM, Schoenhagen P, et al. Effect of intensive compared with moderate lipid-lowering therapy on progression of coronary atherosclerosis. *JAMA.* 2004;291:1071–1080.

33. Schartl M, Bocksch W, Koschyk DH, et al. Use of intravascular ultrasound to compare effects of different strategies of lipid-lowering therapy on plaque volume and composition in patients with coronary artery disease. *Circulation.* 2001;104:387–392.

34. Franco AC, Nissen SE. Coronary intravascular ultrasound: implication for understanding the development and potential regression of atherosclerosis. *Am J Cardiol.* 2001;88:7M–20M.

35. Schoenhagen P, Nissen SE. Coronary atherosclerotic disease burden: an emerging endpoint in progression/regression studies using intravascular ultrasound. *Curr Drug Targets Cardiovasc Haematol Disord.* 2003;3:218–226.

36. Tuzcu EM, Berkalp B, De Franco AC, et al. The dilemma of diagnosing coronary calcification: angiography versus intravascular ultrasound. *J Am Coll Cardiol.* 1996;27:832–838.

37. Mintz GS, Pichard AD, Popma JJ, et al. Determinants and correlates of target lesion calcium in coronary artery disease: a clinical, angiographic and intravascular ultrasound study. *J Am Coll Cardiol.* 1997;29:268–274.

38. Topol EJ, Nissen SE. Our preoccupation with coronary luminology: dissociation between clinical and angiographic findings in ischemic heart disease. *Circulation.* 1995;92:2333–2342.

39. Badak O, Schoenhagen P, Tsunoda T, et al. Characteristics of atherosclerotic plaque distribution in coronary artery bifurcations: an intravascular ultrasound analysis. *Coron Artery Dis.* 2003;14:309–316.

40. Moses JW, Undermir C, Strain JE, et al. Relation between single tomographic intravascular ultrasound image parameters and intracoronary Doppler flow velocity in patients with intermediately severe coronary stenoses. *Am Heart J.* 1998;135:988–994.

41. Takagi A, Tsurumi Y, Ishii Y, et al. Clinical potential of intravascular ultrasound for physiological assessment of coronary stenosis. Relationship between quantitative ultrasound tomography and pressure-derived fractional flow reserve. *Circulation.* 1999;100:250–255.

42. Nishioka T, Amanullah AM, Luo H, et al. Clinical validation of intravascular ultrasound imaging for assessment of coronary stenosis severity. *J Am Coll Cardiol.* 1999;33:1870–1878.

43. Briguori C, Anzuini A, Airoldi F, et al. Intravascular ultrasound criteria for the assessment of the functional significance of intermediate coronary stenoses and comparison with fractional flow reserve. *Am J Cardiol.* 2001;87:136–141.

44. Takayama T, Hodgson JMcB. Prediction of the physiologic severity of coronary lesions using 3-D IVUS: validation by direct coronary pressure measurements. *Cathet Cardiovasc Intervent.* 2001;53:48–55.

45. Fassa A, Wagatsuma K, Higano ST, et al. Intravascular ultrasound-guided treatment for angiographically indeterminate left main coronary artery disease. *J Am Coll Cardiol.* 2005;45:204–211.

46. Jasti V, Ivan E, Yalamanchili V, et al. Correlations between fractional flow reserve and intravascular ultrasound in patients with an ambiguous left main coronary artery stenosis. *Circulation.* 2004;110:2831–2836.

47. Wolfhard GG, Konrza T, Haude M, et al. Intravascular ultrasound (IVUS) examination reverses therapeutic decision from percutaneous

intervention to a surgical approach in patients with alterations of the left main stem. *Thorac Cardiovasc Surg.* 1998;46:281–284.

48. Nishimura RA, Higano ST, Holmes DR. Use of intracoronary ultrasound imaging for assessing left main coronary artery disease. *Mayo Clin Proc.* 1993;68:134–140.

49. Davies SW, Winterton SJ, Rothman MT. Intravascular ultrasound to assess left main stem coronary artery lesion. *Br Heart J.* 1992;68:524–526.

50. Hermiller JB, Buller CE, Tenaglia AN, et al. Unrecognized left main coronary artery disesase in patients undergoing interventional procedures. *Am J Cardiol.* 1993;71:173–176.

51. Tuzcu EM, Hobbs RE, Rincon G, et al. Occult and frequent transmission of atherosclerotic coronary disease with cardiac transplantation: insights from intravascular ultrasound. *Circulation.* 1995;91:1706–1713.

52. Tsutsui H, Ziada KM, Schoenhagen P, et al. Lumen loss in transplant coronary artery disease is a biphasic process involving early intimal thickening and late constrictive remodeling. *Circulation.* 2001;104:653–657.

53. Honye J, Mahon DJ, Jain A, et al. Morphological effects of coronary balloon angioplasty in vivo assessed by intravascular ultrasound imaging. *Circulation.* 1992;85:1012–1025.

54. Fitzgerald PJ, Yock PG. Mechanisms and outcomes of angioplasty and atherectomy assessed by intravascular ultrasound imaging. *J Clin Ultrasound.* 1993;21:579–588.

55. Kimura T, Kaburagi S, Tamura T, et al. Remodeling of human coronary arteries undergoing coronary angioplasty or atherectomy. *Circulation.* 1997;96:475–483.

56. Hoffmann R, Mintz GS, Dussaillant GR, et al. Patterns and mechanisms of instent restenosis. A serial intravascular ultrasound study. *Circulation.* 1996;94:1247–1254.

57. Morino Y, Honda Y, Okura H, et al. An optimal diagnostic threshold for minimal stent area to predict target lesion revascularization following stent implantation in native coronary lesions. *Am J Cardiol.* 2001;88:301–303.

58. De Feyter PF, Kay P, Disco C, et al. Reference chart derived from post-stent-implantation intravascular ultrasound predictors of 6-month expected restenosis on quantitative coronary angiography. *Circulation.* 1999;100:1777–1783.

59. Ziada KM, Kapadia SR, Belli G, et al. Prognostic value of absolute versus relative measures of the procedural result after successful coronary stenting: importance of vessel size in predicting long-term freedom from target vessel revascularization. *Am Heart J.* 2001;1414:823–831.

60. Kasaoka S, Tobis JM, Akiyama T, et al. Angiographic and intravascular ultrasound predictors of in-stent restenosis. *J Am Coll Cardiol.* 1998;32:1630–1635.

61. Castagna MT, Mintz GS, Leiboff BO, et al. The contribution of "mechanical" problems to in-stent restenosis: an intravascular ultrasonographic analysis of 1090 consecutive in-stent restenosis lesions. *Am Heart J.* 2001;142:970–974.

62. Mintz GS, Weissman NJ, Fitzgerald PJ. Intravascular ultrasound assessment of the mechanisms and results of brachytherapy. *Circulation.* 2001;104: 1320–1325.

63. Meerkin D, Tardif JC, Crocker IR, et al. Effects of intracoronary β-radiation therapy after coronary angioplasty. *Circulation.* 1999;99:1660–1665.

64. Fitzgerald PF, Yock PG. Mechanisms and outcomes of angioplasty and atherectomy assessed by intravascular ultrasound imaging. *J Clin Ultrasound.* 1993;21:579–588.

65. Tenaglia AN, Buller CE, Kisslo KB, et al. Mechanisms of balloon angioplasty and directional coronary atherectomy as assessed by intracoronary ultrasound. *J Am Coll Cardiol.* 1992;20:685–691.

66. Mintz GS, Pichard AD, Kent KM, et al. Axial plaque redistribution as a mechanism of percutaneous transluminal coronary angioplasty. *Am J Cardiol.* 1996;77:427–430.

67. Mintz GS, Popma JJ, Prichard AD, et al. Arterial remodeling after coronary angioplasty: a serial intravascular study. *Circulation.* 1996;94:35–51.

68. Dangas G, Mintz GS, Mehran R, et al. Preintervention arterial remodeling as an independent predictor of target-lesion revascularization after non-

stent coronary intervention: an analysis of 777 lesions with intravascular ultrasound imaging. *Circulation.* 1999;99:3149–3154.

69. Okura H, Bayase M, Shimodozono S, et al. Impact of pre-interventional arterial remodeling on subsequent vessel behavior after balloon angioplasty: a serial intravascular ultrasound study. *J Am Coll Cardiol.* 2001;38:2001–2005.

70. Stone GW, Hodgson JMcB, Goar FG, et al. Improved procedural results of coronary angioplasty with intravascular ultrasound guided balloon sizing: The CLOUT Pilot Trial. Clinical outcomes with ultrasound trial (CLOUT) investigators. *Circulation.* 1997;95:2004–2052.

71. Frey AW, Hodgson JMcB, Müller C, et al. Ultrasound-guided strategy for provisional stenting with focal balloon combination catheter: results from the randomized strategy for intracoronary ultrasound-guided PTCA and stenting (SIPS) trial. *Circulation.* 2000;102:2497–2502.

72. Haase KK, Athanasiadis A, Mahrholdt H, et al. Acute and one year follow-up results after vessel size adapted PTCA using intracoronary ultrasound. *Eur Heart J.* 1998;19:263–272.

73. Schroeder S, Baumback A, Haase KK, et al. Reduction of restenosis by vessel size adapted percutaneous transluminal coronary angioplasty using intravascular ultrasound. *Am J Cardiol.* 1999;83:875–879.

74. Abizaid A, Pichard AD, Mintz GS, et al. Acute and long-term results of an intravascular ultrasound-guided percutaneous transluminal coronary angioplasty/provisional stent implantation strategy. *Am J Cardiol.* 1999;84:1298–1303.

75. Mueller C, Hodgson JMcB, Schindler C, et al. Cost-effectiveness of intracoronary ultrasound for percutaneous coronary interventions. *Am J Cardiol.* 2003;91:143–147.

76. Schiele F, Meneveau N, Gilard M, et al. Intravascular ultrasound-guided balloon angioplasty compared with stent: immediate and 6-month results of the multicenter, randomized Balloon Equivalent to Stent Study (BEST). *Circulation.* 2003;107:545–551.

77. Cantor WJ, Peterson ED, Popma JJ, et al. Provisional stenting strategies: systematic overview and implications for clinical decision-making. *J Am Coll Cardiol.* 2000;36:1142–1151.

78. Müller C, Hodgson JMcB, Roskamm H, et al. Single device approach to ultrasound guided PTCA and stenting: initial experience with a combined intracoronary ultrasound/variable diameter balloon. *Cath CV Diag.* 40:393–399.

79. Karvouni E, Standovic G, Albiero R, et al. Cutting balloon angioplasty for treatment of calcified coronary lesions. *Cathet Cardiovasc Intervent.* 2001;54:473–481.

80. Hara H, Nakamura M, Asahara T, et al. Intravascular ultrasonic comparisons of mechanisms of vasodilatation of cutting balloon angioplasty versus conventional balloon angioplasty. *Am J Cardiol.* 2002;89:1253–1256.

81. Montorsi P, Galli S, Fabbiocchi F, et al. Mechanism of cutting balloon angioplasty for in-stent restenosis: An intravascular ultrasound study. *Cathet Cardiovasc Intervent.* 2002;56:166–173.

82. Suneja R, Nair RN, Reddy KG, et al. Mechanisms of angiographically successful directional coronary atherectomy: evaluation by intracoronary ultrasound and comparison with transluminal coronary angioplasty. *Am Heart J.* 1993;126:507–514.

83. Suarez de, Lezo J Romero M, Medina A, et al. Intracoronary ultrasound assessment of directional coronary atherectomy: immediate and follow up findings. *J Am Coll Cardiol.* 1993;21:298–307.

84. Matar FA, Mintz GS, Farb A, et al. The contribution of tissue removal to lumen improvement after directional coronary atherectomy. *Am J Cardiol.* 994;74:647–650.

85. Mintz GS, Potkin BN, Keren G, et al. Intravascular ultrasound evaluation of the effect of rotational atherectomy in obstructive atherosclerotic coronary artery disease. *Circulation.* 1992;86:1383–1393.

86. Albrecht D, Kaspers S, Fussl R, Hopp HW, et al. Coronary plaque morphology affects stent deployment: assessment by intracoronary ultrasound. *Cathet Cardiovasc Diagn.* 1996;38:229–235.

87. Simonton CA, Leon MB, Saim DS, et al. "Optimal" directional coronary atherectomy final results of the optimal atherectomy restenosis study (OARS). *Circulation.* 1998;97:332–339.

88. Baim DS, Cutlip DE, Sharma SK, et al. Final results of the balloon versus optimal atherectomy trial (BOAT). *Circulation.* 1998;97:322–331.

89. Suzuki T, Hosokawa H, Katoh O, et al. Effects of adjunctive balloon angioplasty after intravascular ultrasound-guided optimal directional coronary atherectomy. *J Am Coll Cardiol.* 1999;34:1028–1035.

90. Moussa I, Moses J, Di Mario DC, et al. Stenting after optimal lesion debulking (SOLD) registry. Angiographic and clinical outcome. *Circulation.* 1998;98:1604–1609.

91. Tsuchikane E, Sumitsuji S, Awata N, et al. Final results of the STent versus directional coronary Atherectomy Randomized Trial (START). *J Am Coll Cardiol.* 1999;34:1050–1057.

92. Nakamura S, Colombo A, Gaglione A, et al. Intracoronary ultrasound observations during stent implantation. *Circulation.* 1994;89;2026–2034.

93. Colombo A, Hall P, Nakamura S, et al. Intracoronary stenting without anticoagulation accomplished with intravascular ultrasound guidance. *Circulation.* 1995;91:1676–1688.

94. Maehera A, Takage A, Okura H, et al. Longitudinal plaque redistribution during stent expansion. *Am J Cardiol.* 2000;86:1069–1072.

95. Stone GW, St Goar FG, Hodgson JMcB, et al. Analysis of the relation between stent implantation pressure and expansion. Optimal stent implantation (OSTI) investigators. *Am J Cardiol.* 1999;83:1397–1400.

96. Hur SH, Kitamura K, Morino Y, et al. Efficacy of postdeployment balloon dilatation for current generation stents as assessed by intravascular ultrasound. *Am J Cardiol.* 2001;88:1114–1119.

97. Colombo A, De Gregorio J, Moussa II, et al. Intravascular ultrasound-guided percutaneous transluminal coronary angioplasty with provisional spot stenting for treatment of long coronary lesions. *J Am Coll Cardiol.* 2001;38:1427–1433.

98. Gorge G, Haude M, Ge J, et al. Intravascular ultrasound after low and high inflation pressure coronary artery stent implantation. *J Am Coll Cardiol.* 1995;26:725–730.

99. Shah VM, Mintz GS, Apple S, et al. Background incidence of late malapposition after bare-metal stent implantation. *Circulation.* 2002;106:1753–1755.

100. Hodgson JM. Oh no, even stenting is affected by calcium! *Cathet Cardiovasc Diagn.* 1996;38:236–237.

101. Hoffmann R, Mintz GS, Popma JJ, Satler et al. Treatment of calcified coronary lesions with Palmaz-Schatz stents. An intravascular ultrasound study. *Eur Heart J.* 1998;19:1224–1231.

102. Vavuranakis M, Toutouzas K, Stefanadis C, et al. Stent deployment in calcified lesions: can we overcome calcific restraint with high-pressure balloon inflations? *Cathet Cardiovasc Intervent.* 2001;52:164–172.

103. Hoffmann R, Mintz GS, Kent KM, et al. Comparative early and nine-month results of rotational atherectomy, stents, and the combination of both for calcified lesions in large coronary arteries. *Am J Cardiol.* 1998;81:552–557.

104. Henneke KH, Regar E, Konig A, et al. Impact of target lesion calcification on coronary stent expansion after rotational atherectomy. *Am Heart J.* 1999;137:93–99.

105. von Birgelen C, Gil R, Ruygrok P, et al. Optimized expansion of the Wallstent compared to the Palmaz-Schatz stent: on-line observations with two- and three- dimensional intracoronary ultrasound after angiographic guidance. *Am Heart J.* 1996;131:1067–1075.

106. Okura H, Morino Y, Oshima A, et al. Preintervention arterial remodeling affects clinical outcome following stenting: an intravascular ultrasound study. *J Am Coll Cardiol.* 2001;37:1031–1035.

107. Endo A, Hirayama H, Yoshida O, et al. Arterial remodeling influences the development of intimal hyperplasia after stent implantation. *J Am Coll Cardiol.* 2001;37:70–75.

108. Hibi K, Suzuki T, Honda Y, et al. Quantitative and spatial relation of baseline atherosclerotic plaque burden and subsequent in-stent neointimal proliferation as determined by intravascular ultrasound. *Am J Cardiol.* 2002;90:1164–1167.

109. Shiran A, Weissman NJ, Leiboff B, et al. Effect of preintervention plaque burden on subsequent intimal hyperplasia in stented coronary artery lesions. *Am J Cardiol.* 2000;86:1318–1321.

110. Hoffman R, Mintz GS, Kent KM, et al. Serial intravascular ultrasound predictors of restenosis at the margins of Palmaz-Shatz stents. *Am J Cardiol.* 1997;79:951–953.

111. Hoffman R, Mintz GS, Mehran R, et al. Intravascular ultrasound predictors of angiographic restenosis in lesions treated with Palmaz-Schatz stents. *J Am Coll Cardiol.* 1998;31:43–49.

112. Prati F, Di Mario C, Moussa I, et al. In-stent neointimal proliferation correlates with the amount of residual plaque burden outside the stent: an intravascular ultrasound study. *Circulation.* 1999;99:1011–1014.

113. Hong MK, Park SW, Lee CW, et al. Preintervention arterial remodeling as a predictor of intimal hyperplasia after intracoronary stenting: a serial intravascular ultrasound study. *Clin Cardiol.* 2002;25:11–15.

114. Hong MK, Park SW, Lee CW, et al. Relation between residual plaque burden after stenting and six-month angiographic restenosis. *Am J Cardiol.* 2002;89:368–371.

115. Mintz GS, Popma JJ, Hong MK, et al. Intravascular ultrasound to discern device-specific effects and mechanisms of restenosis. *Am J Cardiol.* 1996;78:18–22.

116. Bauters C, Hubert E, Prat A, et al. Predictors of restenosis after coronary stent implantation. *J Am Coll Cardiol.* 1998;31:1291–1298.

117. Albiero R, Rau T, Schluter M, et al. Comparison of immediate and intermediate-term results of intravascular ultrasound versus angiography-guided Palmaz-Schatz stent implantation in matched lesions. *Circulation.* 1997;96:2997–3005.

118. DeJaegere P, Mudra H, Figulla H, et al. Intravascular ultrasound-guided optimized stent deployment. Immediate and 6-month clinical and angiographic results from the Multicenter Ultrasound Stenting in Coronaries Study (MUSIC study). *Eur Heart J.* 1998;19:1214–1223.

119. Fitzgerald PJ, Oshima A, Hayase M, et al. Final results of the Can Routine Ultrasound Influence Stent Expansion (CRUISE) study. *Circulation.* 2000; 102:523–530.

120. Russo RJ, Attubato MJ, Davidson CJ, et al. Angiography versus intravascular ultrasound-directed stent placement: final results from AVID. *Circulation* (abstr.). 1999;100:I–234.

121. Schiele F, Meneveau N, Vuillemenot A, et al. Impact of intravascular ultrasound guidance in stent deployment on 6-month restenosis rate: a multicenter, randomized study comparing two strategies with and without intravascular ultrasound guidance. RESIST study group. Restenosis after IVUS guided stenting. *J Am Coll Cardiol.* 1998;32:320–328.

122. Mudra H, DiMario C, de Jaegere P, et al. Randomized comparison of coronary stent implantation under ultrasound or angiographic guidance to reduce stent restenosis (OPTICUS study). *Circulation.* 2001;104:1343–1349.

123. Orford JL, Lerman A, Homes DR. Routine intravascular ultrasound guidance of percutaneous coronary intervention. A critical reappraisal. *J Am Coll Cardiol.* 2004;43:1335–1342.

124. Park SW, Lee CW, Hong MK, et al. Randomized comparison of coronary stenting with optimal balloon angioplasty for treatment of lesions in small coronary arteries. *Eur Heart J.* 2000;21:1785–1789.

125. Oemrawsingh PV, Mintz GS, Schalij MJ, et al. Intravascular ultrasound guidance improves angiographic and clinical outcome of stent implantation for long coronary artery stenoses: final results of a randomized comparison with angiographic guidance (TULIP Study). *Circulation.* 2003;107:62–67.

126. Nageh T, De Belder AJ, Thomas MR, et al. Intravascular ultrasound-guided stenting in long lesions: an insight into possible mechanisms of restenosis and comparision of angiographic and intravascular ultrsound data from the MUSIC and RENEWAL trials. *J Interven Cardiol.* 2001;14:397–405.

127. Robinson NM, Balcon R, Layton CA, et al. Intravascular ultrasound assessment of culotte stent deployment for the treatment of stenoses at major coronary bifurcations. *Int J Cardiovasc Intervent.* 2001;4:21–27.

128. Hong MK, Mintz GS, Hong MK, et al. Intravascular ultrasound predictors of target lesion revascularization after stenting of protected left main coronary artery stenoses. *Am J Cardiol.* 1999;83:175–179.

129. Okabe T, Asakura Y, Ishikawa S, et al. Determining appropriate small vessels for stenting by intravascular ultrasound. *J Invasiv Cardiol.* 2000; 12:625–630.

130. Wu Z, McMillan TL, Mintz GS, et al. Impact of the acute results on the long term outcome after the treatment of in-stent restenosis: a serial intravascular ultrasound study. *Cathet Cardiol Intervent.* 2003;60:483–488.

131. Koster R, Hamm CW, Seabra-Gomes R, et al. Laser angioplasty of restenosed coronary stents: Results of a multicenter surveillance trial. *J Am Coll Cardiol.* 1999;34:25–32.

132. Mehran R, Mintz GS, Popma JJ, et al. Mechanisms and results of balloon angioplasty for the treatment of in-stent restenosis. *Am J Cardiol.* 1996;78:618–622.

133. Uren NG, Schwarzacher SP, Metz JA, et al. Predictors and outcomes of stent thrombosis. *Eur Heart J.* 2002;23;124–132.

134. Moussa I, Di Mario C, Reimers B, et al. Subacute stent thrombosis in the era of intravascular ultrasound-guided coronary stenting without anticoagulation: frequency, predictors and clinical outcome. *J Am Coll Cardiol.* 1997;29:6–12.

135. Cutlip DE, Baim DS, Ho KK, et al. Stent thrombosis in the modern era: a pooled analysis of multicenter coronary stent clinical trials. *Circulation.* 2001;103:1967–1971.

136. Mintz GS, Shah VM, Weissman NJ. Regional remodeling as the cause of late stent malapposition. *Circulation.* 2003;107:2660–2663.

137. Hodgson JMcB. Focal angioplasty: theory and clinical application. *Cathet Cardiovasc Diag.* 1997;42:445–451.

138. Hong MK, Mintz GS, Lee CW, et al. Paclitaxel coating reduces in-stent intimal hyperplasia in human coronary arteries: a serial volumetric intravascular ultrasound analysis from the Asian paclitaxel-eluting stent clinical trial (ASPECT). *Circulation.* 2003;107:517–520.

139. Serruys PW, Degertekin M, Tanabe K, et al. Intravascular ultrasound findings in the multicenter randomized double blind RAVEL (Randomized study with the sirolimus-eluting velocity balloon expandable stent in the treatment of patients with de novo native coronary artery lesions) TRIAL. *Circulation.* 2002;106:798–803.

140. Sousa JE, Costa MS, Abizaid A, et al. Lack of neointimal proliferation after implantation of sirolimus-coated stents in human coronary arteries: a quantitative coronary angiography and three-dimensional intravascular ultrasound study. *Circulation.* 2001;103:192–195.

141. Honda Y, Grube E, de la Fuente LM. Novel drug-delivery stent intravascular ultrasound observations from the first human experience with the QP2-eluting polymer stent system. *Circulation.* 2001;140:380–383.

142. Sousa JE, Costa MS, Abizaid AC, et al. Sustained suppression of neointimal proliferation by sirolimus-eluting stents: one-year angiographic and intravascular ultrasound follow-up. *Circulation.* 2001;104:2007–2011.

143. Sonoda S, Morino Y, Ako J, et al. Impact of final stent dimensions on long-term results following sirolimus-eluting stent implantation: serial intravascular ultrasound analysis from the SIRIUS trial. *J Am Coll Cardiol.* 2004;43:1959–1963.

144. Ako J, Morino Y, Honda Y, et al. Late incomplete stent apposition after sirolimus-eluting stent implantation: a serial intravascular ultrasound analysis. *J Am Coll Cardiol.* 2005;46:1002–1005.

145. Virmani R, Liistro F, Standovic G, et al. Mechanism of late in-stent restenosis after implantation of a paclitaxel deriveate-eluting polymer stent system in humans. *Circulation.* 2002;106:2649–2651.

146. Kataoka T, Grube E, Honda Y, et al. 7-hexanoyltaxol-eluting stent for prevention of neointimal growth: an intravascular ultrasound analysis from the Study to COmpare REstenosis rate between QueST and QuaDS–QP2 (SCORE). *Circulation.* 2002;106:1788–1793.

147. Fujii K, Mintz GS, Kobayashi Y, et al. Contribution of stent underexpansion to recurrence after sirolimus-eluting stent implantation for in-stent restenosis. *Circulation.* 2004;109:1085–1088.

148. Beckman JA, Ganz J, Creager MA, et al. Relationship of clinical presentation and calcification of culprit coronary artery stenoses. *Arterioscler Thromb Vasc Biol.* 2001;21:1618–1622.

149. Gyongyosi M, Yang P, Hassan A, et al. Arterial remodeling of native human coronary arteries in patients with unstable angina pectoris: a prospective intravascular ultrasound study. *Heart.* 1999;82:68–74.

150. Nakamura M, Nishikawa H, Mukai S, et al. Impact of coronary artery remodeling on clinical presentation of coronary artery disease: an intravascular ultrasound study. *J Am Coll Cardiol.* 2001;37:63–69.

151. Von Birgelen C, Klinkhart W, Mintz GS, et al. Plaque distribution and vascular remodeling of ruptured and nonruptured coronary plaques in the same vessel: an intravascular ultrasound study in vivo. *J Am Coll Cardiol.* 2001;37:864–870.

152. Takano M, Mizuno K, Okamatsu K, et al. Mechanical and structural characteristics of vulnerable plaques: analysis by coronary angioscopy and intravascular ultrasound. *J Am Coll Cardiol.* 2001;38:99–104.

153. Pasterkamp G, Schoneveld AH, van der Wal AC, et al. Relation of arterial geometry to luminal narrowing and histologic markers for plaque vulnerability: the remodeling paradox. *J Am Coll Cardiol.* 1998;32:655–662.

154. Varnava AM, Mills PG, Davies MJ. Relationship between coronary artery remodeling and plaque vulnerability. *Circulation.* 2002;105:939–943.

155. Smits PC, Pasterkamp G, Quarles Van Ufford MA, et al. Coronary artery disease: arterial remodeling and clinical presentation. *Heart.* 1999;82:461–464.

156. Schoenhagen P, Ziada KM, Kapadia SR, et al. Extent and direction of arterial remodeling in stable versus unstable coronary syndromes: an intravascular ultrasound study. *Circulation.* 2000;101:598–603.

157. Gyongyosi M, Yang P, Hassan A, et al. Intravascular ultrasound predictors of major adverse cardiac events in patients with unstable angina. *Clin Cardiol.* 2000;23:507–515.

158. Schoenhagen P, Tuzcu EM, Ellis SG. Plaque vulnerability, plaque rupture, and acute coronary syndromes: multi-focal manifestation of a systemic disease process. *Circulation.* 2002;106:760–752.

159. Jang IK, Bouma BE, Kang DH, et al. Visualization of coronary atherosclerotic plaques in patients using optical coherence tomography: comparison with intravascular ultrasound. *J Am Coll Cardiol.* 2002;39:604–609.

160. Fuchs S, Stabile E, Mintz GS, et al. Intravascular ultrasound findings in patients with acute coronary syndromes with and without elevated troponin I level. *Am J Cardiol.* 2002;89:1111–1113.

161. Nair A, Kuban BD, Tuzcu EM, et al. Coronary plaque classification with intravascular ultrasound radiofrequency data analysis. *Circulation.* 2002;106: 2200–2206.

162. Rodriguez-Granillo GA, Garcia-Garcia HM, McFadden EP, et al. In vivo intravascular ultrasound-derived thin-cap fibroatheroma detection using ultrasound radiofrequency data analysis. *J Am Coll Cardiol.* 2005:46:2038–2042.

Procedural Techniques

Barry F. Uretsky

CHAPTER 11

Basic Equipment: Guide Catheters, Guide Wires, and Balloons

Michael Ragosta and John S. Douglas Jr.

Guide catheters, guide wires and angioplasty balloons are essential tools of the interventional cardiologist. All coronary interventions require the use of a guide catheter to provide access to the artery and support device delivery. Nearly all current devices necessitate the placement of a guide wire distal to the stenosis. While only occasionally used as the sole treatment device, angioplasty balloons are an indispensable tool for performance of a successful coronary intervention. Thus, it is imperative that the interventionalist have a solid understanding and knowledge of the many choices of the basic equipment available. Often, the difference between an effortless and elegantly performed intervention and one that appears technically challenging lies in the operator's choice of basic equipment.

Guide Catheters

The single most important equipment choice for the performance of a successful intervention is the selection of the appropriate guide catheter. This fact cannot be overstated. This lesson has been repeatedly relearned and many an operator has struggled needlessly with the wrong guide catheter ultimately achieving prompt success only after switching to the proper guide.

Guide catheters differ from diagnostic catheters in several important ways. Guide catheters are stiffer in order to provide support for device passage, but are consequently more difficult to engage than diagnostic catheters and are also more likely to cause trauma to the artery than a diagnostic catheter particularly if there is atherosclerotic disease at the vessel origin. In addition, for any given French (Fr) size, the internal diameter of a guide catheter is larger than a diagnostic catheter allowing easier passage of devices and permitting optimal visualization during contrast injections.

Conventional guide catheter construction is shown in Figure 11–1. The outer layer consists of a polymer such as nylon; the middle layer is typically constructed of braided stainless steel to stiffen the catheter allowing transmission of torque as well as providing support and kink-resistance. The layer lining the lumen usually consists of PTFE (polytetrafluoroethylene) to provide a lubricated coating to facilitate device passage as well as reduce thrombogenicity. A shorter and softer catheter tip prevents trauma to the artery.

The variables involved in selecting a guide catheter include the diameter, the presence of side-holes at the tip, catheter length and curve style and length. Guide catheters are available in outer diameters as small as 5 Fr and as large as 10 Fr (1 Fr = 0.33 mm). The 6- to 8-Fr catheters are the most commonly used with the majority of interventions currently performed with 6- to 7-Fr guide catheters (1). The inner diameter for any given Fr size varies slightly between manufacturers, with current 6-Fr guides having a 0.068 to 0.071 inch inner diameter (ID), 7-Fr guides having a 0.078 to 0.081 inch ID, and 8-Fr guides having a 0.086 to 0.091 inch ID. For most coronary interventions performed with balloons and stents, a 6-Fr guide provides an appropriate inner lumen and adequate support. The smaller diameter of these guides reduces the risk of a vascular complication at the arterial access site and is less traumatic to the coronary artery particularly if there is a need to "deep seat" the catheter (see the subsequent text). There are several circumstances, however, that require the use of larger diameter guide catheters (Table 11–1). These include the use of specialized more bulky devices or when it is desired to use two balloons or stents positioned and inflated simultaneously in the coronary artery as typically employed for the treatment of a bifurcation stenosis ("kissing balloons or stents"). Larger guide catheters are stiffer and provide more support and may be needed to facilitate passage of equipment in some circumstances. Larger diameter guides, however, are more traumatic to the artery and have a higher likelihood of damping or ventricularization of the catheter tip pressure waveform (Fig. 11–2) particularly if there is ostial disease or if the arterial lumen is relatively small as often occurs with the use of an 8-Fr guide in the right coronary artery. Damping and/or ventricularization of the catheter tip pressure indicates obstruction of blood flow by the guide catheter and can lead to ischemia and, if unattended, may result in significant consequences such as arrhythmia or hemodynamic compromise. In addition, vigorous injection of a catheter that is wedged into a coronary artery can lead to dissection. Guide catheters are available with side holes at the catheter tip that restore the pressure waveform. Despite the presence of normal arterial pressure, side holes do not

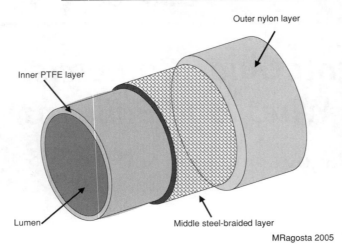

Figure 11–1.
Construction of a typical guide catheter.

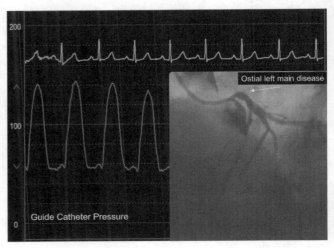

Figure 11–2.
Ventricularization of pressure waveform from guide catheter due to moderate ostial narrowing of the left main coronary artery.

necessarily restore normal hemodynamics to the coronary artery and the maximum flow provided by these side holes is limited (2). Nevertheless, side hole catheters can be helpful when a large bore guide catheter is required and significant damping or ventricularization of the catheter pressure is observed.

Catheter length is typically 100 cm with shorter guides (90 cm) available to allow stents and balloons to reach very distal lesions. This situation may occur when lesions are present distally in a native artery accessed via a saphenous vein or internal mammary bypass graft. A wide variety of standard curve styles, lengths and shapes are available along with several unique, proprietary shapes offered by individual vendors (Table 11–2). A guide catheter should be selected to achieve coaxial engagement and provide support for device delivery. Thus, determining the most appropriate curve style and shape depends on several variables. The *size of the aorta* should be determined. Aortic dilatation requires the use of large guides particularly for the left coronary artery. The *angle of the aortic valve plane* as observed in the left anterior oblique (LAO) view may vary from a horizontal (Fig. 11–3A) to a nearly vertical orientation (Fig. 11–3B) and impacts on the choice of guide catheter.

Table 11–1
Guide Catheter Diameter Requirements

Device	Guide Catheter
Rotational Atherectomy	
Burr Size	
1.25 mm (0.049 in)	6 Fr
1.50 mm (0.059 in)	6 Fr
1.75 mm (0.069 in)	7 Fr
2.00 mm (0.079 in)	8 Fr
2.15 mm (0.085 in)	8 Fr
2.25 mm (0.089 in)	8 Fr
2.50 mm (0.098 in)	9 Fr
Directional Atherectomy	
Vessel Size	
2.5–2.9 mm	7 Fr
3.0–3.4 mm	8 Fr
3.5–4.0 mm	8 Fr
Angiojet	
XMI Catheter	6 Fr
XVG Catheter	7 Fr
Frontrunner Chronic Occlusion Device	8 Fr
Kissing-balloons	7–8 Fr
Kissing stents	8 Fr
Covered stents	7–8 Fr
Stent or Balloon needing extra-support	7–8 Fr

Table 11–2
Examples of Available Guide Catheter Styles and Lengths

Standard Shapes (Curve length in centimeters)
- Right Judkins (3.0, 3.5, 4.0, 4.5, 5.0, 6.0)
- Left Judkins (3.0, 3.5, 4.0, 4.5, 5.0, 6.0)
- Right Amplatz (1, 2)
- Left Amplatz (0.75, 1, 1.5, 2, 3)
- Multi-purpose

Specialty Curves
- Right bypass
- Left bypass
- Internal mammary
- "Q" curve
- Voda curve
- "C' curve (3.0, 3.5, 4.0, 4.5, 5.0)
- Hockey stick
- Transradial curves
- Extra-support right backup
- Extra-support left backup

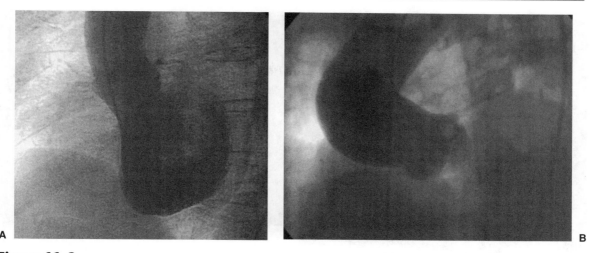

Figure 11–3.

Variations in orientation of the aortic valve plane. **A:** is from a patient with chronic lung disease with a horizontal aortic valve plane. **B:** is from an elderly patient with tortuosity of the aorta and a vertically oriented valve plane.

Similarly, the *angle of coronary artery origin from the aorta* is important to determine and greatly affects the choice of guide catheter. For example, in the case of a superiorly directed origin of the right coronary artery, a right Judkins guide catheter will be inadequate and successful intervention will likely require a left Amplatz shape or one of its variations. Finally, the *degree of support required* for device delivery should be considered. Not all interventions require maximum support, which is obtained from buttressing the guide against the opposite aortic wall. Aggressive guide support is needed to treat lesions in tortuous coronary arteries or beyond sharp angles, in many circumflex arteries and when the artery is rigid or calcified. Similarly, some devices require more back-up for successful delivery including stents, noncompliant balloons or atherectomy devices. Extra support may be accomplished either by the choice of the guide

shape, use of a larger diameter guide or by deeply intubating the coronary (known as "deep-seating," described later).

Several scenarios commonly challenge the interventionalist and require careful guide selection. For the left coronary artery, a long left main stem may lead to great difficulty particularly for lesions in the left circumflex (LCX) since the LCX tends to angle sharply from the left main in this situation. Left Judkins guides are inadequate and cannot be easily deep-seated. Amplatz guides are most useful in such circumstances (Fig. 11–4), but are associated with increased risks (see the subsequent text). Inferiorly directed left main stems are well served with Amplatz guides and superiorly directed left main stems with "C" curves. Treating any lesion in the LCX can be challenging and careful attention to guide choice is important for success. Often a longer Judkins curve is needed; this can be determined

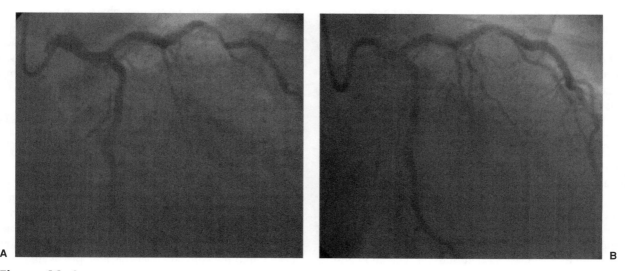

Figure 11–4.

Intervention in the circumflex artery in a patient with a long left main stem **(A)**. An Amplatz guide was required for the intervention **(B)**.

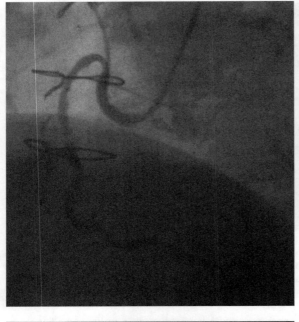

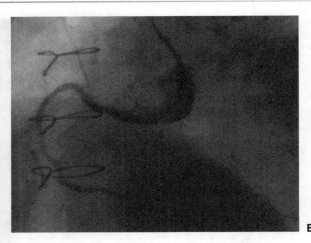

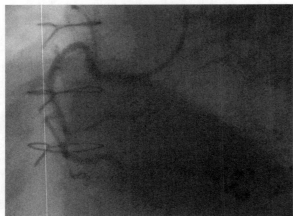

Figure 11–5.
Superiorly directed right coronary artery (Shepherd's crook) **(A)**.
An Amplatz guide was required for success **(B,C)**.

in the LAO caudal view, which shows if the guide is preferentially directed toward the left anterior descending (LAD) or the LCX. Left Amplatz guides or longer "C" curves are particularly helpful for lesions in the LCX. It is sometimes desirable to selectively intubate either the LCX or the LAD in order to optimize guide support for device delivery. When using a left Judkins guide, the catheter should be rotated clockwise to select the LCX or a longer curve length chosen. For the LAD, the catheter should be rotated counterclockwise or a shorter curve length chosen.

For the right coronary artery, there are multiple variations in site and angle of origin from the aorta. Horizontal origins are easy to engage and a right Judkins guide is often adequate unless extra support is required due to lesion characteristics. Inferiorly directed origins are also well managed using either a right Judkins, a right Amplatz or a right bypass guide catheter. It is also easy to "deep-seat" a right Judkins with an inferiorly directed origin. The superiorly directed right coronary artery or "Shepherd's Crook" can be quite challenging. An example is shown in Figure 11–5A. Although a diagnostic right Judkins

catheter is adequate for angiography, it will not provide support for device delivery. A left Amplatz guide catheter was used in this case and provided coaxial engagement and adequate support to successfully perform the intervention (Figs. 11–5B and 11–5C). In addition to an Amplatz guide, there are extra-support curves available. An internal mammary guide catheter may be chosen for its superiorly directed tip but will provide little backup so is generally not recommended. For the anomalously originating right coronary artery that is high and anterior, a left or right Amplatz are usually successfully employed.

The maneuver of deeply intubating the coronary with a guide, or "deep-seating" the guide, is commonly employed when the operator is unable to cross a rigid lesion with a balloon or stent despite coaxial catheter position and reasonable aortic wall support. The guide is gently advanced deeply into the coronary over the angioplasty guide wire until it is just above the lesion facilitating device advancement across the stenosis. An example of the use of a deep-seated catheter position to deliver a stent to a rigid lesion is shown in

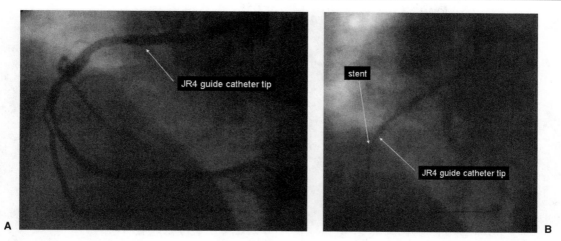

Figure 11–6.
A right Judkins guide catheter in the right coronary was inadequate to support the delivery of a stent to this lesion in the mid-right coronary artery **(A)**. The guide was "deep-seated" allowing success **(B)**.

Figure 11–6. When attempting this technique, it is important that the catheter is coaxial to the artery to minimize the likelihood of arterial dissection and great care should be used if there is evidence of proximal atherosclerotic disease.

It is sometimes necessary to change a guide catheter during an intervention. Often this can be accomplished by simply removing the angioplasty wire and guide and starting anew. Occasionally, however, it is desired to maintain distal wire position during a guide exchange because of the initial difficulty crossing a lesion (e.g., a chronic total occlusion) or because of the presence of an extensive dissection and concern that the artery may abruptly close with an inability to re-cross it with a guide wire. Guide catheter exchange while maintaining distal wire access is technically challenging (3). The guide may be changed over an exchange length (300 cm) 0.014″ wire particularly if an extra-support wire is used but the process can be facilitated by using a 0.035″ exchange wire alongside the 0.014″ wire. As the original guide is withdrawn, it is advantageous to create a redundant loop in the aortic cusp with the 0.014″ guide wire to provide slack and prevent inadvertent removal of the wire.

Guide catheters must be handled with care and several complications may arise from their use particularly when aggressively positioned to increase support. Proximal coronary artery dissections may arise from attempts at deep-seating the guide catheter particularly if a large diameter guide is used or if there is atherosclerotic disease and the catheter is not coaxial to the coronary. Amplatz guide catheters may have a tendency to lunge deeply into the coronary and cause dissection. Rarely, the guide catheter may cause dissection of the aorta (Fig. 11–7). Usually these dissections are small and self-limited, but sometimes they may require surgical intervention if extensive (4). As discussed earlier, ischemia may result if the guide obstructs coronary flow or provokes spasm. An unusual complication may arise when a guide catheter is aggressively buttressed against the opposite aortic wall and tethers the aortic valve open leading to acute aortic insufficiency and hemodynamic compromise (5). This may be recognized by a drop in systolic blood pressure and aortic regurgitation during injections.

Guide Wires

Improvement in wire technology has contributed to the high success rates for coronary intervention seen in contemporary era. The majority of interventions are performed using wires that are 0.014″ in diameter and characterized by highly steerable, flexible, and atraumatic tips. Typically an operator will choose a particular all-purpose wire for the majority of cases (so-called "work horse" wire). Several specialty wires have been designed to overcome specific problems such as vessel tortuosity or highly stenosed lesions and some devices, such as rotational atherectomy, require unique guide wires.

Several characteristics of a guide wire are important to understand. The wire is constructed of a core of stainless steel that provides support for device delivery. The core tapers at the tip with a spring coil welded to it to provide flexibility and "floppiness." The tip strength may vary and stiffer tips provide the ability to penetrate highly stenosed lesions such as chronic occlusions but also have a greater risk of perforation or subintimal wire positioning. A variety of coatings may be applied to the wire to reduce friction. The tip of some wires consists of a hydrophilic polymer, which facilitates the passage down highly tortuous arteries and across highly stenosed lesions. However, care should be used with such wires, because they can more easily lead to perforation if the tip inadvertently strays deeply into a smaller branch. Stiffer cores are also available to increase support and can help straighten tortuous or highly angulated arteries facilitating device delivery.

The wire tip is generally shaped into a gentle curve or "hockey-stick" profile. The wire is advanced in the guide through an introducer in the hemostatic valve to the proximal portion of the coronary. A "torque device" is clamped to the out of body portion of the wire to allow steering. Most guide

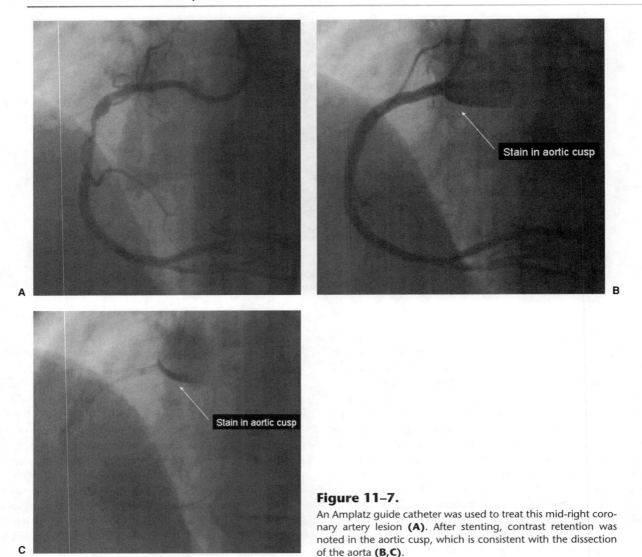

Figure 11–7.

An Amplatz guide catheter was used to treat this mid-right coronary artery lesion **(A)**. After stenting, contrast retention was noted in the aortic cusp, which is consistent with the dissection of the aorta **(B,C)**.

wires have nearly 1:1 torque responsiveness and can be easily advanced to the distal artery. There are several important principles of wire crossing. First, the tip should be free at all times within the lumen of the artery usually accomplished by rotating the wire while advancing. When approaching the lesion, great care should be taken during advancement through the stenosis. The wire tip should never buckle as it approaches or crosses the lesion; this may indicate that the wire tip is burrowing beneath the plaque leading to subintimal positioning. Most wires allow transmission of distal tip sensations to the operator and the wire should be gently withdrawn if there is a sensation of "sticking" or resistance. Once the wire is across the lesion, it should be placed distally in a major arterial segment. Often the wire may stray into a small side-branch; this should be avoided as it may lead to perforation particularly with stiffer tip wires or hydrophilic tips.

In some circumstances when it is difficult to pass a device across a lesion, use of a stiffer, extra-support guide wire or the placement of a second wire alongside the first one may lead to success. This technique is known as the use of a "buddy wire" and is particularly helpful when the artery is highly tortuous or angulated, in the treatment of rigid lesions in noncompliant arteries, or when the there is insufficient guide support (6,7).

Guide wires may result in significant straightening of the artery particularly if the vessel is tortuous and either an extra-support wire or a "buddy-wire" is used. This leads to a characteristic angiographic finding suggesting a coronary lesion and is due to invagination of redundant artery into the arterial lumen. The typical appearance of such a pseudo-lesion is shown in Figure 11–8. The apparent development of a "new lesion" after placement of a guidewire in a previously normal but tortuous or angulated segment should lead the operator to suspect such pseudo-lesions. It is important to recognize these artifacts and the likely setting in which they may occur, because it may lead to unnecessary treatment of that segment. Simply withdrawing to the floppy portion of the guide wire or removing the guide wire altogether restores the vessel to its original configuration and resolves the angiographic finding.

Complications related to guide wires are rare but include several potentially serious conditions such as perforation and

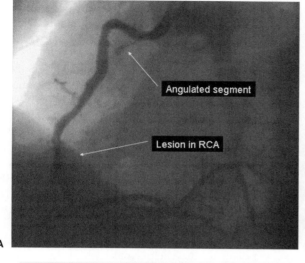

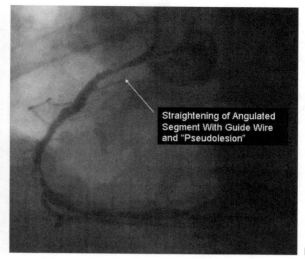

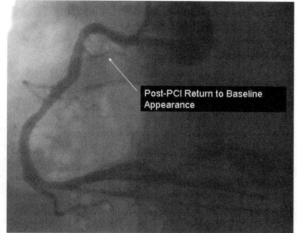

Figure 11–8.
Example of a wire-straightening artifact. The baseline angiogram shows a sharply angulated segment of the proximal RCA and a lesion in the mid-RCA **(A)**. Following the placement of a guide wire, the proximal segment has straightened and there is the appearance of a new "lesion" **(B)**. This represents the artifact from wire straightening. After the intervention, the wire is removed and the vessel returns to its baseline state **(C)**.

coronary artery dissection. In the current era, guide wire perforations are most commonly due to aggressive attempts at crossing chronic occlusions or from inadvertent advancement of the wire tip out of the distal artery or a small branch. Guide wire perforations are especially problematic in the presence of glycoprotein IIb/IIIa inhibitors. Coronary dissections may occur when the wire tip enters the subintimal space and raises an intimal flap or when it strays from the true lumen and boroughs beneath the plaque. In addition, withdrawal of the coronary guide wire should be visualized in order to prevent the guide catheter from being pulled deeply into the coronary ostium leading to possible arterial injury when resistance to withdrawal occurs. Very rare complications include avulsion of the wire tip with distal embolization, or wire entrapment.

Balloon Catheters

Although currently not commonly used as stand alone devices, balloon catheters are indispensable tools for the percutaneous treatment of coronary lesions. Balloons are used as the sole device in only about 20% of coronary interventions (8,9). In the current era, they are typically used as adjuncts to coronary

stents with an important role in predilation before placing a stent or for postdilating the stent after its deployment to achieve full expansion or a larger diameter. Some common reasons for using a balloon alone include treatment of focal in-stent restenosis, treatment of a side branch of a bifurcation after the parent vessel has been stented, treatment of a small caliber (<2.25 mm diameter) artery or treatment of a lesion for which a stent is not deliverable.

The balloon catheter consists of a low-profile shaft designed to enhance its "trackability" and "pushability" without kinking. The shaft contains a lumen leading to the balloon and may have an additional lumen for the guide wire. The balloon is made of one of several different proprietary polymers. The physical characteristics of the balloon material determine the properties and behavior of the balloon. Balloons made of compliant material have the advantage of easily advancing within the artery and crossing a stenosis. Their disadvantage, however, is the fact that the balloon diameter will increase substantially under higher inflation pressures. Thus, if the lesion requires high pressure to dilate, a compliant balloon may greatly increase in both diameter and length resulting in over-sizing and possibly dissection or vessel perforation. Balloon catheters are packaged with a compliance chart that provides the operator with the *in vitro* balloon diameter at various increments of inflation pressure. The listed balloon diameter is the diameter of the balloon when inflated to its nominal pressure, which usually is 6 to 8 atmospheres. The balloon diameter is smaller at inflation pressures below the nominal pressure and is larger at inflation pressures above the nominal pressure. Interventionalists should know the compliance characteristics of the chosen balloon particularly if higher pressures are anticipated. Some compliant balloons may vary greatly at the range of inflation pressures used to dilate lesions. For example, a 3.0-mm diameter, 20-mm long Voyager Balloon (Guidant) is nominal at 8 atmospheres. At 4 atmospheres, it is only 2.66 mm in diameter and at 14 atmospheres it is 3.22 mm. As a general rule, compliant balloons can be quarter-sized up or down from the nominal diameter at the extremes of inflation pressures. It is important to remember that the compliance curve is obtained *in vitro*. Under high pressures in a rigid artery or within the confines of a stent, the balloon may not achieve these idealized diameters. In fact, under such circumstances, a compliant balloon will likely grow substantially in length, rather than in diameter, potentially injuring adjacent segments. In addition to the compliance chart, balloons are provided with a variety of burst pressures. The "burst pressure" is the average pressure required to rupture a balloon and generally exceeds the "rated burst pressure," which is the maximum inflation pressure a balloon is guaranteed not to rupture at a 95% confidence level. Compliant balloons typically have burst pressures of 18 atmospheres and rated burst pressures of 14 atmospheres.

Noncompliant balloons are typically made of polyethylene terephthalate (PET) or nylon and retain their specified diameter regardless of inflation pressure without elongation. For example, a 3.0-mm NC Monorail (Boston Scientific) is nominal at 8 atmospheres and is 2.94 mm at 3 atmospheres, but only 3.09 mm at 16 atmospheres with a rated burst pressure of 18 mm. Noncompliant balloons are very helpful in dilating rigid lesions requiring high atmosphere inflations and are also routinely used in postdilating stents. They are more resistant to puncture and rupture than compliant balloons. However, an undesirable consequence of noncompliant balloon material is the greater difficulty in advancing the balloon in the artery particularly around bends and greater difficulty in crossing lesions. Noncompliant balloons do not re-wrap very well after they are inflated and result in a greater profile, which makes them very difficult to re-use once they have been inflated. Some manufacturers also make semi-compliant balloons that have properties between compliant and noncompliant balloons.

Coronary balloons are available in a wide range of diameters from 1.5 mm up to 5.0 mm and in increments of 0.25 to 0.50 mm. Choosing the optimal balloon diameter is somewhat empiric and based on visual estimation of the diameter of the reference artery. The operator takes into consideration many factors including compliance of the balloon, angulation of the dilated segment, potential for the rigidity of the lesion, and the presence of an adjacent disease. In general, when a balloon alone is contemplated, the balloon size should be slightly greater than the reference segment (i.e., a 1.1 to 1 balloon to artery ratio) (10–12). Undersizing the balloon is preferred when balloons are used to predilate a lesion prior to placement of a coronary stent to minimize dissection and possibly the need for a longer stent.

Balloon catheters are available in an array of lengths from as small as 6 mm to as long as 40 mm. The most commonly used lengths are 15 mm and 20 mm long. Short balloons (<15 mm) may be helpful with very focal lesions particularly if they are on an acute bend, but may be difficult to precisely position and also have a tendency to "spit" proximally or distally during inflation. Balloon length should be carefully considered when dilating a lesion prior to stenting. Use of a balloon longer than the implanted stent may lead to intimal proliferation and restenosis at the injured but un-stented areas or may cause arterial dissection requiring placement of additional stents or a much longer stent than originally planned. Choosing an undersized balloon diameter may help avoid both of these issues. Long balloons (30–40 mm) may be helpful to treat diffuse disease.

Balloon catheters may be over-the-wire, monorail, or consist of a fixed wire at the tip of the balloon. The over-the-wire and monorail balloon catheters are designed to function with a 0.014″ guide wire while the fixed wire at the tip of a balloon style functions as a single unit. There are two lumens running the entire length of over-the-wire balloon catheters. One lumen is for a guide wire and the other is for the balloon. Although this catheter style represents an older technology, over-the-wire balloons remain useful today. Advantages of an over-the-wire balloon include facilitating distal wire positioning in a tortuous artery, providing additional support for crossing chronic occlusions or highly stenosed lesions, and allowing guide wire exchanges without losing distal access. When over-the-wire balloons are used, exchange length wires (300 cm) are necessary to allow exchange for bigger balloon catheters or stent catheters. Catheter exchanges can be cumbersome and are accomplished using the "push-pull" technique where the operator pushes gently on the guide wire with one hand to maintain its distal position while withdrawing the balloon catheter with the other hand usually under fluoroscopic guidance.

Monorail balloons are very popular in the current era. Unlike over-the-wire balloon catheters, the wire lumen of the monorail balloon does not run the entire length of the catheter; instead it involves just the distal 20 to 30 cm. With only a single lumen for the balloon, the catheter is lower profile and the short length of the wire committed to the catheter allows for rapid catheter exchange and catheter exchanges can be made with shorter (190 cm) guide wires reducing procedure time and radiation exposure. However, monorail catheters do not allow for wire exchanges in the event that a more supportive guide wire is needed.

Fixed wire balloons are rarely used. Consisting of just a single lumen for balloon inflation, they are the lowest profile balloons available. Thus, their major role is for the treatment of highly stenosed lesions when neither a small diameter compliant over-the-wire nor monorail balloon catheter crossed the stenosis. The general teaching is that a fixed-wire balloon catheter can cross any stenosis crossed by a 0.014″ guide wire. The major disadvantage of this design lies in the fact that they

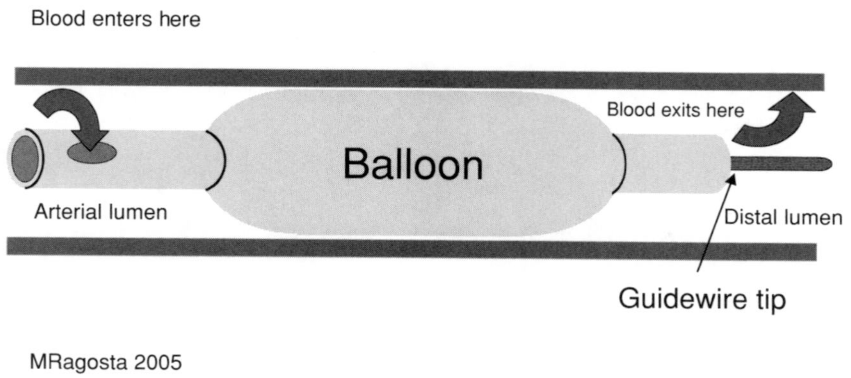

Blood enters here

Figure 11–9.
Schematic representation of an autoperfusion balloon catheter.

can be difficult to steer particularly within tortuous vessels and that they cannot be exchanged leading to the loss of distal arterial access if the balloon requires upsizing.

Perfusion balloons are designed to allow flow to the distal artery during balloon inflation. Rarely used in the current era, they were useful in the pre-stent era to allow prolonged inflations in an attempt to "tack-up" a dissection or to reduce ischemia in cases of abrupt closure destined for emergency bypass surgery. In the current era, perfusion balloons are used to treat dissections when a stent cannot be delivered, in hemodynamically unstable patients who do not tolerate ischemia from balloon inflation, or to allow prolonged inflation to seal a perforation. A schematic representation of a perfusion balloon is shown in Figure 11–9. Blood enters the lumen of the balloon catheter proximal to the balloon, travels along the balloon lumen then exits distally. Blood flow is driven by aortic blood pressure; thus, these catheters are often referred to as "autoperfusion" catheters to distinguish them from catheters designed to provide greater flow rates from active perfusion methods. The rate of blood flow delivered distally from an autoperfusion catheter varies widely dependent on the blood pressure and may be as high as 45 to 50 cc/minutes, which is adequate to maintain myocardial perfusion at basal levels (13–16).

Simply stated, the optimal selection and use of the basic tools differentiate the master from the occasional PCI operator. A few extra minutes spent carefully studying the preintervention angiogram and developing a "game plan" including choice of guide, wire, and balloon will most often lead to a shorter, safer, and more cost-effective coronary intervention.

REFERENCES

1. Ruygrok PN, Ormiston JA, O'Shaughnessy B. Coronary angioplasty in New Zealand 1995-1998: a report from the National Coronary Angioplasty Registry. *NZ Med J.* 2000;113:381–384.
2. DeBruyne B, Stockbroeckx J, Demoor D, et al. Role of side holes in guide catheters: observations on coronary pressure and flow. *Cath Cardiovasc Diagn.* 1994;33:145–152.
3. Selig M, Yazdanfar S. Guide catheter exchange techniques: Bi-coaxial and other methods. *Cathet Cardiovasc Diagn.* 1997;41:442–444.
4. Dunning DW, Kahn JK, Hawkins ET, et al. Iatrogenic coronary artery dissections extending into and involving the aortic root. *Cathet Cardiovasc Intervent.* 2000;51:387–393.
5. Javeed N, Shaikh J, Patel M, et al. Catheter-induced acute aortic insufficiency with hemodynamic collapse during PTCA: an unreported complication. *Cathet Cardiovasc Diagn.* 1997;42:305–307.
6. Saucedo JF, Muller DW, Moscucci M. Facilitated placement of the Palmaz-Schatz stent delivery system with the use of an adjacent 0.018″ stiff wire. *Cathet Cardiovasc Diagn.* 1996;39:106–110.
7. Burzotta F, Trani C, Mazzari MA, et al. Use of a second buddy wire during percutaneous coronary interventions: a simple solution for some challenging situations. *J Inv Cardiol.* 2005;17:171–174.
8. Anderson HV, Shaw RE, Brindis RG, et al. A contemporary overview of percutaneous coronary interventions. The American College of Cardiology-National Cardiovascular Data Registry (ACC-NCDR). *J Am Coll Cardiol.* 2002;39:1096–1103.
9. Williams DO, Holubkov R, Yeh W, et al. Percutaneous coronary intervention in the current era compared with 1985–1986. The National Heart, Lung, and Blood Institute Registries. *Circulation.* 2000;102:2945–2951.
10. Azuma A, Sawada T, Katsume H, et al. Quantitative measurements of balloon-to-artery ratios in coronary angioplasty. *J Cardiol.* 1991;21:879–888.
11. Sharma SK, Israel DH, Kamean JL, et al. Clinical, angiographic, and procedural determinants of major and minor coronary dissection during angioplasty. *Am Heart J.* 1993;126:39–47.
12. Stone GW, Hodgson JM, St Goar FG, et al. Improved procedural results of coronary angioplasty with intravascular-guided balloon sizing: the CLOUT Pilot Trial. *Circulation.* 1997;95:2044–2052.
13. de Muinck ED, Angelini P, Dougherty K, et al. In vitro evaluation of blood flow through autoperfusion balloon catheters. *Cathet Cardiovasc Diagn.* 1993;30:58–62.
14. Quigley PJ, Hinohara T, Phillips HR, et al. Myocardial protection during coronary angioplasty with an autoperfusion balloon catheter in humans. *Circulation.* 1988;78:1128–1134.
15. Turi ZG, Campbell CA, Gottimukkala MV, et al. Preservation of distal coronary perfusion during prolonged balloon inflation with an autoperfusion angioplasty catheter. *Circulation.* 1987;75:1273–1280.
16. Voelker W, Kerkhoffs W, Schmitz B, et al. Comparison of passive and active perfusion catheters: an in vitro study in a pulsatile coronary flow model. *Cathet Cardiovasc Diagn.* 1996;38:421–427.

CHAPTER 12

In-Stent Restenosis

Leo Slavin and Jonathan M. Tobis

Coronary artery disease (CAD) is the leading cause of morbidity and mortality in the United States, accounting for 1 out of every 5 deaths with 13 million Americans estimated to be living with CAD currently (1). In 2001, it was estimated that more than one million individuals suffered a new or recurrent coronary attack. In addition, CAD accounted for approximately $130 billion in total health care expenditures (1).

Percutaneous transluminal coronary balloon angioplasty (PTCA), first preformed in 1977 by Andreas Gruentzig, has revolutionized CAD therapy. Since that time, interventional cardiology has witnessed vast technical improvements and research designed to eliminate some of the limitations of balloon angioplasty (2,3). Restenosis, occurring in approximately 30% to 60% of patients within the first 6 months, has been named the Achilles heel of PTCA (4–6). Restenosis is defined as renarrowing of the vessel that exceeds 50% of the luminal diameter achieved at PTCA (6). The mechanism of restenosis is related to arterial healing response after injury, involving vascular elastic recoil, neointimal proliferation, and negative remodeling (2,3,7). Postballoon angioplasty restenosis primarily results from negative remodeling or vascular contraction accounting for more than 60% of late luminal loss (4,7,8). Bare metal stenting has effectively reduced the restenosis rates to about 15% to 30% by functioning as a mechanical scaffold that eliminates elastic recoil and negative remodeling (4,5,9). The use of stents identified a new problem: restenosis occurring within the stent or in-stent restenosis (ISR). ISR is defined as lumen diameter loss of >50% within the stent. Abnormal coronary reserve can be demonstrated in an artery once the diameter stenosis exceeds 50% (10). The only FDA approved treatment for ISR is intracoronary radiation. Given the prevalence of CAD, the large volume of individuals that will undergo PCI, ISR could continue to be a major problem faced by interventional cardiologists.

Pathogenesis of Restenosis

Postballoon Angioplasty

The comparable size of the coronary arteries, as well as a similar response to injury, makes the porcine coronaries an effective model to demonstrate the pathophysiology and histopathology of restenosis (11). The pathogenesis of restenosis, which is distinct from atherosclerotic plaque formation, is similar to wound healing. The process can be divided into (i) elastic recoil, (ii) neointimal hyperplasia, and (iii) negative vascular remodeling (2,3,7). Elastic recoil is an acute process that is observed within a few minutes after balloon deflation, resulting in a mechanical collapse of the vessel wall. The large quantity of elastic fibers within the tunica media increases the inward recoil force upon balloon inflation, causing an acute luminal collapse following deflation. The recoil force can result in up to 50% loss of cross sectional area and a 33% loss in luminal diameter (12). Neointimal formation and negative remodeling result from direct trauma to the artery.

Neointimal Formation

Balloon inflation increases intravascular pressure, often causing rupture of the medial layer at the junction between the normal segment and the atherosclerotic plaque, leading to a dissection through the tunica media, exposing the subendothelial components (13). The endothelial denudation leads to the loss of antithrombotic factors, such as nitric oxide (NO), prostaglandin (PHI_2), and tissue plasminogen activator (tPA), and promotes platelet adhesion and aggregation. Platelets that are bound to fibrin release cytokines, such as platelet-derived growth factor (PDGF), thromboxane A_2 (TXA_2), and ADP, which signal further platelet aggregation and the formation of thrombus (13,14).

PDGF, transforming growth factor (TGF-b), and epidermal growth factor (EGF) are cytokines released by the platelets that function as mitogens and chemotaxic agents for vascular smooth muscle cells (VSMC) and macrophages (15,16). The macrophages release PDGF and interleukin-6 (IL-6), which further stimulate VSMC. The VSMC normally reside in the tunica media in their quiescent state (15,16). Upon injury, the release of these mediators leads VSMC to phenotypically change into myofibroblasts with synthetic, secretory, proliferative, and migratory functions. These cells exit the G_0 quiescent phase, migrate into the site of injury, and undergo mitosis. In addition, endothelial denudation leads to the loss of heparin-like glycosaminoglycans that normally inhibit the growth of VSMC (17).

Intracellular signaling pathways that govern these changes have been studied in great detail (18). The two major cascades governing the function of VSMC are the tyrosine kinase

From: Slavin L, Chhabra A, Tobis J. Drug-eluting stents: preventing restenosis. *Cardiol Rev.* 2006;14(6). In press.

cascade and the cyclic-AMP pathway (18). Growth factors bind to the receptors and activate tyrosine kinase that leads to a phosphorylation cascade, eventually activating *ras*. *Ras* stimulates *raf* to activate mitogen activated protein kinase kinase (MAPKK), culminating in intranuclear activation of transcription factors that induce proliferation and migration of VSMC (18). The cyclic-AMP pathway leads to the activation of protein kinase A (PKA), which phosphorylates and activates the transcription factor cAMP responsive element binding protein (CREB) (18). In addition, PKA phosphorylates *raf*, inhibiting the other major pathway involved in the activation of VSMC (18). In vitro and in vivo studies demonstrate that the inactivation of *ras* and the activation of the cyclic-AMP pathway leads to a >50% reduction in neointimal formation at 14 days postballoon injury in rat carotid arteries (18,19,20).

The progression of G_0 to G_1 is regulated by a cyclin-dependent kinase (CDK), particularly cyclin D-CDK and cyclin E-CDK-2 (18). The presence of endogenous inhibitors of CDK (CKI) such as p21^{cip1}, p27^{kip1}, and INK4 families regulate the process of entering G_1 and keep VSMC in the G_0 phase (18). Vascular inflammation and injury decreases the level of p27^{kip1} that causes quiescent cells to resume cell division. Activation of cAMP leads to an increase in p27^{kip1} forcing the proliferating cells to exit the cell cycle (18). The complex interplay of intracellular signals leads to the conversion of VSMC to myofibroblasts and migration to the site of injury. Histologic analysis in the porcine model demonstrates that these actin (+) cells colonize the residual thrombus, which forms a cap across the thrombus and proliferates toward the tunica media. The myofibroblasts then degrade the thrombus and replace it with extracellular matrix (ECM), leading to the formation of the neointimal mass (14). The amount of neointima produced is determined by the degree of inflammation generated during vascular injury (21).

Negative Remodeling

Remodeling is a change in arterial size following vascular injury that stems from the ability of the artery to enlarge or contract (22). The process of negative remodeling may be observed 1 to 6 months after balloon angioplasty and accounts for about 60% to 65% of luminal loss observed by intravascular ultrasound (IVUS) (8,22). Wilcox used antibodies against alpha-smooth muscle actin, myosin, and desmin to demonstrate the proliferation of myofibroblasts in the neointima and the adventitia (23). The adventitia is the site with the greatest expression of PDGF and PDGF receptors, which are mediators critical in attracting myofibroblasts to the site of injury (13,23). Upon injury to the vessel, inflammatory cells stimulate conversion of adventitial fibroblasts to myofibroblasts that express alpha-smooth muscle actin and secrete ECM, leading to constriction of the vessel and the formation of a fibrotic scar within the adventitia surrounding the site of injury (23). The combination of elastic recoil, neointimal formation, and negative remodeling accounts for the high restenosis rates after balloon angioplasty.

In-Stent Restenosis

Clinical trials comparing balloon angioplasty versus bare metal stenting demonstrate a reduction in restenosis rates with the use of stents. The introduction of a stent eliminates early elastic recoil and provides a mechanical scaffold that prevents negative remodeling (24). Opposite to initial expectations, studies have demonstrated that stent implantation promotes the development of neointimal hyperplasia (25). Hoffman compared stented and nonstented lesions using serial IVUS studies, confirming the observation that the main mechanism of ISR is due to neointimal hyperplasia rather than negative remodeling (26). The late lumen loss is actually greater with bare metal stents (BMS) than with balloon dilation alone. However, the initial gain in lumen diameter is so much greater with stents that this overcomes the neointimal production to yield a lower restenosis rate (24).

The neointimal formation that occurs in ISR is similar to that following postballoon angioplasty. The exaggerated response seen with stenting occurs secondary to vessel injury and inflammation. Kornowski et al. using a porcine model demonstrated that an increase in vessel injury or vascular inflammation results in an increase in neointimal formation (27). Pigs in which the stent struts perforated the internal elastic lamina and external elastic lamina had greater histologic evidence of inflammatory response and subsequently a larger volume of neointimal formation (27). Other contributing factors to increased inflammatory response may stem from the increased balloon inflation required to place the stent or the irritating reaction to the stent material. Contact allergy to metals including nickel and molybdenum may account for the elevated inflammatory response observed with stents in some patients. Bare metal stents slowly elute metal ions that may stimulate a delayed-type hypersensitivity response within the stented vessel (28). A study was conducted in Germany on 131 patients who after stent implantation underwent cutaneous patch testing to investigate the association of nickel and molybdenum hypersensitivity with ISR. All patients (n = 10) with a positive test result had restenosis (p = 0.03), requiring target vessel revascularization (28). Although the number of patients evaluated in studies investigating the correlation between metal allergy and ISR is small, this intriguing evidence suggests that metallic hypersensitivity may account for a high percentage of restenosis observed with bare metal stenting. In summary, angioplasty with stenting produces the same mechanisms of injury, including endothelial denudation and dissection of the tunica media, but further activates inflammation by increased vascular injury. These events trigger the cellular and molecular cascades described above, eventually leading to neointimal hyperplasia.

Drug-Eluting Stents: Preventing Restenosis

Although bare metal stenting has markedly reduced the incidence of restenosis compared with balloon angioplasty, ISR continues to be a major problem with an incidence of <10% to >30% depending on the lesion length, reference segment diameter, and other characteristics, such as diabetes. Mechanical strategies, systemic pharmacotherapy, and intravascular brachytherapy are methods used to reduce the frequency of ISR. Mechanical strategies include: (i) IVUS-guided high-pressure deployment to achieve larger mean luminal diameter (MLD), (ii) prior debulking therapy, and (iii) avoidance of predilation with "direct" stenting. These strategies may achieve some reduction in restenosis rates in certain cases, but failed to demonstrate a significant benefit in large randomized controlled trials (29–31). The use of stents with thinner struts may reduce restenosis (32). Systemic administration of agents that inhibit specific processes in restenosis has also been suggested as a possible option. Antiplatelet agents, anticoagulants, calcium-channel blockers, ACE inhibitors, statins, and antioxidants have reduced neointimal formation in various animal models. However, the same efficacy has not been observed in randomized trials (32–38). The downside to systemic pharmacotherapy is the inability to deliver a high dose of the agent to the lesion without inducing systemic side effects. Unlike the previous two modalities, intravascular brachytherapy has shown a reduction in neointimal proliferation and ISR in multiple randomized clinical trials (39–41). However, the lack of an optimal radiation dose, the practical difficulty in scheduling the procedure between radiation oncologists and the catherization lab, the edge-effect due to geographic miss leading to in-lesion restenosis, and increased rates of subacute thrombosis have delayed the wide acceptance of intracoronary radiation into clinical practice (42,43).

Drug-impregnated stents that allow a predictable elution of a high dose locally of a therapeutic agent has been shown to be very effective in preventing ISR. The ability of the stent to deliver an agent locally reduces proliferation of VSMC without causing systemic toxicity. The drug can be delivered by the stent through a variety of mechanisms. The first clinical approach used dipping or spraying the drug on to the bare metallic stent (44). This approach lacks the gradual and predictable release that is generated by newer methods, and instead delivers a large bolus immediately into the local area. A second approach coats the metal stent with degradable or nondegradable biopolymers, which are loaded with the drug, and deliver a sustained release of the agent. A drug-free coated polymer layer can be added to function as a diffusion barrier, further controlling the elution kinetics of the agent (45).

The compatibility of the coated polymer with the vessel wall determines the degree of inflammation that is generated upon contact. The majority of polymers utilized for stent coating have introduced a substantial amount of inflammation in experimental models. The major concerns that arise from the use of polymers include chronic inflammation specifically after the elution is complete, direct local toxicity to the vascular tissue, polymer incompatibility with circulating humoral factors, and polymer breakdown and erosion (45). The ideal polymer effectively delivers antirestenotic therapy over an appropriate time course, and in the process remains biologically inert, tolerates mechanical stress, and is not thrombogenic (45).

There have been many agents tested preclinically. The two agents that have repeatedly shown the most success in preclinical and clinical trials are sirolimus and paclitaxel.

Sirolimus-Eluting Stents

Sirolimus (Rapamycin) is a natural macrocyclic lactone with potent immunosuppressive and antimitotic action produced by a fungus, *Streptomyces hygroscopicus*. In 1999, the FDA approved systemic sirolimus for antirejection in renal transplants (46). The agent binds intracellularly to FK binding protein-12 (FKBP-12) forming the immunosuppressive complex that inhibits mammalian target of rapamycin (mTOR), a key regulatory kinase that leads to an increase in the levels of p27^{kip1}. The rise in p27^{kip1} inhibits the cyclin-CDK complex, blocking the G_1-S transition and thereby restricting proliferation of VSMC (47). When bonded to a stent, the effects are achieved locally without the complications of systemic toxicity. The sirolimus-eluting stent generates essentially undetectable sirolimus levels in peripheral blood (48). There have been four pivotal trials conducted with sirolimus-eluting stents (SES) that have led to FDA approval in April 2004 (49–59). The studies used the bare metal Bx-Velocity stent (Johnson and Johnson, New Brunswick, NJ), which is a balloon-expandable design made of tubular grade 316L stainless steel. The platform was coated with 5 mcm consisting of a blend of 33% sirolimus and 67% of non-erodible polymer. The drug-polymer matrix contained 140 mcg/cm^2 of sirolimus. A drug-free polymer coat served as a diffusion barrier to control drug release such that 80% was released in the first 30 days postimplantation and no residual drug was detected beyond 90 days (49–59).

The trials used similar methodology, inclusion and exclusion criteria, and protocols. Patients underwent quantitative angiographic analysis to determine late luminal loss (MLD after procedure – MLD at follow-up), % diameter stenosis, and ISR, defined as diameter stenosis (DS) within the stent of >50%. Major adverse cardiac events (MACE) were defined as death, acute myocardial infarction (MI), total vessel failure (TVF), and target lesion revascularization (TLR). TLR was defined as a repeat PTCA or CABG involving the stented lesion, driven by clinical signs of ischemia in the presence of angiographic restenosis. The first human clinical trial was conducted in Brazil where Sousa and colleagues demonstrated the safety of SES (49–51). The first promising European experience with SES was published shortly thereafter (52,53).

RAVEL Trial

The RAVEL trial was a multicenter, randomized trial of 238 patients to compare the safety and efficacy of BMS (n = 118) and SES (n = 120). The two groups were similar with respect to all clinical variables except for a larger percentage of men in the BMS group. Table 12–1 summarizes the data of the RAVEL and the other major sirolimus trials using the Cypher stent (Johnson and Johnson, New Brunswick, NJ). At 6 months, 211 out of 238 (89%) patients underwent angiographic follow-up and showed a significant reduction in the degree of late luminal

Table 12–1

Summary of Sirolimus Data

	RAVEL	SIRIUS	C-SIRIUS	E-SIRIUS
Number of Patients	238	1058	100	352
Lesion Length (mm)	9.58	14.4	13.6	15.0
RVD (mm)	2.62	2.80	2.63	2.55
DM (%)	19	26	24	23
Follow-up (month)	12	9	9	9
LLL (mm)				
BMS	0.88	1.00	1.02	1.05
SES	−0.01	0.17	0.12	0.20
p-value	<0.001	<0.001	<0.001	<0.0001
ISR (%)				
BMS	28.8	35.4	45.5	41.7
SES	0.0	3.2	0.0	3.9
p-value	<0.001	<0.001	<0.001	<0.0001
TLR				
BMS	25.7*	23.2*	18.0	20.9
SES	6.1	6.8	4.0	8.0
p-value	<0.001	<0.0001	0.05	<0.0001
MACE (%)				
BMS	28.8*	27.4*	18.0	22.6
SES	5.8	12.6	4.0	4.0
p-value	0.002	<0.0001	0.05	<0.0002

Summary of the major randomized, controlled trials involving sirolimus-eluting stents compared to the bare metal stent controls. BMS, bare metal stents; DM, diabetes mellitus; ISR, in-stent restenosis; LLL, late lumen loss; MACE, major adverse cardiac events; RVD, reference vessel diameter; SES, sirolimus-eluting stent; TLR, target lesion revascularization.
*3-year follow-up data.

loss (p <0.001), in-stent % DS (p <0.001), and the rate of ISR (p <0.001) in the sirolimus group. There was a significant decrease in the incidence of TLR (0.8% versus 23.7%, p = 0.001), and MACE (5.8% versus 28.8%, p <0.001) in the SES group versus the BMS group (54). The 3-year follow-up data were recently published demonstrating the continued clinical benefit of SES in 227 (95%) patients. The frequency of TLR was 25.7% in the BMS group and 6.1% in the SES group (p <0.001). The incidence of MACE was 33.1% in the BMS group and 15.8% in the sirolimus cohort (p = 0.002). There was no significant difference between the two groups with regard to death or MI at 9 months and 3 years (55).

SIRIUS Trial

The SIRIUS trial enrolled 1,058 patients in a randomized, double-blind multicenter trial to determine the clinical benefit of SES (n = 533) in comparison to BMS (n = 525). Patients received clopidogrel 75 mg daily for 3 months to reduce the risk of subacute thrombosis. Angiographic follow-up was performed 8 months after the procedure in 703 (66%) patients and demonstrated a significant decrease in the late luminal loss (p <0.001), in the in-stent and in-lesion % DS (p <0.001) in the sirolimus group in comparison to the BMS group. There was a significant reduction in the rate of ISR and in-lesion restenosis (p <0.001) in SES versus BMS. There was

a significant decrease in the incidence of TLR (4.1% versus 16.6%, p <0.001) and MACE (7.1% versus 18.9%, p <0.001) at 9 months (56). The 3-year clinical follow-up data in 985 (93%) patients showed the persistent benefit of SES. The rate of TLR was 23.2% in the BMS group and 6.8% in the SES group (p <0.0001). The frequency of MACE was 27.4% in the BMS group and 12.6% in the SES group (p <0.0001). There was no significant difference between the two groups in terms of death, MI, or stent thrombosis at the 9-month and 3-year follow-up (57).

E-SIRIUS/C-SIRIUS

The E-SIRIUS and the C-SIRIUS trials were randomized, double-blind, multicenter trials that enrolled 352 and 100 patients, respectively, to confirm the successful results found in the RAVEL and SIRIUS trials. Angiographic analysis at the 8-month follow-up was done on 308 (88%) patients in the E-SIRIUS trials and 88 (88%) in the C-SIRIUS trials, and demonstrated a significant reduction in the amount of late luminal loss (p <0.001), in the in-stent and in-lesion % DS (p <0.001) in the SES group as compared to the BMS group. The rate of ISR and in-lesion restenosis was significantly lower in SES versus BMS (Table 12–1). There was also a significant decrease in the frequency of TLR and MACE in the SES group versus the BMS group (p <0.001) at 9 months. There was no significant difference in the frequency of death or MI between the two groups in either of the two trials (58,59).

In summary, the sirolimus trials using the Cypher stent repeatedly demonstrated significant efficacy and safety with the use of SES in the prevention of ISR and the reduction of future requirements for revascularization.

Paclitaxel-Eluting Stents

Paclitaxel is a compound isolated from the bark of the Pacific yew tree of northwestern America (*Taxus brevifolia*). Today the synthetic form of paclitaxel, Taxol, is used systemically as a treatment for breast and ovarian malignancies (60). Paclitaxel exerts its pharmacological effect by inhibiting microtubule depolymerization resulting in the formation of numerous decentralized and unorganized microtubules. This results in inhibition of cellular replication at the G_0/G_1 and G_1/M phase and stops cytokine-mediated induction of cell proliferation and migration (60). The dosage of paclitaxel that is exposed to the vessel wall also determines the type of response that is generated. At high doses, paclitaxel has been shown to cause inflammatory cell loss, medial thinning, and increase in stent thrombosis (61).

Analyzing and comparing the different trials that evaluated the efficacy of paclitaxel-eluting stents (PES) is a challenge due to the variation in the stent platforms used, protocols, dose densities, and techniques. The best approach is to evaluate the trials in subsets that used similar protocols, and more importantly stent platform, coating, and polymer carrier if one was used (62–69).

TAXUS Trials

The first trial in the TAXUS series, TAXUS I, was the first experience in humans with PES using the Taxus stent (Boston Scientific Corp, Minneapolis, MN). The TAXUS trials I to V used a similar protocol (62–66) involving either the NIRx (TAXUS I-III) or the Express stent platform (TAXUS IV, TAXUS V) that was coated with a proprietary coating and containing a polymer carrier on the surface. The copolymer system provides homogenous coverage upon stent deployment and assures predictable pharmacokinetics of drug delivery. The proprietary coating forms a biphasic release of paclitaxel with an initial burst in the first few days and a second release completed by the tenth day. The dose used was 1 mcg/mm^2. Other specifics about trial methodology and protocol have been described elsewhere (62–66). The relevant data involving paclitaxel polymer coated stents is shown in Table 12–2.

TAXUS I was a prospective, double-blind, multicenter trial that randomized 61 patients into either the TAXUS or the BMS

Table 12–2

Summary of the Polymer-Coated Paclitaxel Data

	TAXUS I	TAXUS II-MR	TAXUS II-SR	TAXUS IV	TAXUS V
Number of Patients	61	269	267	1314	1156
Lesion Length (mm)	11.3	10.5	10.6	13.4	17.3
RVD (mm)	2.97	2.70	2.80	2.75	2.69
DM (%)	18.1	15.5	13.5	32.3	30.8
Follow-up (month)	12	12	12	9	9
LLL (mm)					
BMS	0.71	0.77	0.79	0.92	0.90
PES	0.36	0.30	0.31	0.39	0.49
p-value	0.008	<0.0001	<0.0001	<0.001	<0.001
ISR (%)					
BMS	10.0	20.2	17.9	24.4	31.9
PES	0.0	4.7	2.3	5.5	13.7
p-value	NS	0.0002	0.0002	<0.001	<0.0001
TLR (%)					
BMS	13.3	14.6	12.0	17.4*	15.7
PES	0.0	3.1	4.6	5.6	8.6
p-value	NS	0.002	0.04	<0.0001	<0.0003
MACE (%)					
BMS	10.0	21.4	22.0	24.9*	21.2
PES	3.0	9.9	10.9	14.7	15.0
p-value	NS	0.017	0.02	<0.0001	0.008

Summary of the major randomized, controlled trials involving the polymer-coated paclitaxel-eluted stents in comparison to their matched controls. BMS, bare metal stents; DM, diabetes mellitus; ISR, in-stent restenosis; LLL, late luminal loss; MACE, major adverse cardiac events; MR, moderate-release; PES, paclitaxel-eluting stent; RVD, reference vessel diameter; SR, slow-release; TLR, target lesion revascularization.
*2-year follow-up data.

group using the same stent platform without medication. Angiography at 6-months showed a significant decrease in the late luminal loss (p = 0.008) and% DS (p <0.001) in the PES group in comparison to the BMS group. However, due to insufficient power of the study, the incidence of ISR, TLR, and MACE was not significantly different (62).

The TAXUS II trial was a randomized, double-blind, multicenter trial that randomized patients into two separate PES groups. Both the slow-release (SR) and the moderate-release (MR) paclitaxel formulations had their respective controls that were matched for clinical and angiographic variables. At the 6-month follow-up, there was a significant decrease in the late luminal loss (p <0.0001) and in-stent % DS (p <0.0001) in both the SR and MR groups when compared to their respective controls. The rate of ISR and in-lesion restenosis was significantly lower in both PES groups compared to their respective controls (Table 12–2). The 12-month incidence of MACE was significantly lower in the TAXUS groups versus their matched controls (p = 0.02). There was no significant difference in the rate of MI or death between either of the paclitaxel-eluting stent formulations with their respective BMS groups (63).

TAXUS IV was a randomized, double-blind, multicenter trial that enrolled 1,314 patients with similar clinical and angiographic variables to determine the efficacy and safety of PES (n = 662) versus BMS (n = 652). Clopidogrel was administered for 6 months after the procedure. Five hundred and fifty-nine (43%) patients underwent follow-up angiography that demonstrated a significant reduction in the amount of late lumen loss (p <0.001), in-stent % DS (p <0.001), and the rate of ISR (p <0.001) in the PES group as compared with the BMS group. The incidence of TLR (3% versus 11.3%) and MACE (8.5% versus 15%) was significantly lower in PES versus BMS group (p <0.001). There was no significant difference in the frequency of death from cardiac causes, MI, or stent thrombosis (64). The 2-year follow-up clinical data in 1,238 (94%) patients demonstrated the continued benefit of PES. The rate of TLR was 17.4% in the BMS group and 5.6% in the PES group (p <0.0001). The incidence of MACE was 24.9% in the BMS group and 14.7% in the PES group (p <0.0001). There was no significant difference in the incidence of cardiac death, MI or stent thrombosis between the two groups (65).

TAXUS V was a double-blind, multicenter trial that randomized 1,172 patients to determine the efficacy of PES in more complex lesions. In the 990 (75%) patients that underwent angiographic follow-up at 9-months, there was a significant decrease in the rate of ISR and in-lesion restenosis in the PES group (p <0.001). Clinically, there was a significant decrease in the frequency of TLR (p <0.0003) and MACE (p = 0.008) in the PES group in comparison to the BMS group. There was no significant difference in the incidence of MI or cardiac death between the two cohorts. However, there was an increase in the incidence of MI (8.3% versus 3.3%, n = 376) at 30-days in the PES versus BMS subgroup that received multiple stents (p = 0.047). Although the subset analysis was underpowered, the data prompted further studies involving more complex lesions (66).

ASPECT/ELUTES/DELIVER Trials

The ASPECT trial was a randomized, multicenter, controlled, double-blind study that evaluated the utility of PES to reduce ISR. The results of this trial and the other trials that did not utilize a polymer coating system are shown in Table 12–3. The trial also attempted to show a dose-dependent reduction in restenosis by utilizing two groups of PES with a dosage of 3.1 mcg/mm^2 and 1.3 mcg/mm^2 with the same controls. One hundred and seventy-seven patients were randomized into three groups: (i) 60 into the 3.1-PES group, (ii) 58 into the 1.3-PES group, and (iii) 59 into the BMS group. Unlike the TAXUS trial, the ASPECT trial did not utilize a polymer carrier, but used a proprietary process to bond paclitaxel on to the abluminal surface of the Supra-G stent (Cook Inc, Bloomington, IN). Antiplatelet therapy was not standardized with some patients receiving cilostazol in place of clopidogrel. Angiographic analysis conducted in 172 (97%) patients demonstrated a significant dose-dependent reduction in late lumen loss (p <0.001) and % DS (p <0.001). The incidence of ISR was 4% in the 3.1-PES group, 12% in the 1.3-PES group, and 27% in the BMS group (p <0.001). The rate of TLR was 3.4% in all three groups, and the frequency of MACE at 6-months was 5.2% in the BMS and 1.3-PES groups, and 11.9% in the

Table 12–3

Summary of the Nonpolymer-Coated Paclitaxel Data

	ASPECT	ELUTES	DELIVER
Dose (mcg/mm^2)	3.1	2.7	3.0
Number of Patients	177	190	1041
Lesion Length (mm)	10.9	10.8	11.4
RVD (mm)	2.92	2.96	2.81
DM (%)	20	15.8	28.8
Follow-up (month)	6	12	9
LLL (mm)			
BMS	1.04	0.73	0.98
PES	0.29	0.11	0.81
p-value	<0.001	0.002	0.0025
ISR (%)			
BMS	27.0	20.6	20.6
PES	4.0	3.2	14.9
p-value	<0.001	0.056	0.02
TLR (%)			
BMS	3.4	15.8	11.3
PES	3.4	5.4	8.1
p-value	NS	NS	NS
MACE (%)			NR
BMS	5.2	18.4	
PES	11.9	13.5	
p-value	NS	NS	

Summary of the major randomized, controlled trials involving the nonpolymer-coated paclitaxel-eluted stents in comparison to their matched controls. BMS, bare metal stents; DM, diabetes mellitus; ISR, in-stent restenosis; LLL, late luminal loss; MACE, major adverse cardiac events; NR, not reported; PES, paclitaxel-eluting stent; RVD, reference vessel diameter; TLR, target lesion revascularization.

3.1-PES group. The increase in MACE was attributed to an increase in subacute thrombosis in the 3.1-PES group, specifically in the patients that received cilostazol (67).

The ELUTES trial was a randomized, double-blind, controlled trial that evaluated the efficacy and safety of PES without a polymer coating. The cohort of patients was randomized into five groups (BMS, 0.2 mcg/mm^2, 0.7 mcg/mm^2, 1.4 mcg/mm^2, 2.7 mcg/mm^2) with similar clinical variables except for a significant difference in age between the 0.2 and the 2.7-PES groups (p = 0.02). The V-Flex Plus stent (Cook Inc, Bloomington, IN) was prepared similarly to the method used in the ASPECT trial. Angiography at the 6-month follow-up showed a significant reduction in late luminal loss (p = 0.002),% DS (p = 0.006), and the rate of ISR (p = 0.056) only in the 2.7-PES group compared with the BMS group. The lower dosage PES had no significant difference in any variables in comparison to the BMS. The rates of TLR and MACE were not significantly different between the five groups (68).

The DELIVER trial was a prospective, randomized, blinded, placebo-control trial that randomized 1,043 patients with similar clinical variables into the paclitaxel-coated (3.0 mcg/mm^2) ACHIEVE stent (Guidant Corp, Santa Clara, CA) (n = 522) versus the Rx ML PENTA stainless steel stent (Guidant Corp, Santa Clara, CA) (n = 519). Angiography at 8-months in 442 (42%) patients demonstrated a significant decrease in the late lumen loss (p = 0.002), in-stent (p = 0.02) and in-lesion % DS (p = 0.04) in PES in comparison to BMS. There was no significant difference in the incidence of ISR, in-lesion restenosis, and TLR between the two groups (69).

Sirolimus versus Paclitaxel-Eluting Stent Trials

The TAXi trial was the first prospective, randomized trial that compared the efficacy of SES (CYPHER) versus PES (TAXUS). Two hundred and two patients with similar demographics were randomized into two groups: the SES (n = 102) group and the PES (n = 100) group. Although the data showed no significant difference in MACE between SES and PES at 6-months, the trial was limited in its sample size to determine any clinical superiority between the two drug-eluting stents (DES) (70).

REALITY Trial

The REALITY trial was a large prospective, randomized trial that compared the polymer-coated Cypher SES against the polymer-coated Taxus PES in terms of safety and efficacy. The study randomized 1,353 patients with similar angiographic and clinical variables into SES (n = 684) and PES (n = 669) groups with the primary endpoint of the in-lesion restenosis rate at 8-months. The data from the REALITY trial, as well as other PES versus SES trials, are shown in Table 12–4. The trial demonstrated a significant decrease in the in-stent, in-lesion % DS, and late luminal loss in patients treated with SES in comparison to PES (p <0.001). However, the incidence of

in-lesion, ISR, TLR, MACE, MI, or cardiac death was not significantly different between the two groups at 9-months. Interestingly, the rate of vessel thrombosis at 30 days was significantly lower (0.4% versus 1.8%, p = 0.02) in the SES versus the PES group. The decrease in 30-day vessel thrombosis with SES raised concern about the long-term safety of PES versus SES, but this may have been a statistical aberrancy (71).

SIRTAX Trial

SIRTAX was a prospective, randomized trial that compared the efficacy of SES against PES. The study randomized 1,012 patients with similar clinical and angiographic variables into an SES group (n = 503) and a PES group (n = 509) with the primary end-point of MACE at 9 months. Follow-up angiography in 540 (53.4%) patients showed a significant decrease in late lumen loss (p <0.001) in the SES group. The rate of ISR and in-lesion restenosis was significantly lower in the SES group (p <0.02) at 9 months. The incidence of TLR was 4.8% in SES and 8.3% in PES (p = 0.025), and the frequency of MACE was 6.2% in the sirolimus and 10.8% in the paclitaxel group (p = 0.009). There was no significant difference in the rates of death, cardiac death, MI, or stent thrombosis between the two groups (72).

ISAR-DESIRE/ISAR-DIABETES Trials

In distinction to the previous trials that assessed DES to prevent restenosis, ISAR-DESIRE was a prospective, randomized, controlled trial that assessed the efficacy of DES in the treatment of ISR in comparison to conventional balloon angioplasty. Three hundred patients with similar clinical variables and documented angiographic ISR were randomized to receive either SES (n = 100), PES (n = 100), or balloon angioplasty (n = 100). Angiographic analysis preformed in 275 (92%) patients showed a significant decrease in rates of restenosis in both DES cohorts in comparison to balloon angioplasty at 9 months. A secondary analysis comparing the two DES cohorts showed a significant decrease in late lumen loss (p = 0.004) and in-stent % DS (p = 0.004) in the SES versus the PES group. There were lower rates of in-stent, in-lesion restenosis, and MACE that did not reach significance in the SES group. There was no significant difference in the incidence of death or MI across all three groups (73).

ISAR-DIABETES was a randomized trial that evaluated whether PES showed similar efficacy as SES in the management of patients with diabetes. Two hundred and fifty patients were randomized 1:1 to receive either SES or PES. The trial showed a significant decrease in late lumen loss (p <0.001), % DS (p = 0.004) in the SES group. There was a significant decrease in the incidence of ISR and in-lesion restenosis (p = 0.02) in the SES versus the PES group. The frequency of TLR was 6.4% in the SES group and 12% in the PES group. Although the rate of TLR in the PES group was almost double that of the SES, it lacked statistical significance probably due to small sample size. There was no significant difference in the incidence of death or MI in the two treatment arms (74).

Table 12–4

Summary of Sirolimus (CYPHER) versus Paclitaxel (TAXUS) Data

	REALITY	SIRTAX	ISAR-DESIRE	ISAR-DIABETES
Number of Patients	1353	1012	200	250
Lesion Length (mm)	17.1	12.9	11.95	13.1
RVD (mm)	2.40	2.83	2.60	2.73
DM (%)	27.9	19.9	21.5	100
Follow-up (month)	8	9	12	9
LLL (mm)				
SES	0.09	0.12	0.10	0.19
PES	0.31	0.25	0.26	0.46
p-value	<0.001	<0.001	0.009	<0.001
ISR (%)				
SES	7.0	3.2	11.0	4.9
PES	8.3	7.5	18.5	13.6
p-value	NS	0.013	NS	0.02
TLR (%)				
SES	5.0	4.8	8.0*	6.4
PES	5.4	8.3	19.0	12.0
p-value	NS	0.025	NS	NS
MACE (%)				NR
SES	9.2	6.2	11.0	
PES	10.6	10.8	22.0	
p-value	NS	0.009	NS	

Summary of the randomized clinical trials comparing the efficacy of sirolimus to paclitaxel-eluting stents. DM, diabetes mellitus; ISR, in-stent restenosis; LLL, late lumen loss; MACE, major adverse cardiac events; NR, not reported; PES, paclitaxel-eluting stent; RVD, reference vessel diameter; SES, sirolimus-eluting stents; TLR, target lesion revascularization.
*Target vessel revascularization.

Sirolimus-Eluting Stents versus Coronary Artery Bypass Graft Trial

ARTS II Trial

The ARTS II was a multicenter, nonrandomized, open-label trial that evaluated the effectiveness of SES in the prevention of future revascularization and major adverse cardiac and cerebrovascular events (MACCE) in patients with multivessel disease. A group of 607 patients that received SES was compared to the CABG cohort (n = 602) from the ARTS I trial. This was a historical control group and not a contemporary randomized trial. Nevertheless, the surgical results of the ARTS I Trial were excellent compared with other CABG trials. At 1-year follow-up the rate of percutaneous revascularization was 5.4% in the SES group and 3.0% in the CABG group (p = NS). Surgical revascularization was 2.0% in the SES group and 0.7% in the CABG group (p = NS). The incidence of MACCE was 10.2% in the SES group and 11.6% in the CABG cohort (p = NS). The rate of death, stroke, and MI was significantly lower with SES in comparison to CABG (p <0.001). Although the trial used a historical control, it suggests that SES may provide a safer alternative to surgery with equivalent efficacy in patients with multivessel disease. Prospective, randomized, controlled trials will be required to directly compare the effectiveness of angioplasty with drug-eluting stent implantation at decreasing revascularization while simultaneously reducing the cardiovascular morbidity associated with surgery (75). These preliminary results are encouraging and suggest that percutaneous intervention may have finally reached the goal of providing a true alternative to bypass surgery for the majority of patients with coronary artery disease.

Discussion and Conclusion

Restenosis has been a limiting factor to the clinical success of PCI. The introduction of stents significantly reduced rates of restenosis by eliminating elastic recoil and negative remodeling. However, the augmented inflammatory response that leads to an increase in neointimal hyperplasia associated with stenting, initiated a new challenge in interventional cardiology: ISR. Understanding the pathophysiology of restenosis, and specifically ISR, on a cellular and molecular level allowed for the development of targeted therapy. The DES delivers antiproliferative agents at effective doses to an area that experiences intense inflammation thus reducing neointimal formation without any systemic effects (48). Some of the earlier concerns surrounding

DES pertained to its increased propensity to cause coronary aneurysms based on experimental animal data (76). There were warnings that the drug or the polymer could damage the vessel leading to progressive luminal dilation, aneurysm formation, and predispose the vessel to thrombosis or rupture (76). However, none of the major clinical trials that compared either SES or PES to BMS showed a significant difference in aneurysm formation between the two groups (54,56,58,59,62–65). The wide-use of DES has brought forth another concern of subacute stent thrombosis that may result in a later catastrophic cardiac event. The use of ASA and clopidogrel is crucial in preventing subacute stent thrombosis (77). The major clinical trials involving sirolimus and paclitaxel demonstrated a total thrombosis rate of 0.4% and 0.6%, respectively (56,64). However, the majority of the patients in these trials presented with relatively simple lesions. With the increased utility of DES in patients with acute MI, bifurcation lesions, treatment for ISR, the rate of subacute stent thrombosis may increase. A recent prospective, observational study that enrolled a total of 2,229 consecutive patients with complicated lesions who underwent stenting with either SES or PES to evaluate stent thrombosis (78). At the 9-month follow-up, 29 (1.3%) patients had stent thrombosis and 14 (0.6%) patients developed subacute thrombosis with a case-fatality rate of 45% (78). The most common predictor of stent thrombosis was premature discontinuation of antiplatelet therapy. Early discontinuation of antiplatelet therapy is associated with a 30-fold increase in incidence of stent thrombosis (79). Other independent predictors included renal failure, bifurcation lesions, diabetes, low ejection fraction, and stent length (78). Although the rate of stent thrombosis in this observational study was significantly higher, the absolute number of cases is still low. Given the consequences of stent thrombosis, it is critical that patients and their physicians are educated regarding continuing their antiplatelet therapy with ASA and clopidogrel. The duration of therapy may need to be increased in patients with more complicated lesions, though that conclusion will have to be drawn from further randomized controlled trials.

In reviewing the data from major randomized trials involving SES and PES, one can appreciate the potential of drug-eluting stents. Approximately 3,160 patients were evaluated in the Bx-Velocity SES, and 4201 were evaluated in studies involving the TAXUS stent. The angiographic data are impressive. SES produces a remarkable reduction in late luminal loss, diameter stenosis, and neointimal hyperplasia demonstrating the effectiveness of sirolimus in inhibiting rapidly proliferating VSMC. The reduction in ISR to <5% of the lesions underlines the success sirolimus stents have at keeping the vessel patent. Clinically, SES was successful in significantly reducing MACE by decreasing the requirement for revascularization. In none of the sirolimus trials was there a mortality benefit or a significant reduction in the incidence of MI. The efficacy and safety of sirolimus up to 4-years of follow-up indicates that the coated polymer stent loaded with 1 mcg/mm^2 of sirolimus serves as an effective agent in the prevention of ISR. The coated polymer controls the release kinetics to provide an initial burst of sirolimus at the time of a high rate of proliferation and a basal elution for inhibition of neointimal formation within the critical window of the first month.

The paclitaxel trials can be divided into two groups. The first is the TAXUS trials (62–66), which used a coated polymer and repeatedly demonstrated significant reduction in late lumen loss, diameter stenosis, and neointimal hyperplasia. The reduction in the incidence of ISR is not as dramatic as observed in the sirolimus trials but is significant. The rate of MACE at the 1-year follow-up was again reduced significantly by decreasing the need for revascularization; however, there was no reduction in the incidence of MI or cardiac mortality. The second group of trials (ASPECT, ELUTES, DELIVER) (67–69) did not use a polymer-coated stent and failed to demonstrate a clinical benefit in terms of MACE or prevention of future revascularization. The trials also showed that an increased paclitaxel dose was required to produce a significant angiographic benefit that was comparable to the TAXUS or sirolimus groups. The controlled-release of the drug with the coated polymer generates a greater angiographic benefit and more favorable clinical outcomes. The lack of polymer requires the use of higher doses of antiproliferative agents that perhaps induced injury to the vessel wall reducing the benefit of PES and, thus, does not show improvement in clinical outcomes.

Although the use of DES has been shown to be safe, there are numerous unresolved issues. The number of study patients who received these stents is still relatively small. The lesions treated in these trials are relatively simple in the sense that the lesion length is short, the reference vessel diameter is large, and the percentage of patients with diabetes is small, which are all factors that will lower the rate of restenosis. In addition, the majority of the trials enrolled patients without previous interventions. The TAXUS III trial treated a cohort of 28 patients with ISR without controls. The repeat restenosis rate was 16%. The benefit in terms of late lumen loss and MACE was reduced compared with the results reported in previous trials involving PES (80). The issue of edge-restenosis appears to be resolved. Previously, there was a concern that the uneven distribution of the agent would deliver less of the drug to the edges, thus reducing ISR but increasing in-lesion restenosis (81). The studies that reported the in-lesion % DS and incidence of in-lesion restenosis demonstrated that there was no significant difference in edge restenosis between DES and the BMS group (81). Stent malapposition is another potential problem detected by IVUS that is increased in the SES group in comparison to the controls in the SIRIUS and RAVEL trials at 6-months (54,56). Such findings were not observed in the TAXUS-II trial (63). However, these observations have not been associated with any adverse events to date.

In addition, there are only limited data involving DES in complex lesion subsets that include acute MI, bifurcation lesions, left main disease, and saphenous vein grafts. The majority of the clinical trials excluded patients that presented such therapeutic challenges. Recently, some of these subsets have been investigated in clinical trials. The STRATEGY trial was the first randomized, single-center trial that randomized 175 patients to evaluate the effectiveness of SES versus BMS in acute MI. The trial demonstrated significant reduction in late lumen loss, ISR (7.5% versus 28%, p = 0.01), in-lesion restenosis, and TLR (6% versus 20%, p = 0.006) in the SES versus BMS group at 8 months. There was no significant difference in the rate of death, reinfarction, or stent thrombosis at 30 days and 8 months (82). The data are comparable to the RESEARCH registry that showed a significant decrease in MACE (9.4% versus 17%, p = 0.02) and TVR (1.1% versus 8.2%, p <0.01) in the SES versus the BMS group at the 10-month follow-up. Again there was no significant difference in the incidence of stent thrombosis, death, or reinfarction at 30 and 300 days (83). The preliminary clinical data suggest that SES is as safe as BMS when used during acute MI and appear to produce less restenosis in this setting as well.

Another unresolved issue is the role of DES in the treatment of bifurcation lesions. Historically, stenting of the side branch (SB) has yielded a high restenosis rate (30%) (84). Prospective, as well as retrospective data involving either SES or PES has been unable to show any angiographic or clinical benefit with stenting of the SB compared with provisional stenting (85–88). Stent malapposition, breakage of polymer secondary to the overlap of multiple strut layers and uneven distribution of struts may account for the lack of benefit with SB stenting (85). Potentially newer implantation techniques, such as the "crush" technique, reduce stent malapposition and may show improvement in clinical and angiographic parameters (87). One of the main concerns regarding stenting both the main branch (MB) and the SB is the increased risk of both post-procedural and subacute stent thrombosis (85–88). The failure to use periprocedural glycoprotein IIb/IIIA inhibitors and premature discontinuation of antiplatelet therapy was largely responsible for an increased incidence of stent thrombosis (85–88). Only large randomized trials involving bifurcation lesions will establish the appropriate procedural technique, the benefit of SB stenting, and the ideal duration of antiplatelet therapy.

The use of DES as treatment for unprotected left main (LM) disease is another unresolved area of DES. Traditionally, unprotected LM lesions are an indication for surgical revascularization (89). Recently, retrospective and small prospective studies have demonstrated the safety of DES in the treatment of unprotected LM disease (89–91). In comparison to historical BMS controls, DES showed a reduction in the rates of MI, MACE, and TVR at 6-months and 1-year, calling for a randomized trial comparing DES (89,91).

The use of DES in the treatment of saphenous vein graft (SVG) lesions is beginning to be explored. Past studies estimate that at least 50% of SVG lesions will develop stenosis or occlusion within 10 years of implantation (92). Given the higher morbidity and mortality associated with repeat surgical revascularization, PCI is a preferred option (92). Although BMS improved outcomes in SVG lesions compared with balloon angioplasty, the rates of ISR remain elevated (20%–37%) (92). A retrospective analysis that compared DES versus historical BMS controls showed a reduction in restenosis (10% versus 26.7%, p = 0.03), TLR and MACE at 6-months, demonstrating the safety of DES in these lesions (92). Given that 4% to 7% of stented SVG lesions developed late occlusion, the safety of DES will be evaluated only with long-term follow-up and more clinical trial data (92).

Other questions, such as whether DES only delay eventual restenosis, can only be answered with longer follow-up. The 3-year follow-up data from the RAVEL trial suggest that the reduction in TLR and MACE obtained from SES is attenuated at 3 years compared with 1 year. However, the SIRIUS trial showed persistent benefits at the 3-year follow-up in reducing the incidence of TLR and MACE in the SES group. This discrepancy will be resolved with further follow-up from both the sirolimus and paclitaxel groups. In addition, the long-term compatibility of the coated polymer with the vessel remains to be seen. Early polymers were pro-inflammatory within the vasculature, exaggerating neointimal hyperplasia (45). It is conceivable that the polymer may produce a chronic hypersensitivity vasculitis that could lead to neointimal proliferation and vessel occlusion. Only long-term follow-up will be able to determine if such problems will arise.

The lack of a mortality benefit may be a concern for practitioners in the community. However, the absence of a mortality benefit in drug-eluting stent clinical trials is consistent with the fact that angioplasty has repeatedly failed to show improvement in mortality in patients with stable CAD. This is attributed to the high crossover of medically treated patients to PTCA once they become unstable. Angioplasty, as an extension of medical therapy, reduces angina, limitation of activities of daily living, decreases hospitalization, and provides a less invasive alternative to surgical revascularization. These benefits need to be balanced with the excess cost to the health care system that comes with the usage of these stents (93).

Another issue that will continue to evolve with the introduction of new drug-eluting stent platforms and pharmaceuticals is to decide which coated stent is clinically superior and should be used as the mainstream therapy for CAD. A recent meta-analysis attempted to resolve the conflict of which stent provides the most benefit (94). Although the sirolimus-eluting stent was superior in reducing the rates of restenosis and TVR, the incidence of death, MI, or stent thrombosis was similar (94). Further follow-up and more studies will address which drug-eluting stent maybe clinically superior.

The cost of DES has also been a major limiting factor to the wide use of this intervention. Based on the cost analysis conducted by Cohen, it is estimated that there is approximately a $2,000 cost difference when DES are used as opposed to BMS. Thus, an extra 2.4 billion would be added in procedural costs yearly if any DES are used. However, the reduction in the need for further PCI or CABG reduces that amount to 1.5 billion each year (95,96). Well-informed patients understand the clinical and angiographic benefits of drug-eluting stents that have been demonstrated in large-scale randomized clinical trials. Patients request these stents that provide a preventive strategy to ISR. Perhaps as newer antiproliferative agents and improved stent platforms are approved by the FDA, the cost of DES will be appreciably reduced.

REFERENCES

1. American Heart Association. Heart Disease Stroke Statistics – 2003 Update. Dallas: American Heart Association; 2002.

2. Lowe HC, Oesterle SN, Khachigian LM. Coronary in-stent restenosis: current status and future strategies. *J Am Coll Cardiol.* 2002;39:183–193.

3. Schwartz RS. Animal models of human coronary restenosis. In: Topol EJ, ed. *Textbook of Interventional Cardiology.* 2nd ed. Philadelphia: WB Saunders; 1994:365–381.

4. Serruys PW, de Jaegere P, Kiemeneij F, et al. A comparison of balloon-expandable-stent implantation with balloon angioplasty in patients with coronary artery disease. Benestent Study Group. *N Engl J Med.* 1994;331:489–495.

5. Fischman DL, Leon MB, Baim DS, et al. A randomized comparison of coronary-stent placement and balloon angioplasty in the treatment of coronary artery disease. *N Engl J Med.* 1994;331:496–501.

6. Holmes DR Jr., Vlietstra RE, Smith HC, et al. Restenosis after percutaneous transluminal coronary angioplasty (PTCA): a report from the PTCA Registry of the National Heart, Lung, and Blood Institute. *Am J Cardiol.* 1984;53:77C–81C.

7. Mintz GS, Popma JJ, Pichard AD, et al. Arterial remodeling after coronary angioplasty: a serial intravascular ultrasound study. *Circulation.* 1996;94:35–43.

8. Kimura T, Kaburagi S, Tashima Y, et al. Geometric remodeling and intimal regrowth as mechanisms of restenosis: observations from serial ultrasound analysis of restenosis (SURE) trial. *Circulation.* 1995;92:I–76.

9. Sigwart U, Puel J, Mirkovitch V, et al. Intravascular stents to prevent occlusion and restenosis after transluminal angioplasty. *N Engl J Med.* 1987;316:701–706.

10. Gould K, Lipscomb K, Hamilton GW. Physiological basis for assessing critical coronary stenosis: instantaneous flow response and regional distribution during coronary hyperemia as measures of coronary flow reserve. *Am J Cardiol.* 1974;33:87–94.

11. Garas SM, Huber P, Scott NA. Overview of therapies for prevention of restenosis after coronary interventions. *Pharmacol Ther.* 2001;92:165–178.

12. Rensing BJ, Hermans WR, Beatt KJ, et al. Quantitative angiographic assessment of elastic recoil after percutaneous transluminal coronary angioplasty. *Am J Cardiol.* 1990;66:1039–1044.

13. Scott NA, Cipolla GD, Ross CE, et al. Identification of a potential role for the adventitia in vascular lesion formation after balloon overstretch injury of porcine coronary arteries. *Circulation.* 1996;93:2178–2187.

14. Schwartz RS, Henry TD. Pathophysiology of coronary artery restenosis. *Rev Cardiovasc Med.* 2002;3:S4–S9.

15. Grant MB, Wargovich TJ, Ellis EA, et al. Localization of insulin-like growth factor I and inhibition of coronary smooth muscle cell growth by somatostatin analogues in human coronary smooth muscle cells. A potential treatment for restenosis? *Circulation.* 1994;89:1511–1517.

16. Reidy MA, Fingerle J, Lindner V. Factors controlling the development of arterial lesions after injury. *Circulation.* 1992;86:III43–III46.

17. Castellot JJ Jr, Addonizio ML, Rosenberg R, et al. Cultured endothelial cells produce heparin-like inhibitor of smooth muscle growth. *J Cell Biol.* 1981;90:372–377.

18. Indolfi C, Mongiardo A, Curcio A. Molecular mechanisms of in-stent restenosis and approach to therapy with eluting stents. *Trends Cardiovasc Med.* 2003;13:142–148.

19. Indolfi C, Avvedimento EV, Rapacciuolo A, et al. Inhibition of cellular RAS prevents smooth muscle cell proliferation after vascular injury in vivo. *Nat Med.* 1995;6:541–545.

20. Indolfi C, Avvedimento EV, Rapacciuolo A, et al. In vivo gene transfer: prevention of neointima formation by inhibition of mitogen-activated protein kinase kinase. *Basic Res Cardiol.* 1997;92:378–384.

21. Grewe PH, Deneke T, Machraoui A, et al. Acute and chronic tissue response to coronary stent implantation: pathologic findings in human specimen. *J Am Coll Cardiol.* 2000;35:157–163.

22. Mintz GS, Popma JJ, Pichard AD, et al. Arterial remodeling after coronary angioplasty: a serial intravascular ultrasound study. *Circulation.* 1996;94:35–43.

23. Wilcox JN, Waksman R, King SB, et al. The role of the adventitia in the arterial response to angioplasty: the effect of intravascular radiation. *Int J Radiat Biol Phys.* 1996;36:789–796.

24. Kuntz RE, Gibson CM, Nobuyoshi M, et al. Generalized model of restenosis after conventional balloon angioplasty, stenting and directional atherectomy. *J Am Coll Cardiol.* 1993;21:15–25.

25. Gordon PC, Gibson CM, Cohen DJ, et al. Mechanisms of restenosis and redilation within coronary stents-quantitative angiographic assessment. *J Am Coll Cardiol.* 1993;21:1166–1174.

26. Hoffmann R, Mintz GS, Dussaillant GR, et al. Patterns and mechanisms of in-stent restenosis. A serial intravascular ultrasound study. *Circulation.* 1996;94:1247–1254.

27. Kornowski R, Hong MK, Tio FO, et al. In-stent restenosis: contributions of inflammatory responses and arterial injury to neointimal hyperplasia. *J Am Coll Cardiol.* 1998;31:224–230.

28. Koster R, Vieluf D, Kiehn M, et al. Nickel and molybdenum contact allergies in patients with coronary in-stent restenosis. *Lancet.* 2000;356:1895–1897.

29. Fitzgerald PJ, Oshima A, Hayase M, et al. Final results of the Can Routine Ultrasound Influence Stent Expansion (CRUISE) study. *Circulation.* 2000;102:523–530.

30. Bittl JA, Chew DP, Topol EJ, et al. Meta-analysis of randomized trials of percutaneous transluminal coronary angioplasty versus atherectomy, cutting balloon atherotomy, or laser angioplasty. *J Am Coll Cardiol.* 2004;43:936–942.

31. Martinez-Elbal L, Ruiz-Nodar JM, Zueco J, et al. Direct coronary stenting versus stenting with balloon pre-dilation: immediate and follow-up results of a multicenter, prospective, randomized study. The DISCO trial. *Eur Heart J.* 2002;23:633–640.

32. Kastrati A, Mehilli J, Dirschinger J, et al. Intracoronary stenting and angiographic results: strut thickness effect on restenosis outcome (ISAR-STEREO) trial. *Circulation.* 2001;103:2816–2821.

33. Takagi T, Akasaka T, Yamamuro A, et al. Troglitazone reduced neointimal tissue proliferation after coronary stent implantation in patients with non-insulin dependent diabetes mellitus. *J Am Coll Cardiol.* 2000;36:1529–1535.

34. Holmes DR Jr, Savage M, LaBlanche JM, et al. Results of Prevention of REStenosis with Tranilast and its Outcomes (PRESTO) trial. *Circulation.* 2002;106:1243–1250.

35. Walter DH, Schachinger V, Elsner M, et al. Effect of statin therapy on restenosis after coronary stent implantation. *Am J Cardiol.* 2000;85:962–968.

36. Tanabe Y, Ito E, Nakagawa I. Effect of cilostazol on restenosis after coronary angioplasty and stenting in comparison to conventional coronary artery stenting with ticlopidine. *Int J Cardiol.* 2001;78:285–291.

37. Kozuma K, Hara K, Yamasaki M. Effects of cilostazol on late lumen loss and repeat revascularization after Palmaz-Schatz coronary stent implantation. *Am Heart J.* 2001;141:124–130.

38. Park S, Lee CW, Kim H, et al. Effects of cilostazol on angiographic restenosis after coronary stent placement. *Am J Cardiol* 2000;86:499–503.

39. Raizner AE, Oesterle SN, Waksman R, et al. Inhibition of restenosis with beta-emitting radiotherapy: report of the Proliferation Reduction with Vascular Energy Trial (PREVENT). *Circulation.* 2000;102:951–958.

40. Sabate M, Pimentel G, Prieto C, et al. Intracoronary brachytherapy after stenting de novo lesions in diabetic patients: results of a randomized intravascular ultrasound study. *J Am Coll Cardiol.* 2004;44:520–527.

41. Coen V, Serruys P, Sauerwein W, et al. Reno, a European postmarket surveillance registry, confirms effectiveness of coronary brachytherapy in routine clinical practice. *Int J Radiat Oncol Biol Phys.* 2003;55:1019–1026.

42. Amols HI, Zaider M, Weinberger J, et al. Dosimetric consideration for catheter-based beta and gamma emitters in the therapy of neointimal hyperplasia in human coronary arteries. *Int J Radiat Oncol Biol Phys.* 1996;36:913–921.

43. Sabate M, Costa MA, Kozuma K, et al. Geographic miss: a cause of treatment failure in radio-oncology applied to intracoronary radiation therapy. *Circulation.* 2000;103:E65–E66.

44. Heldman AW, Cheng L, Jenkins GM, et al. Paclitaxel stent coating inhibits neointimal hyperplasia at 4 weeks in a porcine model of coronary restenosis. *Circulation.* 2001;103:2289–2295.

45. van der Giessen WJ, Lincoff AM, Schwartz RS, et al. Marked inflammatory sequelae to implantation of biodegradable and nonbiodegradable polymers in porcine coronary arteries. *Circulation.* 1996;94:1690–1697.

46. Saunders RN, Metcalfe MS, Nicholson ML. Rapamycin in transplantation: a review of the evidence. *Kidney Int.* 2001;59:3–16.

47. Poon M, Marx SO, Gallo R, et al. Rapamycin inhibits vascular smooth muscle cell migration. *J Clin Invest.* 1996;98:2277–2283.

48. Suzuki T, Kopia G, Hayashi S, et al. Stent-based delivery of sirolimus reduces neointimal formation in a porcine coronary model. *Circulation.* 2001;104:1188–1193.

49. Sousa JE, Costa MA, Abizaid A, et al. Lack of neointimal proliferation after implantation of sirolimus-coated stents in human coronary arteries. A quantitative coronary angiography and three-dimensional intravascular ultrasound study. *Circulation.* 2001;103:192–195.

50. Sousa JE, Costa MA, Abizaid A, et al. Sustained suppression of neointimal proliferation by sirolimus-eluting stents. One-year angiographic and intravascular ultrasound follow-up. *Circulation.* 2001;104:2007–2011.

51. Sousa JE, Costa MA, Sousa A, et al. Two-year angiographic and intravascular ultrasound follow-up after implantation of sirolimus-eluting stents in human coronary arteries. *Circulation.* 2003;107:381–383.

52. Rensing BJ, Vos J, Smits PC, et al. Coronary restenosis elimination with sirolimus eluting stent. First European human experience with 6-month angiographic and intravascular ultrasound follow-up. *Eur Heart J.* 2001; 22:2125–2130.

53. Degertekin M, Serruys PW, Foley DP, et al. Persistent inhibition of neointimal hyperplasia after sirolimus-eluting stent implantation. Long-term (up to 2 years) clinical, angiographic, and intravascular ultrasound follow-up. *Circulation.* 2002;106:1610–1613.

54. Morice MC, Serruys P, Sousa JE, et al. A randomized comparison of a sirolimus-eluting stent with a standard stent for coronary revascularization. *N Engl J Med.* 2002;346:1773–1780.

55. Fajadet J, Morice MC, Bode C, et al. Maintenance of long-term clinical benefit with sirolimus-eluting coronary stents. Three-year results of the RAVEL trial. *Circulation.* 2005;111:1040–1044.

56. Moses JW, Leon MB, Popma JJ, et al. Sirolimus-eluting stents versus standard stents in patients with stenosis in a native coronary artery. *N Engl J Med.* 2003;349:1315–1323.

57. Leon MB for the SIRIUS Trial Investigators. Long-term clinical benefit of CYPHER sirolimus-eluting coronary stents: 3-year follow-up of the SIRIUS study. Presented at: 54th Annual Scientific Session of the American College of Cardiology; March, 2005; Orlando, FL.

58. Schofer J, Schluter M, Gershlick AH, et al. Sirolimus-eluting stents for treatment of patients with long atherosclerotic lesions in small coronary arteries: double-blind, randomized controlled trial (E-SIRIUS). *Lancet.* 2003;362:1093–1099.

59. Schampaert E, Cohen EA, Schluter M, et al. The Canadian study of sirolimus-eluting stent in the treatment of patients with long de novo lesions in small native coronary arteries (C-SIRIUS). *J Am Coll Cardiol.* 2004; 43:1110–1115.

60. Rowinsky EK, Donehower RC. Paclitaxel (taxol). *N Engl J Med.* 1995; 332:1004–1014.

61. Farb A, Heller PF, Shroff S, et al. Pathological analysis of local delivery of paclitaxel via a polymer-coated stent. *Circulation.* 2001;104:473–479.

62. Grube E, Silber S, Hauptmann KE, et al. TAXUS I: Six- and twelve-month results from a randomized, double-blind trial on a slow release paclitaxel-eluting stent for de novo coronary lesions. *Circulation.* 2003;107: 38–42.

63. Colombo A, Drzewiecki J, Banning A, et al. Randomized study to assess the effectiveness of slow- and moderate-release polymer-based paclitaxel-eluting stents for coronary artery lesions. *Circulation.* 2003;108:788–794.

64. Stone GW, Ellis SG, Cox DA, et al. A polymer-based, paclitaxel-eluting stent in patients with coronary artery disease. *N Engl J Med.* 2004;350: 221–231.

65. TAXUS IV US Pivotal Trial data at 24-months. Available at: http://www.bostonscientific.com.

66. Stone GW, Ellis SG, Cannon L, et al. Comparison of a polymer-based paclitaxel-eluting stent with a bare metal stent in patients with complex coronary artery disease. *JAMA.* 2005;294:1215–1223.

67. Park SJ, Shim WH, Ho DS, et al. A paclitaxel-eluting stent for prevention of coronary restenosis. *N Engl J Med.* 2003;348:1537–1545.

68. Gershlick A, De Scheerder I, Chevalier B, et al. Inhibition of restenosis with a paclitaxel-eluting, polymer-free coronary stent (ELUTES). *Circulation.* 2004;109:487–493.

69. Lansky AJ, Costa RA, Mintz GS, et al. Non-polymer-based paclitaxel-coated coronary stents for the treatment of patients with de novo coronary lesions. Angiographic follow-up of the DELIVER clinical trial. *Circulation.* 2004;109:1948–1954.

70. Goy JJ, Stauffer JC, Siegenthaler M, et al. A prospective randomized comparison between paclitaxel and sirolimus stents in the real world of interventional cardiology. *J Am Coll Cardiol.* 2005;45:308–311.

71. Morice MC for the REALITY Trial Investigators. REALITY: a prospective, randomized, multi-center comparison study of the CYPHER sirolimus-eluting and TAXUS paclitaxel-eluting stent systems. Presented at: 54th Annual Scientific Session of the American College of Cardiology; March 2005; Orlando, FL.

72. Windecker S, Remondino A, Eberli F, et al. Sirolimus-eluting and paclitaxel-eluting stents for coronary revascularization. *N Engl J Med.* 2005;353:653–662.

73. Kastrati A, Mehilli J, von Beckerath N, et al. Sirolimus-eluting stent or paclitaxel-eluting stent vs balloon angioplasty for prevention of recurrences in patients with coronary in-stent restenosis: a randomized controlled trial. *JAMA.* 2005;293:165–171.

74. Dibra A, Kastrati A, Mehilli J, et al. Paclitaxel-eluting or sirolimus-eluting stents to prevent restenosis in diabetic patients. *N Engl J Med.* 2005;353:663–670.

75. Serruys PW. Arterial revascularization therapies study part II of the sirolimus-eluting stent in the treatment of patients with multivessel de novo coronary artery lesions. Presented at: 54th Annual Scientific Session of the American College of Cardiology; March, 2005; Orlando, FL.

76. Vik-Mo H, Wiseth R, Hegbom K. Coronary aneurysm after implantation of a paclitaxel-eluting stent. *Scand Cardiovasc. J* 2004;38:349–352.

77. Steinhubl SR, Berger PB, Mann JT, et al. Clopidogrel for the reduction of events during observation. *JAMA.* 2002;288:2411–2420.

78. Iakovou I, Schmidt T, Bonizzoni E, et al. Incidence, predictors, and outcome of thrombosis after successful implantation of drug-eluting stents. *JAMA.* 2005;293:2126–2130.

79. Jeremias A, Sylvia B, Bridges J, et al. Stent thrombosis after successful sirolimus-eluting stent implantation. *Circulation.* 2004;109:1930–1932.

80. Tanabe K, Serruys PW, Grube E, et al. TAXUS III Trial. In-stent restenosis treated with stent-based delivery of paclitaxel incorporated in a slow-release polymer formulation. *Circulation.* 2003;107:559–564.

81. Babapulle MH, Joseph L, Belisle P, et al. A hierarchical Bayesian meta-analysis of randomized clinical trials of drug-eluting stents. *Lancet.* 2004;364:583–591.

82. Valgimigli M, Percoco G, Malagutti P, et al. Tirofiban and sirolimus-eluting stent vs abciximab and bare-metal stent for acute myocardial infarction. *JAMA.* 2005;293:2109–2117.

83. Lemos PA, Saia F, Hofma S, et al. Short- and long-term clinical benefit of sirolimus-eluting stents compared to conventional bare stents for patients with acute myocardial infarction. *J Am Coll Cardiol.* 2004;43:704–708.

84. Melikian N, Airoldi F, Di Mario C. Coronary bifurcation stenting. Current techniques, outcomes and possible future developments. *Minera Cardioangiol.* 2004;52:365–378.

85. Colombo A, Moses JW, Morice MC, et al. Randomized study to evaluate sirolimus-eluting stents implanted at coronary bifurcation lesions. *Circulation.* 2004;109:1244–1249.

86. Pan M, Suarez de Lezo J, Medina A, et al. Rapamycin-eluting stents for the treatment of bifurcated coronary lesions: A randomized comparison of a simple versus complex strategy. *Am Heart J.* 2004;148:857–864.

87. Ge L, Airoldi F, Iakovou I, et al. Clinical and angiographic outcome after implantation of drug-eluting stents in bifurcation lesions with the crush stent technique. Importance of final kissing balloon post-dilation. *J Am Coll Cardiol.* 2005;46:613–620.

88. Ge L, Tsagalou E, Iakovou I, et al. In-hospital and nine-month outcome of treatment of coronary bifurcational lesions with sirolimus-eluting stent. *Am J Cardiol.* 2005;95:757–760.

89. Valgimigli M, van Mieghem CAG, Ong AT, et al. Short- and long-term clinical outcomes after drug-eluting stent implantation for the percutaneous treatment of left main coronary artery disease. *Circulation*. 2005;11:1383–1389.

90. Arampatzis CA, Lemos PA, Hoye A, et al. Elective sirolimus-eluting stent implantation for left main coronary artery disease: six-month angiographic follow-up and 1-year clinical outcome. *Cathet Cardiovasc Interv*. 2004;62:292–296.

91. Chieffo A, Stankovic G, Bonizzoni E, et al. Early and mid-term results of drug-eluting stent implantation in unprotected left main. *Circulation*. 2005;111:791–795.

92. Ge L, Iakovou I, Sangiorgi GM, et al. Treatment of saphenous vein graft lesions with drug-eluting stents. *J Am Coll Cardiol*. 2005;45:989–994.

93. Cohen DJ, Breall JA, Ho KK, et al. Economics of elective coronary revascularization. Comparison of costs and charges for conventional angioplasty, directional atherectomy, stenting and bypass surgery. *J Am Coll Cardiol*. 1993;22:1052–1059.

94. Kastrati A, Dibra A, Eberle S, et al. Sirolimus-eluting stents vs paclitaxel-eluting stents in patients with coronary artery disease. Meta-analysis of randomized trials. *JAMA*. 2005;294:819–825.

95. Cohen DJ, Bakhai A, Shi C, et al. Cost-effectiveness of sirolimus-eluting stents for treatment of complex coronary stenoses: results from the Sirolimus-Eluting Balloon Expandable Stent in the Treatment of Patients With De Novo Native Coronary Artery Lesions (SIRIUS) trial. *Circulation*. 2004;110:508–514.

96. Lemos PA, Serruys PW, Sousa JE. Drug-eluting stents: cost versus clinical benefit. *Circulation*. 2003;107:3003–3007.

Procedures and Management

Barry F. Uretsky

CHAPTER 13

Secondary Prevention

Arun Kuchela

The diagnosis of coronary artery disease (CAD) carries a high risk of future ischemic cardiac events (1,2). Although primary prevention is targeted at modifying risk factors in an effort to prevent the development of coronary heart disease (CHD), secondary prevention focuses on both controlling risk factors and directing therapies to prevent disease progression and future events (3). The AHA/ACC guidelines for secondary prevention list several goals, which will be reviewed (Table 13–1) (4).

Risk factors may be divided into four categories: predisposing factors (age, gender, family history, and genetics), risk-modifying behaviors (smoking, diet, physical activity, and alcohol), metabolic risk factors (hypertension, diabetes, dyslipidemias, obesity, and metabolic syndrome) and disease markers (abnormal noninvasive or invasive tests and biomarkers) (5). Some of these risk factors can be modified, either by lifestyle changes or drug therapy.

Lifestyle Changes

Several CAD guidelines list nine lifestyle and dietary recommendations (6) (Table 13–2).

Smoking

Smoking is one of the conventional cardiac risk factors in the Framingham study and is associated with a relative risk (RR) or odds ratio (OR) of at least 1.5 to 3.0. A systematic review of 20 studies showed a 36% reduction in the crude relative risk with smoking cessation in patients with prior MI or angina regardless of age, gender, index event, country, or year of study (7). A more recent systematic review conservatively estimated the mortality risk reduction of smoking cessation at 35% in patients with CAD (6).

Physical Activity

Physical activity has been known for sometime to be associated with fewer ischemic cardiac events. It is unclear whether this is by a direct effect or by the associated effects on other cardiac risk factors (lower blood pressure, less insulin resistance, less obesity, or improved lipid profile) (8). The previously mentioned review estimated a 25% reduction in all-cause mortality with regular exercise (6). The American Heart Association (AHA) scientific statements on exercise and cardiac rehabilitation both discuss the importance of physical activity and the former recommends a prescription for 30 minutes or more of daily moderate-intensity physical activity (8,9).

Lipid Lowering

Lipid lowering therapy, especially with statins, is an important focus of secondary prevention and is extensively studied, but not fully answered. LDL reduction with statin therapy is directly proportional to the decrease in cardiac events (10) (Fig. 13–1).

The Scandinavian Simvastatin Survival Trial (4S) established the benefit of lipid lowering for secondary prevention in patients with hypercholesterolemia. It randomized 4,444 patients with documented coronary artery disease (angina or previous MI) and total cholesterol between 200 to 300 mg/dL to simvastatin 20 to 40 mg/day or placebo. The primary end point was all-cause mortality and the median follow-up was 5.4 years. Simvastatin reduced total cholesterol by 25%, LDL by 35%, and raised HDL by 8%. There was a 30% relative risk reduction (RRR) in overall mortality (8.2% versus 11.5%; $P = 0.0003$), 39% fewer nonfatal MI's, 41% fewer coronary deaths, 34% fewer coronary events, and 37% lower risk of revascularization (11).

The benefit of lipid lowering for secondary prevention in patients with average cholesterol was evaluated in the Cholesterol and Recurrent Events (CARE) Study. It randomized 4,159 patients with a MI at least 3 months prior and total cholesterol <240 mg/dL, LDL between 115 to 147 mg/dL and triglycerides <350 mg/dL to pravastatin 40 mg/day versus placebo. The primary end point was coronary death and nonfatal MI, with a median follow-up of 5 years. Pravastatin treatment reduced the primary endpoint by 24% (13.2% versus 10.2%; p = 0.003). There was a 25% reduction in MI's (p = 0.006), 31% reduction in stroke (p = 0.03), and 27% less revascularization with pravastatin. However, there was a nonsignificant 9% reduction in all-cause mortality (p = 0.37) and a 20% reduction in cardiovascular death (p = 0.10) with treatment. The reduction in events was greatest with higher LDL levels (35% reduction for LDL >150 mg/dL, 26% reduction for 125 to 150 mg/dL, and 3% increase for LDL <125 mg/dL). Thus, CARE demonstrated

---

Table 13–1

AHA/ACC Secondary Prevention Goals for Patients with Coronary and Other Vascular Disease

Smoking	Complete cessation
BP Control	<140/90 mm Hg or
	<130/85 mm Hg if CHF or renal insufficiency
	<130/80 mm Hg if diabetes
Lipid Management	Primary goal LDL <100 mg/dL
Physical Activity	Minimum of 30 minutes 3 to 4 days/week;
	Optimally, on a daily basis
Weight Management	BMI 18.5 to 24.9 kg/m^2
Diabetes Management	HbA1c <7%
Anti-platelet Agents	Aspirin 75 to 325 mg/d indefinitely, Clopidogrel 75 mg/d or warfarin if aspirin contraindicated
ACE inhibitors	All patients indefinitely post-MI. Consider for all other coronary or vascular disease patients
Beta Blockers	Indefinitely for all post-MI and ACS. Use as needed for angina, rhythm, or BP.

Adapted from: Smith SC Jr, et al. AHA/ACC scientific statement: AHA/ACC guidelines for preventing heart attack and death in patients with atherosclerotic cardiovascular disease: 2001 update: a statement for healthcare professionals from the American Heart Association and the American College of Cardiology. *Circulation.* 2001;104:1577–1579, with permission.

---

a clear nonmortality benefit to secondary prevention with pravastatin in patients with average cholesterol (12).

The long-term intervention with pravastatin in ischemic disease (LIPID) trial also evaluated the effect of lipid lowering in patients with CAD and average cholesterol. It randomized 9,014 patients with prior MI or unstable angina and total cholesterol between 155 to 271 mg/dL to pravastatin 40 mg/day or placebo for a mean follow-up of 6.1 years. The primary end point of coronary heart disease death was reduced from 8.3% to 6.4% (RRR 24%; p < 0.001) with pravastatin. In addition, total all-cause mortality was reduced by 22% (P < 0.001), MI's by 29% (p < 0.001), strokes by 19% (p = 0.048), and revascularization by 20% (p < 0.001) (13). The large Heart Protection Study (HPS), which randomized 20,536 patients in the United Kingdom with CAD, DM, or other vascular disease to either simvastatin 40 mg/day or placebo, showed a significant reduction in all-cause mortality (12.9% versus 14.7%; p = 0.0003) with lipid lowering over 5 years. There was also a significant 18% reduction in coronary artery death (p = 0.0005). Consistent with other studies, it showed a proportional risk reduction of 25% for vascular events for every 1 mmol/L reduction in LDL (14).

The AVERT study compared aggressive lipid lowering to balloon angioplasty (PTCA) and usual care, including lipid lowering, in patients with stable one or two vessel CAD and moderate angina. The study randomized 341 patients with normal left ventricular (LV) function and an LDL ≥115 mg/dL to either atorvastatin 80 mg/day or PTCA for a follow-up period of 18 months. The primary end point of ischemic events was reduced by 36% in the atorvastatin group (13% versus 21%; p = 0.048 which was not significant after adjusting for interim analyses), which had a 46% reduction in LDL (72 mg/dL) compared with an 18% reduction in the PTCA group (199 mg/dL). The results of AVERT were quite controversial and the study was felt to have significant limitations. However, the results suggest that aggressive lipid lowering is reasonable in patients with stable angina and should be complementary to percutaneous interventions (15).

The MIRACL study randomized 3,086 patients with unstable angina or non-Q-wave MI to atorvastatin 80 mg/day or placebo for 16 weeks. The primary end point of death, nonfatal

---

Table 13–2

Lifestyle and Dietary Factor Recommendations to Improve Prognosis in Patients with Coronary Artery Disease (CAD)

1. Stop smoking
2. Engage in regular moderate intensive physical activity
3. Use alcohol in moderation
4. Maintain healthy body weight (BMI <25 kg/m^2)
5. Limit saturated fat intake (max 10 energy%) and trans fatty acid (max 1 energy%)
6. Consume fish regularly (1 to 2 portions of oily fish per week)
7. Sufficient consumption of fruits and vegetables (≥400 g/day)
8. Use fiber containing grain products, legumes, and or nuts (≥3 U/d)
9. Reduce salt intake to maximum of 2400 mg/d

From: Iestra JA, et al. Effect size estimates of lifestyle and dietary changes on all-cause mortality in coronary artery disease patients: a systematic review. *Circulation.* 2005;112:924–934, with permission.

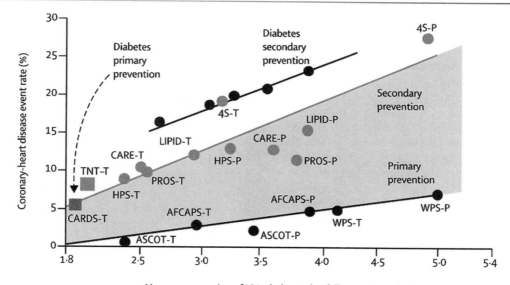

Figure 13–1.

Relationship between LDL cholesterol reduction and coronary events (P, placebo; T, treatment). (From: Opie LH, Commerford PJ, Gersh BJ. Controversies in stable coronary artery disease. *Lancet.* 2006;367:69–78, with permission.)

MI, cardiac arrest or recurrent symptomatic ischemia occurred in 14.8% of the atorvastatin group compared with 17.4% in the placebo group (RR 0.84; P = 0.048), and was driven primarily by less symptomatic ischemia in the treatment group (6.2% versus 8.4%; P = 0.02) (16).

The effect of the intensity of lipid lowering therapy was assessed in the REVERSAL Trial. The study evaluated 502 patients randomized to pravastatin 40 mg versus 80 mg of atorvastatin for 18 months. The primary end point of IVUS determined percentage change in atheroma volume was lower in the intensive lipid-lowering (atorvastatin) group than in the moderate lipid lowering group (0.4% versus 2.7% respectively; P = 0.02), with no significant change in atheroma burden with the former. The intensity of lipid lowering was associated with proportional LDL and CRP lowering (17).

The timing and intensity of lipid lowering was examined in the A to Z Trial. The study randomized 4,497 patients with ACS to either 40 mg/day of simvastatin for 1 month followed by 80 mg/day or placebo for 4 months followed by simvastatin 20 mg/day. Patients were followed for between 6 to 24 months with a primary end point composite of cardiovascular death, nonfatal MI, readmission for ACS, and stroke. There was no significant difference in the primary end point (16.7% in the delayed versus 14.4% in the early/intensive; P = 0.14) when examined at 4 months, but it was significantly reduced in the early/intensive group from 4 months onwards. There was also a reduction in cardiovascular death with the early/intensive regimen (4.1% versus 4.4%; P = 0.05) (18).

The PROVE IT-TIMI 22 study also looked at the intensity of lipid lowering in ACS patients. It randomized 4,162 patients to either pravastatin 40 mg/day or atorvastatin 80 mg/day for 18 to 36 months. The LDL was significantly reduced with atorvastatin (62 mg/dL vs 95 mg/dL; P < 0.001), as was the primary end point composite of all-cause mortality, MI, unstable angina, or revascularization (22.4% versus 26.3%; P = 0.005). It concluded that early intensive lipid lowering to levels below the current standard was protective against major cardiovascular event (MACE) (19). A comparison of A to Z and PROVE It revealed several factors that could explain the disparate results, especially the intensity of therapy in the early phase, the effect on C-reactive protein and differences in early revascularization. Taken together, they were felt to support early intensive statin therapy with revascularization in ACS (20).

The Treating to New Targets (TNT) Trial examined the efficacy and safety of intensive lipid lowering in 10,001 patients with clinically evident CHD. Patients with LDL levels <130 mg/dL were randomized to either 10 mg or 80 mg per day of atorvastatin and were followed for 4.9 years. The primary end point of first major cardiovascular event (MACE) was reduced by 22% (p < 0.001) in the high dose group, with no difference in overall mortality. The mean LDL in the high dose group was 77 mg/dL, versus 101 mg/dL in the lower dose group, with a significant increase in persistent liver aminotransferase levels (19).

The effect of intensive lipid lowering for secondary prevention after an acute MI was evaluated in the IDEAL (Incremental Decrease in End Points through Aggressive Lipid Lowering) Study which randomized 8,888 patients to either atorvastatin 80 mg or simvastatin 20 mg for a median follow-up of 4.8 years. The primary end point of major coronary event occurred in 10.4% of the simvastatin patients versus 9.3% of the atorvastatin group (p = 0.07). There was a statistically significant decrease in nonfatal MI with atorvastatin 80 mg vs simvastatin 20 mg, but no difference in cardiovascular or overall mortality (21).

A meta-analysis of 14 trials, including 90,056 participants, found a 12% proportional reduction in all-cause mortality for every mmol/L reduction in LDL (p < 0.0001). This included a 19% reduction in coronary mortality (p < 0.0001) and a 21% reduction in major vascular events (MI, revascularization, and stroke) (p < 0.0001). This study estimated an overall reduction in major vascular events of one fifth per mmol/L LDL reduction, which translated into 48 fewer patients per 1,000 with CHD having events (22).

The National Cholesterol Education Program (NCEP) Adult Treatment Panel III identifies LDL cholesterol as the major cause of CHD and is the primary target of lipid-lowering therapy. The initial report listed the target for LDL lowering in patients with CHD or CHD risk equivalents (e.g., diabetes) as <100 mg/dL. Therapeutic lifestyle changes should by instituted for any LDL above 100 mg/dL, and drug therapy for any LDL ≥130 mg/dL. Drug therapy was optional for LDL between 100 to 129 mg/dL. Based on the results of more current trials, such as HPS and PROVE IT, the NCEP issued an update with inclusion of a target LDL <70 mg/dL for very high risk persons (CHD plus multiple major risk factors, severe and poorly controlled risk factors, multiple risk factors of the metabolic syndrome, or acute coronary syndromes). For high risk patients (CHD or equivalents) the threshold for considering drug therapy is an LDL ≥100 mg/dL (23).

Hypertension

Blood pressure is a direct and continuous risk factor for CHD (24,25). Evidence from antihypertensive clinical trials suggests a substantial reduction in cardiovascular events of between 20% to 40% (26). The Seventh Joint National Committee on Prevention, Detection, Evaluation and Treatment of High Blood Pressure (JNC 7) defines three categories: normal (systolic <120 mm Hg and diastolic <80 mm Hg), prehypertension (systolic 120 to 139 mm Hg or diastolic 80 to 89 mm Hg), and hypertension (systolic ≥140 mm Hg or diastolic ≥90 mm Hg). The goal blood pressure is <140/90 mm Hg, or <130/80 with diabetes or chronic kidney disease. While thiazide-type diuretics are the recommended drug of first choice, persons with ischemic heart disease, heart failure, and post MI have compelling reasons for angiotensin converting enzyme inhibitors (ACEI), angiotensin receptor blockers (ARBs), and beta blockers from clinical trial evidence (25).

The benefit of ACEI post MI and with LV dysfunction was established by several trials, including SAVE, CONSENSUS I, and SOLVD (27–30). The Heart Outcomes Prevention Evaluation Study (HOPE), using ramipril, and the EUROPA study of perindopril found a significant reduction in cardiovascular events with ACEIs in patients with known CHD or at high risk, but without LV dysfunction (31,32). The PEACE Trial of trandolapril in patients with stable CAD, normal LV function, and lower risk found no benefit with the addition of an ACEI in terms of cardiovascular morality, MI, or revascularization (33). The LIFE trial demonstrated a significant reduction in cardiovascular events in patients with essential hypertension and LV hypertrophy from losartan compared with atenolol (34). Beta blockers have been shown to improve survival following MI

and with LV dysfunction. They receive a class 1 recommendation for these indications in the ACC/AHA guidelines (35,36).

Antithrombotic Therapy

A meta-analysis of 287 studies, involving 135,000 patients showed that among high risk patients, anti-platelet therapy reduces non-fatal MI, stroke, or vascular death by a significant 22%, which in absolute terms is the prevention of 36 events per 1,000 patients with prior MI. Aspirin was the most widely studied, in doses of 75 to 150 mg per day, and is an effective regimen for long-term use (37). It receives a class one indication in the ACC/AHA guidelines (35,38).

Clopidogrel is presently recommended for those allergic or intolerant to aspirin therapy. The CAPRIE trial randomized high risk patients with either prior MI, stroke or peripheral vascular disease to clopidogrel 75 mg a day or aspirin 81 mg a day. There was a statistically significant 8.7% reduction (P = 0.043) in the composite primary end point of stroke, MI, or vascular death at 2 years with clopidogrel (vs aspirin) (39). The CURE trial of clopidogrel and aspirin versus aspirin alone in patients with NSTEMI showed a 20% reduction in the composite primary end point of cardiovascular death, MI, or stroke (40). However, the recently published CHARISMA trial of clopidogrel and low-dose aspirin versus aspirin alone in patients with CVD or multiple risk factors showed no significant benefit to the combination therapy (41).

Summary

Secondary prevention of CHD events is an extremely important aspect of the care of patients with coronary disease. There are well established recommendations for risk factor modification and evolving strategies with drug therapy. The key recommendations from the European guidelines are (a) lifestyle changes, (b) prescription of aspirin and a statin, and (c) drug therapy (10) (Table 13–3).

Table 13–3

Essential Recommendations from the ESC Guidelines for Management of Patients with CHD

- Lifestyle changes
  - Stop smoking
  - Healthy food choices
  - Increase physical activity
- Aspirin and statin
- Consider additional drug therapy
  - Antihypertensive agents
  - Beta blockers
  - ACE inhibitors

Adapted from: Opie LH, Commerford PJ, Gersh BJ. Controversies in stable coronary artery disease. *Lancet.* 2006;367:69–78., with permission.

REFERENCES

1. D'Agostino RB, Russell MW, Huse DM, et al. Primary and subsequent coronary risk appraisal: new results from the Framingham study. *Am Heart J.* 2000;139:272–281.

2. Executive summary of the Third Report of The National Cholesterol Education Program (NCEP) expert panel on detection, evaluation, and treatment of high blood cholesterol in adults (adult treatment panel III). *JAMA.* 2001;285:2486–2497.

3. Grundy SM, Balady GJ, Criqui MH, et al. Primary prevention of coronary heart disease: guidance from Framingham: a statement for healthcare professionals from the American Heart Association task force on risk reduction. *Circulation.* 1998;97: 1876–1887.

4. Smith SC Jr, Blair SN, Bonow RO, et al. AHA/ACC scientific statement: AHA/ACC guidelines for preventing heart attack and death in patients with atherosclerotic cardiovascular disease: 2001 update: a statement for healthcare professionals from the American Heart Association and the American College of Cardiology. *Circulation.* 2001;104:1577–1579.

5. Gaziano JM, Manson JE, Ridker PM, Primary and secondary prevention of coronary heart disease. In: Zipes D, Libby P, Bonow RO, et al, eds. *Braunwald's heart disease: a textbook of cardiovascular medicine.* Elsevier Saunders: Philadelphia; 2005:1057–1084.

6. Iestra JA, Kromhout D, van der Schouw, et al. Effect size estimates of lifestyle and dietary changes on all-cause mortality in coronary artery disease patients: a systematic review. *Circulation.* 2005;112:924–934.

7. Critchley JA, Capewell S, Mortality risk reduction associated with smoking cessation in patients with coronary heart disease: a systematic review. *JAMA.* 2003;290:86–97.

8. Thompson PD, Buchner D, Pina IL, et al. Exercise and physical activity in the prevention and treatment of atherosclerotic cardiovascular disease: a statement from the Council on Clinical Cardiology (Subcommittee on Exercise, Rehabilitation, and Prevention) and the Council on Nutrition, Physical Activity, and Metabolism (Subcommittee on Physical Activity). *Circulation.* 2003;107:3109–3116.

9. Leon AS, Franklin BA, Costa F, et al. Cardiac rehabilitation and secondary prevention of coronary heart disease: an American Heart Association scientific statement from the Council on Clinical Cardiology (Subcommittee on Exercise, Cardiac Rehabilitation, and Prevention) and the Council on Nutrition, Physical Activity, and Metabolism (Subcommittee on Physical Activity), in collaboration with the American association of Cardiovascular and Pulmonary Rehabilitation. *Circulation.* 2005;111:369–376.

10. Opie LH, Commerford PJ, Gersh BJ, Controversies in stable coronary artery disease. *Lancet.* 2006;367:69–78.

11. Randomised trial of cholesterol lowering in 4,444 patients with coronary heart disease: the Scandinavian Simvastatin Survival Study (4S). *Lancet.* 1994;344:1383–1389.

12. Sacks FM, Pfeffer MA, Moye LA, et al. The effect of pravastatin on coronary events after myocardial infarction in patients with average cholesterol levels. Cholesterol and recurrent events trial investigators. *N Engl J Med.* 1996;335:1001–1009.

13. Prevention of cardiovascular events and death with pravastatin in patients with coronary heart disease and a broad range of initial cholesterol levels. The long-term intervention with pravastatin in ischaemic disease (LIPID) study group. *N Engl J Med.* 1998;339:1349–1357.

14. MRC/BHF heart protection study of cholesterol lowering with simvastatin in 20,536 high-risk individuals: a randomised placebo-controlled trial. *Lancet.* 2002;360:7–22.

15. Pitt B, Waters D, Brown WV, et al. Aggressive lipid-lowering therapy compared with angioplasty in stable coronary artery disease. Atorvastatin versus revascularization treatment investigators. *N Engl J Med.* 1999;341:70–76.

16. Schwartz GG, Olsson AG, Ezekowitz MD, et al. Effects of atorvastatin on early recurrent ischemic events in acute coronary syndromes: the MIRACL study: a randomized controlled trial. *JAMA.* 2001;285:1711–1718.

17. Nissen SE, Tuzcu EM, Schoenhagen P, et al. Effect of intensive compared with moderate lipid-lowering therapy on progression of coronary atherosclerosis: a randomized controlled trial. *JAMA.* 2004;291:1071–1080.

18. de Lemos JA, Blazing MA, Wiviott SD, et al. Early intensive vs a delayed conservative simvastatin strategy in patients with acute coronary syndromes: phase Z of the A to Z trial. *JAMA.* 2004;292:1307–1316.

19. Cannon CP, Braunwald E, McCabe CH, et al. Intensive versus moderate lipid lowering with statins after acute coronary syndromes. *N Engl J Med.* 2004;350:1495–1504.

20. Wiviott SD, de Lemos JA, Cannon CP, et al. A tale of two trials: a comparison of the post-acute coronary syndrome lipid-lowering trials A to Z and PROVE IT-TIMI 22. *Circulation.* 2006;113:1406–1414.

21. Pedersen TR, Faergeman O, Kastelein JJ, et al. High-dose atorvastatin vs usual-dose simvastatin for secondary prevention after myocardial infarction: the IDEAL study: a randomized controlled trial. *JAMA.* 2005;294:2437–2445.

22. Baigent C, Keech A, Kearney PM, et al. Efficacy and safety of cholesterol-lowering treatment: prospective meta-analysis of data from 90,056 participants in 14 randomised trials of statins. *Lancet.* 2005;366:1267–1278.

23. Grundy SM, Cleeman JI, Merz CN, et al. Implications of recent clinical trials for the National Cholesterol Education Program Adult Treatment Panel III guidelines. *Circulation.* 2004;110:227–239.

24. Lewington S, Clarke R, Qizilbash N, et al. Age-specific relevance of usual blood pressure to vascular mortality: a meta-analysis of individual data for one million adults in 61 prospective studies. *Lancet.* 2002;360:1903–1913.

25. Chobanian AV, Bakris GL, Black HR, et al. The seventh report of the Joint National Committee on Prevention, Detection, Evaluation, and Treatment of High Blood Pressure: the JNC 7 report. *JAMA.* 2003;289:2560–2572.

26. Neal B, MacMahon S, Chapman N. Effects of ACE inhibitors, calcium antagonists, and other blood-pressure-lowering drugs: results of prospectively designed overviews of randomised trials. Blood Pressure Lowering Treatment Trialists' Collaboration. *Lancet.* 2000;356:1955–1964.

27. Effects of enalapril on mortality in severe congestive heart failure. Results of the Cooperative North Scandinavian Enalapril Survival Study (CONSENSUS). The CONSENSUS Trial Study Group. *N Engl J Med.* 1987; 316:1429–1435.

28. Effect of enalapril on survival in patients with reduced left ventricular ejection fractions and congestive heart failure. The SOLVD Investigators. *N Engl J Med.* 1991;325:293–302.

29. Pfeffer MA, Braunwald E, Moye LA, et al. Effect of captopril on mortality and morbidity in patients with left ventricular dysfunction after myocardial infarction. Results of the survival and ventricular enlargement trial. The SAVE Investigators. *N Engl J Med.* 1992;327:669–677.

30. Swedberg K, Held P, Kjekshus J, et al. Effects of the early administration of enalapril on mortality in patients with acute myocardial infarction. Results of the Cooperative New Scandinavian Enalapril Survival Study II (CONSENSUS II). *N Engl J Med.* 1992;327:678–684.

31. Yusuf S, Sleight P, Pogue J, et al. Effects of an angiotensin-converting-enzyme inhibitor, ramipril, on cardiovascular events in high-risk patients. The Heart Outcomes Prevention Evaluation Study Investigators. *N Engl J Med.* 2000;342:145–153.

32. Fox KM. Efficacy of perindopril in reduction of cardiovascular events among patients with stable coronary artery disease: randomised, double-blind, placebo-controlled, multicentre trial (the EUROPA study). *Lancet.* 2003;362:782–788.

33. Braunwald E, Domanski MJ, Fowler SE, et al. Angiotensin-converting-enzyme inhibition in stable coronary artery disease. *N Engl J Med.* 2004;351:2058–2068.

34. Dahlof B, Devereux RB, Kjeldsen SE, et al. Cardiovascular morbidity and mortality in the Losartan intervention for endpoint reduction in hypertension study (LIFE): a randomised trial against atenolol. *Lancet.* 2002;359:995–1003.

35. Gibbons RJ, Abrams J, Chatterjee K, et al. ACC/AHA 2002 guideline update for the management of patients with chronic stable angina—summary article: a report of the American College of Cardiology/American Heart Association Task Force on Practice Guidelines (Committee on the Management of Patients with Chronic Stable Angina). *Circulation.* 2003;107:149–158.

36. Hunt SA, Abraham WT, Chin MH, et al. ACC/AHA 2005 guideline update for the diagnosis and management of chronic heart failure in the adult: a report of the American College of Cardiology/American Heart Association Task Force on Practice Guidelines (Writing Committee to Update the 2001 Guidelines for the Evaluation and Management of Heart Failure). *J Am Coll Cardiol.* 2005;46:1–82.

37. Collaborative meta-analysis of randomised trials of anti-platelet therapy for prevention of death, myocardial infarction, and stroke in high risk patients. *BMJ.* 2002;324:71–86.

38. Antman EM, Anbe DT, Armstrong PW, et al. ACC/AHA guidelines for the management of patients with ST-elevation myocardial infarction—executive summary. A report of the American College of Cardiology/American Heart Association Task Force on Practice Guidelines (Writing Committee to revise the 1999 guidelines for the management of patients with acute myocardial infarction). *J Am Coll Cardiol.* 2004;44:671–719.

39. A randomised, blinded, trial of clopidogrel versus aspirin in patients at risk of ischaemic events (CAPRIE). CAPRIE Steering Committee. *Lancet.* 1996;348:1329–1339.

40. Yusuf S, Zhao F, Mehta SR, et al. Effects of clopidogrel in addition to aspirin in patients with acute coronary syndromes without ST-segment elevation. *N Engl J Med.* 2001;345:494–502.

41. Bhatt DL, Fox KA, Hacke W, et al. Clopidogrel and aspirin versus aspirin alone for the prevention of atherothrombotic events. *N Engl J Med.* 2006;354:1706–1717.

CHAPTER 14

Procedures and Management: Multivessel Angioplasty

Hussam N. Hamdalla and David J. Moliterno

Over the past three decades, advances in the field of interventional cardiology have allowed the broadening of lesion types and acuities to include treatment of more patients with acute coronary syndromes and those with multivessel coronary artery disease (MVD). Several early randomized trials comparing medical, surgical, and percutaneous therapy among patients with MVD were performed to discern any relative advantages of the different approaches. Each of the treatment options have continued to evolve. In 2002, an estimated 1,200,000 angioplasty procedures and 515,000 bypass procedures were performed in the United States (1). According to past SCAI (The Society for Cardiovascular Angiography and Interventions) and NHLBI (National Heart, Lung, and Blood Institute) registries, approximately 40% to 60% of patients undergoing percutaneous revascularization have had MVD (2,3). Two-vessel disease was present in more than half of these patients, mostly involving the left anterior descending artery and right coronary artery (3,4). Roughly one-third underwent multisite intervention, and this portion has remained unchanged over the past decade (4,5).

Several different definitions of MVD have been used in the literature. The most common definitions are (a) ≥70% stenosis in ≥2 coronary arteries; (b) ≥70% stenosis in one coronary artery and ≥50% stenosis in a second coronary artery; and (c) ≥50% stenosis in ≥2 coronary arteries (6,7). The definition used has important implications for clinical practice and long-term outcome. In this chapter, we review the procedural and clinical outcome of MVD-PCI.

Clinical Profile

When approaching a patient with MVD, there are many factors that should be considered. Not surprisingly, these patients are more likely to have multiple comorbid conditions, including diabetes, renal insufficiency, prior myocardial infarction (MI), and reduced left ventricular (LV) function as compared with those who have single-vessel coronary artery disease. They are more likely to require complex procedures due to anatomical reasons such as calcified lesions, chronic total occlusions, and diffusely diseased and smaller vessels. All these clinical, anatomic, and procedural variables influence decisions regarding the revascularization method. In current practice, a percutaneous revascularization approach is more likely for patients with 2-vessel disease compared with a surgical revascularization preference for patients with 3-vessel disease (8).

Patient-Related Factors

Age

Beyond being a risk factor for coronary artery disease (CAD) and comorbidities in general, advanced age is an important predictor of outcome following PCI and more so following coronary artery bypass graft surgery (CABG). In the NHLBI dynamic registry, patients of advanced age (>80 years old) were twice as likely to have 3-vessel CAD compared with younger (<65 years) patients (38% versus 20%) (9). They were also more likely to have calcified arteries (40% versus 20%) and undergo multivessel PCI (40% versus 30%). Many clinical trials have excluded patients >75 years old, and we remain wary of broadly extrapolating trial data to the elderly population. Although coronary surgery can be safely performed in selected octogenarians, such patients are at particularly high risk for in-hospital mortality and postoperative stroke (9% and 5%, respectively) (10). Thus, percutaneous revascularization may be a preferable approach even for the elderly with MVD. Again, this presumption is confounded by a paucity of data regarding the benefit of PCI and the risk of bleeding with polypharmacy anticoagulation. Klein et al. studied >8,000 patients with a mean age of 83 years from the American College of Cardiology-National Cardiovascular Data Registry (ACC-NCDR) who underwent PCI and reported a good procedural success and acceptable mortality (11). Multisite PCI was performed in 35%, and angiographic success was high (93%), with stents placed in 75% of patients. Indications for PCI in this registry were most commonly acute MI (33%) and unstable angina (56%), rather than elective stable angina (11%). Thus, when medical therapy fails to control anginal symptoms, PCI can be performed with a high success rate, and >90% of long-term survivors indicate a high level of satisfaction with their quality-of-life and health status (12).

Elderly patients do have more procedural complications and worse long-term outcome after PCI compared with younger patients. Sadeghi et al. evaluated the safety of glycoprotein (GP) IIb/IIIa inhibitors in almost 1,400 patients ≥80 years old undergoing PCI (13). They found that GP IIb/IIIa inhibitor use was associated with increased access site bleeding (26% versus 20%) and major bleeding (7.8% versus 4.2%) compared to no GP IIb/IIIa inhibitor use, but was not associated with increased risk of transfusion or intracranial hemorrhage. Elderly (>65 years) patients undergoing PCI had a higher in-hospital (4.6% versus 0.6%) and 1-year mortality (11% versus 2.1%) compared to younger patients (9). In-hospital mortality was further increased if the patients were admitted with acute MI (reaching 14%) and was high as 43% if they were admitted with cardiogenic shock (11). Data are not readily available for elderly patients undergoing multivessel intervention versus single-vessel intervention, though it is plausible that those with multivessel disease are at particularly high risk for adverse events with PCI, though possibly less than with CABG.

LV Dysfunction

Of patients undergoing PCI, approximately 5% to 15% will have left ventricular dysfunction with an ejection fraction (EF) <40% (5,14). LeFeuvre et al. studied 194 patients who had multivessel PCI and found LV function to be the only independent predictor of cardiac death at 7-year follow-up (15). Likewise, O'Keefe et al. followed 700 patients who underwent multivessel PCI and found LV function (EF <40%) to be a powerful predictor of both in-hospital mortality and long-term outcome (16). Survival at 5-year follow-up was significantly better among those with preserved LV function (89% versus 81%, $p = 0.05$). Ellis and colleagues reported a 2-year follow-up on 350 patients following multivessel angioplasty and noted that LV ejection fraction of >40% correlated significantly with overall survival (Fig. 14–1) (17). Survival benefit

seems to be related to viable myocardium in these high-risk patients regardless of the method of revascularization. Allman et al. performed a meta-analysis on patients with LV dysfunction who underwent revascularization following a viability study (18). The benefit of revascularization among patients with LV dysfunction was achieved only in patients with documented myocardial viability (Fig. 14–2). Patients with preserved LV function tend to tolerate acute complications better, likely resulting in better in-hospital outcome. Transient ischemia during balloon inflations and abrupt vessel closure in an artery supplying the remaining viable myocardium are not tolerated well among patients with severe LV dysfunction.

Diabetes

Diabetic patients represent 20% to 25% of patients undergoing revascularization, and they are more likely to have diffuse CAD, multivessel involvement, and LV dysfunction than nondiabetic patients (19,20). Diabetics more often have 3-vessel CAD compared with nondiabetic patients (44.7% versus 25.4% $p = 0.002$) (20). The BARI (Bypass Angioplasty Revascularization Investigation) trial compared PCI with CABG in the management of patients with MVD and found a survival advantage with surgical revascularization among diabetic patients (21). Five-year survival for diabetics assigned to PTCA was 65.5% compared with 80.6% for those assigned to CABG. The survival benefit was evident in patients who had at least one internal mammary artery used as a conduit. This observation has led the ACC/AHA committee to designate a Class IIb indication for PCI among patients with MVD with significant proximal LAD and treated diabetes (22). However, the ARTS (Arterial Revascularization Therapies Study) trial recruited 208 patients with diabetes among the patients randomized to either PCI with stent or CABG. In this study there was no significant

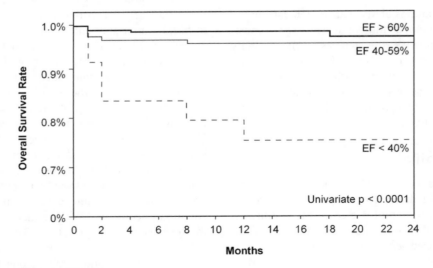

Figure 14–1.

Correlates of outcome between ventricular ejection fraction (EF) and overall survival. (Reproduced from: Ellis SG, Cowley MJ, and Disciascio G, et al. Determinants of 2-year outcome after coronary angioplasty in patients with multivessel disease on the basis of comprehensive preprocedural evaluation: implications for patient selection. *Circulation.* 1991;83:1905–1914, with permission.)

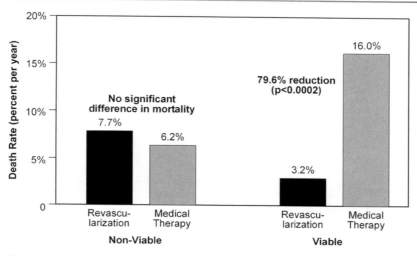

Figure 14–2.

Death rates for patients with and without myocardial viability treated by revascularization or medical therapy. (Reprinted from: Allman KC, et al. Myocardial viability testing and impact of revascularization on prognosis in patients with coronary artery disease and left ventricular dysfunction: a meta-analysis. *J Am Coll Cardiol.* 2002;39:1151–1158, with permission.)

difference in survival between the arms at 5-years (23). The more recent introduction of the DES was associated with further reduction in restenosis among different cohorts of patients including diabetic patients. Early data suggest a reduction in revascularization seen with the sirolimus and paclitaxel coated stents in the diabetic patients with near equivalency to that seen in the surgical arms. It remains unclear if these findings will hold in randomized trials and more information is needed before reaching a more definite conclusion. The equivalency of percutaneous versus surgical revascularization is being re-evaluated in the FREEDOM trial (Future Revascularization Evaluation in Patients with Diabetes Mellitus: Optimal Management of Multivessel Disease), which is a multicenter, prospective randomized trial comparing CABG with PCI stenting using sirolimus-eluting stents in diabetic patients with multivessel disease.

Renal Insufficiency

Cardiac disease accounts for 50% of the mortality among hemodialysis patients. In particular, among patients with significant renal insufficiency, >70% will have MVD on angiography (20,24,25). Patients with severe renal insufficiency are more likely to be older, female, diabetic, and hypertensive. In addition, they more frequently have MVD, vein graft disease, complex lesions, and had been more frequently treated with rotational atherectomy in past registries. Best et al. detailed the association between the degree of renal insufficiency and cardiovascular outcome from the Mayo Clinic PCI registry and the PRESTO (Prevention of REStenosis with Tranilast and its Outcomes) trial (26,27). After successful PCI, 1-year mortality was 1.5% among those with a creatinine clearance ≥70 mL/min (n = 2,558), 3.6% for a clearance of 50 to 69 mL/min (n = 1,458), 7.8% for a clearance of 30 to 49 mL/min

(n = 828), and 18.3% for a clearance of <30 mL/min (n = 141) (Fig. 14–3).

Chronic renal insufficiency impacts two aspects of patients with MVD: long-term outcome with increased risk of cardiovascular mortality and concern of worsening renal function with contrast-induced nephropathy. Pharmacotherapy dose adjustment is needed with renal insufficiency especially for therapy given for more than several half-lives (i.e., extended infusion). Many anticoagulants, such as small molecule GP IIb/IIIa inhibitors, heparins, and some direct thrombin inhibitors, are renally excreted. Unfractionated heparin may be a better choice compared with low-molecular-weight heparin, because of easier monitoring and adjustment using activated partial thromboplastin time or activated clotting time. Patients with chronic renal insufficiency should undergo a staged procedure in an attempt to avoid contrast-induced nephropathy.

Acute Myocardial Infarction

Multivessel CAD is a key predictor of increased mortality and reduced global LV systolic function after ST-elevation myocardial infarction (STEMI) (28,29). Almost half of patients presenting with an acute MI have multivessel disease. In the pre-stent era, balloon angioplasty was associated with a relatively high incidence of abrupt vessel closure due to thrombus and dissections. As such, this led to an exclusive focus on the infarct-related artery in the acute setting of myocardial infarction. Patients with acute MI and MVD compared with patients with acute MI and single-vessel disease (SVD) have higher mortality rates (7.5% versus 2.5% p = 0.005) and re-infarction rates (3.2% versus 0.6% p = 0.02) at early (30-day) follow-up (30,31). Furthermore, patients who undergo staged PCI before hospital discharge continue to a have higher rate

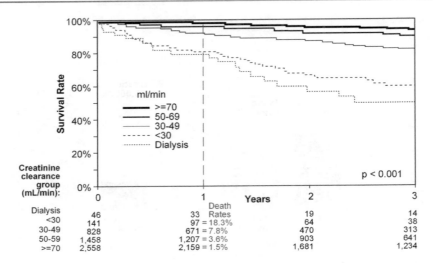

Figure 14–3.

All-cause mortality after successful percutaneous coronary intervention in patients based on their estimated creatinine clearance. (Reproduced from: Best PJM, et al. The impact of renal insufficiency on clinical outcomes in patients undergoing percutaneous coronary interventions. *J Am Coll Cardiol.* 2002;39:1113–1119, with permission.)

of reinfarction compared with patients who have infarct artery PCI alone when assessed at 1 year (15% versus 2.8% p < 0.001). Even with many advances in the management of MI and improvements in primary angioplasty, immediate multivessel PCI may still not be safe during MI. The current guidelines still list noninfarct artery PCI as a Class III indication in this setting (36).

TIMI (Thrombolysis in Myocardial Infarction) flow is known to be slower than normal in all coronary arteries (i.e., including the nonculprit artery) during an acute MI. Nonculprit artery flow on average has a corrected TIMI frame count (CTFC) of 30.9 ± 15.0 frames compared with normal flow in the absence of MI (CTFC 21 ± 3.1, p < 0.0001) (32). The severity of lumen obstruction of nonculprit lesions can also change in the setting of MI. Hanratty et al. studied angiograms from patients undergoing catheterization during an MI and compared them with follow-up angiograms which were performed 6 months later. They observed that roughly one-fifth of nonculprit vessels which had >50% diameter stenosis at the time of MI, had a <50% narrowing at late follow-up angiography (33). An exaggerated estimate of the severity of stenosis during MI or heightened vascular tone (vasoconstriction) may lead to unnecessary revascularization procedures.

In contrast, patients with cardiogenic shock during or shortly following STEMI may be a unique subgroup that derives particular benefit from complete revascularization during index PCI. In the SHOCK trial there was a significantly lower 30-day mortality among patients <75 years (41.4% to 56.8% p = 0.01) who underwent early revascularization, either PCI or surgical (34). Multivessel revascularization, therefore, may be useful if ischemia is due to MVD, and disease in the nonculprit artery is impeding a compensatory hypercontractile response in nonculprit territory (35). ACC/AHA guidelines provide a Class I indication for multivessel PCI some patients with STEMI and cardiogenic shock. Specifically, for patients <75 years who present within 36 hours of MI, and are suitable for revascularization within 18 hours of shock onset, multivessel revascularization should be performed.

Unstable Angina/Non-ST Elevation MI

Patients presenting with unstable angina (UA) who have multivessel CAD are managed differently from STEMI patients. A sub-analysis from the ARTS trial compared patients with unstable versus stable angina who underwent multivessel revascularization. At 1-year follow-up, the respective rates of MI (5.2% versus 5.1%), death (2.7% versus 2.4%), or revascularization (16.8% versus 16.9%) were similar (37). In TARGET (do Tirofiban And Reopro Give similar Efficacy Trial) patients with ACS and undergoing multivessel revascularization had similar 1-year mortality and target vessel revascularization (TVR) at 1-year compared with patients undergoing single-vessel revascularization. The multivessel revascularization group did have a higher rate of periprocedural MI (HR 1.47; 95% CI 1.12 to 1.92; p = 0.005) (38). These two posthoc analyses suggest unstable angina patients with multivessel revascularization have a similar long-term outcome compared with patients undergoing single-vessel revascularization. Likewise, Brener et al. demonstrated the safety and efficacy of multivessel PCI compared to culprit-lesion only PCI among patients with ACS and MVD from the TACTICS-TIMI 18 (Treat Angina with aggrastat and determine Cost of Therapy with an Invasive or Conservative Strategy-Thrombolysis In Myocardial Infarction 18) trial (39). The group of patients who underwent multivessel PCI had similar rates for mortality and MI at 30 days and 6 months compared with the culprit-lesion only group; however, they had a significantly lower rate of subsequent revascularization at 6 months (1.5% versus 6.3%).

As such, the current ACC/AHA practice guidelines designate a Class I indication for single- or multivessel PCI in ACS patients provided there is a high likelihood of success; the procedure-related morbidity and mortality risk is low, the vessel(s) to be dilated subtend(s) a moderate or large area of viable myocardium, and have "high-risk" by noninvasive testing (40).

Lesion-Related Factors

Among the considerations in treating patients with MVD is deciding whether complete revascularization is a key goal, and which lesions should be treated. This decision process must take into account anatomical features, including lesion complexity, presence of left main disease, bifurcation lesions, and chronic total occlusions. Although complete anatomical revascularization may not be the objective in all patients with MVD, functionally adequate revascularization should be the aim to realize comparable outcome to surgical revascularization. The ability to attain revascularization comparable to CABG may be quite challenging in some cases since it requires successful treatment of all stenoses compromising vessels ≥1.5 mm, which supply viable myocardium (41).

Complete versus Incomplete Revascularization

The concept of complete cardiac revascularization for patients with MVD has been of ongoing interest in interventional cardiology. The benefit of complete revascularization has been proved in surgical series where patients with a bypass graft placed at all ischemic territories have shown improved outcomes compared to similar patients in whom some territories were not grafted. The "standard" definition of complete revascularization is achieved when all stenoses ≥50% in vessels ≥1.5 mm in diameter is reduced to <50% diameter stenosis. In older surgical series, in which the duration of patient follow-up was 1 to 5 years, 68% to 78% of patients with complete revascularization were asymptomatic, whereas only 42% to 58% of patients with incomplete revascularization were asymptomatic (42–44). In the Multivessel Angioplasty Prognosis Study (MAPS), complete revascularization was achieved in only 25% of patients (45). The reasons for incomplete revascularization were untreated stenosis <70% (40%), jeopardized territory ≤10% (30%), untreated chronic total occlusion (20.5%), akinetic associated myocardium (12.6%), high-risk stenosis (10.8%), residual stenosis after coronary angioplasty ≥50% (8.6%), failure to cross lesion with a wire or a balloon (4.3%), and failed angioplasty of chronic total occlusion (3.6%).

In the BARI trial angiographic assessment was made before patient randomization to determine the suitability of intended complete revascularization or intended incomplete revascularization (7). In those undergoing a percutaneous revascularization, despite an overall worse clinical and angiographic baseline profile in the incomplete revascularization group, freedom from death, MI, and repeat revascularization (CABG/angioplasty) was similar to the complete revascularization group. Not surprisingly, patients who had surgical revas-

cularization were more likely to be free of angina at 5 years and the need for repeat revascularization was substantially greater in the incomplete revascularization angioplasty arm. This was supported by similar findings in the ARTS trial in which complete revascularization was achieved in 84.1% of bypass surgery patients and in 70.5% of the stented patients (p < 0.001) (6).

The decision to perform complete revascularization procedures should not be based on anatomical assessment only, but rather in combination with functional assessment especially for lesions of borderline severity. It is important to appreciate that visual assessment of coronary stenosis severity has important limitations. Fractional flow reserve (8) using a pressure-wire can be readily performed in the catheterization laboratory and may be more accurate than a scintigraphic stress test in assessing hemodynamic significance of coronary artery stenosis. Berger et al. studied patients with MVD and performed immediate PCI if FFR was <0.75 or deferred PCI if FFR was >0.75 (46). At a 3-year follow-up there was no increased risk of MI in the deferred vessels and only 6% required PCI.

Achieving complete revascularization may not be imperative in all cases since it is dependent on viability of the downstream myocardium. Complete revascularization may also be a reflection of baseline characteristics: less severe disease and better left ventricular function, rather than the revascularization strategy itself.

Left Main Disease

Left main (LM) disease classically has been viewed as a "surgical disease." This approach was established by the Veterans Administration Cooperative study documenting the survival benefit with surgical revascularization versus medical therapy (47) and the early poor outcomes of the balloon angioplasty (48). Tan et al. reported a better outcome from the unprotected LM (ULTIMA) registry using stents and atherectomy compared with earlier reports using balloon angioplasty (49). The event-free survival inversely correlated with LV systolic function ≤30%, severe mitral regurgitation, cardiogenic shock, serum creatinine ≥2.0 mg/dL, and severe lesion calcification. Noticeably, there was an increased rate of sudden cardiac death (10.6%) within the first 6 months after hospital discharge. Although 1-year mortality was high (20% to 24%), this most likely reflected the high risk for surgery or inoperable patients who were "selected" for PCI. When patients were stratified into a low-risk group (age <65, LVEF >30%, and absence of cardiogenic shock) the 1-year mortality was 3.4%. One of the biggest limitations of percutaneous revascularization of the LM has been target vessel revascularization (TVR); which may be addressed with drug-eluting stents (DES). The RESEARCH (Rapamycin-Eluting Stent Evaluated At Rotterdam Cardiology Hospital) and T-SEARCH (Taxus-eluting Stent Evaluated At Rotterdam Cardiology Hospital) registries showed a decrease in TVR of LM from 23% with bare metal stents (BMS) to 6% with DES (50). The standard of care for patients with LM disease, despite the new breakthroughs with restenosis, continues to be surgical revascularization. The ACC/AHA guidelines designate a Class I for bypass surgery for patients with significant LM and Class III for percutaneous revascularization if they are acceptable candidates for surgery.

Bifurcation Lesion

Many MVD lesions involve bifurcations in the coronary arteries and are limiting in achieving long-term success. Except for the left main CAD, both the main branch and side branch are considered as one vessel (e.g., left anterior descending artery and diagonal branch). Bifurcation lesions pose a technical challenge to the interventional cardiologist and yield lower rates of procedural success (87%–97%) and higher rates of complications (51,52). Likewise, long-term success is confounded by a higher rate of restenosis mainly at the side branch (20%–45%) and stent thrombosis (5%). Whether to double wire (using separate simultaneous wires) the main artery and side branch depends on the size of the side branch and myocardium it supplies, the extent of side branch, ostial disease, and perhaps the angle of side branch origination. Strategies have ranged from stenting the main branch with or without balloon angioplasty of the side branch to stenting both branches. Different techniques, including kissing balloon angioplasty, T-stenting, Y-stenting, and Culotte stenting of the bifurcation lesion, continue to challenge the interventional cardiologist. Initial reports on use of DES in bifurcation lesions revealed an improvement in the restenosis rates; however, the benefit has not been as pronounced as in nonbifurcation DES cases. The use of DES and dedicated bifurcation stents continues to be explored to improve long-term outcome (52a).

Chronic Total Occlusion

Chronic total occlusion (CTO) is present in almost 30% of MVD and is one of the most technically challenging and limiting steps in achieving complete revascularization (53). Revascularizing CTOs has two primary challenges, the first being recanalization of the artery. Different devices have been used over the past decade to achieve recanalization, including stiffer wires, rotational atherectomy, laser wires, optical coherence reflectometry, and the Safe-Cross radiofrequency wire. Most of these devices were met with technical failure and high complication rates. The second challenge is a high rate of restenosis and reocclusion using balloon angioplasty and bare metal stents. Early data with drug-eluting stents appear promising in decreasing the restenosis rate (2%–8%) once recanalization is achieved compared to that with bare metal stents (30%–40%) (54,55). In the presence of a CTO that supplies a larea of viable myocardium attempts to recanalize the occluded artery should be made first, and failure to do so merits reevaluation of the bypass surgery option to achieve complete revascularization.

Procedure-Related Factors

The technical success of MVD is dependent on lesion and procedural factors that affect the immediate outcome. Using balloon angioplasty the procedural success of multivessel PCI was 82% to 89% with a major complications rate (death, MI, or CABG) of 3% to 9% at 30 days (56–58). This has improved with the advent of better antiplatelet therapy (GP IIb/IIIa inhibitors and thienopyridines) and drug-eluting stents.

Antiplatelet Therapy

Instrumentation of coronary arteries can result in thrombotic complications due to plaque rupture, vessel dissection, platelet activation and slow antegrade flow. This can manifest as abrupt vessel closure, side branch occlusion, and frank thrombus formation. Even without these major complications, a rise in periprocedural CK and CK-MB (consistent with MI) is associated with a higher risk of death and subsequent MI during short- and long-term follow-up. Patients undergoing multivessel intervention are at an increased risk of periprocedural MI compared to single vessel patients even with the most current antiplatelet therapy. Kornowski et al. studied 398 consecutive MVD patients treated with stents and compared them to 1,941 patients with SVD from the Cardiology Research Foundation Angioplasty Database (59). Procedural success was comparable between MVD (96%) and SVD intervention (97%). Despite a similar in-hospital outcome between both groups, periprocedural MI with a CK-MB ≥ 3 was significantly higher in MVD patients (23% versus 18% p = 0.02).

Adjunctive pharmacotherapy in the early days of balloon angioplasty was limited to aspirin and heparin. Introduction of GP IIb/IIIa inhibitors and thienopyridines has changed the procedural outcome considerably. This has translated into a significant decrease in abrupt vessel closure, thrombus formation, and periprocedural MI. Although the improved procedural outcome with the current drug therapy is seen in both MVD- and SVD-PCI, those who undergo MVD-PCI remain at a relatively higher risk of periprocedural MI. Shishehbor et al. compared MVD to SVD in the TARGET trial where all patients received a GP IIb/IIIa inhibitor, either abciximab or tirofiban (38). The rates of periprocedural MI remained significantly elevated in patients with MVD (9.1% versus 5.5%).

Data on the benefit of clopidogrel among patients with MVD from randomized trials are limited. In the Intracoronary Stenting and Antithrombotic Regimen–Rapid Early Action for Coronary Treatment (ISAR-REACT) (60) and the Intracoronary Stenting and Antithrombotic Regimen: is abciximab a Superior Way to Eliminate Elevated Thrombotic risk in diabetics (ISAR-SWEET) (61) trials, patients were randomized to abciximab or placebo. They were all pretreated with 600 mg clopidogrel >2 hours before the procedure.

Drug-Eluting Stents

In-stent restenosis and target vessel revascularization remain the major limitations of long-term results following percutaneous revascularization. Within the past few years, drug-eluting stents have substantially reduced the in-stent restenosis rate and TVR. Several registries considering DES in multivessel intervention have demonstrated low MI rates

Table 14–1

Pooled Data of Drug Eluting Stents in Patients with MVD

Series	N	Months	MACE		
			MI	Death	TVR
Serruys, et al. (63)	150	6	—	—	3.3%
Arampatzis, et al. (68)	99	9	1.0%	1.0%	9.0%
Mikhail, et al. (69)	281	6	0.4%	2.5%	13.2%
Orlic, et al. (70)	155	6	3.6%	2.7%	16.1%
STENT (71)	527	9	1.2%	1.8%	2.3%
ARTS II (72)	607	12	1.2%	1%	8.5%
Pooled	1,819	6–12	1.2%	1.5%	7.7%

STENT (Strategic Transcatheter Evaluation of New Therapies), ARTS (Arterial Revascularization Therapies Study Part II).

(1% to 3%), mortality (1% to 3%), and TVR (9% to 16%) (Table 14–1). The ARTS II trial is a multicenter, nonrandomized, open-label trial comparing sirolimus-eluting stent implantation in patients with multivessel disease to the surgical group of ARTS I (63). Although 1-year revascularization in the DES arm was still higher than the historical CABG arm (8.5% versus 4.1%, p = 0.003), drug-eluting stents are closing the gap on surgery (64). SYNTAX (SYNergy between PCI with TAXus and cardiac surgery) is a large randomized multicenter trial comparing PCI with paclitaxel-eluting stents to CABG among patients with multivessel coronary artery disease. Enrollment is ongoing, and it will reevaluate the equivalency of PCI using drug-eluting stents versus surgery.

Summary

Nearly a century ago, Herrick wrote, "The clinical manifestations of coronary obstruction will evidently vary greatly, depending on the size, location and number of vessels occluded. The symptoms and end-results must also be influenced by blood pressure, by the condition of the myocardium not immediately affected by the obstruction, and by the ability of the remaining vessels properly to carry on their work, as determined by their health or disease. No simple picture of the condition can, therefore, be drawn" (65). Likewise today, no simple recommendation can be made on the treatment of multivessel coronary artery disease. The risk-benefit ratio of multivessel revascularization should be carefully assessed for each patient. Percutaneous intervention should be weighed against surgical revascularization being mindful of the completeness of revascularization and long-term outcome considering the cardiac and noncardiac health of the patient. The role of balloon angioplasty in multivessel disease has been carefully evaluated by several randomized trials of PTCA versus CABG. The trials convincingly demonstrated that the hard end points of death and Q-wave myocardial infarction were not different between these two modalities at 1- to 5-year follow-up. MVD-PCI has the advantage of lower in-hospital mortality compared to

surgery (8). However, the shortcoming of MVD intervention has been increased revascularization procedures secondary to restenosis. The advent of DES was a landmark achievement in interventional cardiology, as it has narrowed the difference in TVR between percutaneous and surgical revascularization. While single-vessel intervention is often aimed at relieving angina, MVD-PCI in some cases may improve left ventricular function and long-term survival. Compared with SVD patients, MVD patients have a worse short-term outcome as observed in the ACC-NCDR with an in-hospital mortality of 1.9% versus 0.8% (4). MVD-PCI has been associated with increased risk of periprocedural MI which adversely affects long-term outcome (38,59). The ACC/AHA guidelines designates a Class I indication for MVD-PCI in two- or three-vessel disease among patients with anatomy suitable for percutaneous revascularization, normal LV function, and who do not have diabetes (22). Multivessel PCI should only be performed by an experienced interventionist after considering all the options and outcomes with the patient.

When approaching MVD intervention, a complete assessment of the comorbid conditions and LV functions is imperative. Viability assessment is sometimes needed to assist in discerning which target lesions are to be treated. Adequate prehydration and staging the intervention are prudent in the presence of renal insufficiency to decrease the risk of nephropathy. The benefit of the intra-aortic balloon pump (IABP) is clear in patients with cardiogenic shock which is further enhanced with revascularization (34,66). Patients undergoing revascularization of an artery supplying a large area of viable myocardium or with LV dysfunction are at risk of developing hemodynamic compromise and an additional arterial line for expedited intra-aortic balloon pump insertion should be considered. The established benefit of an IABP in patients undergoing percutaneous revascularization is limited in the absence of cardiogenic shock, malignant ventricular arrhythmias or post-MI mechanical complication (67). The order of which stenoses are treated can directly impact the safety of multivessel intervention (Fig. 14–4). A large area of viable myocardium supplied by a chronic total occlusion should be targeted first. In the absence of chronic total occlusion, the artery supplying

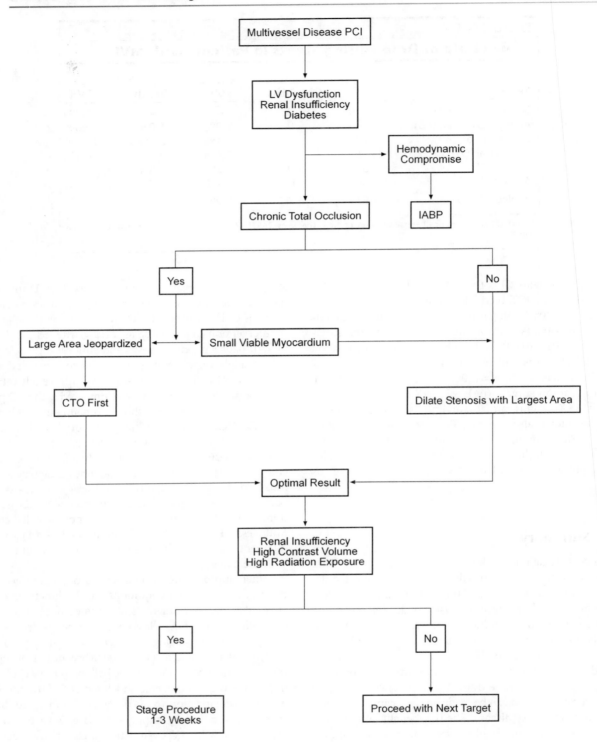

Figure 14–4.

A suggested approach to percutaneous revascularization of multivessel disease. This may vary depending on lesion complexity and anatomical difficulty. (PCI percutaneous coronary intervention, IABP intra-aortic balloon pump, CTO chronic total occlusion, LV left ventricle.)

the largest area of viable myocardium should be attempted first provided the lesion is not overly complex. Before attempting the second artery, reassessment of contrast use and radiation exposure to determine the need for a staged procedure should be made. In the setting of STEMI, dilation of nonculprit vessel stenosis should be deferred unless the patient is presenting with cardiogenic shock and hemodynamic stability is not attained with the culprit vessel PCI.

The procedural and long-term outcome of MVD-PCI continues to be refined and improved with better deliverability of drug-eluting stents. Different medicated stents, including bio-absorbable stents are being evaluated that may further narrow the difference between percutaneous and surgical revascularization.

REFERENCES

1. AHA. *Heart Disease and Stroke Statistics.* 2005.

2. Laskey WK, et al. Changes in the practice of percutaneous coronary intervention: a comparison of enrollment waves in the National Heart, Lung, and Blood Institute (NHLBI) Dynamic Registry. *Am J Cardiol.* 2001;87:964–969.

3. Laskey WK, Kimmel S, Krone RJ. Contemporary trends in coronary intervention: a report from the Registry of the Society for Cardiac Angiography and Interventions. *Cath Cardiovasc Intervent.* 2000;49:19–22.

4. Anderson HV, et al. A contemporary overview of percutaneous coronary interventions. The American College of Cardiology-National Cardiovascular Data Registry (ACC-NCDR). *J Am Coll Cardiol.* 2002;39:1096–1103.

5. McGrath PD, et al. Changing outcomes in percutaneous coronary interventions: a study of 34,752 procedures in northern New England, 1990 to 1997. Northern New England Cardiovascular Disease Study Group. *J Am Coll Cardiol.* 1999;34:674–680.

6. van den Brand MJ, et al. The effect of completeness of revascularization on event-free survival at one year in the ARTS trial. *J Am Coll Cardiol.* 2002;39:559–564.

7. Bourassa MG, et al. Is a strategy of intended incomplete percutaneous transluminal coronary angioplasty revascularization acceptable in non-diabetic patients who are candidates for coronary artery bypass graft surgery? The Bypass Angioplasty Revascularization Investigation (BARI). *J Am Coll Cardiol.* 1999;33:1627–1636.

8. Hannan EL, et al. Long-term outcomes of coronary-artery bypass grafting versus stent implantation. *N Engl J Med.* 2005;352:2174–2183.

9. Cohen HA, et al. Impact of age on procedural and 1-year outcome in percutaneous transluminal coronary angioplasty: a report from the NHLBI dynamic registry. *Am Heart J.* 2003;146:513–519.

10. Baskett R, et al. Outcomes in octogenarians undergoing coronary artery bypass grafting. *Cmaj.* 2005;172:1183–1186.

11. Klein LW, et al. Percutaneous coronary interventions in octogenarians in the American College of Cardiology-National Cardiovascular Data Registry: development of a nomogram predictive of in-hospital mortality. *J Am Coll Cardiol.* 2002;40:394–402.

12. Little T, et al. Late outcome and quality of life following percutaneous transluminal coronary angioplasty in octogenarians. *Cath Cardiovasc Intervent.* 1993;29:261–266.

13. Sadeghi HM, et al. Percutaneous coronary interventions in octogenarians. glycoprotein IIb/IIIa receptor inhibitors' safety profile. *J Am Coll Cardiol.* 2003;42:428–432.

14. Weintraub WS, et al. Changing use of coronary angioplasty and coronary bypass surgery in the treatment of chronic coronary artery disease. *Am J Cardiol.* 1990;65:183.

15. Le Feuvre C, et al. Five- to ten-year outcome after multivessel percutaneous transluminal coronary angioplasty. *Am J Cardiol.* 1993;71:1153–1158.

16. O'Keefe JH Jr, et al. Multivessel coronary angioplasty from 1980 to 1989: procedural results and long-term outcome. *J Am Coll Cardiol* 1990;16:1097–1102.

17. Ellis SG, et al. Determinants of 2-year outcome after coronary angioplasty in patients with multivessel disease on the basis of comprehensive preprocedural evaluation. Implications for patient selection. The Multivessel Angioplasty Prognosis Study Group. *Circulation.* 1991;83:1905–1914.

18. Allman KC, et al. Myocardial viability testing and impact of revascularization on prognosis in patients with coronary artery disease and left ventricular dysfunction: a meta-analysis. *J Am Coll Cardiol.* 2002;39:1151–1158.

19. Natali A Coronary atherosclerosis in Type II diabetes: angiographic findings and clinical outcome. *Diabetologia.* 2000;43:632–641.

20. Ammann P, et al. Coronary anatomy and left ventricular ejection fraction in patients with type 2 diabetes admitted for elective coronary angiography. *Cath Cardiovasc Intervent.* 2004;62:432–438.

21. Influence of diabetes on 5-year mortality and morbidity in a randomized trial comparing CABG and PTCA in patients with multivessel disease: the Bypass Angioplasty Revascularization Investigation (BARI). *Circulation.* 1997;96:1761–1769.

22. Gibbons RJ, et al. ACC/AHA 2002 guideline update for the management of patients with chronic stable angina: a report of the American College of Cardiology/American Heart Association Task Force on practice guidelines (Committee on the Management of Patients with Chronic Stable Angina). Available from: http://www.acc.org/clinical/guidelines/stable/stable_clean.pdf.

23. Serruys PW, et al. Five-year outcomes after coronary stenting versus bypass surgery for the treatment of multivessel disease: the final analysis of the Arterial Revascularization Therapies Study (ARTS) randomized trial. *J Am Coll Cardiol* 2005;46:575–581.

24. System URD. *USRDS 2004 Annual data report.* In: National Institutes of Health, ed. National Institutes of Diabetes and Digestive and Kidney Diseases. Bethesda, MD; 2004.

25. Joki N, et al. Onset of coronary artery disease prior to initiation of haemodialysis in patients with end-stage renal disease. *Nephrol Dial Transplant.* 1997;12:718–723.

26. Best PJ, et al. The impact of renal insufficiency on clinical outcomes in patients undergoing percutaneous coronary interventions. *J Am Coll Cardiol* 2002;39:1113–1119.

27. Best PJ, et al. Impact of mild or moderate chronic kidney disease on the frequency of restenosis: results from the PRESTO trial. *J Am Coll Cardiol.* 2004;44:1786–1791.

28. Muller DW, et al. Multivessel coronary artery disease: a key predictor of short-term prognosis after reperfusion therapy for acute myocardial infarction. Thrombolysis and Angioplasty in Myocardial Infarction (TAMI) Study Group. *Am Heart J.* 1991;121:1042–1049.

29. Kahn JK, et al. Timing and mechanism of in-hospital and late death after primary coronary angioplasty during acute myocardial infarction. *Am J Cardiol.* 1990;66:1045–1048.

30. Corpus RA, et al. Multivessel percutaneous coronary intervention in patients with multivessel disease and acute myocardial infarction. *Am Heart J.* 2004;148:493–500.

31. Roe MT, et al. Initial experience with multivessel percutaneous coronary intervention during mechanical reperfusion for acute myocardial infarction. *Am J Cardiol.* 2001;88:170–173.

32. Gibson CM, et al. Impaired coronary blood flow in nonculprit arteries in the setting of acute myocardial infarction. *J Am Coll Cardiol.* 1999;34:974.

33. Hanratty CG, et al. Exaggeration of nonculprit stenosis severity during acute myocardial infarction: implications for immediate multivessel revascularization. *J Am Coll Cardiol.* 2002;40:911–916.

34. Hochman JS, et al. Early revascularization in acute myocardial infarction complicated by cardiogenic shock. SHOCK Investigators. Should we emergently revascularize occluded coronaries for cardiogenic shock. *N Engl J Med.* 1999;341:625–634.

35. Grines CL, et al. Prognostic implications and predictors of enhanced regional wall motion of the noninfarct zone after thrombolysis and angioplasty therapy of acute myocardial infarction. The TAMI Study Groups. *Circulation.* 1989;80:245–253.

36. Antman EM, et al. ACC/AHA guidelines for the management of patients with ST-elevation myocardial infarction; A report of the American College of Cardiology/American Heart Association Task Force on Practice Guidelines (Committee to revise the 1999 Guidelines for the management of patients with acute myocardial infarction). *J Am Coll Cardiol.* 2004;44:E1–E211.

37. de Feyter PJ, et al. Bypass surgery versus stenting for the treatment of multivessel disease in patients with unstable angina compared with stable angina. *Circulation.* 2002;105:2367–2372.

38. Shishehbor M, et al. Clinical outcome of multivessel coronary intervention in the contemporary percutaneous revascularization era. In press.

39. Brener SJ, et al. Efficacy and safety of multivessel percutaneous revascularization and tirofiban therapy in patients with acute coronary syndromes. *Am J Cardiol*. 2002;90:631–633.

40. Smith SC Jr, et al. ACC/AHA guidelines of percutaneous coronary interventions (revision of the 1993 PTCA guidelines)—executive summary. A report of the American College of Cardiology/American Heart Association Task Force on Practice Guidelines (committee to revise the 1993 guidelines for percutaneous transluminal coronary angioplasty). *J Am Coll Cardiol*. 2001;37:2215–2239.

41. Faxon DP, et al. The degree of revascularization and outcome after multivessel coronary angioplasty. *Am Heart J*. 1992;123:854–859.

42. Cukingnan RA, et al. Influence of complete coronary revascularization on relief of angina. *J Thorac Cardiovasc Surg*. 1980;79:188–193.

43. Lavee J, et al. Does complete revascularization by the conventional method truly provide the best possible results? Analysis of results and comparison with revascularization of infarct-prone segments (systematic segmental myocardial revascularization): the Sheba Study. *J Thorac Cardiovasc Surg*. 1986;92:279–290.

44. Lawrie GM, et al. The influence of residual disease after coronary bypass on the 5-year survival rate of 1,274 men with coronary artery disease. *Circulation*. 1982;66:717–723.

45. Cowley MJ, et al. Is traditionally defined complete revascularization needed for patients with multivessel disease treated by elective coronary angioplasty? Multivessel Angioplasty Prognosis Study (MAPS) Group. *J Am Coll Cardiol*. 1993;22:1289–1297.

46. Berger A, et al. Long-term clinical outcome after fractional flow reserve-guided percutaneous coronary intervention in patients with multivessel disease. *J Am Coll Cardiol*. 2005;46:438–442.

47. Takaro T, et al. The VA cooperative randomized study of surgery for coronary arterial occlusive disease II. Subgroup with significant left main lesions. *Circulation*. 1976;54:III107–III117.

48. O'Keefe JH Jr, et al. Left main coronary angioplasty: early and late results of 127 acute and elective procedures. *Am J Cardiol*. 1989;64:144–147.

49. Tan WA, et al. Long-term clinical outcomes after unprotected left main trunk percutaneous revascularization in 279 patients. *Circulation*. 2001;104:1609–1614.

50. Valgimigli M, et al. Short- and long-term clinical outcome after drug-eluting stent implantation for the percutaneous treatment of left main coronary artery disease: insights from the Rapamycin-eluting and taxus stent evaluated at Rotterdam Cardiology Hospital registries (RESEARCH and T-SEARCH). *Circulation*. 2005;111:1383–1389.

51. Pan M, et al. Simple and complex stent strategies for bifurcated coronary arterial stenosis involving the side branch origin. *Am J Cardiol*. 1999;83:1320–1325.

52. Al Suwaidi J, et al. Immediate and long-term outcome of intracoronary stent implantation for true bifurcation lesions. *J Am Coll Cardiol*. 2000;35:929–936.

52a. Hoye A, Iakovou I, Ge L, et al. Long-term outcomes after stenting of bifurcation lesions with the "crush" technique: predictors of an adverse outcome. *JACC* 2006 May 16;47(10):1949–1958.

53. Rogers WJ, et al. Bypass Angioplasty Revascularization Investigation (BARI): baseline clinical and angiographic data. *Am J Cardiol*. 1995;75:9C–17C.

54. Nakamura S, et al. Impact of sirolimus-eluting stent on the outcome of patients with chronic total occlusions. *Am J Cardiol*. 2005;95:161.

55. Werner GS, et al. Prevention of lesion recurrence in chronic total coronary occlusions by paclitaxel-eluting stents. *J Am Coll Cardiol*. 2004;44:2301.

56. Ellis SG, et al. Coronary morphologic and clinical determinants of procedural outcome with angioplasty for multivessel coronary disease. Implications for patient selection. Multivessel Angioplasty Prognosis Study Group. *Circulation*. 1990;82:1193–1202.

57. Deligonul U, et al. Coronary angioplasty: a therapeutic option for symptomatic patients with two and three vessel coronary disease. *J Am Coll Cardiol* 1988;11:1173–1179.

58. Myler RK, et al. Multiple vessel coronary angioplasty: classification, results, and patterns of restenosis in 494 consecutive patients. *Cathet Cardiovasc Diagn*. 1987;13:1–15.

59. Kornowski R, et al. Procedural results and late clinical outcomes following multivessel coronary stenting. *J Am Coll Cardiol*. 1999;33:420–426.

60. Kastrati A, et al. A clinical trial of abciximab in elective percutaneous coronary intervention after pretreatment with clopidogrel. *N Engl J Med*. 2004;350:232–238.

61. Mehilli J, et al. Randomized clinical trial of abciximab in diabetic patients undergoing elective percutaneous coronary interventions after treatment with a high loading dose of clopidogrel. *Circulation*. 2004;110:3627–3635.

62. Kastrati A. *Personal communication*. 2005.

63. Serruys PW, Lemos PA, van Hout BA. Sirolimus eluting stent implantation for patients with multivessel disease: rationale for the arterial revascularisation therapies study part II (ARTS II). *Heart*. 2004;90:995–998.

64. Serruys PW. Arterial Revascularisation Therapies Study II. Presented at ACC meeting 2005; Orlando, FL.

65. Herrick J. Clinical features of sudden obstruction of the coronary arteries. *J Am Med Assoc*. 1912;59:2010–2015.

66. Sanborn TA, et al. Impact of thrombolysis, intra-aortic balloon pump counterpulsation, and their combination in cardiogenic shock complicating acute myocardial infarction: a report from the SHOCK Trial Registry. *J Am Coll Cardiol*. 2000;36:1123.

67. Stone MD, Marsalese MD, Brodie MD. A prospective, randomized evaluation of prophylactic intraaortic balloon counterpulsation in high risk patients with acute myocardial infarction treated with primary angioplasty. *J Am Coll Cardiol*. 1997;29:1459.

68. Arampatzis CA, et al. Elective sirolimus-eluting stent implantation for multivessel disease involving significant LAD stenosis: one-year clinical outcomes of 99 consecutive patients–the Rotterdam experience. *Cath Cardiovasc Intervent*. 2004;63:57–60.

69. Mikhail GW, et al. The use of drug eluting stents in single and multivessel disease: results from a single centre experience. *Heart*. 2004;90:990–994.

70. Orlic D, et al. Treatment of multivessel coronary artery disease with sirolimus-eluting stent implantation: immediate and mid-term results. *J Am Coll Cardiol*. 2004;43:1154–1160.

71. Simonton C, et al. Clinical efficacy and safety of drug-eluting stents in multi-lesion and multi-vessel procedures: results from the Strategic Transcatheter Evaluation of New Therapies (STENT) Group. (abstr) *Am J Cardiol*. 2005;96:178.

72. Serruys PW. ARTS II: Arterial Revascularization Therapies Study Part II–sirolimus-eluting stents vs PCI and CABG at 1 Year. In: Orlando, FL: American College of Cardiology; 2005.

CHAPTER 15

Device Approaches to Special Circumstances; Thrombus-Containing Lesions, Aorto-Ostial Lesions, Saphenous Vein Grafts, and Chronic Total Occlusions

Christopher J. White

Specific circumstances or special situations arise during the catheter-based management of patients which in turn dictate the use of specific devices or strategies to maximize success. These situations include: (a) thrombus-containing lesions, (b) aorto-ostial lesions, (c) saphenous vein grafts, and (d) chronic total occlusions (CTO). The devices, in addition to conventional balloon angioplasty, available for use in these special circumstances include stents, atherectomy devices, lasers, and thrombectomy devices (Table 15–1).

Thrombus-Containing Lesions

Intracoronary thrombus is most commonly found in patients presenting with an acute coronary syndrome (ACS) (i.e., unstable angina [UA], non-ST-elevation myocardial infarction [NSTEMI], or ST-elevation myocardial infarction [STEMI]) representing a continuous spectrum of coronary occlusion caused by sequential atherosclerotic plaque rupture, platelet aggregation, and thrombosis. Thrombus containing lesions are associated with an increase in the complication rate for percutaneous coronary intervention (PCI). The diagnosis or identification of thrombus-containing lesions is best with direct visualization using an angioscope (1). Radiographic contrast angiography has poor sensitivity and specificity for thrombus containing lesions when compared to angioscopy (2). A typical finding at the time of angiography is contrast staining or a filling defect. Intravascular ultrasound (IVUS) also has poor sensitivity and specificity for intraluminal thrombus because fresh thrombus often has an acoustic signature very similar to blood.

Despite its poor sensitivity and specificity for intraluminal thrombus, angiographic intracoronary thrombus is associated with adverse outcomes during percutaneous coronary inter-

vention (3). Patients with evidence of intracoronary thrombus had a greater likelihood of death, myocardial infarction, and abrupt closure following intervention. In the IMPACT-II study, the use of a IIb/IIIa antiplatelet agent reduced the overall angiographic complication rate following PCI, with a trend toward fewer instances of residual thrombus with a IIb/IIIa antiplatelet agent 2.1% compared to 3.2% with placebo (P = 0.09) (4). There was no difference regarding distal embolization between the IIb/IIIa treated group and the placebo group.

In clinical trials of directional atherectomy (DCA), its use has been associated with increased complications in thrombus-containing lesions. Specifically, thrombus-containing lesions have been associated with a decreased success rate, increased risk of embolization, increased risk of no/slow flow, and an increase in major adverse cardiac events (MACE). The recommendation is to avoid the use of DCA in thrombus-containing lesions.

Another form of atherectomy, or debulking, uses the transluminal extraction catheter (TEC). This device has also been shown to be associated with increased complications after PCI including an increased incidence of no/slow flow, myocardial infarction, and increased distal embolization (5). These results have led to a recommendation to avoid using this catheter in thrombus-containing lesions. Rotational atherectomy has met with great problems in thrombus-containing lesions and is not recommended for use in these lesions.

The excimer laser catheter was associated with a sixfold increase in failure rate in thrombus-containing lesions (6,7). Intracoronary thrombus has been associated with a greater risk of embolization and a marked decrease in clinical success.

Rheolytic thrombectomy (RT) using the AngioJet® catheter (Possis Medical, Inc., Minneapolis, MN) has been shown to

Table 15-1	
Available Devices for Thrombus Treatment	
PTCA	THROMBECTOMY
DCA	Angiojet
TEC	X-ciser
LASER	Acolysis
STENT	Catheter aspiration

PTCA, percutaneous transluminal coronary angioplasty; DCA, directional coronary atherectomy; TEC, transluminal extraction catheter; LASER, light amplification by stimulated emission radiation.

be an effective method for removing intravascular thrombus in the coronary and the peripheral arterial circulation (8–10). Isolated case reports have suggested RT may also be a promising percutaneous method for treating coronary stent thrombosis (11,12). The AngioJet LF 140 system consists of a 5.0 Fr, dual lumen, over-the-wire (0.014″–0.018″) RT catheter with an external pump console that provides pressurized saline to the catheter tip (13). Multiple high-velocity saline jets exit from the distal catheter tip and are directed retrograde across a small gap, toward the more proximal opening of a separate evacuation lumen. The jets create a localized low-pressure zone (Bernoulli Effect) that draws thrombus into the gap where the jets pulverize it into small particles. The jets are also used to propel the thrombus debris through the catheter evacuation lumen and out of the body. Preclinical studies have shown that the catheter produces minimal or no vessel wall damage (13).

The Vegas-II trial was a randomized trial in which 349 patients with thrombus containing lesions were treated with intracoronary thrombolysis (urokinase) and definitive PCI, compared to mechanical thrombectomy (AngioJet) with definitive PCI. The primary endpoint of the trial included: (a) freedom from MACE at 30 days, (b) <50% residual diameter stenosis, (c) ≥20% improvement in lesion diameter stenosis, and (d) TIMI-3 flow (8). There were fewer bleeding complications in

the RT group (Fig. 15–1) than the intracoronary thrombolysis group. The 30-day outcome demonstrated a significantly lower MACE for the RT group of 15.1% compared to 32.1% for the thrombolysis group (P <0.001). However, there was no difference for the primary endpoint of the trial. The conclusion was that RT was safer than intracoronary thrombolysis with fewer in-hospital MACE, fewer vascular complications, and fewer bleeding complications. There was also more rapid thrombus removal with RT and a reduced length of hospital stay.

A more recent trial (X-TRACT) of another mechanical thrombectomy device (x-sizer, ev3, Plymouth, MN) in thrombus containing vein grafts has been reported (14). In this trial, 839 thrombus containing native coronary arteries or saphenous vein grafts were randomized to stent implantation with or without prior thrombectomy. The 30-day outcomes for MACE, MACE-native, and MACE-SVG were not different. There was a trend toward fewer death and myocardial infarctions in the x-sizer group (6.3%) compared to the stent-alone group (9.8%, P = 0.07). However, after the first year, there was no difference in MACE, death or myocardial infarction, or target lesion revascularization (Fig. 15–2). There was no evidence that mechanical thrombectomy with x-sizer improved early or late event-free survival compared to bare metal stents alone.

The ATLAS trial was a multicenter trial of ultrasound ablation (acolysis) compared to abciximab in thrombus containing lesions of native and saphenous vein grafts (15). The primary endpoint of the trial was procedure success, TIMI-3 flow, and freedom from MACE at 30-days. This trial was stopped early do to an excess of adverse events in the acolysis arm (Fig. 15–3).

Aorto-Ostial Lesions

Aorto-ostial lesions are technically challenging and are associated with a lower procedural success rate, increased complication rate, and an increased restenosis rate after PCI.

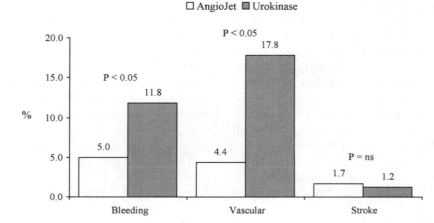

Figure 15–1.
Bar graph showing the complication rate for mechanical thrombectomy compared to the thrombolysis (8).

X-TRACT Trial

□ X-SIZER ■ STENT

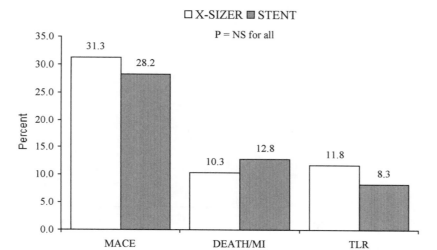

Figure 15–2.

Bar graph of the X-sizer trial for thrombus containing native coronary arteries and saphenous vein grafts (MACE, major adverse cardiac events; MI, myocardial infarction; TLR, target lesion revascularization) (14).

Strategies to improve outcomes have included debulking strategies with excision of plaque (DCA) or excimer-laser (ELCA) ablation. Stents have been employed to overcome elastic recoil and undilatable lesions have been approached with cutting balloons and rotational atherectomy (Rotoblator). The use of adjunctive devices has been associated with a high success rate, but DCA, ELCA, and Rotablator have been associated with a high restenosis rate, 40% to 55%, compared to 23% to 35% for stents (16–18).

In a series of 340 consecutive patients with aorto-ostial SVG lesions, a debulking strategy of either ELCA or DCA with stent was compared to stent alone. There was no advantage (i.e., procedure success, acute complications, or late patency) for the strategy of debulking plus stent placement compared to stent alone (19).

Saphenous Vein Grafts

Following aorto-coronary bypass surgery (CABG), patients often develop accelerated atherosclerosis of their saphenous vein grafts (SVGs) (20–23). Graft failure contributes significantly to morbidity and mortality in these patients (24). Treatment

ATLAS TRIAL

□ Acolysis ■ Abciximab

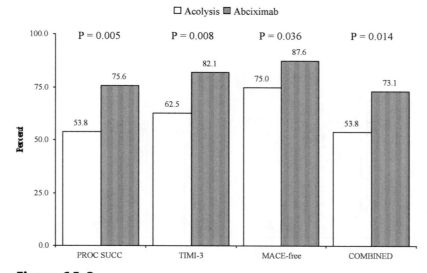

Figure 15–3.

Bar graph showing outcomes of the ATLAS trial (Proc Succ, procedure success; TIMI, thrombolysis in myocardial infarction; MACE, major adverse cardiac events) (15).

SAFER TRIAL

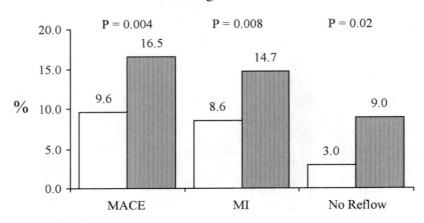

Figure 15–4.
Bar graph of the SAFER trial, embolic protection trial in SVG's (MACE, major adverse cardiac event; MI, myocardial infarction) (28).

options are limited for these individuals. Repeat CABG is unattractive due to higher mortality and morbidity including a perioperative myocardial infarction rate of up to 10% (25).

In an attempt to improve the acute success rate for PCI of SVGs, several trials investigating the potential benefit of platelet glycoprotein (GP) IIb/IIIa receptor antagonists have been performed. In the EPIC trial, which included 101 SVGs, the abciximab bolus plus infusion group had a statistically lower rate of embolization (3%) compared to the abciximab bolus alone group (6%) and the the control group (18% P = 0.017) (26). In a pooled analysis from five randomized trials, in SVGs there was no benefit regarding the 6-month outcomes of death, myocardial infarction, or target vessel revascularizaiton for platelet GP IIb/IIIa receptor inhibition (27).

There are two trials that have demonstrated benefit for embolic protection devices in SVGs (28–30). In the SAFER trial, distal emboli protection with the Percusurge distal occlusion balloon was compared to a control group. The embolic protection group had a statistically better outcome than the controls (Fig. 15–4). Of interest, in the SAFER trial, was a statistically significant benefit for the group of SVG patients treated with platelet GP IIb/IIIa receptor antagonists with emboli protection compared to those without distal protection. The FIRE trial randomized the Percusurge device against the Filterwire and found no difference between the two methods of embolic protection (Fig. 15–5) (30).

Attempts to use debulking devices, such as the TEC or DCA, in diseased SVGs have met with problems (31–33). The major

FIRE TRIAL

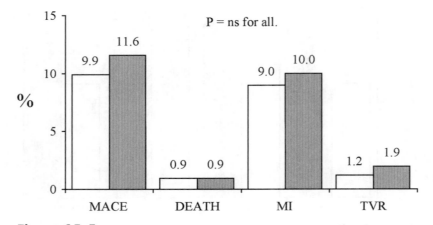

Figure 15–5.
Bar graph showing results of the FIRE trial (MACE, major adverse cardiac events; MI, myocardial infarction; TLR, target lesion revascularization) (30).

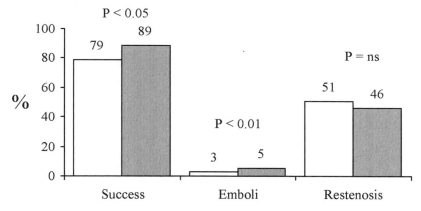

Figure 15–6.
Results of the CAVEAT-II trial comparing DCA to PTCA outcomes in SVG (34).

difficulty with these devices has been the creation of embolic complications with a lower procedure success rate and more complications (Fig. 15–6) (34). The Saphenous Vein De Novo Trial (SAVED) compared PTCA versus bare metal stents (BMSs) in 220 de novo SVG lesions (35). Stents were associated with a higher procedural success rate and a higher event-free survival rate, but they did not lower the restenosis rate in SVG compared to PTCA alone (Table 15–2). In the Randomized Evaluation of PTFE Covered Stent (RE-COVERS) trial, the use of covered stents did not improve the outcomes compared to BMSs in SVGs (Fig. 15–7) (36). The negative data were confirmed in the Stents in Graphs (STING) trial using a PTFE covered JoMed® stent (37). Preliminary data suggest that DES are superior to BMSs in SVG for reducing restenosis. A series of consecutive SVGs treated before the availability of DES were compared to consecutive patients treated with DES and showed a significantly lower MACE rate at the 6-month follow-up (Table 15–3) (38). In summary, the periprocedural event rate is increased when treating SVGs that are older grafts, acute coronary syndromes, thrombus-containing lesions, diffuse disease, and vessel diameter.

Table 15–2

A Comparison of BMS and PTCA in SVG's (SAVED)

	PTCA	BMS	P Value
Procedure success	69	92	<0.001
Restenosis	46	37	0.24
Event-free survival	58	73	0.03
TLR	26	17	0.09

PTCA, percutaneous transluminal coronary angioplasty; BMS, bare metal stent; TLR, target lesion revascularization. (From: Savage MP, Douglas JS, Jr., Fischman DL, et al. Stent placement compared with balloon angioplasty for obstructed coronary bypass grafts. Saphenous Vein De Novo Trial Investigators. *N Engl J Med.* 1997;337:740–747, with permission.)

Chronic Total Occlusions

Chronic total occlusions are identified in up to 20% of patients undergoing coronary angiography. Catheter-based therapy of chronic total occlusions (CTO) has traditionally been associated with longer procedure time and increased radiation exposure, equipment cost, lower success rate, and complication rates. The primary indication for the treatment of a CTO is limiting angina pectoris refractory to maximally tolerated medical therapy, a large area of viable myocardium subtended by the occlusion, and an angiographically "favorable" appearance of the CTO. The expected success rate for a CTO is about 70%.

The most common causes of failed attempt are inability to cross the occlusion with a guidewire (80%), failure to cross with a balloon (15%), and inability to dilate the lesion (5%) (Table 15–4) (39). The first randomized trial of excimer laser-assisted angioplasty for total coronary occlusions demonstrated no benefit for the laser group (40,41). Delivering laser energy through a "laserwire" to cross CTOs demonstrated a success rate of only 50% to 60%, a perforation rate of 21%, and perforation with tamponade in 1% (42,43).

The recanalization of a CTO is hampered by a high rate of lesion recurrence. Several randomized trials demonstrated the superiority of BMSs to PTCA (Fig. 15–8) (44,45). The use of paclitaxel-eluting stents in CTOs in a strategy of extensive stent coverage and the optional use of additional BMSs was studied in two groups of patients. Eighty-two consecutive patients with a CTO (duration >2 weeks) were compared with 82 clinically and lesion-matched patients treated by BMSs. Periprocedural adverse events were 3.3% with Taxus and 3.3% with BMSs, but 12 months MACE was significantly lower in the group with exclusive use of Taxus (13.3% versus 56.7%; P < 0.001), mainly due to a lower target lesion revascularization of 10.0% as compared to 53.4% (P < 0.001).

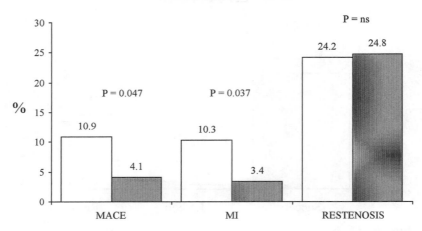

Figure 15–7.

The RECOVERS trial, comparing covered stents (JOMED) to BMS in SVG's (MACE, major adverse cardiac events; MI, myocardial infarction) (36).

Table 15–3			
A Nonrandomized Comparison of SVG's Treated with DES vs BMS at 6 Months			
	DES	**BMS**	**P Value**
MACE	11.5	28.1	0.02
Restenosis	10	26.7	0.03
TVR	4.9	23.1	0.003

From: Ge L, Iakovou I, Sangiorgi GM, et al. Treatment of saphenous vein graft lesions with drug-eluting stents: immediate and midterm outcome. *J Am Coll Cardiol.* 2005;45:989–994, with permission.

Table 15–4
Multivariate Predictors of PCI Failure
• CTO length >15 mm
• Duration >180 days
• Moderate to severe calcification
• Stump morphology not definable

From: Olivari Z, Rubartelli P, Piscione F, et al. Immediate results and one-year clinical outcome after percutaneous coronary interventions in chronic total occlusions: data from a multicenter, prospective, observational study (TOAST-GISE). *J Am Coll Cardiol.* 2003;41:1672–1678, with permission.

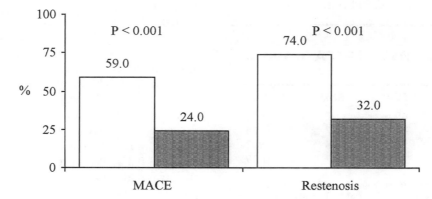

Figure 15–8.

The SICCO trial randomized BMS versus PTCA for CTO's with follow-up at 33 ± 6 months. (MACE, major adverse cardiac events) (45).

There was only one late reocclusion with Taxus (1.7%) as compared to 21.7% with BMSs (P < 0.05). DES resulted in an 80% reduction of target vessel failure as compared to BMSs, with a lower risk of late reocclusions without increased acute adverse events in CTOs. However, diffuse atherosclerosis in CTOs should be covered completely by the drug-eluting stents (46–48).

REFERENCES

1. White CJ, Ramee SR, Collins TJ, et al. Percutaneous coronary angioscopy: applications in interventional cardiology. *J Interv Cardiol.* 1993;6:61–67.
2. White CJ, Ramee SR, Collins TJ, et al. Coronary thrombi increase PTCA risk. Angioscopy as a clinical tool. *Circulation.* 1996;93:253–258.
3. Singh M, Reeder GS, Ohman EM, et al. Does the presence of thrombus seen on a coronary angiogram affect the outcome after percutaneous coronary angioplasty? An Angiographic Trials Pool data experience. *J Am Coll Cardiol.* 2001;38:624–630.
4. Blankenship JC, Sigmon KN, Pieper KS, et al. Effect of eptifibatide on angiographic complications during percutaneous coronary intervention in the IMPACT–(Integrilin to Minimize Platelet Aggregation and Coronary Thrombosis) II Trial. *Am J Cardiol.* 2001;88:969–973.
5. Dooris M, Hoffmann M, Glazier S, et al. Comparative results of transluminal extraction coronary atherectomy in saphenous vein graft lesions with and without thrombus. *J Am Coll Cardiol.* 1995;25:1700–1705.
6. Estella P, Ryan TJ, Jr., Landzberg JS, et al. Excimer laser-assisted coronary angioplasty for lesions containing thrombus. *J Am Coll Cardiol.* 1993;21:1550–1556.
7. Baumbach A, Oswald H, Kvasnicka J, et al. Clinical results of coronary excimer laser angioplasty: report from the European Coronary Excimer Laser Angioplasty Registry. *Eur Heart J.* 1994;15:89–96.
8. Kuntz RE, Baim DS, Cohen DJ, et al. A trial comparing rheolytic thrombectomy with intracoronary urokinase for coronary and vein graft thrombus (the Vein Graft AngioJet Study [VeGAS 2]). *Am J Cardiol.* 2002;89:326–330.
9. Silva JA, Ramee SR, Cohen DJ, et al. Rheolytic thrombectomy during percutaneous revascularization for acute myocardial infarction: experience with the AngioJet catheter. *Am Heart J.* 2001;141:353–359.
10. Silva JA, Ramee SR, Collins TJ, et al. Rheolytic thrombectomy in the treatment of acute limb-threatening ischemia: immediate results and six-month follow-up of the multicenter AngioJet registry. Possis Peripheral AngioJet Study AngioJet Investigators. *Cathet Cardiovasc Diagn.* 1998;45:386–393.
11. Scott LR, Silva JA, White C, et al. Rheolytic thrombectomy: a new treatment for stent thrombosis. *Catheter Cardiovasc Interv.* 1999;47:97–101.
12. Waksman R, Bhargava B, Leon MB. Late thrombosis following intracoronary brachytherapy. *Catheter Cardiovasc Interv.* 2000;49:344–347.
13. Henry TD, Setum CM, Wilson GJ, et al. Preclinical evaluation of a rheolytic catheter for percutaneous coronary artery/saphenous vein graft thrombectomy. *J Invasive Cardiol.* 1999;11:475–484.
14. Stone GW, Cox DA, Babb J, et al. Prospective, randomized evaluation of thrombectomy prior to percutaneous intervention in diseased saphenous vein grafts and thrombus-containing coronary arteries. *J Am Coll Cardiol.* 2003;42:2007–2013.
15. Singh M, Rosenschein U, Ho KK, et al. Treatment of saphenous vein bypass grafts with ultrasound thrombolysis: a randomized study (ATLAS). *Circulation.* 2003;107:2331–2336.
16. Boehrer JD, Ellis SG, Pieper K, et al. Directional atherectomy versus balloon angioplasty for coronary ostial and nonostial left anterior descending coronary artery lesions: results from a randomized multicenter trial. The CAVEAT-I investigators. Coronary Angioplasty versus Excisional Atherectomy Trial. *J Am Coll Cardiol.* 1995;25:1380–1386.
17. Stephan WJ, Bates ER, Garratt KN, et al. Directional atherectomy of coronary and saphenous vein graft ostial stenoses. *Am J Cardiol.* 1995;75:1015–1018.
18. Rocha-Singh KJ, Morris N, Wong S, et al. Coronary stenting for treatment of ostial stenoses of native coronary arteries of aorto-coronary venous grafts. *Am J Cardiol.* 1995;75:26–29.
19. Ahmed JM, Hong MK, Mehran R, et al. Comparison of debulking followed by stenting versus stenting alone for saphenous vein graft aortoostial lesions: immediate and one-year clinical outcomes. *J Am Coll Cardiol.* 2000;35:1560–1568.
20. Ip JH, Fuster V, Badimon L, et al. Syndromes of accelerated atherosclerosis: role of vascular injury and smooth muscle cell proliferation. *J Am Coll Cardiol.* 1990;15:1667–1687.
21. Bulkley BH, Hutchins GM. Accelerated "atherosclerosis". A morphologic study of 97 saphenous vein coronary artery bypass grafts. *Circulation.* 1977;55:163–169.
22. Ratliff NB, Myles JL. Rapidly progressive atherosclerosis in aortocoronary saphenous vein grafts. Possible immune-mediated disease. *Arch Pathol Lab Med.* 1989;113:772–776.
23. Kalan JM, Roberts WC. Morphologic findings in saphenous veins used as coronary arterial bypass conduits for longer than 1 year: necropsy analysis of 53 patients, 123 saphenous veins, and 1,865 five-millimeter segments of veins. *Am Heart J.* 1990;119:1164–1184.
24. Lytle BW, Loop FD, Taylor PC, et al. Vein graft disease: the clinical impact of stenoses in saphenous vein bypass grafts to coronary arteries. *J Thorac Cardiovasc Surg.* 1992;103:831–840.
25. Fitzgibbon GM, Kafka HP, Leach AJ, et al. Coronary bypass graft fate and patient outcome: angiographic follow-up of 5,065 grafts related to survival and reoperation in 1,388 patients during 25 years. *J Am Coll Cardiol.* 1996;28:616–626.
26. Mak KH, Challapalli R, Eisenberg MJ, et al. Effect of platelet glycoprotein IIb/IIIa receptor inhibition on distal embolization during percutaneous revascularization of aortocoronary saphenous vein grafts. EPIC Investigators. Evaluation of IIb/IIIa platelet receptor antagonist 7E3 in Preventing Ischemic Complications. *Am J Cardiol.* 1997;80:985–988.
27. Roffi M, Mukherjee D, Chew DP, et al. Lack of benefit from intravenous platelet glycoprotein IIb/IIIa receptor inhibition as adjunctive treatment for percutaneous interventions of aortocoronary bypass grafts: a pooled analysis of five randomized clinical trials. *Circulation.* 2002;106:3063–3067.
28. Baim DS, Wahr D, George B, et al. Randomized trial of a distal embolic protection device during percutaneous intervention of saphenous vein aorto-coronary bypass grafts. *Circulation.* 2002;105:1285–1290.
29. Stone GW, Rogers C, Ramee S, et al. Distal filter protection during saphenous vein graft stenting: technical and clinical correlates of efficacy. *J Am Coll Cardiol.* 2002;40:1882–1888.
30. Stone GW, Rogers C, Hermiller J, et al. Randomized comparison of distal protection with a filter-based catheter and a balloon occlusion and aspiration system during percutaneous intervention of diseased saphenous vein aorto-coronary bypass grafts. *Circulation.* 2003;108:548–553.
31. Safian RD, Grines CL, May MA, et al. Clinical and angiographic results of transluminal extraction coronary atherectomy in saphenous vein bypass grafts. *Circulation.* 1994;89:302–312.
32. Popma JJ, Brogan WC, 3rd, Pichard AD, et al. Rotational coronary atherectomy of ostial stenoses. *Am J Cardiol.* 1993;71:436–438.
33. Popma JJ, Leon MB, Mintz GS, et al. Results of coronary angioplasty using the transluminal extraction catheter. *Am J Cardiol.* 1992;70:1526–1532.
34. Holmes DR, Jr., Topol EJ, Califf RM, et al. A multicenter, randomized trial of coronary angioplasty versus directional atherectomy for patients with saphenous vein bypass graft lesions. CAVEAT-II Investigators. *Circulation.* 1995;91:1966–1974.
35. Savage MP, Douglas JS, Jr., Fischman DL, et al. Stent placement compared with balloon angioplasty for obstructed coronary bypass grafts. Saphenous Vein De Novo Trial Investigators. *N Engl J Med.* 1997;337:740–747.
36. Stankovic G, Colombo A, Presbitero P, et al. Randomized evaluation of polytetrafluoroethylene-covered stent in saphenous vein grafts: the Randomized Evaluation of polytetrafluoroethylene COVERed stent in

Saphenous vein grafts (RECOVERS) Trial. *Circulation*. 2003;108:37–42.

37. Schachinger V, Hamm CW, Munzel T, et al. A randomized trial of polytetrafluoroethylene-membrane-covered stents compared with conventional stents in aortocoronary saphenous vein grafts. *J Am Coll Cardiol*. 2003;42:1360–1369.

38. Ge L, Iakovou I, Sangiorgi GM, et al. Treatment of saphenous vein graft lesions with drug-eluting stents: immediate and midterm outcome. *J Am Coll Cardiol*. 2005;45:989–994.

39. Olivari Z, Rubartelli P, Piscione F, et al. Immediate results and one-year clinical outcome after percutaneous coronary interventions in chronic total occlusions: data from a multicenter, prospective, observational study (TOAST-GISE). *J Am Coll Cardiol*. 2003;41:1672–1678.

40. Appelman YE, Koolen JJ, Piek JJ, et al. Excimer laser angioplasty versus balloon angioplasty in functional and total coronary occlusions. *Am J Cardiol*. 1996;78:757–762.

41. Appelman YE, Piek JJ, Strikwerda S, et al. Randomized trial of excimer laser angioplasty versus balloon angioplasty for treatment of obstructive coronary artery disease. *Lancet*. 1996;347:79–84.

42. Hamburger JN, Serruys PW, Scabra-Gomes R, et al. Recanalization of total coronary occlusions using a laser guidewire (the European TOTAL Surveillance Study). *Am J Cardiol*. 1997;80:1419–1423.

43. Schofer J, Rau T, Schluter M, et al. Short-term results and intermediate-term follow-up of laser wire recanalization of chronic coronary artery occlusions: a single-center experience. *J Am Coll Cardiol*. 1997;30:1722–1778.

44. Buller CE, Dzavik V, Carere RG, et al. Primary stenting versus balloon angioplasty in occluded coronary arteries: the Total Occlusion Study of Canada (TOSCA). *Circulation*. 1999;100:236–242.

45. Sirnes PA, Golf S, Myreng Y, et al. Sustained benefit of stenting chronic coronary occlusion: long-term clinical follow-up of the Stenting in Chronic Coronary Occlusion (SICCO) study. *J Am Coll Cardiol*. 1998;32:305–310.

46. Werner GS, Schwarz G, Prochnau D, et al. Paclitaxel-eluting stents for the treatment of chronic total coronary occlusions: A strategy of extensive lesion coverage with drug-eluting stents. *Catheter Cardiovas Interv*. 2006;67:1–9.

47. Buellesfeld L, Gerckens U, Mueller R, et al. Polymer-based paclitaxel-eluting stent for treatment of chronic total occlusions of native coronaries: results of a Taxus CTO registry. *Catheter Cardiovasc Interv*. 2005;66:173–177.

48. Ge L, Iakovou I, Cosgrave J, et al. Immediate and mid-term outcomes of sirolimus-eluting stent implantation for chronic total occlusions. *Eur Heart J*. 2005;26:1056–1062.

CHAPTER 16

Complications in the Current Era of PCI

Warren K. Laskey

Major adverse clinical events (MACE) following percutaneous coronary intervention (PCI) include death, peri-procedural myocardial infarction, emergent coronary artery bypass graft surgery (CABG), significant vessel dissection or perforation, cerebrovascular accident, or vascular complication (1). The combined incidence of the first three of these adverse events has decreased over time, in large part due to improved technology, pharmacology, and operator experience (2). Although the advent of coronary stents has led to a decrease in overall in-hospital MACE, complications unique to their use have also developed. The advent of potent anti-coagulant and anti-platelet agents has also resulted in a decrease in peri-procedural thrombotic events with, however, an increase in the risk of bleeding. An additional serious complication of PCI, radiographic contrast media-associated nephropathy (CAN), is discussed in the section on contrast media. Finally, lethal, albeit rare, complications of contemporary PCI are discussed for completeness.

In-Hospital MACE

The clinical trial literature has consistently defined MACE as one or more of the following serious events occurring in the postprocedural period but prior to hospital discharge: death, myocardial infarction, and urgent/emergent CABG (3). In recent years, the inclusion of peri-procedural cerebrovascular events has expanded the acronym to MACCE (major adverse cardiac and cerebrovascular event) although the peri-procedural stroke rate in recent observational and clinical trial settings remains <0.5%. In-hospital MACE rates have consistently declined over the past decade (2), which is mostly due to the decreased rate of emergent CABG and the attendant risk of perioperative myocardial infarction. Reported rates of in-hospital mortality average 1% to 2%, urgent/emergent CABG is generally <2%, and rates of Q-wave myocardial infarction are 1% to 2%. These *average* in-hospital MACE rates will, naturally, differ from group-specific and condition-specific MACE rates (e.g., elderly patients, ST segment elevation myocardial infarction, and shock). Currently, in-hospital composite MACE (death, Q-wave myocardial infarction, and urgent/emergent

CABG) rates average 4% to 5%. Risk factors for in-hospital MACE are outlined in Table 16–1.

Importantly, MACE rates have been noted to be lower than historical averages in older, increasingly complex patients and patients with extensive comorbidities such that contemporary in-hospital MACE rates compare favorably to corresponding adverse outcome rates in the balloon angioplasty era (2,4). Nevertheless, MACE rates reported from the clinical trial literature are often a "best-case scenario" with MACE rates from "real world" observational series and registries generally higher (5).

Peri-Procedural Myocardial Infarction

The advancement of the concept of peri-procedural myonecrosis along with the increased sensitivity (for cell necrosis) with biomarkers such as troponin has resulted in variable, albeit increased, rates of peri-procedural myocardial infarction, depending on the specific criteria used (6,7). There is little debate over the prognostic importance of *substantial* postprocedural increases in CK or CK-MB levels or the development of a Q-wave myocardial infarction (8). The majority of these substantial increases in biomarkers or the development of Q-wave myocardial infarction occurs in the setting of evident intraprocedural complications. Risk factors for peri-procedural myocardial infarction are outlined in Table 16–2. In approximately 20% to 25% of otherwise "uncomplicated" PCI procedures (no intraprocedural events, for example, side branch occlusion, abrupt vessel closure, or significant dissection), CK-MB determinations has been noted to be significantly elevated over baseline (≥3x normal). The rate of postprocedural increase of the more sensitive marker of myocardial injury, troponin, approaches 50%. The clinical significance of these increases in postprocedural markers of myocardial injury, particularly with small, (i.e., <3-fold, increases), continues to be debated (7). However, when extent, or burden, of atherosclerotic disease is taken in account, the predictive importance of these minor increases in postprocedural biomarker release diminishes (9). Of clinical relevance is the consistent decrease in the rate of postprocedural biomarker release with the use of platelet glycoprotein IIb/IIIa receptor antagonists (10) as well as with the pre-procedural administration of thienopyridines (11).

Table 16–1
Risk Factors for In-Hospital MACE

Clinical Factors	Procedural Factors
Multi-vessel disease	Lesion characteristics
Decreased LV function	• Length
• shock	• Associated thrombus
Comorbidity	• Bifurcation
• renal insufficiency	Procedural circumstances
• peripheral vascular disease	• Urgent/emergent
Age	Intra-procedural complications
? Gender	abrupt vessel closure
Myocardial infarction within 24 hours	significant dissection

Distal Thromboembolism

An important contributor to peri-procedural myonecrosis and biomarker release is distal embolization of target site plaque and/or thrombus material (12). Initially ascribed to the ablative interventions, (e.g., PTCRA and DCA), increasingly sensitive techniques for the detection of myocardial injury/necrosis have suggested that such distal embolization may occur in as many as 50% of all PCIs. Evidence in support of this important etiology of procedural complication ranges from magnetic resonance imaging detection of areas of subclinical infarction (13) to the retrieval of macroscopic material from distal protection devices deployed during PCI (14). A further proof of concept lies in the reduction of the peri-procedural myocardial infarction rate in the treatment arms of clinical trials evaluating distal protection devices (15).

Predictors of In-Hospital MACE in the Current Stent Era

Many of the predictors of in-hospital MACE in the current stent era are identical to those of the balloon angioplasty era and reflect, predominantly, the clinical condition of the patient and procedural circumstances (16). The *relative* importance of relationship between specific lesion characteristics and procedural outcome (in contrast to risk of MACE), while critical in the balloon angioplasty era (17), has diminished in the stent era. Because many lesion characteristics are associated with underlying clinical factors (18), multivariate analyses of the predictors of adverse outcomes predominantly reflect these clinical variables (19). However, one lesion characteristic—associated thrombus—continues to confer an increased risk of procedural complication in the current stent era (20).

Early (Procedure-30 Day) Stent Thrombosis

Shortly after the introduction of bare metal stents into the general practice of PCI, the hazard of acute stent thrombosis was immediately recognized. Despite a complex, and lengthy, anticoagulation regimen, rates of early stent thrombosis exceeded 5% with associated increased risks of myocardial infarction and death (21). The bimodal temporal pattern of the risk of stent thrombosis (24–48 hours; 72–96 hours) reflected several key procedural variables (i.e., residual dissection and the absence of anti-platelet therapy, respectively). It was not until the introduction of the thienopyridine agents (ticlopidine and clopidogrel) that these unacceptable rates and risks were controlled (22,23). In the current era of PCI with routine administration of thienopyridines the overall risk of early clinical stent thrombosis (procedure to 30 days) is 0.9% (24). This risk is highest in the 1- to 2-day period following stent implantation (24) and is accompanied by a greater than 60% risk of death or myocardial infarction. The appropriate management of this true emergency condition requires prompt recognition of the etiology of the acute thrombosis and expeditious restoration of antegrade flow.

Risk factors for early stent thrombosis are the presence of significant untreated dissection, poor or inadequate stent deployment, compromised outflow distal to the stented segment, residual thrombus, length of the stented vessel, and cessation of treatment with a dual anti-platelet regimen (Table 16–3). The risk of early stent thrombosis seen with drug-eluting stents is similar to that of bare metal stents (25).

Late (>30 Day) Stent Thrombosis

Available data on the long-term (>30 day) risk of bare metal stent thrombosis indicates a continuing risk of thrombosis

Table 16–2
Risk Factors for Peri-Procedural Myocardial Infarction

Thrombus-associated lesion	Coronary embolization
Saphenous vein graft intervention	Transient abrupt closure
Ablative procedures	Complex lesions
DCA	Large dissections
PTCRA	Large plaque burden
	Acute coronary syndromes

Table 16–3
Risk Factors for Early (<30 Day) Stent Thrombosis

Significant residual dissection
Stent length >25 mm
MLD <3.0 mm
Sub-optimal stent deployment
Age >60 years
Abrupt/threatened closure
Premature discontinuation of anti-platelet therapy

Adapted from: Cutlip DE, Baim DS, Ho KK, et al. Stent thrombosis in the modern era. A pooled analysis of multi-center coronary stent clinical trials. *Circulation.* 2001;103:1967–1971, with permission.

albeit considerably lower than the early risk (24). Given the recommendations for extended (beyond 30 days) administration of dual anti-platelet treatment following drug-eluting stent implantation, it is important to note that the longer-term risk, (i.e., >6 months), of stent thrombosis observed in the pivotal randomized clinical trials was similar to that associated with bare metal stents (the sirolimus-eluting stent thrombosis rate at 1 year was 0.4% and the paclitaxel-eluting stent thrombosis rate at 9 months was 0.9%).

Recently, however, the rate of stent thrombosis at 9 months in an observational study of patients receiving drug-eluting stents was reported to be 1.3% with an equal distribution of early stent thrombosis (i.e., within 30 days; rate = 0.6%) and delayed stent thrombosis (i.e., 30 days to 9 months; rate = 0.7%) (26). The mortality rate associated with stent thrombosis was 45% and the critical role of premature anti-platelet therapy discontinuation was again confirmed. Currently, the FDA-mandated labeling for the use of drug-eluting stents carries the recommendation for the extended use of anti-platelet therapy, for example, 6 months or longer (at the physician's discretion).

Cerebrovascular Complications of PCI

Cerebrovascular complications of contemporary PCI can be categorized as embolic (nonhemorrhagic) or hemorrhagic (Table 16–4). Although the overall procedural-related stroke rate in the PCI literature is <0.5%, this rate varies substantially with age, clinical setting and the vigor of anti-coagulation and anti-platelet therapy. Although the use of platelet GP IIb/IIIa receptor antagonists does not, by itself, confer an increased risk of stroke (27), the conjunctive use of standard dose heparin along with such platelet inhibitors is associated with a significant increase in the risk of hemorrhagic stroke. The use of the newer adjunctive anti-coagulants—low molecular weight heparin (28) and bivalirudin (29)—during contemporary PCI do not appear to be associated with an increased risk of stroke when evaluated in randomized controlled trial settings. However, the overall rate of procedural-related stoke in the

Table 16–4
Cerebrovascular Complications of PCI with Adjunctive Abciximab

	Abciximab (%)	Placebo (%)
All strokes	15/4680 (0.32)	9/3023 (0.30)
Intracranial bleed/ hemorrhagic stroke	7/4680 (0.15)	3/3023 (0.10)
Nonhemorrhagic stroke	8/4680 (0.17)	6/3023 (0.20)

Adapted from: Akkerhuis KM, Deckers JW, Lincoff AM, et al. Risk of stroke associated with abciximab among patients undergoing percutaneous coronary intervention. *JAMA*. 2001;286:78–82, with permission.

Table 16–5
TIMI Classification System for Procedural-Related Bleeding

Major bleeding	Hemorrhagic stroke or Hematocrit decrease >15 point or Hematocrit decrease 10–15 points with clinical bleeding
Minor bleeding	Hematocrit decrease <10 points with clinical bleeding or Hematocrit decrease 10–15 points without clinical bleeding

SYNERGY trial was 1% by 30 days and contrasts with procedural stroke rates of 0% and <1% in the PCI arms of ERACI-2 and ARTS, respectively.

Hemorrhagic Complications of PCI

Peri-procedural bleeding, including access site bleeding, is the most frequent complication of PCI. However, differences in definition and criteria for severity make comparisons over time and between studies difficult. The development of a standardized set of criteria for assessing the severity of procedural-related bleeding, the TIMI risk score, is now the most widely used metric of this complication (Table 16–5). Rates of TIMI-grade significant bleeding complications in the current era of stent deployment, adjunctive anti-platelet therapy, and thrombin-specific anti-coagulants average <1%, whereas composite (major + minor TIMI grade) rates of bleeding average <4% (30). There is also a significant (direct) relationship between the risk of hemorrhage and the activated clotting time (30). Important predictors of significant hemorrhagic complications of PCI include age, weight (BSA), female sex, platelet glycoprotein receptor inhibitor use, intra-procedural hypotension, intra-aortic balloon insertion, and chronic renal insufficiency.

An important caveat in the era of GP IIb/IIIa use is the incidence of thrombocytopenia and associated significant bleeding. The overall risk of thrombocytopenia with platelet GP IIb/IIIa receptor antagonists is 3% and is more prevalent with abciximab (2.4%) than with small molecule inhibitors (0.5%) (31). Severe bleeding is more frequently encountered in the setting of thrombocytopenia and the latter is itself a risk marker for adverse outcomes. The management of significant hemorrhage with GP IIb/IIIa receptor antagonists involves immediate cessation of the infusion, reversal of systemic anti-coagulation, platelet transfusion in patients receiving abciximab and observation and supportive means for patients receiving small molecule inhibitors.

Rare but Life-Threatening Complications of PCI

The presence of ongoing myocardial ischemia and delayed antegrade flow in the epicardial coronary arterial circulation in

Table 16–6

Recommendations for the Management of No-Reflow

First-line management	Adenosine (10–20 mcg bolus)
	Verapamil (100–200 mcg bolus)
	Nitroprusside (50–100 mcg bolus)
Alternatives	Rapid, forceful injections of saline or blood
	Diltiazem (0.5–2.5 mg)
	Papaverine (10–20 mcg)
	Nicardipine (200 mcg)
	Nicorandil (2 mcg)
	Epinephrine (50–100 mcg)
Ineffective/contra-indicated regimens	i.c. nitroglycerin
	CABG
	Stent placement with successful result thrombolytics

Adapted from: Klein LW, Kern MJ, Berger P, et al. Society of Cardiac Angiography and Interventions: Suggested management of the no-reflow phenomenon in the cardiac catheterization laboratory. *Cathet Cardiovasc Interv.* 2003;60:194–201, with permission.

the absence of proximal, upstream conduit vessel obstruction defines the no-reflow phenonmenon (32). Although infrequent (0.6%–2%) in the overall PCI experience, the no-reflow event occurs more frequently during older saphenous vein graft interventions, intervention on lesions with considerable plaque bulk, interventions during acute coronary syndromes, and during rotational atherectomy. Common to all procedures is the liberation and distal embolization of significant amounts of plaque coupled with vasoconstriction of the distal arterial bed. No-reflow carries a 30% risk of myocardial infarction and a 5% to 15% risk of procedural mortality (33). Accordingly, strategies to prevent, and treat, no-reflow have evolved, albeit anecdotally and without rigorous clinical testing (34). Pharmacologic regimens for prophylaxis are inconsistent in their efficacy, except for the setting of rotational atherectomy, and the incidence of no-reflow with use of distal protection devices as well as thombectomy devices exceeds 10% (34). Appropriate management presumes early recognition and the systematic administration of distal arteriolar vasodilators (Table 16–6). Success rates vary widely in this anecdotal literature but, as noted previously, this complication of PCI confers a 10% risk of procedural mortality.

Another life threatening complication of PCI is coronary arterial perforation. Initially seen with the advent of new PCI modalities, particularly ablative techniques (35), perforation remains an infrequent complication overall (~0.5%). However, ablative (debulking) techniques, advanced age and female gender remain risk factors for this complication. Perforation with frank bleeding into the pericardial sac is a bona fide emergency requiring immediate attention: anti-coagulation must be immediately reversed; elimination of the extravasation of blood by proximal occlusion or placement of a covered stent over the culprit area; relief of hemodynamic compromise, if

present; and platelet transfusion for patients receiving abciximab. The risk of procedural mortality ranges from 5% to 10% (36). Despite successful management, delayed manifestations beyond 24 hours have been reported and support the need for close observation of these patients.

REFERENCES

1. Smith SC, Jr., Dove JT, Jacobs AK, et al. ACC/AHA guidelines for percutaneous coronary intervention (revision of the 1993 PTCA guidelines)-executive summary: a report of the American College of Cardiology/American Heart Association task force on practice guidelines (Committee to revise the 1993 guidelines for percutaneous transluminal coronary angioplasty) endorsed by the Society for Cardiac Angiography and Interventions. *Circulation.* 2001;103:830–835.
2. Williams DO, Holubkov R, Yeh W, et al. Percutaneous coronary intervention in the current era compared with 1985–1986: the National Heart, Lung and Blood Institute Registries. *Circulation.* 2000;102:2945–2951.
3. Dorros G, Cowley MJ, Simpson J, et al. Percutaneous transluminal coronary angioplasty: report of complications from the National Heart, Lung and Blood Institute PTCA Registry. *Circulation.* 1983;67:723–730.
4. Shaw RE, Anderson V, Brindis RG, et al. Development of a risk adjustment mortality model using the American College of Cardiology National Cardiovascular Data Registry (ACC-NCDR) experience: 1998–2000. *J Am Coll Cardiol.* 2002;39:1101–1112.
5. Moscucci M, O'Connor GT, Ellis SG, et al. Validation of risk-adjustment models for in-hospital percutaneous transluminal coronary angioplasty mortality on an independent data set. *J Am Coll Cardiol.* 1999;34:692–697.
6. Califf RM, Abdelmeguid AE, Kuntz RE, et al. Myonecrosis after revascularization procedures. *J Am Coll Cardiol.* 1998;31:241–251.
7. Bhatt DL, Topol EJ, Cutlip DE, et al. Does creatine kinase-MB elevation after percutaneous coronary intervention predict outcomes in 2005? *Circulation.* 2005;112:906–923.
8. Stone GW, Mehran R, Dangas G, et al. Differential impact on survival of electrocardiographic Q-wave versus enzymatic myocardial infarction after percutaneous intervention: a device specific analysis of 7,147 patients. *Circulation.* 2001;104:642–647.
9. Mehran R, Dangas G, Mintz GS, et al. Atherosclerotic plaque burden and CK-MB enzyme elevation after coronary interventions: intravascular ultrasound study of 2,256 patients. *Circulation.* 2000;101:604–610.
10. Madan M, Berkowitz SD, Tcheng JE. Glycoprotein IIb/IIIa integrin blockade. *Circulation.* 1998;98:2629–2635.
11. Chew DP, Bhatt DL, Robbins MA, et al. Effect of clopidogrel added to aspirin before percutaneous coronary intervention on the risk associated with C-reactive protein. *Am J Cardiol.* 2001;88:672–674.
12. Topol EJ, Yadav JS. Recognition of the importance of embolization in atherosclerotic vascular disease. *Circulation.* 2000;101:570–580.
13. Ricciardi MJ, Wu E, Davidson CJ, et al. Visualization of discrete microinfarction after percutaneous coronary intervention associated with mild creatine kinase-MB elevation. *Circulation.* 2001;103:2780–2783.
14. Bhatt DL, Topol EJ. Peri-procedural myocardial infarction and emboli protection. In: Topol EJ, ed. *Textbook of Interventional Cardiology.* 4th ed. Philadelphia, PA: Saunders; 2003:251–266.
15. Baim DS, Wahr D, George B, et al. Randomized trial of a distal embolic protection device during percutaneous intervention of saphenous vein aorto-coronary bypass grafts. *Circulation.* 2002;105:1285–1290.
16. Holmes DR, Berger PB, Garratt KN, et al. Application of the New York State PTCA mortality model in patients undergoing stent implantation. *Circulation.* 2000;102:517–522.
17. Ellis SG, Vandormael MG, Cowley MJ, et al. Coronary morphologic and clinical determinants of procedural outcome with angioplasty for multivessel disease. Multivessel Angioplasty Prognosis Study Group. *Circulation.* 1990;82:1193–1202.
18. Krone RJ, Kimmel SE, Laskey WK, et al. Evaluation of the Society for Cardiac Angiography and Interventions' lesion classification system in

14,133 patients with percutaneous coronary interventions in the current stent era. *Cathet Cardiovasc Inter.* 2002;55:1–7.

19. Block PC, Peterson ED, Krone RJ, et al. Identification of variables needed to risk-adjust outcomes of coronary interventions: evidence-based guidelines for efficient data collection. *J Am Coll Cardiol.* 1998;32:275–282.

20. Singh M, Berger PB, Ting HH, et al. Influence of coronary thrombus on outcome of percutaneous coronary angioplasty in the current era (the Mayo Clinic experience). *Am J Cardiol.* 2001;88:1091–1096.

21. Schomig A, Neumann F-J, Kastrati A, et al. A randomized comparison of anti-platelet and anti-coagulant therapy after the placement of coronary artery stents. *N Engl J Med.* 1996;334:1084–1089.

22. Bertrand ME, Rupprecht HJ, Urban P, et al. Double-blind study of the safety of clopidogrel with and without a loading dose in combination with aspirin compared to ticlopidine in combination with aspirin after coronary stenting: the clopidogrel aspirin stent international cooperative study (CLASSICS). *Circulation.* 2000;102:624–649.

23. Leon MB, Baim DS, Popma JJ, et al. A clinical trial comparing three anti-thrombotic drug regimens after coronary artery stenting. Stent Anticoagulation Restenosis Study Investigators. *N Engl J Med.* 1998;339:1665–1671.

24. Cutlip DE, Baim DS, Ho KK, et al. Stent thrombosis in the modern era. A pooled analysis of multi-center coronary stent clinical trials. *Circulation.* 2001;103:1967–1971.

25. Moreno R, Fernandez C, Hernandez R, et al. Drug-eluting stent thrombosis. Results from a pooled analysis including 10 randomized studies. *J Am Coll Cardiol.* 2005;45:954–959.

26. Iakovou I, Schmidt T, Bonizzoni E, et al. Incidence, predictors and outcome of thrombosis after successful implantation of drug-eluting stents. *JAMA.* 2005;293:2126–2130.

27. Akkerhuis KM, Deckers JW, Lincoff AM, et al. Risk of stroke associated with abciximab among patients undergoing percutaneous coronary intervention. *JAMA.* 2001;286:78–82.

28. The SYNERGY Trial Investigators. Enoxaparin vs unfractionated heparin in high-risk patients with non-ST-segment elevation acute coronary syndromes managed with an intended early invasive strategy. Primary results of the SYNERGY randomized trial. *JAMA.* 2004;292:45–54.

29. Lincoff AM, Bittl JA, Harrington RA, et al. Bivalirudin and provisional glycoprotein IIb/IIIa blockade compared with heparin and planned glycoprotein IIb/IIIa blockade during percutaneous coronary intervention (REPLACE-2 randomized trial). *JAMA.* 2003;289:853–863.

30. Brener SJ, Moliterno DJ, Lincoff AM, et al. Relationship between activated clotting time and ischemic or hemorrhagic complications. *Circulation.* 2004;110:994–998.

31. Merlini PA, Rossi M, Menozzi A, et al. Thrombocytopenia caused by abciximab or tirofiban and its association with clinical outcome in patients undergoing coronary stenting. *Circulation.* 2004;109:2203–2206.

32. Bates ER, Krell MJ, Dean EN, et al. Demonstration of the "no-reflow" phenomenon by digital coronary arteriography. *Am J Cardiol.* 1986;57:177–178.

33. Piana RN, Paik GY, Moscucci M, et al. Incidence and treatment of no-reflow after percutaneous coronary intervention. *Circulation.* 1994;89:2514–2518.

34. Klein LW, Kern MJ, Berger P, et al. Society of Cardiac Angiography and Interventions: Suggested management of the no-reflow phenomenon in the cardiac catheterization laboratory. *Cathet Cardiovasc Interv.* 2003;60:194–201.

35. Ellis SG, Ajluni S, Arnold AZ, et al. Increased coronary perforation in the new device era. Incidence, classification, management and outcome. *Circulation.* 1994;90:2725–2730.

36. Fasseas P, Orford JL, Panetta CJ, et al. Indidence, correlates, management and clinical outcome of coronary perforation: analysis of 16,298 procedures. *Am Heart J.* 2004;147:140–145.

CHAPTER 17

Vascular Access and Hemostasis

Barry F. Uretsky and Christopher J. White

Vascular access and hemostasis are required on all percutaneous procedures. As such, mastery of these technical aspects is essential for any invasive and interventional cardiologist (1–3). Access complications, although uncommon, still are the most frequently encountered problem from invasive and interventional procedures. Planning the access on the basis of the patient's history, physical examination and anticipated cardiovascular diagnosis with attention to technical details reduces procedure time and complications. Anticipation and knowledge of potential complications and their treatment allow rapid response should any of these problems develop. This chapter will discuss the basics of access techniques, special considerations in certain patient subgroups and situations, and complications and their treatment.

▓ Arterial Access

Patient History

As in most areas of medicine, patient history is important in determining the appropriate site and technique for access. A history of peripheral arterial disease (PAD) and/or vascular surgery should be routinely sought as should any difficulty from previous procedures. Knowledge of the technical aspects of previous vascular surgical procedures can aid in planning the appropriate access approach.

Physical Examination

Body habitus, particularly extreme obesity may urge the operator to consider an upper extremity approach. All pulses should be palpated for presence and strength and ausculted for bruits. For radial artery access, the Allen's test should be performed to assure adequacy of the ulnar artery in the event of radial artery occlusion. The general appearance of the limb should be noted as well as any signs of PAD. Any differences in blood pressure between the upper extremities should be noted.

Technical Issues: General Principles of Access

Whenever possible a front wall only needle puncture should be employed. This is particularly important with common femoral artery (CFA) and brachial artery (BA) access. In the former, posterior wall puncture increases the risk of posterior bleeding including development of retroperitoneal hematoma which may cause intravascular volume depletion and hypotension, not infrequently before bleeding is recognized clinically. In the case of brachial access, bleeding into the closed fascial compartment can produce a "compartment syndrome" and may produce brachial nerve injury and compression of the brachial artery with hand ischemia.

Reliable landmarks are important in accessing the artery, particularly the CFA, which is the appropriate vessel for inguinal area access. If one locates the anterior superior spine and the symphysis pubis, the point of maximal arterial impulse is about half-way between these two points in over 90% of cases and accessing the CFA at this point is ideal (Fig. 17–1A). This point is typically slightly below the inguinal ligament and is for all intents and purposes always at or above the inguinal crease. In fact, the inguinal crease is an unreliable landmark for access and is increasingly so in obese patients. Another useful landmark for access is the radiographic femoral head. If the femoral head is divided into quadrants, the inferior medial quadrant (3 o'clock–6 o'clock) should be the area where the femoral artery is accessed (Fig. 17–1B).

Access requires a cooperative patient. If the patient cannot lie flat, it must be ascertained prior to the procedure at what angle the patient can lie still during the procedure. As that angle increases, so does the difficulty in accessing the CFA. Based on the operator's experience, level of comfort, and the procedure to be performed, consideration of upper extremity artery access should be entertained.

Fluoroscopic guidance in advancing the guide wire should be used routinely. Fluoroscopy prevents inadvertent entry of a guide wire into a branch where it may cause vascular injury, even with use of "atraumatic" wires. Another useful guide wire technique from the femoral artery is that once the artery is accessed, a long guide wire is passed to the level of the diaphragm where the first catheter diagnostic or guide catheter is advanced. All subsequent wire exchanges may be performed with the wire tip at the diaphragm level. This approach circumvents inadvertent guide wire injury in an atherosclerotic infra-renal aorta.

Tips to Aid in Vascular Access

1. **Operator control of access site and hemostasis** while inserting the needle, wire, and sheath are of paramount

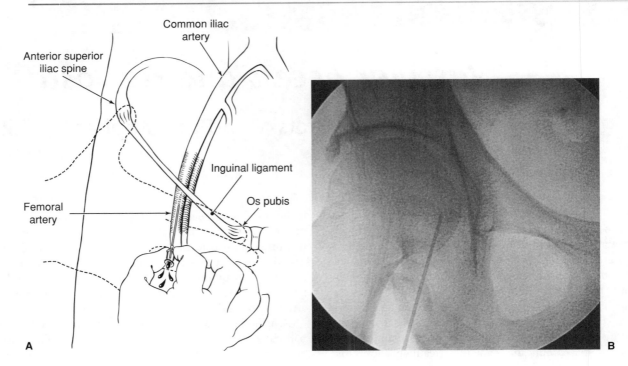

Figure 17–1.
Accessing the femoral artery. **A:** An imaginary line between the anterior superior spine of the hip and the symphysis pubis is constructed. This imaginary line usually corresponds to the course of the inguinal ligament. The location along this line where the pulse is maximal is an excellent site to access the common femoral artery (CFA). **B:** The inferior medial quadrant of the femoral head on x-ray for needle entry is also a good landmark for CFA entry. (From: Uretsky BF. *Cardiac Catheterization*. Malden, MA: Blackwell Science; 1997, with permission.)

importance in preventing bleeding. The third and fourth fingers can be used to palpate and compress the artery above and near the needle puncture and the second finger and thumb can be used to hold the needle (Fig. 17–2). It is important to emphasize that while only the guide wire is in the artery, the arterial hole is larger than the guidewire. If

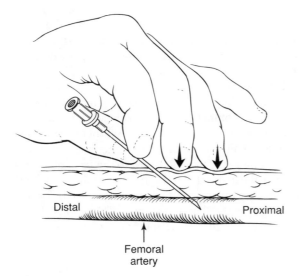

Figure 17–2.
The position of the hand and needle allows the operator to control hemostasis and hold the needle. (From: Uretsky BF. *Cardiac Catheterization*. Malden, MA: Blackwell Science; 1997, with permission.)

adequate pressure is not applied proximal to the hole, blood loss into the subcutaneous tissue increases the likelihood of hematoma development.

2. **Pulsatile bleedback** through the needle proportionate to the systolic and pulse pressures and degree of vascular obstruction should always be present before threading a wire in order to avoid vascular injury on entry. If the operator believes he has entered the vessel through the anterior wall but flow is not good, the operator may then advance the needle further which may improve flow or produce resistance from the periosteum. If the latter occurs, the operator knows he has traversed the posterior wall and that heightened anticipation regarding posterior bleeding should be kept in mind for the rest of the procedure. On withdrawal, flashback should be brisk. An alternative approach to poor bleedback is to simply withdraw the needle and try again. A minute or so of firm pressure is applied prior to the next attempt.

3. **The angle of entry between skin and needle** can vary from almost perpendicular to horizontal although 45 degrees is a reasonable starting point. An advantage to a 60-degree angle is the minimal distance between skin and artery. The disadvantage is that the wire may advance directly to the back wall of the artery and not traverse smoothly into the vessel. Should that occur, the wire should be removed and the needle angle decreased assuring that pulsatile flow is maintained; the wire can then be reintroduced. Conversely, the shallower angle usually allows for the guide wire to

advance easily, but does increase the distance between skin and artery, which may make accessing more difficult, particularly in obese patients.

4. **The long axis of the needle** should be directed parallel to the assumed course of the artery. This technique decreases the risk that other structures are inadvertently traumatized.

5. With the guide wire in place, the **sheath** should be advanced with the wire fixed and a slight twisting motion to the sheath advancement. Movement should be like a "knife through butter."

6. The **guide wire** should never be advanced against significant resistance. The wire should be withdrawn, good bleed-back confirmed, and then gently readvanced. If resistance occurs at the same point, the wire should be withdrawn and small amounts of contrast injected through the sheath to understand the anatomic basis of the resistance. If there is complete occlusion of the vessel, then another site should be accessed. If resistance is due to tortuosity or to severe but not critically occlusive atherosclerotic disease, then use of a hydrophilic guide wire often allows for wire passage into the central aorta.

7. A skin incision and generous spreading of the subcutaneous tissue ("**nick and tunnel**") can facilitate entry of catheters and sheaths. It is the authors' approach to perform this maneuver prior to needle entry to minimize any difficulties in sheath advancement.

8. If **both arterial and venous veins** from the femoral site are being accessed, the operator should consider accessing the artery first. A missed arterial attempt may enter the vein allowing for venous access. The opposite approach rarely nets an artery.

Access in PAD Patients or Patients with Aortofemoral Bypass Grafts

One can expect increased difficulties in the above groups and consideration should be given to utilizing the brachial artery (BA) or radial artery (RA). It should be emphasized that patients with vascular disease may also have tortuous and diseased upper extremity vessels and extensive manipulation may increase embolic stroke risk. Thus, decision-making as to access site should be individualized. If any radiographic studies have been performed such as contrast or MR angiography, these studies should be reviewed, if possible, prior to accessing the vessel. Access through a bypass graft is possible but probably should be avoided in the early postoperative period. Occlusion of the superficial femoral artery is not a contraindication to CFA access, but care should be taken to obtain access at the appropriate landmarks to avoid puncturing the deep femoral artery which represents the only direct circulation to the distal leg.

Arterial Complications and Their Treatment

Femoral Artery

Although its large size increases ease of access, its use is associated with a somewhat higher incidence of complications compared with the radial approach and similar to the brachial approach, but the risk of serious hemorrhage is highest using the femoral approach.

Bleeding from the vascular site, either from the anterior puncture site or through a posterior needle pass is the most frequent serious adverse access site complication. Incidence of this complication varies in multiple series with a need for transfusion in interventional series averaging 3% (3). The medical literature describes multiple risk factors for this complication. Although there is no universal agreement on any single risk factor, the most frequently cited include female gender, low body surface area, obesity, hypertension, over- or prolonged anticoagulation or Gp IIb/IIIa inhibitors with full-dose heparin, use of intravenous thrombolytic agents, elevated serum creatinine, larger sheath size, prolonged time of sheath in the artery, older age, low platelet count, intra-aortic balloon pump, concomitant venous sheath, peripheral artery disease, and repeat intervention (3). Prevention of bleeding includes use of the smallest possible sheath size, decreasing the dose of intravenous heparin (70 U/kg) with concomitant Gp Ib/IIIa use, sheath removal as soon as possible with activated clotting time (ACT) of 150 to 170 seconds or less, particularly with manual compression, and not using anticoagulants after the procedure. Bleeding around a sheath may be due to a fairly inelastic artery with puncture directly through an atherosclerotic plaque or frank trauma during sheath insertion. One method to control the bleeding is to upsize the sheath by one French size, which is usually adequate for hemostasis. If bleeding persists, albeit at a slow rate, then manual compression can usually reduce bleeding until the case is finished at which time a decision regarding the use of a closure device vs manual compression must be made. Should anticoagulation be able to be stopped or reversed, this maneuver may be invaluable in terminating active bleeding.

Groin hematoma can be treated conservatively unless the amount of blood loss is severe, bleeding doesn't stop, or the hematoma becomes tense. The size of the hematoma usually recedes within 1 to 2 weeks. Should the amount of blood loss produce a substantial drop (3–4 gm%) in hemoglobin or a moderate decrease (1–2 gm%) in a compromised patient, particularly as the hemoglobin drops below 9 to 10 gm%, transfusion should be considered. If the bleeding does not stop, the same measures as described for retroperitoneal hematoma should be undertaken. Should the hematoma become tense compromising distal arterial flow, venous outflow, neural function, or skin viability, then surgical decompression is necessary.

One particularly dreaded bleeding event is **retroperitoneal hematoma** (3). It is quite unusual with diagnostic catheterization (<0.15%) but somewhat higher (0.5%–2%) with interventional procedures. It should be suspected when there is hypotension without groin swelling to suggest a hematoma. Flank pain and abdominal fullness, although helpful in making the diagnosis, develop in less than half of cases. The risk of bleeding into the retroperitoneal space is increased with a "high" femoral puncture (above the inguinal ligament) and a back wall puncture of the vessel. As shown in Figure 17–1, knowledge of the femoral vascular and inguinal anatomy is helpful in minimizing this risk. The goal is to access the common femoral artery in its middle third, corresponding to the vascular segment overlying the medial third of the femoral head.

If the suspicion of retroperitoneal hematoma is high, fluid and blood resuscitation should be begun before definitive diagnosis by CT scanning or abdominal/pelvic ultrasound is performed (3). Stopping or reversing heparin anticoagulation using protamine is important. If the patient has received the Gp IIb/IIIa receptor blocker abciximab, then platelet transfusions can be given. The same does not apply to the small molecule platelet glycoprotein IIb/IIIa inhibitors, eptifibatide and tirofiban. These small molecules are competitive inhibitors, not tightly bound to the receptor, leaving excess free drug available to inhibit the transfused platelets. However, their shorter half-life allows the antiplatelet effects to wear off after several hours. Most patients can be treated conservatively, but a percentage may require further intervention to stop the bleeding. There is no antidote for direct thrombin inhibitors for drugs such as bivalirudin and argotraban; as such, supportive care should be provided as the effect of these drugs wear off.

If bleeding persists and causes hemodynamic embarrassment, a percutaneous approach by internal balloon tamponade from contralateral access may avoid the need for surgery. Once the bleeding site has been identified angiographically, tamponade of the bleeding with an angioplasty balloon can stabilize the patient. Use of a covered stent may also be considered but the location of the access site in a place of frequent flexion may produce strut fracture or stent distortion and is not routinely recommended. Open surgical repair may also be considered (3).

Pseudoaneurysm is an accumulation of blood contained by the surrounding tissue adjacent to the arterial puncture. Its continuity with the arterial lumen differentiates it from a hematoma. Unlike simple hematoma, pseudoaneurysm is pulsatile and a bruit may be heard over the site. Physical examination alone is an unreliable method of distinguishing between hematoma and pseudoaneurysm. Pseudoaneurysm may occur in 1% to 3% of cases clinically and the incidence varies widely in clinical series. However, the incidence by systematic ultrasound evaluation is probably twice this figure, demonstrating that there is frequent spontaneous closure of small pseudoaneurysms. Risk factors described in the literature, particularly after manual compression for hemostasis, include obesity, older (>70 years) females, diabetes, and a relatively low (>2 cm below the inguinal ligament) access site. Patients with pseudoaneurysms often present with pain at the access site several days following the procedure. On physical examination, a pulsatile mass may be present with a systolic bruit. Pseudoaneurysm may be complicated by rupture with significant, even life-threatening bleeding, thromboembolism, or extrinsic compression of nearby neurovascular structures.

Management of a femoral pseudoaneurysm is dependent upon its size, severity of symptoms and need for continued anticoagulation. Small (<2 cm) pseudoaneurysms may be observed and followed without treatment; they frequently thrombose or close spontaneously, particularly in the absence of chronic anticoagulation. Larger aneurysms can be treated with compression of the pseudoaneurysm neck as defined by Doppler flow on ultrasound, thrombin directly injected into the pseudoaneurysm, endovascular coil insertion, or by placement of a covered stent. Ultrasound compression causes thrombosis of the pseudoaneurysm by compressing the pseudoaneurysm neck with the ultrasound probe. Variable success rates, ranging from 55% to 90%, have been reported (3–5). It is, however, time-consuming, uncomfortable to the patient often requiring sedation and analgesia, and labor intensive. Compression time may vary from 10 minutes to as long as 300 minutes, with 30 minutes being the average compression time. If patients must continue anticoagulation after successful compression, close follow-up is necessary as the risk of recurrence or rupture of the pseudoaneurysm is increased. Predictors of failure include obesity, large pseudoaneurysm size, concomitant anticoagulation therapy, and groin discomfort (3). Ultrasound guided compression is unattractive or contraindicated in the presence of infection, a tense hematoma, or limb threatening ischemia.

Multiple series have reported success rates of 86% to 97% for treatment of femoral artery pseudoaneurysms with bovine thrombin (500 U–10,000 U) under sonographic guidance (3,6). A risk associated with thrombin injection is that the injected thrombin may exit the pseudoaneurysm, enter the native circulation, and cause distal extremity thrombosis (35). The risk of distal embolization can be minimized by directing the needle away from the neck of the pseudoaneurysm thereby minimizing the risk of injecting thrombin into the native circulation. Ultrasound-guided thrombin instillation is also associated with the failure to occlude the pseudoaneurysm in 3% to 14% and may require repeat injection for failed therapy (2%–4%). Another technique to prevent distal thrombin embolization is the use of angioplasty balloon occlusion of the femoral artery at the site of the pseudoaneurysm neck during thrombin injection to prevent embolization. Patients who have had previous exposure to thrombin or bovine proteins are at risk of immunologic cross reactivity with side effects including hypotension, bradycardia, anaphylaxis, and inhibition of coagulation. It may be helpful for patients who have had prior exposure to bovine thrombin to undergo skin testing to detect possible allergy.

Covered stents have been used successfully to exclude femoral artery pseudoaneurysms (3). The use of covered stents are not ideal if the pseudoaneurysm involves the bifurcation of the common femoral artery into the superficial femoral artery and the profunda femoris artery, as it will cause occlusion of the branch vessels. Placement of a self-expanding covered stent into the common femoral artery may preclude future vascular access at this site. Covered stents may also be associated with an increased risk of subacute stent thrombosis and late stent occlusion, especially when deployed in a common femoral artery with poor run off.

Successful closure of pseudoaneurysms has been reported with coil embolization. Coil embolization of femoral pseudoaneurysms appears to be effective, but can be time consuming.

Other disadvantages include the potential for persistent flow between loosely packed coils. If the coils are placed superficially, local discomfort and pressure necrosis of the overlying skin may occur.

Surgical repair of pseudoaneurysms is usually reserved for the failure of less invasive approaches. Disadvantages include post-operative discomfort, increased costs, and prolonged hospital stay.

Arteriovenous fistula (AVF) occurs in <0.5% of cases and is typically related to accessing the superficial or deep femoral artery with the needle having tracked through an adjacent vein (3). The risk of creating an AVF is increased by either a high or low femoral puncture, multiple puncture attempts, and prolonged clotting times. Fistulae may not be clinically evident for several days following the procedure. Clinically, AVF is characterized by a continuous to-and-fro murmur over the access site. The diagnosis can be confirmed by Doppler ultrasound studies. Most fistulae are small, are diagnosed as an incidental finding, and remain stable in size or close over time. Rarely a fistula will be large and cause swelling and tenderness due to venous dilation and in extreme cases, arterial insufficiency due to a steal phenomenon.

A symptomatic AVF requires closure to prevent increased shunting and distal swelling and tenderness. Ultrasound guided compression and the use of covered stents on the arterial side of the fistula have been successful in small numbers of patients. One significant disadvantage related to the use of covered stents for closure of an AVF is the increased incidence (12%–17%) of stent thrombosis. Percutaneous coil embolization has also been described in a small number of patients. However, experience with this technique remains limited. Surgical repair is usually reserved for those patients who fail a less invasive approach.

Arterial occlusion from dissection or thrombosis is very unusual occurring in <0.5% of cases (8). It is usually related to a large sheath relative to vessel size such as what one may find in patients with severe peripheral arterial disease. It has also been related to advanced age, cardiomyopathy, the presence of a hypercoagulable state (e.g., protein C or S deficiency, lupus anticoagulant), iatrogenic arterial dissection, or development of thrombus in and around the indwelling sheath or related to intraarterial material as part of a closure device. Development of leg ischemia is a medical urgency and requires intervention. Traditionally, surgical correction has been the mainstay of treatment but percutaneous methods can also be employed immediately in the cath lab. If it is felt that the cause of the ischemia is thrombus then intra-arterial thrombolysis, rheolytic thombectomy, or aspiration thrombectomy can be employed after obtaining access from the contralateral femoral artery.

Signs and symptoms are those typically found with acute extremity ischemia (5 P's): pain, pallor, paresthesia, pulseless, and polar (cold). The diagnosis of ischemia is suggested by the physical examination and may be confirmed by duplex ultrasound. Patients with symptomatic limb ischemia following vascular access should undergo angiography to characterize the anatomic basis for the ischemia. Treatment options include balloon angioplasty to restore flow with or without a selective infusion of thrombolytic therapy, stents or catheter thrombectomy. If percutaneous methods fail, surgical thrombectomy and repair are usually required.

Iatrogenic dissection of the femoral or iliac artery from PCI ranges from 0.01% to 0.4%. Vascular access dissection may contribute to the development of distal extremity ischemia, pseudoaneurysm, or thrombus formation. The recognition of a vascular dissection should be followed by angiography to characterize the extent of the dissection. Treatment may include balloon angioplasty or endovascular stent placement or surgical repair to stabilize a flow limiting dissection. If the dissection is small, observation may be all that is necessary as the intraluminal pressure may "tack down" a small intimal flap.

Infection is a rare complication and frequently is not found in large series of patients reported in the literature. However, groin infections tend to manifest several days after the procedure and are likely underreported in all but the most comprehensive quality improvement programs, which include a 30-day follow-up. Risk factors reported in the literature include diabetes, repeat intervention at the same site, long indwelling sheath time, and the use of most of the hemostasis devices. The most common organisms isolated are *Staphylococcus aureus* and epidermis. Pyrogenic reactions following cardiac catheterization generally occur within 1 hour of the procedure and manifest as fever, chills, and lethargy.

Nerve injury has been reported in at least three circumstances. With a very large retroperitoneal hematoma there can be compression of the lumbar plexus. More frequently, there may be femoral nerve palsy, usually transient, from nerve compression due to a large tense hematoma at the access site or direct femoral nerve injury from an errant needle stick. This complication usually needs no specific treatment and recedes with time (7).

Brachial Artery

The current popularity for the use of the brachial approach has waned for several reasons. First arterial cannulation by cutdown access (Sones technique) has been replaced by the percutaneous approach. The radial artery has become, in turn, the favored percutaneous approach because of a decrease in type and severity of complications. Brachial artery access still has utility in some cases as the size of the artery is larger than the radial artery which will allow larger-diameter sheaths and catheters to be used. Also, the shorter distance to the heart and less likelihood of vessel spasm may allow easier catheter manipulation. Anticoagulation should routinely be given in view of the relatively small size of the artery and the consequences of profound hand ischemia from thrombosis.

The brachial artery is accessed at the elbow crease where the pulsation is strongest. The artery in this location is in a compartment with the brachial vein and median nerve. Bleeding into that area can cause a compartment syndrome with ischemic injury to the median nerve and ischemia to the hand from decreased blood flow. A relatively high stick above the compartment is difficult as the artery becomes deep within the muscles. An unsuccessful attempt in this area which produces bleeding may be difficult to control and may also produce a compartment syndrome, requiring surgery for decompression. The possibility of thrombosis appears to be higher than femoral access, although both techniques demonstrate a relatively low incidence.

If a pulse deficit or other ischemic symptom suggests thrombosis after cannulation of the brachial artery, local thrombolysis or catheter thrombectomy may be performed. If the problem is an intimal flap or dissection, angioplasty or stent placement may be required to restore antegrade flow. If these invasive measures are not successful, surgical repair is usually required.

Radial Artery

Radial artery is accessed near the wrist where the pulse is strongest, usually 1 cm or so proximal to the styloid process. It has become popular because it allows rapid ambulation and decreases the risk of severe bleeding. The artery can be successfully cannulated in over 95% of cases. An Allen's test should be performed prior to entry to ascertain that ulnar artery circulation is adequate in case the radial artery occludes after the procedure. This complication, almost always without clinical consequences, may occur in 1% to 5% of cases.

Although the radial artery is small in size, the availability of low profile catheters and devices makes it possible to perform coronary interventions using small (5–6 Fr) sheaths. The transradial approach allows immediate post-procedural ambulation resulting in increased patient comfort. The disadvantages of the transradial approach include more frequent access failure than for the femoral approach, and the inability to perform procedures requiring larger-sized sheaths.

In the one study that compared the radial artery with the brachial and femoral access sites, radial artery access was associated with the lowest incidence of complications (4).

Arterial Hemostasis

There are various methods for vascular hemostasis. The standard against which other methods have been tested is manual hemostasis.

Manual Compression

The proper technique for manual compression is essential. At the femoral or brachial access site, some degree of distal flow should be assured. This aspect is particularly important in manual compression of the femoral artery in patients with PAD. Should a foot pulse not be palpable prior to the procedure, a Doppler signal should be verified prior to the procedure and checked during manual hemostasis. Likewise, if access is obtained through a bypass graft, manual compression should be adequate to stop bleeding with a foot pulse or Doppler signal present. The proper method of manual compression is to tamponade the vessel slightly above and on the access site with direct fingertip pressure. Digital pressure should be applied by fingertips only, such as that applied by a musician to the keys of a piano or strings of a violin (Fig. 17–3).

Prior to compression, one heart pulsation without pressure should be allowed to send blood preferentially through the skin. Such a maneuver improves the possibility that bleeding will track through the skin, allowing the operator to be aware of bleeding recurrence. The length of time for compression varies according to sheath size and presence and level of anticoagulation. Each lab should have its own protocol but in general 10 to 20 minutes for the femoral site, 10 to 15 minutes for the brachial site, and 5 to 10 minutes at the radial site in the absence of anticoagulation are usually adequate. The use of pressure dressings is not recommended to control bleeding as no study has demonstrated their safety and the dressings themselves may obscure bleeding. Also, the purported value of

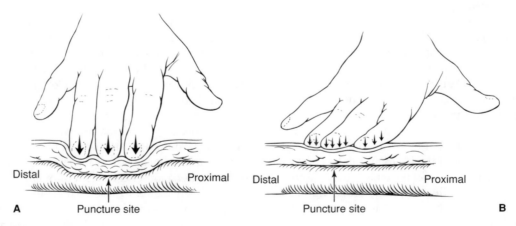

Figure 17–3.
Application of digital pressure. **A:** This panel shows the correct technique of confining full force to a small area. **B:** This panel demonstrates poor technique, spreading force diffuse so that pressure (force/area) is less at each point. (From: Uretsky BF. *Cardiac Catheterization*. Malden, MA: Blackwell Science; 1997, with permission.)

the dressing, namely its ability to tamponade the vessel while freeing up an individual from compression, actually is a major danger to the patient as the patient should be observed until hemostasis is assured. The length of bed rest after femoral sheath removal has not been standardized. With larger sheaths, a period of 6 hours has been traditionally recommended (standard rule: 1 hour compression/French size). With smaller sheaths and use of chemically impregnated pads to aid in manual hemostasis, the length of bed rest may be significantly decreased. Each cath lab should have a standardized protocol in this regard.

Manual Compression with Chemically-Impregnated Pads

The use of chemically-impregnated pads has allowed a decrease in time to hemostasis using the manual method. It offers the other advantage of relatively lower direct cost than closure devices and the lowering of indirect cost by freeing ancillary personnel from performing manual hemostasis.

External Clamps

The advantage of this method is that clamps free up ancillary personnel and are inexpensive. Clamps are relatively uncomfortable for the patient and do not decrease compression time, are difficult to use in certain patients for practical reasons such as in the obese patient, and still require intermittent observation. Severe bleeding in a patient with a clamp which is either applied poorly or moves in an unobserved patient is a formula for disaster.

Closure Devices

Closure devices as a group have the distinct advantage of decreasing the time required for hemostasis and length of stay. In these regards all currently available devices in the United States have shown favorable results. Decreasing hemostasis time increases patient comfort and frees up ancillary personnel. They do add a new cost to the procedure which is only partially offset by freeing up ancillary personnel. Complication rates for both diagnostic and interventional procedure appear similar to manual compression. To date, no prospective randomized clinical trial has shown that any device decreases complication rates compared with manual compression. It should be emphasized that because complications with manual compression are relatively low, a very large sample size typically in the several thousand patient range would be required to show a difference in favor of the closure device (9). Currently available devices include a collagen plug applied on the outer arterial surface of the puncture site (VasoSeal), an external collagen plug firmly attached to the outside of the vessel by a suture and an intravascular "anchor" (Angio-Seal), and a suture based system (Perclose). Newer systems are likely to be introduced in the near future.

Venous Access, Hemostasis, and Complications

Patient History

The operator should be aware of any venous disease before accessing the venous system. If the femoral vein is used, certainty that a vena caval filter has not been implanted is important as is knowledge that recent lower leg thrombosis is not present. Knowledge of previous internal jugular venous access may help to avoid extensive exploration of a previous thrombosed vein. Ultrasound examination of the internal jugular vein is often quite helpful in this regard.

Operational Venous Anatomy and Access Technique

Femoral Vein

The femoral vein runs parallel and medial to the femoral artery at the inguinal ligament area. The femoral vein is usually larger in diameter than the artery. The vein is compressible and because of low pressure cannot be palpated. When accessing both the artery and vein, the vein should be ideally accessed about 1 cm medially and below the arterial puncture site. This separation decreases the probability of developing an arteriovenous fistula.

Internal Jugular Vein

The internal jugular vein is positioned lateral to the carotid artery, medial to the external jugular vein, and usually just lateral to the outer edge of the medial head of the sternocleidomastoid muscle. To identify landmarks, patients are instructed to lie supine without a pillow under the head, and in the case of the right internal jugular, with the head turned 30° to the left. Patients with a low venous pressure may be placed in the Trendelenburg position or may perform a Valsalva maneuver to engorge the extrathoracic veins.

A standard access approach utilizes landmarks (Fig. 17–4). In short, the two heads of the sternocleidomastoid and clavicle create a triangle. The needle should be position near the medial border of the lateral head of the muscle at least half-way up the triangle with a 45- to 60-degree angle to the horizontal. A more acute angle allows the needle tip to go further caudad, increasing the risk of pnemothorax.

An alternate approach is to utilize a specially configured ultrasound probe with a needle holder. The angle between skin and holder is about 60 degrees, which will cause the needle to intersect the internal jugular vein at 1.5 cm below the skin surface. This technique virtually eliminates the risk of pneumothorax; as such, a Valsalva maneuver can be used to increase the diameter of the internal jugular during accessing (Fig. 17–5).

Subclavian Vein

Pertinent procedural anatomy is shown (Fig. 17–6). The proximal subclavian vein and artery are hidden behind the first rib,

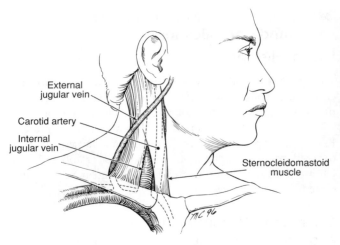

Figure 17–4.

Internal jugular vein access by landmarks. The patient is placed flat and the head is directed to the left for right vein access. The lateral and medial heads of the sternocleidomastod muscle and clavicle form a triangle within, which the internal jugular vein and carotid artery traverse. The carotid artery can usually be palpated. The internal jugular vein is usually just lateral to the carotid artery and just beneath the medial border of the lateral head of the muscle. The site of entry should be at least one third of the way from the clavicle to the jaw to ensure that the apex of the lung is not nicked by the needle and that if the carotid artery is entered, it can be compressed. (From: Uretsky BF. *Cardiac Catheterization*. Malden, MA: Blackwell Science; 1997, with permission.)

proximal clavicle, and sternum. The vein is more superficially located. The vessels emerge at approximately the midpoint of the clavicle. The vein is relatively accessible at this point. Toward its lateral border, the vessel is extrathoracic and travels in a somewhat deeper location.

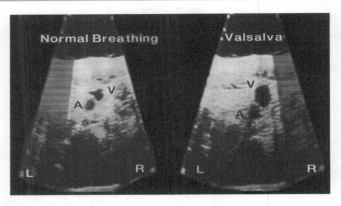

Figure 17–5.

Transverse view of ultrasound of the right internal jugular vein at baseline (*left panel*) and during a Valsalva maneuver (*right panel*). Note the carotid artery below and slightly medial to the vein (V). (From: Uretsky BF. *Cardiac Catheterization*. Malden, MA: Blackwell Science; 1997, with permission.)

There is no accessing technique that has been universally accepted. One method is to consider the clavicle as divided into equal-length sections (Fig. 17–6). The medial end of the most lateral segment will be the place where the needle passes through the skin. After local anesthesia, the needle should be directed to the sternal notch, "hugging" the clavicle. The needle tip should probably not advance further than 2 to 3 cm for fear of the needle hitting the lung with consequent pneomothorax. In theory, the lateral aspect of the subclavian has appeal because it is extrathoracic; it runs deeper and has less well defined landmarks in that location, however, making access more problematic.

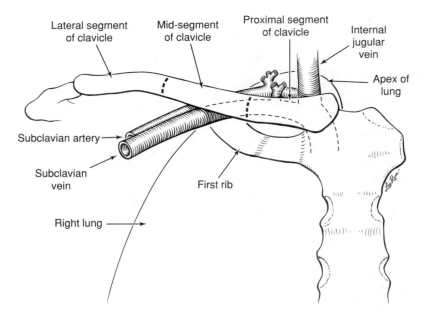

Figure 17–6.

Operational anatomy for accessing the right subclavian vein (see text for further explanation). (From: Uretsky BF. *Cardiac Catheterization*. Malden, MA: Blackwell Science; 1997, with permission.)

Concern about pneumothorax, particularly in compromised patients, and the inability to directly compress the subclavian artery and vein has made the subclavian approach less attractive for invasive (nondevice implanting) cardiologists.

REFERENCES

1. Uretsky BF. *Cardiac Catheterization*. Malden, MA: Blackwell Science; 1997.
2. Kern MJ. *The Cardiac Catheterization Handbook*. St Louis, MO: Mosby; 2003.
3. Wiley JM, White CJ, Uretsky BF. Noncoronary complications of coronary inmtervention. *Cath Cardiovasc Intervent*. 2002;57:257–265.
4. Kiemeneij F, Laarman GJ, Odekerken D, et al. A randomized comparison of percutaneous transluminal coronary angioplasty by the radial, brachial and femoral approaches: the ACCESS study. *J Am Coll Cardiol*. 1997; 29:1269–1275.
5. Sheiman, RG, Brophy, DP. Treatment of iatrogenic femoral pseudoaneurysms with percutaneous thrombin injection: experience in 54 patients. *Radiology*. 2001;219:123–112.
6. Morrison SL, Obrand DA, Steinmetz OK, et al. Treatment of femoral artery pseudoaneurysms with percutaneous thrombin injection. *Ann Vasc Surg*. 2000;14:634–639.
7. Jarosz JM, McKeown B, Reidy JF. Short-term femoral nerve complications following percutaneous transfemoral procedures. *J Vasc Interv Radiol*. 1995;6:351–353.
8. Toursarkissian B, Mejia A, Smilanich RP, et al. Changing patterns of access site complications with the use of percutaneous closure devices. *Vasc Surg*. 2001;35:203–206.
9. Nikolsky N, Mehran R, Halkin A, et al. Vascular complications associated with arteriotomy closure devices in patients undergoing percutaneous coronary procedures. *J Am Coll Cardiol*. 2004;44:1200–1209.

CHAPTER 18

Postinterventional Management

Joseph D. Babb

Although much emphasis is given technical aspects of percutaneous coronary intervention (PCI) performance in the catheterization laboratory, the short and long-term success of PCI is as strongly related to postinterventional management as it is to technical performance in the catheterization laboratory. Attention to details regarding management decisions in the time between the catheterization laboratory door and the hospital discharge door can greatly influence the ultimate outcome of the patient. The intention of this chapter is to review these issues and highlight critical areas of decision making.

The postinterventional period can be divided temporally into acute, subacute, and long term issues. It can also be viewed by topic (e.g., antithrombotic/anti-platelet management, access site management, etc.) For purposes of this discussion, the topical approach has been chosen.

Anti-Platelet and Antithrombin Management

Oral Anti-Platelet Therapy

The critical importance of proper patient preparation is the subject of more extensive discussion in other chapters in this book. The essential importance of aspirin administration was highlighted by Barnathan et al. (1). In this study, done in the balloon angioplasty era, patients were stratified by whether they had received aspirin and dipyridamole pre-procedure, in the cath lab, or never received at all. To assess the role these oral anti-platelet agents played in controlling thrombosis post-PCI, they kept the patients on the catheter table for a 30-minute postprocedure angiogram and evaluated for the presence of intracoronary thrombus. They found that when both agents were given pre-procedure, there was no evidence of post-PCI thrombus compared to an 11.8% incidence with ASA with or without dipyridamole (a commonly used anti-platelet agent of that era, since abandoned for PCI use) given postprocedure and a 14.8% incidence when no ASA was given. Thus, proper management of an agent as basic as ASA can influence the outcome of highly technical PCI procedures. While the development of more potent anti-platelet agents for oral and intravenous use may seem to supersede such data, the fact remains that remembering to give ASA even postprocedure improved outcomes compared to no ASA at all. Therefore, before the patient leaves the cath lab, we have one last chance to correct

pre-procedure oversights and check for administration of aspirin.

Certainly in the current era, thienopyridine administration has become of paramount importance, particularly in patients undergoing stenting. These agents have superseded the use of dipyridamole and oral antithrombins based upon clinical trial data. Again, as with aspirin, proper pre-procedure dosing is optimal. However, if the patient has come to the catheterization laboratory emergently/urgently without adequate time for full preparation, there is one last chance to correct such oversights by checking medication administration before the patient leaves the laboratory. In the United States today, clopidogrel is generally used preferentially over ticlopidine, not because of better efficacy but because of the improved side effect profile (2). Data from PCI-CURE demonstrated the improved outcomes associated with pretreatment with clopidogrel before PCI followed by long-term therapy (3). CREDO showed that optimal results with clopidogrel loading doses of 300 mgm orally requires at least 15 hours to be seen (4). If less time is available, 600 mgm orally is preferred. Once again, postprocedure but before the patient leaves the catheterization laboratory, once should check for administration of the proper dose of thienopyridine to optimize outcomes.

Postprocedure Heparin

Although many operators now utilize low molecular weight heparins (LMWH) for intra-procedural management, a large proportion of operators still prefer unfractionated heparin (UFH) due to its ease of administration, easy assay, and easy reversibility when necessary. In the early days of PCI, it was routine to administer intravenous UFH for up to 24 hours to all patients and to delay sheath removal until the heparin was discontinued. In that era of balloon only angioplasty, unrecognized dissections and/or uncontrolled thrombotic tendencies led to subacute closure in a significant number of patients. This was the rationale behind the practice of continued antithrombotic therapy for 24 hours. This was the era before glycoprotein IIb/IIIa inhibitors, thienopyridine drugs, and stents; however, these are therapies that provide improved sealing of dissections and control of coagulation. This practice of postprocedure heparin was abandoned because of data that demonstrated no benefit from such prolonged heparin, but a definite increase in postprocedure bleeding (5). Today, there is no reason to continue UFH postprocedure on a routine basis. Special cases, such as intra-coronary lytic infusion, resolution of demonstrable intra-coronary thrombus, and the like, may dictate its use on a case-by-case basis, however.

Intravenous Glycoprotein Receptor Blocking IIb/IIIa Agents

Intravenous glycoprotein IIb/IIIa receptor blocking agents (Gp IIb/IIIa) have been demonstrated to be of substantial benefit in many patient subsets. With the advent of more potent oral anti-platelet regimens, their usage appears to be declining somewhat but still remains widespread. Data regarding selection of agent, dosage, and patient subsets are presented elsewhere in this volume.

Relative to postprocedure management, the issues of greatest concern revolve around postprocedure bleeding and the need for urgent postprocedure surgery. Postprocedure bleeding may be related to access site problems (v.i.), but when it is related to gastrointestinal, retroperitoneal, genitourinary, or other cavitary or organ bleeding, cessation of Gp IIb/IIIa therapy is generally immediately advisable.

When the patient develops an acute need for surgery postprocedure during the same time the GpIIb/IIIa is infusing or when effects of the drug are still present, then distinct management algorithms are needed. These algorithms are based on the stoichiometry of the drugs. If the agent used is the monoclonal antibody abciximab, the stoichiometry is such that there are fewer molecules of abciximab in the system than there are IIb/IIIa receptors. Therefore, there is no reservoir of free abciximab in the plasma. In this case, giving the patient platelet transfusions will dilute the receptor occupancy of the IIb/IIIa receptors and allow return of platelet function. Such transfusions should be given prior to beginning surgery if cardiopulmonary bypass is not to be used. If, however, cardiopulmonary bypass is planned, such transfusions should be deferred until the patient is ready to come off bypass. In this way, the transfused platelets are not destroyed by the bypass itself and are immediately available and functional. If, however, the Gp IIb/IIIa agent is one of the small molecules (tirofiban or eptifibatide), the stoichiometry is different. In this case, there is a large plasma reservoir of the free Gp IIb/IIIa blocking drug, and administered platelets will simply be inactivated by this free drug. Therefore, recovery of platelet function is best achieved by patient waiting. Given the half life of these agents, recovery of platelet function can generally be expected in 3 to 5 hours postdrug discontinuance. Because both agents are dialyzable, in extreme cases dialysis can be used to regain platelet function.

Thrombocytopenia is a postprocedure management issue occasionally seen and may be related to heparin, Gp IIb/IIIa agents, or thienopyridines. Of the three currently available intravenous Gp IIb/IIIa blocking agents, abciximab is the only one which is a monoclonal antibody and has the highest reported incidence of postadministration thrombocytopenia. The incidence rate, defined as a platelet count falling below 100,000/mm^3, has been reported to be between 2.5% and 6%

in a number of clinical trials (6). In such patients, platelet transfusions were reported in 0.9% to 6% of patients. The other two IV Gp IIb/IIIa agents are small molecules relatively speaking. Eptifibatide is a cyclic heptapeptide and has been associated with platelet counts <100,000 mm^3 in 1.2% to 6.8% of patients in clinical trials. Tirofiban is a nonpeptide molecule and has the lowest reported frequency of platelet counts below 100,000 mm^3, occurring in 0.2% to 0.5% of the study patients. Because all three agents may be associated with clinically significant thrombocytopenia, platelet counts should be monitored in any patient exposed to these agents. Baseline counts should be obtained as well as counts 2 to 4 hours postexposure and 24 hours later (6).

It is important to differentiate thrombocytopenia from pseudothrombocytopenia in such patients. Pseudothrombocytopenia is rare and occurs as a result of artifactual clumping of platelets in vitro. When processed through the standard platelet counters used in clinical laboratories, the result is a falsely low reported platelet count. The correct procedure to diagnose pseudotrombocytopenia and differentiate it from true thrombocytopenia is to draw three tubes of blood, one each with citrate, heparin, and ethylenediaminetetraacetic acid (EDTA) as anti-coagulants. Additionally, a smear should be sent for analysis. If the platelet count is normal in any one of the three tubes and the smear shows clumped platelets, pseudothrombocytopenia is diagnosed. Because this is a laboratory finding and not a true low platelet count, no therapy is needed.

Therapy for true thrombocytopenia is open to some debate. There is some evidence that intravenous corticosteroids may be of some benefit, but the data supporting the use of intravenous immunoglobin are conflicting. In general, corticosteroids alone or, in severe cases, in conjunction with IV immunoglobin is the recommended therapy (6). Of course, platelet transfusions should be considered if the count drops to very low levels. Unfortunately, there is no generally agreed upon threshold to trigger platelet transfusion, in part because the process is seemingly immune mediated. As such, exposure of banked platelets to the patient's serum may inactivate them and, if the drug is stopped promptly, restoration of platelet count is expected in from 3 to 14 days with abciximab and 1 to 5 days with eptifibatide and tirofiban. Thus, the crucial elements are to check the platelet count postexposure, correctly diagnose true thrombocytopenia as described previously, and discontinue the offending agent immediately. It is worth noting that the risk of recurrent thrombocytopenia with re-exposure of abciximab has been studied and found in about 50% of the original patients and in many of them, a more severe degree of thrombocytopenia occurred (7).

If heparin is the suspected offending agent, heparin antibody tests can be ordered in most clinical laboratories today. After finding a positive test, one should immediately suspend all forms of heparin administration.

Chest Pain

In the early prestent and pre-Gp IIb/IIIa days of PCI, postprocedure chest pain was seen in up to 50% of patients (8). Acute vessel closure occurred in 2% to 7% of patients, about 50% in the laboratory and another 25% to 33% within the first 24 hours postprocedure (6). Procedure variables (dissection >15 mm, use of advanced devices (DCA 4.2%–8% in CAVEAT, 11% TEC, up to 6% ELCA), omission of anti-platelet agents (9) and patient variables (female gender, LVEF <30%, age >70) were found to relate to increased incidence of post-PCI ischemic events. Fortunately, the advent of stents, Gp IIb/IIIa, improved oral anti-platelet therapy, and greater operator experience has markedly reduced this problem. Nonetheless, proper response to the post-PCI patient with chest pain remains crucial.

Chest pain with associated ST segment elevation is an obvious indication of acute closure and a call for immediate return to the catheterization laboratory for repeat intervention. Here there is little doubt and time is of the essence. Of particular concern is the patient whose interventional artery is the circumflex. In one study, <50% of patients with balloon occlusion of the circumflex artery demonstrated intracoronary ECG changes (10). This observation is consistent with the well-known clinical axiom that circumflex artery ischemia is often electrocardiographically silent. Thus, in such a patient with circumflex intervention, a high level of suspicion must be maintained if post-PCI chest pain occurs. The cardiac ultrasound may provide useful evidence of a new lateral wall motion abnormality if the LV had previously documented normal motion. But, absent such data, it may be necessary to re-angiogram the patient whose story is compelling for ischemic chest discomfort. Other patients for whom one needs to have a high index of suspicion and a low threshold for repeat angiography include the elderly, females, those with a potentially large ischemic burden in case of closure (e.g., proximal vessel disease), those with a low EF, and patients with a recent acute MI. Waiting to assess enzymatic changes may allow profound ischemia and LV failure to develop. The preferred biomarker in such circumstances is a CK MB, particularly if a prior troponin abnormality has been documented.

Hypotension

Postprocedure hypotension can be an indicator of a serious problem. It should not be dismissed as trivial and inconsequential except by process of exclusion. The first concern is that hypotension is a manifestation of postprocedure ischemia. The patient must be carefully questioned about symptoms, typical or atypical, which might represent ischemia. An ECG may be needed to exclude heart block or ST-T changes suggestive of ischemia. Other testing such as bedside echocardiography looking for new wall motion abnormalities may also be warranted. If ischemia is not a likely component, then bleeding is the most likely serious problem. In this regard, it is vital to know if arterial access was smooth, uncomplicated, and achieved by a single front wall only puncture, or if difficulties were experienced. The latter greatly enhances the chances of post-PCI access site bleeding. Also, the use of intravenous IIb/IIIa agents or the presence of residual lytic agents will increase the likelihood of bleeding. If heparin has been administered,

one must immediately check the ACT or aPTT for heparin effect and discontinue IV administration until excessive anticoagulation is excluded. The IV IIb/IIIb agent should also be discontinued if bleeding is occurring. Depending upon the type of agent used, platelet transfusions may or may not be indicated.

Initial therapy when bleeding is suspected is always volume expansion. It is crucial, however, not to be lulled into a false sense of security by restoration of blood pressure immediately upon volume administration. More than one patient has suffered from the premature termination of assessment when BP was quickly restored and other assessments not undertaken. If bleeding is suspected, it is imperative to determine the site and extent of the bleeding. Depending upon the facilities available and the skill set of the interventional practitioner, assessment may be best done by ultrasound, CT scanning, or direct arteriography. In any case, once a suspicion of bleeding is raised, a full assessment of whether or not it is occurring and appropriate response to those findings is essential. Most retroperitoneal bleeding auto-tamponades and does not require other therapy. Nonetheless, if this is found, it is often advisable to consult the available vascular surgery personnel to follow the patient with you. If access site bleeding is shown or an arterial laceration is detected, this may require open surgical therapy or percutaneous coil embolization or other treatment, depending upon the training, skills, and resources available to the interventionalist.

Postprocedure Biomarkers

The first study to raise significant concern regarding development of cardiac biomarker positivity was the EPIC trial (11). In this study of high risk patients undergoing PCI with the use of abciximab, an increase in late mortality was seen when the CK ratio became >3x upper limit of normal and rose progressively with further increases in CK. This was also found to be true in interventions on saphenous vein grafts (SVG) with CK-MB >5x ULN having an 11.7% 1-year mortality compared to 4.8% for no increase in CK-MB (12). These observations caused considerable controversy and debate about their relevance, because no study confirmed an acute increase in mortality, only a late increase. A large retrospective review by Stone et al. in over 7,000 patients showed an inflection point for increased adverse outcomes at 1 and 2 years at a threshold of 8x ULN CK-MB (13). In this study, CPK-MB >8x UNL was the second most powerful indicator (after Q-wave MI) of in-hospital death. This seemed to confirm the importance of these post-PCI biomarker abnormalities and lent substance to the recommendations made in 1998 to obtain pre- and postprocedure CK-MBs and treat those with elevations as having a small NSTEMI with delayed discharge and increased surveillance (14). The mechanism of this delayed effect remains a matter of discussion, but current thinking is that such elevations, in the absence of documented major vessel occlusion, are probably markers for a more extensive atherosclerotic process with microembolization occurring at the time to PCI. Late death is likely the result of this more extensive atherosclerosis and not the small NSTEMI in the peri-procedural period.

Contrast Nephropathy

The important topic of contrast induced nephropathy (CIN) is covered extensively elsewhere in this volume. Relative to post-procedure management, it is important to carefully monitor the patient at risk for 48 to 72 hours postcontrast exposure to detect evidence of this serious problem. Patients at risk include those with elevated serum creatinine, low creatinine clearance, and those receiving large volumes of contrast (e.g., >3 cc/kg body weight). Patients who are volume contracted at the time of contrast exposure are also at risk. Traditional thinking has been that diabetes is not an independent risk factor for postcontrast nephropathy but is an additive one in the present of renal dysfunction. More recent multivariable analysis by Mehran and colleagues (15) suggests that diabetes may be an independent risk factor but that renal dysfunction remains by far the most critical one.

In the past, there was great concern about the presence of metformin in a patient undergoing radiographic contrast administration. Deferral of catheterization for 24 to 48 hours has been recommended to allow clearance of the drug pre-catheterization (16). More recently, it has been recommended that for elective catheterization, it is still advisable to withhold metformin therapy while for urgent/emergent one, it is appropriate to proceed with the needed study. Of critical importance, however, is withholding the drug for 2 to 4 days postprocedure to be certain there is no rise in the serum creatinine. Increases of ≥0.5 mgm/dL or 25% above baseline define CIN. In such a case, metformin must be withheld until the serum creatinine returns to baseline. Since creatinine tends to peak about 3 days postcontrast exposure, it is wise to wait at least this long before concluding that the risk period has passed.

In the current era of multivessel PCI and staged procedures for the same, it is very important to give sufficient time for contrast effects to abate before re-exposing the patient. The only good data we have relative to the risk of re-exposure comes from the ionic contrast era (17). In this study, there was a 40% increase in risk of CIN of contrast was re-administered within 72 hours. Although the use of non-ionic and isosmolar contrasts should reduce this risk, we have nothing other than anecdotal data to indicate re-exposure within 72 hours is as safe as waiting >72 hours. Therefore, it would seem prudent in the absence of demonstrable clinical urgency to defer repeat procedures, particularly in the patient at increased risk (borderline creatinine, reduced creatinine clearance, coexistent diabetes, large volume of contrast on the initial study, etc.).

A full discussion about preventive measures for CIN and management of CIN is seen in the appropriate chapter. Suffice to say that the most potent preventive measure is pre-procedure isotonic saline hydration.

Statins and Lipid Management

A substantial body of evidence is now available to indicate that statins produce pleiotropic effects beyond those of reducing serum LDL cholesterol. Inflammatory markers, such as IL6, and hs-CRP, may be reduced. These effects occur within hours of drug administration and are seen well before measurable reductions in LDL cholesterol. It is likely these pleiotropic effects account for the reported improved outcomes in patients who receive statins pre-procedure as opposed to later (17a). What is quite clear is that unless there is demonstrable, and unequivocal evidence of serious statin side-effects, they should not be discontinued post-PCI. These data come from a study by Heeschen and colleagues in which adverse combined end-points were almost quadrupled at 48 hours in patients whose statins were discontinued compared to those in whom they were continued (18). Of note is that patients in whom statins were discontinued actually had an almost twofold higher incidence of adverse events at 48 hours than those in whom statins had never been given, suggesting a form of rebound. Similar but less striking results were seen at 48 hours and 7 days.

Certainly, treatment with statins and other appropriate dyslipidemic therapy is of great benefit. Numerous studies have shown improved long term outcomes with use of these agents, even when the LDL was not markedly elevated (19,20). While some debate has occurred relative to the optimal dosing of these drugs, the key factor appears to be achieving a LDL cholesterol of about 60 mgm/dL through whatever means are needed (21).

Glycemic Control

Evidence is now available that improved glycemic control translates to reduction in macrovascular events. This has been well known to be so for microvascular disease, but only more recently has been shown for macrovascular disease such as CAD.

The DIGAMI trial compared outcomes in acute MI patients with diabetes who were randomly assigned to an aggressive management strategy with intravenous glucose-insulin acutely for 24 hours followed by insulin therapy for 3 or more months compared to continued standard therapy for that patient (22). Over 80% of patients in both groups were Type 2 diabetics. The mortality at 3.4 years of average follow-up was 44% in the control (standard therapy) group versus 33% in the insulin group (p = 0.011).

More recently, there is evidence that improved glycemic control with hemoglobin A1c levels of <7% is associated with reduced rates of target vessel revascularization (TVR) at 12 months (15% for optimal, 34% for non-optimal, p = 0.02) (22). Although this is a small study, it lends substance to other observations about the importance of optimal glycemic control relative to macrovascular atherosclerotic disease manifestations. In this case, the modification may be to minimize the documented enhanced intimal hyperplasia seen in diabetic patients, although this is hypothetical at present. What evidence now exists that improved glycemic control is related to improved long-term outcomes post-PCI (23).

Smoking Cessation

The link between cigarette smoking and atherosclerosis is well established. As part of an organized, comprehensive long-term management plan, it is therefore essential that smoking cessation be assertively addressed. Failure to do so compromises not only the long-term success of the PCI, but also the long-term health of the patient. It is not acceptable to defer this important action to another (primary) physician.

Life Style Modification

Embracing a healthy life style is also part of postinterventional management. Having had a serious cardiovascular event of sufficient magnitude to warrant PCI, the patient likely has lowered his/her defenses and is open to discussions that might otherwise be rejected. It is important that the interventional physician take advantage of this opportunity to discuss issues such as increased physical activity, reducing alcohol intake, stress modification, healthier eating habits, and the like. Once the patient has recovered and is feeling better, it is more likely that normal defense mechanisms will be back in place and such discussions may be rejected and come to naught. The interventional physician has an obligation to the patient to make the best effort to enjoin changes for a healthier life style.

Although it is difficult at first to remember to address all of the relevant life style issues postintervention, it is essential to do so in order to enhance the changes of both acute and long-term success. Some have suggested using a simple mnemonic such as ABCDE:

1. Activity, alcohol
2. Blood pressure, beta blockers
3. Cigarette cessation
4. Diet
5. Exercise

Resumption of Long-Term Antithrombotic (Coumadin) Therapy

In the early years of PCI and stenting, an antithrombotic strategy was employed to reduce postprocedure clotting and stent thrombosis. Two large trials, ISAR (23) and STARS (24) demonstrated conclusively that an anti-platelet strategy was superior to an anti-coagulant strategy. Part of the difficulty created by the anti-coagulant strategy was the pro-coagulant phase patients go through in the first few days of therapy before anti-coagulation takes place. This is due to the early reduction in Factor V and VII levels before Factor II levels are reduced.

This same concern exists when coumadin therapy is resumed early post-PCI before full endothelialization of the balloon or stent site occurs. Although no clear guideline document or consensus statement currently exists to guide practitioners, the current pattern of practice is summarized as follows. If the patient is deemed to be a relatively low risk of thromboembolic event for the next few weeks or months, coumadin therapy should be deferred until full endothelialization has occurred (i.e., 4 to 6 weeks for a bare metal stent and 3 to 6 months for a drug eluting stent). If, on the other hand, the patient is deemed to be at high risk of near term thromboembolism (e.g., mechanical mitral prosthesis in presence of AF and large

left atrium), then coumadin anti-coagulation should be done under cover of full heparin anti-coagulation until a therapeutic INR is achieved. Note that to use self-administered LMWH at home is outside of FDA guidelines for LMWH utilization. Therefore, a safer course of action is probably to administer the full dose IV UFH in a hospital setting with ACT/aPTT control until a therapeutic INR is achieved.

Post-PCI Stress Testing

The issue of routine post-PCI stress testing to assess for recurrent ischemia is the subject of considerable discussion and strong opinion. Early stress testing within the first days to weeks post-PCI was shown to give misleading information and a high rate of false positive studies many years ago (25). This was felt to be secondary to insufficiently recovered microcirculation post-PCI giving rise to residual abnormal microperfusion, even in the presence of a satisfactory PCI result. In the pre-DES era, because ischemia may be silent and restenosis was frequent, some advocated routine stress testing several weeks to a few months post-PCI. The 2002 guideline update for exercise testing favored a more selective evaluation of high-risk patients only, however, because the "prognostic benefit of controlling silent ischemia needs to be proved" (26). In the era of DES with a markedly reduced incidence of restenosis, this position seems reasonable and prudent for the overwhelming majority of patients.

Publications from the American Diabetes Association have suggested a high level of surveillance for diabetic patients because of their known propensity for silent ischemia (27). They recommend that even in the asymptomatic patient with diabetes, if there are two or more concomitant risk factors for CAD, stress testing should be performed. A more recent article suggests that a more aggressive diagnostic approach employing coronary arteriography in asymptomatic diabetics with ≤ 1 associated risk factors and a positive stress echocardiogram (28). Both of these suggestions applied to patients without pre-existing PCI, however, so one must be cautious attempting to extrapolate these recommendations to the patient population under discussion here. Indeed, there is no current justification based on available evidence to indicate that diabetic patients should be treated any differently than non-diabetic ones relative to post-PCI stress testing.

REFERENCES

1. Barnathan ES, Schwartz JS, Taylor L, et al. Aspirin and dipyridamole in the prevention of acute coronary thrombosis complicating coronary angioplasty. *Circulation.* 1987;76:125–134.
2. Bertrand ME, Rupprecht HJ, Urban P, et al. Double-blind study of the safety of clopidogrel with and without a loading dose in combination with aspirin compared with ticlopidine in combination with aspirin after coronary stenting: the clopidogrel aspirin stent international cooperative study (CLASSICS). *Circulation.* 2000;102:624–629.
3. Mehta SR, Yusuf S, Peters RJ, et al. Effects of Effects of pretreatment with clopidogrel and aspirin followed by long-term therapy in patients undergoing percutaneous coronary intervention: the PCI-CURE study. *Lancet.* 2001;358:527–533.

4. Steinhubl SR, Berger PB, Brennan DM, et al. Optimal timing for the initiation of pretreatment with 300 mg clopidogrel before percutaneous coronary intervention. *J Amer Coll Cardiol.* 2006;47:939–943.

5. Friedman HZ, Cragg DR, Glazier SM, et al. Randomized prospective evaluation of prolonged versus abbreviated intravenous heparin therapy after coronary angioplasty. *J Am Coll Cardiol.* 1994;24:1214–1219.

6. Huxtable JM, Tafreshi MJ, Rakkar. Frequency and management of thrombocytopenia with the glycoprotein IIb/IIIa receptor antagonists. *Amer J Cardio.* 2006;97:426–429.

7. Tcheng JE, Kereiakes DJ, Lincoff AM, et al. Abciximab readministration: results of the ReoPro Readministration Registry. *Circulation.* 2001;104: 870–875.

8. O'Meara JJ, Dehmer G, Care of the patient and management of complications after percutaneous coronary artery interventions. *Ann Int Med.* 1997;127:458–471.

9. Bertrand ME, Allain H, Lablanche JM, et al. and investigators for the TACT Trial: Results of a randomized trial of ticlopidine versus placebo for prevention of acute closure and restenosis after coronary angioplasty (PTCA): The TACT Study (abstract), *Circulation.* 82:III-190 (abstract 754), 1990.

10. Pande AK, Meier B, Urban P, et al. Intracoronary electrocardiogram during coronary angioplasty. *Am Heart J.* 1992;124:337–341.

11. Narins CR, Miller DP, Califf RM, et al. The relationship between periprocedural myocardial infarction and subsequent target vessel revascularization following percutaneous coronary revascularization: insights from the EPIC trial. Evaluation of IIb/IIIa platelet receptor antagonist 7E3 in Preventing Ischemic Complications. *J Am Coll Cardiol.* 1999;33:647–653.

12. Hong MK, Mehran R, Dangas G, Creatine kinase-MB enzyme elevation following successful saphenous vein graft intervention is associated with late mortality. *Circulation.* 1999;100:2400–2405.

13. Stone GW, Mehran R, Dangas G, et al. Differential impact on survival of electrocardiographic Q-wave versus enzymatic myocardial infarction after percutaneous intervention: a device-specific analysis of 7147 patients. *Circulation.* 2001;104:642–647.

14. Califf R, Abdelmedguid AE, Kuntz RE, et al. Myonecrosis after revascularization procedures. *J Am Coll Cardiol.* 1998;31:241–251.

15. Mehran R, Aymong ED, Nikolsky E, et al. A simple risk score for prediction of contrast-induced nephropathy after percutaneous coronary intervention: development and initial validation. *J Am Coll Cardiol.* 2004;44:1393–1399.

16. Heupler FA. Guidelines for performing angiography in patients taking metformin. Members of the Laboratory Performance Standards Committee of the Society for Cardiac Angiography and Interventions. *Cathet Cardiovasc Diagn.* 1998;43:121–123.

17. Taliercio CP, Vlietstra RE, Fisher LD, et al. Risks for renal dysfunction with cardiac angiography. *Ann Intern Med.* 1986;104:501–504.

17a. Pasceri V, Patti G, Nusca A, et al. Randomized trial of atorvastatin for reduction of myocardial damage during coronary intervention: results from the ARMYDA (Atorvastatin for Reduction in MYocardial Damage during Angioplasty) Study, *Circulation.* 2004;110:674–678.

18. Heeschen C, Hamm CW, Laufs U, et al. Withdrawal of statins increases event rates in patients with acute coronary syndromes. *Circulation.* 2002;105:1446–1452.

19. Heart Protection Study Collaborative Group, MRC/BHF Heart Protection Study of cholesterol-lowering with simvastatin in 20536 high risk individuals: a randomized placebo-controlled trial, *Lancet.* 2002;360: 7–22.

20. Cannon CP, Braunwald E, McCabe CH, et al. Intensive versus moderate lipid lowering with statins after acute coronary syndromes. *New Engl J Med.* 2004;350:1495–1504.

21. Malmberg K, Norhammar A, Wedel H, et al. Glycometabolic state at admission: important risk marker of mortality in conventionally treated patients with diabetes mellitus and acute myocardial infarction: long-term results from the Diabetes and Insulin-Glucose Infusion in Acute Myocardial Infarction (DIGAMI) study. *Circulation.* 1999;99:2626–2632.

22. Corpus RA, George PB, House JA, et al. Optimal glycemic control is associated with a lower rate of target vessel revascularization in treated type II diabetic patients undergoing elective percutaneous coronary intervention. *J Am Coll Cardiol.* 2004;43:8–14.

23. Schomig A, Neumann FJ, Kastrati A, et al. A randomized comparison of antiplatelet and anticoagulant therapy after the placement of coronary-artery stents. *N Engl J Med.* 1996;334:1084–1089.

24. Leon MB, Baim DS, Popma JJ, et al. A clinical trial comparing three antithrombotic-drug regimens after coronary-artery stenting. Stent Anticoagulation Restenosis Study Investigators. *N Engl J Med.* 1998;339:1665–1671.

25. Manyari DE, Knudtson M, Kloiber R, et al. Sequential thallium-201 myocardial perfusion studies after successful percutaneous transluminal coronary artery angioplasty: delayed resolution of exercise-induced scintigraphic abnormalities. *Circulation.* 1988;77:86–95.

26. Gibbons RJ, Antman EM, Alpert JS, et al. ACC/AHA 2002 guideline update for exercise testing: summary article: a report of the American College of Cardiology/American Heart Association Task Force on Practice Guidelines (Committee to Update the 1997 Exercise Testing Guidelines). *Circulation.* 2002;106:1883–1892.

27. Barrett EJ, Ginsberg HN, Pauker SG, et al. Consensus development conference on the diagnosis of coronary heart disease in people with diabetes: 10–11 February 1998, Miami, Florida. American Diabetes Association. *Diabetes Care.* 1998;21:1551–1559.

28. Scognamiglio R, Negut C, Ramondo A, et al. Detection of coronary artery disease in asymptomatic patients with type 2 diabetes mellitus. *J Am Coll Cardiol.* 2006;47:65–71.

Approaches to Complex Clinical Subsets

Lloyd W. Klein

CHAPTER 19

Approach to Coronary Artery Disease: Medical Therapy (Including Risk-Factor Modification), Coronary Artery Bypass Graft Surgery, and Percutaneous Coronary Intervention Including Complex PCI

Douglass A. Morrison, David J. Moliterno, and George W. Vetrovec

An important pathopysiologic insight that is supported by a variety of research lines of evidence is the concept that acute coronary syndromes (ACS) derive from plaque rupture and release into the local coronary lumen of substances which can elicit local thrombosis, distal embolization, and both large and small-vessel vasospasm (1–3). In this context, ACS includes acute myocardial infarction (MI), both ST-elevation myocardial infarction (STEMI) and non-STEMI, unstable angina without myocardial necrosis, and most cases of sudden cardiac death (SCD) (1–3). Conversely, stable coronary syndromes include stable angina, stable ischemic cardiomyopathy, and CAD patients, who have either silent ischemia, or no documented ischemia (4).

Historically, coronary angiography, and coronary artery bypass graft (CABG) surgery were introduced prior to the recognition of plaque rupture and its attendant mechanistic insights (5–8). Although three trials comparing medical therapy with CABG were limited to stable patients and two were conducted among patients with unstable angina, patients with MI were excluded from all early CABG trials (5,7–13). During this period, the main classification scheme for CAD focused on a number of main coronary arteries with a high-grade obstruction (>70% of left anterior descending, circumflex, and provider of pos-

terior descending, usually right coronary artery), plus the left ventricular ejection fraction (albeit that patients with LVEF <.35 were also systematically excluded from revascularization trials) (5,9–13). As important and useful as this categorization has been, review of the randomized clinical trials of therapy for CAD (Tables 19–1 through 19–6) demonstrates that a more useful categorization today is based upon the primary division of CAD patients into Stable versus Unstable syndromes (5–8).

As one reviews the evidence, particularly randomized clinical trial (RCT) evidence, two additional classification concepts that will become useful are (a) symptomatic versus asymptomatic and (b) "medically refractory" (7,8). Although exertional chest pressure or throat discomfort (i.e., classic angina) is usually considered first (and is the focus of the Canadian Symptom Classification), dyspnea, often referred to as "angina equivalent" is also a frequent symptom of reversible myocardial ischemia. Both categories of symptoms are often treated with antianginal medications (such as nitrates, beta-blockers, and/or calcium blockers) and appropriate risk-factor modification, such as statins and blood pressure control. Symptoms that remain after medical therapy has been optimized are said to be medically refractory. Relief of symptoms is among the

Table 19–1

Randomized Clinical Trials of Medical Therapy Versus CABG

Trial	n	Major Outcome	Primary Result	Patient Exclusions	Subgroups with Survival Benefit
VA Cooperative Study 1972–1974	686	5-year survival	No difference	Recent MI CHF Severe LV dysfunction	Left main, three-vessel LVEF <0.50
European Cooperative European centers 1973–1976	768	7-year survival	CABG better	LVEF <0.50 Left main	Improvement of Ischemia: Patients with LAD and ECG
CASS NIH 1975–1979	780	5-year survival	No difference	Left main	Three-vessel CAD
NHLBI NIH 1972–1976	288	30-month survival	No difference	Left main LVEF <0.30	Three-vessel CAD
VA Cooperative Study 1976–1978	468	5-year survival	No overall difference	Left main LVEF <0.30	Three-vessel CAD

best-documented benefits of cardiac revascularization, using either CABG or PCI (5,6).

With the recognition that STEMI meant complete thrombotic occlusion of a major epicardial coronary (88% in Spokane series, versus non-STEMI where ~75% of patients had some antegrade filling through the "infarct-related artery"), and the demonstration of therapeutic benefit of reperfusion strategies for patients with STEMI (but not non-STEMI, at least to the same extent), this distinction became an additional useful addition to our classification scheme (1–3).

◼ Treatment Options for CAD Patients

Medical therapy for CAD includes five categories of that randomized clinical trials have shown to be associated with improved survival: aspirin, statins, clopidogrel, beta-blockers, and angiotensin-converting enzyme inhibition (ACE-I) and/or angiotensin receptor blockers (ARB) (14). Risk-factor modification, specifically smoking cessation, blood pressure control,

lipid lowering, diabetes control, and exercise are also associated with improved outcomes among CAD patients. Accordingly, all patients with CAD should receive targeted risk factor modification and survival enhancing medical therapy. For patients who continue to have symptoms despite medical therapy (medically refractory), there are two broad categories of revascularization: CABG and PCI (which is used to imply balloon dilatation with or without stents and/or atheroablative technologies). Both CABG and PCI are associated with relief of regional myocardial ischemia and relief of angina in most patients for whom they are technically feasible (5,6).

There are no compelling data to support the hypothesis that either CABG or PCI prevent myocardial infarction in stable patients; both procedures can be complicated by new infarction in a small number of cases (5,6). Based upon the medical therapy versus CABG trials of the early 1970s, the notion has persisted that CABG of patients with three-vessel CAD, left main CAD, and two-vessel CAD, which includes proximal involvement of the left anterior descending artery, can prolong life. The

Table 19–2

Randomized Clinical Trials of Stable Coronary Artery Disease Patients Receiving Medical Therapy Versus PCI

Trial	n	Major Outcome	Result	Caveats/Comments
ACME USA 1987–1990	212	Exercise tolerance	PCI better	pre-stent
ACME USA 1987–1990	101	Exercise tolerance	No difference	pre-stent
RITA-2 UK, Ireland 1992–1996	1,018	Death or MI	PCI better PCI had less angina	9% with stents
AVERT USA, Europe 1995–1996	341	Any ischemic event	No difference	39% of PCI with stents 25% of PCI with no lipid lowering
ACIP USA, Canada, UK 1991–1993	558	2-year mortality	No difference	Revascularization by CABG or PCI Revascularization gave better event free survival Angina-guided; ischemia-guided revascularization
MASS Brazil 1988–1991	214	Event-free survival	CABG	Revascularization by CABG or PCI Patients with LAD only

Table 19–3

PTCA Versus CABG Survival Trials: Pre-Stent/Pre-Glycoprotein IIb/IIA Inhibitor/Pre-Dual Anti-Platelet Therapy

Trial	Screened	Enrolled	Age	LVEF	MI	Diabetes	Angina Grade 3/4	Survival Period	Mortality PCI	Mortality CABG
BARI 1988–1991	12,530	1829 (15%)	61	0.57	55	25%	64%	5 year	14%	11%
CABRI 1988–1993	23,047	1054 (5%)	60	0.63	42	12%	62%	1 year	4%	2%
EAST 1987–1990	5,118	392 (8%)	62	0.61	41	23%	80%	3 years	7%	6%
GABI 1986–1991	8,981	359 (4%)	59	0.56	47	13%	—	1 year	2%	5%
RITA 1 1989–1991	27,975	1011 (4%)	57	—	43	6%	59%	2.5 years	3%	4%
ERACI I 1988–1990	1,409	127 (9%)	57	0.61	50	11%	100%	1 year	5%	5%
MASS I 1988–1991		142	56	0.75	0	23%	—	3 years	1%	1%
Lausanne		134	56	—	—	12%	78%			
Toulouse		152	67		38	13%	53%			

medical therapy of the 1970s never included statins, clopidogrel, ACE-I or ARBs; and neither aspirin nor beta-blockers were routinely employed. Accordingly, it is an extrapolation to consider that a stable patient treated to blood pressure and lipid targets with contemporary medical therapy would enjoy a survival benefit, especially if such a patient were asymptomatic and/or had no documented myocardial ischemia.

What is the Randomized Clinical Trial Data to Support Revascularization of Specific CAD Patient Subsets?

The medical therapy versus CABG trials are listed in Table 19–1 (7,8); there were three trials limited to stable angina patients and two trials of unstable patients, all completed in the 1970s (9–13). In addition to the limited medical therapy available at the time, specific patient groups that were excluded from all of these trials included: patients with on-going or recent MI, hemodynamic instability, severe left ventricular dysfunction (defined as LVEF <.30) prior to CABG, and severe comorbidity. These trials constitute the Randomized Clinical Trial (RCT)

database from which the concepts of survival prolongation among patients with left main >50% stenosis, three-vessel CAD, and two-vessel CAD with involvement of the left anterior descending artery have all been inferred (5,9–13).

Further support for these hypotheses is derived from nonrandomized registries such as the state of New York registry and the Duke Database, which is cited in CATHSAP (5). The fundamental noncausal alternatives present in nearly all cohort studies, and most nonrandomly allocated studies, are relevant to the interpretation of registry data; they are selection bias, confounding, and information bias (15). Each of these systematic sources of error may be present in registry data. For example, if the prevailing attitude or culture asserts that in general, patients with three-vessel CAD derive a survival advantage from CABG, what kinds of patients with three-vessel CAD would not be referred for CABG? It is likely that operating with such an attitude physicians would favor CABG for otherwise healthy patients, deferring on CABG in the case of high-risk patients such as the elderly, severely comorbid, or demented. Under the conditions of such a selection bias, the finding of worse outcomes for patients with three-vessel disease who were managed medically could be a "self-fulfilling

Table 19–4

Non-ST-Elevation Myocardial Infarction/Unstable Angina Strategy Trials

Trial	Number Patients	Proportion Undergoing Revascularization Conservative	Proportion Undergoing Revascularization Invasive	Death or MI 6 to 12 Months Conservative	Death or MI 6 to 12 Months Invasive	Death 6 to 12 Months Conservative	Death 6 to 12 Months Invasive
TIMI-IIIb 1989–1992 USA	1,473	50%	63%	12%	11%	—	—
VANQWISH 1993–1996 US VA	920	33%	44%	14%	23%	8%	14%
FRISC-II 1996–1998 Scandinavia	2,457	9%	71%	14%	10%	4%	2%
TACTICS-TIMI 18 1997–1999 USA	2,200	36%	61%	10%	7%	4%	3%
RITA-3 1997–2001 UK	1,810	10%	44%	8%	8%	4%	5%

Table 19–5
Acute ST-Elevation MI PCI Versus Thrombolytic Trials

| First Author | Number | | Lytic | Stent | GPIIb/IIIa | Death | | Total Stroke | |
	PCI	Lytic				PCI	Lytic	PCI	Lytic
Zilstra	152	149	SK	No	No	1%	7%	0.7%	2%
Ribeiro	50	50	SK	No	No	6%	2%	0	0
Grinfeld	54	58	SK	No	No	9%	14%	—	—
Zilstra	47	53	SK	No	No	2%	2%	2%	4%
Akhras	42	45	SK	No	No	0	9%	—	—
Widimsky	101	99	SK	Yes	No	7%	14%	0	1%
deBoer	46	41	SK	Yes	No	7%	22%	2%	7%
Widimsky	429	421	SK	Yes	Yes	7%	10%	—	—
DeWood	46	44	Duteplase	No	No	7%	5%	—	—
Grines	195	200	TPA 3 hr	No	No	3%	7%	0	4%
Gibbons	47	56	Duteplase	No	No	4%	4%	0	0
Ribichini	55	55	Acc. tPA	No	No	2%	6%	0	0
Garcia	95	94	Acc. tPA	No	No	3%	11%	—	—
GUSTO IIB	565	573	Acc. tPA	No	No	6%	7%	1%	2%
LeMay	62	61	Acc. tPA	Yes	Yes	5%	3%	2%	3%
Bonnefoy	421	419	Acc. tPA	Yes	Yes	5%	4%	0	1%
Schomig	71	69	Acc. tPA	Yes	Yes	4%	7%	—	—
Vermeer	75	75	Acc. tPA	Yes	No	7%	7%	3%	3%
Andersen	790	782	Acc. tPA	Yes	NA	7%	8%	1%	2%
Kastrati	81	81	Acc. tPA	Yes	Yes	3%	6%	1%	1%
Aversano	225	226	Acc. tPA	Yes	Yes	5%	7%	1%	4%
Grines	71	66	Acc. tPA	Yes	Yes	8%	12%	0	5%
Hochman	152	150	Acc. tPA	Yes	Yes	47%	56%	3%	1%

Adapted from: Keeley EC, Boura JA, Grines CL: Primary angioplasty versus intravenous thrombolytic therapy for acute myocardial infarction: a quantitative review of 23 randomized trials. *Lancet.* 2003;361:13–20, with permission.

prophecy." Similarly, given that reading a coronary angiogram is highly subjective, it is at least possible that readers might under-read coronary narrowings in patients deemed highly unfavorable for CABG, and perhaps over-read patients who are otherwise favorable, thereby introducing a "mixing of effects" or confounding. Finally, misclassification or information bias could occur if follow-up were differential between patients sent for CABG and those who were, for one reason or another, turned down. These alternative explanations suggest the need for caution in trying to attribute cause and effect to cohort or registry studies (15).

Despite the fact that much of the early exponential growth of PCI came in low-risk patients who had been managed medically prior to PCI's inception, the medical therapy versus PCI randomized trial database is limited (Table 19–2) (6,16–20). These trials enrolled relatively small numbers of low-risk patients who were primarily single-vessel CAD with normal LVEF. Medical therapy was almost as limited, as in the previously mentioned CABG trials, and most high-risk groups were systematically excluded. The categories of complex anatomy, which are discussed later (Table 19–9 compares the roles of bare metal and drug-eluting stents in these subsets), were uniformly excluded in these trials. The conclusion of these trials is that PCI can relieve myocardial ischemia and ischemia-related symptoms with additional improvement in functional capacity. There is no case to be made for either prevention of MI or survival benefit among these groups, by PCI (6,16–20).

There were nine major RCTs comparing balloon angioplasty or PTCA with CABG in the late 1980s and early 1990s (Table 19–3) (7,21,22). As in the first two categories of randomized trials, a major issue relevant to generalizability of RCT results to patients seen in clinical practice is the consistent finding that these trials all enrolled <10% of the screened patients. The majority of angiographic exclusions for these trials were by the interventionists, based upon anatomy that was unfavorable for PTCA. In addition, as in the previous two categories of trials, most high-risk clinical and angiographic features constituted systematic reason for exclusion. Based upon the clinical inclusion criteria of mostly young, healthy subjects with normal LV function, favorable anatomy, and absent major comorbidity, the survival in both the CABG and PCI groups were good, and not significantly different. As mentioned previously, these trials continue to provide support for the generic concepts that both PCI and CABG can relieve myocardial ischemia (5,6).

There have been two major high-risk subsets from which RCT data has emerged consistently to support revascularization: STEMI and non-STEMI (otherwise known as high-risk or troponin positive unstable angina) (Tables 19–4 and 19–5) (23–27,28–40). Both STEMI and non-STEMI are subsets of acute coronary syndromes; both are likely due to plaque rupture in the vast majority of cases; both are *higher risk* than stable patients, and as such, have higher event rates with which to compare therapies. *These two datasets also provide evidence for reducing subsequent re-infarction or extension of MI with PCI* (23–40).

Table 19-6

PCI Versus CABG Trials in the Stent-Era

Trial	Screened n	Enrolled (%)	Age	LVEF	Prior MI	Diabetes	Two- to Three-Vessel	Unstable Angina	Exclusions	Follow-up	Death PCI	Death CABG
ARTS 1997–1998	1,205		61	0.60	44%	17%	98%	37%	LVEF <0.30	1 year	6%	3%
SoS 1996–1999	988		62	0.57	45%	14%	100%	24%	MI <48 hours	2 years (median)	5%	2%
MASS II 2000	611	3% to 6%	60	0.68	44%	30%	0	—	Only single-vessel LAD included	1 year	2%	1%
ERACI II 1996–1998	5,619	16%	61		29%	17%	95%	92%		25 months	1%	4%
AWESOME 1995–2000	2,431	19% of clinically eligible	67	0.45	71%	33%	82%	100%	Only "medically refractory" included	3 year	20%	21%

Table 19–7

Potential Benefits of Revascularization by Either CABG or PCI

	Trials showing benefit of CABG versus medical therapy	Trials showing benefit of PCI versus medical therapy
Relieve Stable Ischemia	VA Cooperative, European Cooperative, CASS	ACME, RITA-2, ACIP TIME
Relieve Unstable Ischemia (ACS)	VA Cooperative, NHLBI Cooperative	TIMI-IIIb, VANQWISH, FRISC-II, TACTICS TIMI-18, RITA-3, AWESOME PAMI, GUSTO IIb, Mayo, PRAGUE,
Relieve Symptoms	Nearly every trial that compared CABG with alternative therapy	Nearly every trial which compared PCI with alternative therapy
Improve Functional Capacity		ACME
Improve Ventricular Function		None
Prevent Myocardial Infarction	None	STEMI and non-STEMI trials
Prolong Life in Stable Patients	European Cooperative, metaanalysis of VA Coop, European, and CASS	None
Prolong Life in Unstable patients		FRISC-II, TACTICS TIMI-18, RITA-3, PAMI, GUSTO IIb, Mayo, PRAGUE,

Revised from: Minerva Cardioangiologica 2005, with permission.

Patients with unstable angina were enrolled in five RCT, that attempted to compare a so-called conservative strategy, which favored contemporary medical management, against an invasive strategy, which favored coronary angiography and revascularization (Table 19–4) (23–27). Most revascularization was performed by PCI, particularly in the three most recent trials (FRISC II, TACTICS-TIMI 18, and RITA 3), which also included more contemporary antiplatelet medications (25–27). There was also a greater difference between the proportions that underwent revascularization in the conservative and invasive strategies, in the more recent trials. In aggregate, these trials found hard clinical outcome differences (including survival and re-infarction) in favor of an invasive strategy for the portion of patients with high-risk features, specifically ECG abnormalities and/or biomarker positivity, both of which are additional diagnostic criteria for necrosis or MI (25–27).

STEMI trials of thrombolytic reperfusion randomized against primary angioplasty or emergency PCI were summarized and meta-analyzed in a seminal paper by Keeley and coworkers, from which Table 19–5 was modified (28). In aggregate, these trials of nearly 8,000 randomly allocated patients suggest that excellent emergency PCI can be associated with survival benefit and reduction of all-cause stroke, as well as reduction in recurrent infarctions, when compared with contemporary medical therapy (28–40). This is among the most compelling evidence that PCI can enhance survival in a high-risk cohort (28–40).

There is a general unifying theme between the subset analyses of the medical therapy versus CABG trials of the 1970s and the more contemporary STEMI and non-STEMI medical therapy versus PCI trials, namely that it is only among patients at *higher risk* that revascularization is associated with a survival benefit compared to the medical therapy of the time (9–13,25–40). More importantly the risk category that sup-

ports a survival benefit with revascularization against *contemporary* medical therapy is acute coronary syndromes, *with acute MI*. The data in Tables 19–4 and 19–5 support the application of emergency PCI (door-to-balloon time <90 minutes) for STEMI (28–40) and urgent PCI (<72 hours) for non-STEMI (23–27).

The additional use of stents, as part of PCI has been compared with CABG in five trials (Table 19–6): ERACI II and AWESOME were primarily focused on ACS patients (41–45), whereas MASS, ARTS, and SoS primarily included stable patients with lower risk profiles (46,47). Besides showing a narrowing of the difference in repeat revascularization rates between CABG and PCI with stents, compared with the PTCA trials of Table 19–3, these trials also included significantly higher proportions of screened patients, because stents have allowed a major widening of the acceptable anatomy that can be approached with PCI (7,22,41–47,48–87).

Table 19–7 summarizes the randomized trial data for both CABG and PCI (7,8). It emphasizes that both methods, by relieving myocardial ischemia, are well suited to relieve symptoms, improve functional capacity, and enhance quality-of-life. Neither CABG nor PCI have been shown to prevent MI in stable patients, although both the STEMI and non-STEMI trials suggest re-infarction and extension of MI can be reduced with PCI. *The most compelling evidence for prolonging life with PCI comes with acute MI patients, and the most compelling evidence for prolonging life with CABG comes with multivessel disease among symptomatic and highly ischemic patients* (25–40).

What are the Different Advantages and Disadvantages of CABG and PCI?

One of the consequences of designing and interpreting trials comparing CABG with PCI has been the tendency to view

Table 19–8

Advantages and Disadvantages of CABG and PCI

Percutaneous Coronary Intervention (PCI)
Advantages
- Less morbid than CABG
- More rapid reperfusion in ACS

Disadvantages
- Less control than CABG
- Restenosis
- Cannot revascularize many chronic totals (CTO)

Coronary Artery Bypass Graft (CABG) Surgery
Advantages
- Complete revascularization
- More durable results, especially with arterial conduits

Disadvantages
- Morbidity of general anesthesia
- Morbidity of intubation and mechanical ventilation
- Morbidity and mortality of heart-lung bypass

Morbidity and mortality of sternotomy, pericardiotomy, thoracotomy

them similarly. As emphasized in Table 19–8, these two revascularization methods have very different advantages and disadvantages (8). Specifically, given that patients must undergo a diagnostic coronary angiogram before either CABG or PCI, and time-to-reperfusion is so important, immediate PCI has an advantage for STEMI. In addition, because most of the total occlusions in acute MI, especially STEMI, are acute thrombotic occlusions, this is a favorable anatomic subset for PCI; even incomplete revascularization may stabilize multivessel disease patients, allowing them to undergo complete revascularization by CABG at a time (>7 days out) when the risk of CABG associated mortality is significantly less. The advantages afforded by stents do not include any improvement in the treatment of chronic total occlusions, that cannot be crossed with a wire, balloon, or a stent. CABG can be ideally suited for many of those patients. Accordingly, the presence of one or more large vessels with chronic total occlusions (CTO) tends to favor CABG.

Complex Anatomy Means Lower Likelihood of Success and Higher Likelihood of Complications: Stents have Reduced the Complexity

Diffuse Disease

Early in their experience with CABG, surgeons learned that diffuse disease frequently would not support long-term patency of a graft (5). Diffuse disease is one of the most frequent angiographic reasons for surgeons to refuse patients for CABG; it has also been one of the most difficult to unambiguously define and

quantify. Similarly, interventionists soon learned that PTCA of long lesions, or diffuse disease, had worse short and long-term outcomes than PTCA of discrete narrowings (6). In the original NHLBI PTCA anatomic risk score, lesions <10 mm in length were class A; lesions >10 but <20 mm were class B; lesions >20 mm were class C lesions (48–51). Nonetheless, a number of reports from the balloon era suggested that long lesions could be dilated and often the patients would have a long-term favorable outcome. With the advent of stenting, long stents and overlapping stents were used in selected patients with refractory ischemia. Ultrasound taught that some stents were underdeployed, and that in some cases the actual vessel size was underestimated by the angiographic lumenogram; this allowed for larger dilatation and improved clinical and angiographic outcomes (52–58). Restenosis studies demonstrated the differences between diffuse in-stent restenosis, edge dissection, and discrete in-stent re-narrowings (e.g., at underdeployed segments), all of which allowed for some improvements in technique. The advent of drug-eluting stents provided for both an overall reduction in restenosis and a specific decrease in the long, diffuse restenosis, which was the most difficult to treat. A number of registry experiences, notably C-SIRIUS, support the application of DES to long lesions (88–94). Case series have reported relief of myocardial ischemia for prolonged periods with multiple overlapping stents, dubbed "full-metal-jacket" stenting. There is no question that with BMS and DES many more patients with diffuse CAD are being considered for PCI clinical care and research than even one decade ago. Although nearly every registry report of DES suggests longer stent length, some of that greater length is attributable to a systematic difference in approach; namely with BMS, operators tried to minimize stent length so as to avoid in-stent thrombosis or restenosis, whereas with DES, operators want to cover the entire area that has been pre-dilated so as to avoid edge dissections or "candy-wrapper" restenosis (48–100).

Small Caliber Vessels

Small caliber vessel, usually defined as either <3.0 mm or <2.5 mm, has been recognized as a risk factor for acute occlusive syndromes and restenosis in the balloon angioplasty era. Bare metal stents reduced the rates of both complications in early trials and registry experiences, but trials often excluded patients with artery diameters less than one or both of these criteria. As of 2004, Moreno and colleagues found reports of 11 randomized clinical trials comparing balloon angioplasty with bare metal stenting in patients whose "normal" segment was felt to be <3.0 mm; included were trials with the acronyms ISAR-SMART, SISCA, BESMART, SISA, COAST, RAP, LASMAL, SVS, CHIVAS, and COMPASS (66). These trials used a variety of BMS in vessels down to 2.0 mm. Elective stenting appeared to be effective in improving outcomes relative to PTCA. In the RESEARCH registry experience, 2.25 mm stents were used and approximately one-third of the patients had nominal diameters <2.25 mm; despite the inclusion of these patient groups, overall restenosis rates are much lower than the historic controls with bare metal stents (48–51,58–66).

Table 19-9

Complex PCI Means Lower Likelihood of Acute and/or Long-Term Success and/or Higher Likelihood of Complication; How Bare Metal Stents, and Drug-Eluting Stents Have Changed PCI for the Better

Anatomic Feature or Clinical Feature	Bare-Metal Stent Helpful?	Drug-Eluting Stent Helpful?
2.5 mm to 3.5 mm; <20 mm long; Without calcium, thrombus, tortuosity or bifurcation	STRESS, BENESTENT	RAVEL, SIRIUS, TAXUS IV Babapulle et al., meta-analysis of DES, ISAR-DESIRE
Diffuse	BENESTENT II	RESEARCH registry C-SIRIUS
Small caliber	ISAR-SMART, SISCA, BESMART, COMPASS, CHIVAS, SVS, SISA, COAST, RAP, LASMAL	RESEARCH registry
Osteal	Cohort	Cohort
Bifurcation	Cohorts using: T stent, Y stent, V stent, kissing stents, "culotte"	Cohort s using: Crush, kissing stents
Heavy calcium	Cohort s including both rotablator and excimer laser registries	Cohort
Tortuous		
Saphenous vein	SAVED	Cohort
Chronic total	SICCO, GISSOC, TOSCA, SARECCO, SPATCO	RESEARCH registry
Thrombus containing	EPISTENT	
Clinical Feature		
STEMI	Stent-PAMI, PASTA, GRAMI, FRESCO, CADILLAC	RESEARCH registry
Non-STEMI	EPISTENT	RESEARCH registry
Shock	Cohort	
On-going Ischemia!		

Revised from: Antonucci et al., *Minerva Cardioangiologica*, 2005; Park et al., with permission.

Ostial Lesions

From the balloon-era, osteal lesions have been found to be associated with more frequent acute occlusive syndromes, and less favorable acute and long-term success rates. For this particular anatomic subset, recoil of more elastic aortic tissue was thought to be part of the problem. This perception led to the attempts to debulk tissue using laser or rotablator for lesions with attendant calcium and directional atherectomy for lesions thought to be more fibrotic; if an intravascular ultrasound (IVUS) probe could be passed, these anatomic speculations could be solidified based upon the vessel tomography. Bare-metal stents provided a means of preventing vessel recoil even without prior debulking. For example, Ahmed and coworkers from the Washington Hospital Center reported in 2000 on the application of BMS to 320 consecutive cases of Ostial vein graft lesions, concluding that prior debulking was rarely necessary (70). Subsequently, drug-eluting stents have been applied to Ostial lesions and have been accompanied by comparable low rates of acute complications with improved long-term outcomes secondary to reduced restenosis rates; an example is a study of 32 patients with aorto-ostial lesions treated with sirolimus-eluting stents and compared with BMS in 50 consecutive cases of aorto-ostial lesions reported by Iakovou and coworkers from Milan in 2004 (71).

Bifurcation Disease

Lesions involving coronary artery bifurcations have been problematic from the beginning of PTCA (6). The first considerations are whether the side-branch or so-called daughter is large enough to merit consideration (e.g., if this patient were going to CABG, would a surgeon place a graft in it?). If the side-branch is too small to graft perhaps the best approach is simply to treat the main vessel. Among the complicating issues are whether the size of the territory supplied by the daughter is large, especially in a patient who already has left ventricular systolic dysfunction; under these circumstances, occlusion of the side-branch may be poorly tolerated. The answers to these questions have relevance to choosing CABG or support device, such as an intra-aortic balloon pump for PCI (72–74).

If the daughter branch is large and important and the decision is made to try to treat with PCI, the next consideration is whether by virtue of involvement in the lesion or the probability that dilatation of the main vessel will lead to plaque shift or "snow-plowing" down the side, one should place wires in both vessels (double-wire). As a generality, when these issues are in doubt, it is probably best to err on the side of control by placing two wires. Similarly, most series from the balloon-era support the concept of simultaneously inflating a balloon in both branches, so-called kissing balloons. Clearly, as portions of both balloons are sitting in the parent (prebifurcation) segment, one should err on the side of undersizing balloons so as not to overstretch the parent segment.

The advent of stenting has led to a variety of creative attempts to avoid recoil and shift into segments after dilatation (72–74). Based upon at least one randomized trial and a number of cohort experiences, most operators favor trying to get by initially with stenting the main branch and perhaps finishing, as one started with kissing balloon inflations. Additional stent strategies have included: a stent in the daughter abutting a stent in the parent to create a T configuration; two separate stents in the two daughters simulating a V configuration; a Y configuration when the angle of the daughters is substantially <90 degrees; kissing stents to create a double-barrel Y; and a stent through the side of another to make little pants, or culotte, configuration (74).

With the advent of drug-eluting stents (DES) the rules changed slightly again; specifically one wants to cover the area that is potentially injured by dilatation with drug. Accordingly, after pretreatment with kissing balloons, one wants to avoid even small gaps created by T or V stents, which fail to cover part of the dilated areas. One creative solution was to crush the portion of the side-branch stent, which overlapped the area beyond the side-branch ostium, which is covered by the main branch stent. Another is to emphasize either double-barrel kissing stents (which can be difficult to position, especially with relatively small branches) or culotte stenting. Another is to emphasize main branch stenting, with treatment of the side branch only if "one has to," and then by passing the stent through a dilated side unit of the main branch stent. An excellent recent review, complete with very clear diagrams, by Iakovou and Columbo summarizes these options (74).

One extremely important point is that even with DES, a tight bifurcation lesion of two very important branches, the primary example of which is a tight bifurcation unprotected left main, is still a good reason to consider the CABG alternative (5,6).

Heavy Calcium

Calcified vessels are often a subset of diffuse disease and/or small caliber vessels. However, in addition to the features of those conditions, the presence of heavy calcium, especially in the innermost layers (intima and media) may render the lesion difficult to dilate. Some calcified lesions will not allow for passage of even a low profile balloon. The risks of high-pressure dilatation can include creation of a large potentially occlusive dissection flap and/or perforation. Although many flaps can be sealed with stents and some perforations can be sealed with covered stents, it is not always possible to pass a stent even after

enough balloon inflation to create a flap or perforation. Truly undilatable lesions call for some adjunctive procedure; rotablator, lasers, and cutting balloons have all been tried with some reported successes among "undilatable lesions." The primary remaining technology for these cases is rotablator, because it can usually cross lesions which cutting balloon may not, and its rate of perforation is probably less than laser.

Particularly with long lesions, current standards of rotablator therapy include: lesion modification with only one or two burrs (as opposed to attempting stand-alone rotablation) followed by stenting; reduced speed and duration of runs to avoid both overheating and embolization of large amounts of ground up material (68,69).

Chronic Total Occlusions

The first issue with total occlusions is passing the wire. In lesions known to be more than 3-months-old, and particularly if there is a long segment of occlusion and angiographic bridging collaterals, which suggests chronicity and fibrosis, wire passage may be accomplished in <50% of cases as opposed to more like 70% with short, recent occlusions and >90% of acute STEMI cases. Even when a wire is passed and clear evidence of being in the true lumen distally is obtained, there are additional cases where either a balloon or a low profile stent (after predilatation) cannot be passed. In cases where this point is achieved, a number of prospective trials support an improvement in long-term outcomes with BMS. Studies such as SICCO, GISSOC, TOSCA, SARECCO, and SPATCO have all been reported in peer-reviewed literature to support this concept. Hoye et al. reported further reduction in long-term adverse outcomes with sirolimus-eluting stents over BMS from the RESEARCH registry (75–79).

Saphenous Vein Grafts

A number of early series documented distal embolization and "no-reflow" after balloon angioplasty of old vein grafts. Most operators are particularly worried about SVGs with what appears to be thrombotic lesions, friable margins and diffuse patulous segments, but studies have suggested it is often hard to predict, based on the angiographic appearance, which procedures will be complicated by "no-reflow" (defined as a widely patent segment, with no antegrade flow, presumably secondary to distal embolization with or without distal small vessel spasm). Both the SAFER and FIRE trials suggest distal protection, with either a filter device or a balloon-occlusion system, can reduce this complication. A number of small observational studies suggest that local administration of small vessel dilators, such as adenosine, nitroprusside, verapamil or nicardipine, can often partially or completely relieve this syndrome.

The SAVED trial supports the application of BMS to SVG cases. Registry experiences including the Rotterdam RESEARCH registry with sirolimus-eluting-stents support the use of DES (80–83).

Thrombus Containing Lesions, Especially STEMI

The efficacy of glycoprotein IIb/IIIa receptor antagonists as adjuncts to PCI has focused on patients with acute syndromes, and is likely skewed in favor of patients who are clinically likely to be thrombotic as in EPIC, EPILOGUE, and CAPTURE. EPISTENT extended this effectiveness to include patients treated with BMS. At least five trials of STEMI have been concordant in showing abciximab to be specifically advantageous: RAPPORT, ADMIRAL, ACE, CADILLAC, and GUSTO IVb (84–89).

Drug-Eluting Stents: A Further Advance in Reducing Restenosis

The effectiveness of Drug-Eluting Stents (DES) in further reducing repeat revascularization procedures, among patients with favorable anatomy (2.5–3.5 mm diameter; length <20 mm, not heavily calcified or tortuous, no angiographic thrombus or acute coronary syndromes) were provided by the seminal RAVEL and SIRIUS trials for sirolimus-eluting stents and the TAXUS series of trials for the paclitaxel-eluting stents (90–93). Two changes in approach have included (longer stent lengths) in an effort to cover all territory that has been injured with balloon predilatation and prolonged (3–6 months or longer) dual anti-platelet therapy with aspirin plus a thienopyridine, usually clopidogrel. Registry experiences are rapidly accumulating to demonstrate the safety and short-term efficacy of using DES for many different anatomic and clinical subsets, especially acute coronary syndromes, where thrombus-containing lesions present a particular cause for concern regarding both metal and delayed endothelialization. As of this time, both sirolimus and paclitaxel eluting stents appear to be applicable in these contexts (93–98).

Summary of Approach to CAD Therapy in 2005

In marked contrast to the revascularization trials (both CABG and PCI) previously cited, the majority of the trials of aspirin, statins, clopidogrel beta-blocking agents and angiotensin-converting-enzyme inhibition (ACE-I) or angiotensin receptor blocking agents (ARB) for coronary artery disease (CAD) patients:

- Did not exclude the majority of clinically eligible subjects from randomization
- Were conducted double-blind
- Included contemporary control arms (for example, the control arm of most ACE-I or ARB trials included patients on aspirin and beta-blockers and in many cases, statins).

Consequently, good data from well-done randomized clinical trials (RCT) support the application of most of these categories of drugs, in RCT doses, to CAD patients, regardless of whether they are going to, or already have received either PCI or CABG (8,14). Similarly, the available secondary prevention trial data

support the ACC/AHA targets for blood pressure control, lipid management, diabetes management, smoking cessation and physical activity, regardless of whether patients are to receive, or have received PCI or CABG.

The first critical factor in the decision to go to coronary angiography and consider for cardiac revascularization, is whether the patient in question is stable or unstable, from the standpoints of ischemia and hemodynamics. For patients determined to be having an acute coronary syndrome (ACS) or unstable ischemia, an electrocardiogram (ECG) should be obtained within 10 minutes of arrival for purposes of identifying patients with ST-elevation myocardial infarction (STEMI). Patients with STEMI have an indication for emergent reperfusion, and where it is available, this means coronary angiography and PCI, with the goal door-to-balloon time of <90 minutes. Patients with ACS and non-STEMI have an indication for urgent, meaning within this hospital stay and/or <72 hours, coronary angiography and revascularization, most often by PCI. Patients who are hemodynamically unstable (cardiogenic shock or acute pulmonary edema) secondary to myocardial ischemia also have an emergent indication for coronary angiography and revascularization.

Patients with either stable ischemia or nonhigh-risk (meaning essentially no MI) unstable ischemia can be assessed further, after titration of all appropriate medical therapy and risk factor modification, for potential benefit with revascularization. Symptoms referable to ischemia, which are refractory to medical management, are among the best indicators for revascularization. The rationale of prolonging life with revascularization of stable patients is an extrapolation from the 1970s medical therapy versus CABG trials, among the subsets with three-vessel CAD, left main involvement, and/or two-vessel CAD including left anterior descending, especially with mild/moderate degrees of left ventricular dysfunction. Given the extraordinary progress in medical management since those trials were completed, this extrapolation is relatively weak for patients without large areas of reversible myocardial ischemia and/or medically refractory symptoms.

Once the decision is made that a patient is likely to benefit from revascularization, it is well to consider his/her anatomy and clinical picture from the perspective of advantages/disadvantages of CABG and PCI. PCI provides a much more rapid means of reperfusion for the unstable patient, at much lower morbidity, and perhaps, acute mortality. CABG provides much more complete revascularization (chronic total occlusions) and perhaps more durable results (when arterial conduits are compared perhaps even against DES). It is not yet know if multiple DES is a better or worse option for diffuse CAD or small vessel CAD.

Finally, as previously mentioned, the completion of either PCI or CABG should be accompanied by redoubled efforts to both optimize medical management and minimize risk factors.

REFERENCES

1. Ryan TJ, Antman EM, Brooks NH, et al. ACC/AHA guidelines for the management of patients with acute myocardial infarction: 1999 update: a

report of the American College of Cardiology/American Heart Association Task Force on Practice Guidelines (Committee on Management of Acute Myocardial Infarction). *J Am Coll Cardiol.* 1999;34:890–911.

2. Braunwald E, Antman EM, Beasley JW, et al. ACC/AHA guidelines for the management of patients with unstable angina and non-ST-segment elevation myocardial infarction: a report of the American College of Cardiology/American Heart Association Task Force on Practice Guidelines (Committee on the Management of Patients with Unstable Angina). *J Am Coll Cardiol.* 2000;36:970–1062.

3. Braunwald E, Antman EM, Beasley JW, et al. ACC/AHA guideline update for the management of patients with unstable angina and non-ST segment elevation myocardial infarction: summary article; a report of the American College of Cardiology/American Heart Association Task Force on Practice Guidelines. (Committee on the Management of Patients with Unstable Angina). *J Am Coll Cardiol.* 2002;40:1366–1374.

4. Gibbons RJ, Chatterjee K, Daley J, et al. ACC/AHA/ACP-ASIM guideline for the management of patients with chronic stable angina. *J Am Coll Cardiol.* 1999;33:2093–2197.

5. Eagle KA, Guyton RA, Davidoff R, et al. ACC/AHA guidelines for coronary artery bypass graft surgery: a report of the American College of Cardiology/American Heart Association Task Force on Practice Guidelines (Committee to revise the 1991 Guidelines for Coronary Artery Bypass Graft Surgery). *J Am Coll Cardiol.* 1999;34:1262–346.

6. Smith SC Jr, Dove JT, Jacobs AK, Kennedy JW, et al. ACC/AHA guidelines for percutaneous coronary intervention: a report of the American College of Cardiology/American Heart Association Task Force on practice guidelines (Committee to revise the 1993 Guidelines for Percutaneous Coronary Transluminal Angioplasty). *J Am Coll Cardiol.* 2001;37:2239i–lxvi.

7. Morrison DA, Sacks J. Balancing benefit against risk in the choice of therapy for coronary artery disease. Lessons from prospective, randomized, clinical trials of percutaneous coronary intervention and coronary artery bypass graft surgery. *Minerva Cardioangiologica.* 2003;51:585–597.

8. Morrison DA. Multivessel percutaneous coronary intervention (PCI): a new paradigm for a new century. *Minerva Cardioangiol.* 2005. In press.

9. The Veterans Administration Coronary Artery Bypass Surgery Cooperative Study Group, Eleven-year survival in the Veterans Administrations randomized trial of coronary bypass surgery for stable angina. *N Engl J Med.* 1984;319:332–337.

10. Varnauskas E and the European Coronary Surgery Study Group. Twelve-year follow-up of survival in the randomized European Coronary Surgery study. *N Engl J Med.* 1988;319:332–337.

11. Coronary Artery Surgery Study (CASS) Group. CASS: a randomized trial of coronary bypass surgery. *Circulation.* 1983;68:939–950.

12. Luchi RJ, Scott SM, Deupree RH and the principal investigators and their associates of the Veterans Administration Cooperative Study No. 28. Comparison of medical and surgical treatment for unstable angina pectoris. *N Engl J Med.* 1987;316:977–984.

13. Russell RO, Moraski RE, Kouchoukos N, et al. Unstable angina pectoris: National Cooperative Study Group to compare surgical and medical therapy II. In-hospital experience and initial follow-up results in patients with one, two, and three vessel disease. *Am J Cardiol.* 1978;42:839–848.

14. Morrison DA, Sacks J. What constitutes medically refractory in the new millennium? In: Morrison DA, Serruys PW, eds. *High-Risk Cardiac Revascularization and Clinical Trials.* Martin Dunitz: London; 2002:11–24.

15. Rothman KJ, Greenland S. *Modern Epidemiology.* 2nd ed. Philadelphia: Lippincott Williams & Wilkins; 1998.

16. Parisi AF, Folland ED, Hartigan P, Veterans Affairs ACME Investigators. A comparison of angioplasty with medical therapy in the treatment of single-vessel coronary artery disease. *N Engl J Med.* 1992;326:10–16.

17. RITA-2 trial Participants. Coronary angioplasty versus medical therapy for angina: the second randomized intervention treatment of angina (RITA-2) trial. *Lancet.* 1997;350:461–468.

18. Pitt B, Waters D, Brown WV, et al. for the Atorvastatin versus Revascularization Treatment Investigators. Aggressive lipid-lowering therapy compared with angioplasty in stable coronary artery disease. *N Engl J Med.* 1999;341:70–76.

19. Bourassa MG, Knatterud GL, Pepine CJ, et al. for the ACIP Investigators. Asymptomatic Cardiac Ischemia Pilot (ACIP) Study Improvement of Car-diac Ischemia at 1 year after PTCA and CABG. *Circulation.* 1995;92(suppl II):II, 1–7.

20. Pfisterer M, Buser P, Osswald S, et al. for the Trial of Invasive versus Medical Therapy in Elderly patients (TIME) investigators. Outcome of elderly patients with chronic symptomatic coronary artery disease with an invasive vs. optimized medical treatment strategy. One-year results of the randomized TIME Trial. *JAMA.* 2003;289:1117–1123.

21. Yusuf S, Zucker D, Peduzzi P, et al. Effect of coronary artery bypass graft surgery on survival: overview of 10-year results from randomised trials by the Coronary Artery Bypass Graft Surgery Trialists Collaboration. *Lancet.* 1994;344:563–570.

22. Pocock SJ, Henderson RA, Rickards AF, et al. Meta-analysis of randomized trials comparing Coronary Angioplasty with bypass Surgery. *Lancet.* 1995;346:1184–1189.

23. The TIMI IIIB Investigators. Effects of tissue plasminogen activator and a comparison of early invasive and conservative strategies in unstable angina and non-Q-wave myocardial infarction. *Circulation.* 1994;89:1545–1556.

24. Boden WE, O'Rourke RA, Crawford MH, et al. for the Veterans affairs Non-Q-Wave Infarction Strategies in Hospital (VANQWISH) Trial Investigators. Outcomes in patients with acute non-Q-wave myocardial infarction randomly assigned to an invasive strategy as compared with a conservative mangement strategy. *N Engl J Med.* 1998;338:1785–1792.

25. Fragmin and Fast Revascularization during Instability in Coronary Artery Disease Investigators. Invasive compared with non-invasive treatment in unstable coronary artery disease: FRISC II prospective randomized multicentre study. *Lancet.* 1999;3554:708–715.

26. Cannon CP, Weintraub WS, Demopoulos LA et al for the TACTICS-Thrombolysis in Myocardial Infarction 18 Investigators. Comparison of early invasive and conservative strategies in patients with unstable coronary syndromes treated with the glycoprotein IIb/IIIa inhibitor tirofiban. *N Engl J Med.* 2001;344:1879–1887.

27. Fox KAA, Poole-Wilson PA, Henderson RA et al for the Randomized Intervention Trial of Unstable Angina (RITA) Investigators. Interventional versus conservative treatment for patients with unstable angina or non-ST-elevation myocardial infarction: the British Heart Foundation RITA 3 randomized trial. *Lancet.* 2002;360:743–751.

28. Keeley EC, Boura JA, Grines CL. Primary angioplasty versus intravenous thrombolytic therapy for acute myocardial infarction: a quantitative review of 23 randomized trials. *Lancet.* 2003;361:13–20.

29. Zijlstra F, de Boer MJ, Hormtje JC, et al. A comparison of immediate angioplasty with intravenous streptokinase in acute myocardial infarction. *N Engl J Med.* 1993: 328:680–684.

30. Grines CL, Browne KF, Marco J, et al. A comparison of immediate angioplasty with thrombolytic therapy for acute myocardial infarction. *N Engl J Med.* 1993;328:673–679.

31. Gibbons RJ, Holmes DR, Reeder GS, et al. Immediate angioplasty compared with the administration of a thrombolytic agent follwed by conservative treatment for myocardial infarction. *N Engl J Med.* 1993;328:685–691.

32. Ribbichini F, Steffinino G, Dllavalle A, et al. Comparison of thrombolytic therapy and primary coronary angioplasty with liberal stenting for inferior myocardial infarction with precordial ST-segment depression: immediate and long-term results of a randomized study. *J Am Coll Cardiol.* 1998;32:1687–1694.

33. Garcia E, Elizaga J, Soriano J, et al. Primary angioplasty versus systemic thrombolysis in anterior myocardial infarction. *J Am Coll Cardiol.* 1999;33:605–611.

34. The Global Use of Strategies to Open Occluded Arteries in Acute Coronary Syndromes (GUSTO IIb) Angioplasty Substudy Investigators. A clinical trial comparing primary coronary angioplasty with tissue plasminogen activator for acute myocardial infarction. *N Engl J Med.* 1997;336:1621–1628.

35. Le May MR, Labinaz M, Davies RF, et al. Stenting versus thrombolysis in acute myocardial infarction (STAT). *J Am Coll Cardiol.* 2001;37:985–991.

36. Bonnefoy E, Lapostelle F, Leizoroviccz A, et al. Primary angioplasty versus prehospital fibrinolysis in acute myocardial infarction; a randomized study. *Lancet.* 2002;360:825–829.

37. Schomig A, Kastrati A, Dirschinger J, et al. Coronary stenting plus platelet glycoprotein IIb/IIIa blockade compared with tissue plasminogen activator in acute myocardial infarction. *N Engl J Med.* 2000;343:385–391.

38. Andersen H, Nielsen TT, Rasmussen K, et al for the DANAMI-2 investigators. A comparison of coronary angioplasty with fibrinolytic therapy in acute myocardial infarction. *N Engl J Med.* 2003;349:733–742.

39. Kastrati A, Mehilli J, Dirschinger J, et al. Myocardial salvage after coronary stenting plus abciximab versus fibrinolysis plus abciximab in patients with acute myocardial infarction: a randomized trial. *Lancet.* 2002;359:920–925.

40. Hochman JS, Sleeper LA, Webb JG, et al. Early revascularization in acute myocardial infarction complicated by cardiogenic shock. *N Engl J Med.* 1999;341:625–634.

41. Morrison DA, Sethi G, Sacks J, et al. Percutaneous coronary intervention versus coronary artery bypass graft surgery for patients with medically refractory myocardial ischenia and risk factors for adverse outcomes with bypass: a multicenter, randomized trial. *J Am Coll Cardiol.* 2001;38:143–149.

42. Morrison DA, Sethi G, Sacks J, et al. A Multi-center, randomized trial of percutaneous coronary intervention versus bypass surgery in high-risk unstable angina patients. The VA AWESOME Multicenter Registry: comparison with the randomized clinical trail. *J Am Coll Cardiol.* 2002;39:266–273.

43. Morrison DA, Sethi G, Sacks J, et al. for the Investigators of the Department of Veterans Affairs Cooperative Study #385, the Angina with Extremely Serious Operative Mortality Evaluation (AWESOME). Percutaneous coronary intervention versus repeat bypass surgery for patients with medically refractory myocardial ischemia AWESOME randomized trial and registry experience with post-CABG Patients. *J American Coll Cardiol.* 2002;40:1951–1954.

44. Sedlis, S, Morrison, DA, Lorin, J, et al. for the Investigators of the Department of Veterans Affairs Cooperative Study #385, the Angina with Extremely Serious Operative Mortality Evaluation (AWESOME). Percutaneous coronary intervention versus coronary bypass graft surgery for diabetic patients with unstable angina and risk factors for adverse outcomes with bypass; outcome of diabetic patients in the AWESOME randomized trial and registry. *J Am Coll Cardiol.* 2002;40:1555–1566.

45. Rodriguez A, Bernardi V, Navia J, et al. Argentine randomized study: Coronary angioplasty with stenting versus coronary bypass surgery in patients with multiple-vessel disease (ERACI II): 30-day and one-year follow-up results. *J Am Coll Cardiol.* 2001;37:51–58.

46. Serruys PW, Unger F, Sousa JE, et al. for the Arterial Revascualrization Therapies Study Group. Comparison of coronary-artery bypass surgery and stenting for the treatment of multivessel disease. *N Engl J Med.* 2001;344:1117–1124.

47. Coronary artery bypass surgery versus percutaneous coronary intervention with stent implantation in patients with multivessel coronary artery disease (the Stent or Surgery trial): a randomized controlled trial. *Lancet.* 2002;360:965–970.

48. Moushmoush B, Kramer B, Hsieh AM, et al. Does the AHA/ACC task force grading system predict outcome in multivessel coronary angioplasty? *Cath CV Diag.* 1992;27:97–105.

49. Tan K, Sulke N, Taub N, et al. Clinical and lesion morphologic determinants of coronary angioplasty success and complications: current experience. *J Am Coll Cardiol.* 1995;25:855–865.

50. Krone RJ, Laskey WK, Johnson C, et al. for the Registry Committee of the Society for Cardiac Angiography and Interventions. A simplified lesion classification for predicting success and complications of coronary angioplasty. *Am J Cardiol.* 2000;85:1179–1184.

51. Krone RJ, Kimmel SE, Laskey WK, et al. for the Registry Committee of the Society for Cardiac Angiography and Interventions. Evaluation of the Society for Cardiac Angiography and Interventions' lesion classification system in 14,133 patients with percutaneous coronary interventions in the current stent era. *Cath CV Intervent.* 2002;55:1–7.

52. Hall p, Nakamura S, Maiello L, et al. A randomized comparison of combined ticlopidine and aspirin therapy versus aspirin therapy alone after successful intravascular ultrasound-guided stent implantation. *Circulation.* 1996;93:215–222.

53. Schomig A, Neumann FJ, Kastrati A, et al. A randomized comparison of antiplatelet and anticoagulant therapy after the placement of coronary-artery stents. *N Engl J Med.* 1996;334:1084–1089.

54. Leon MB, Baim DS, Popma JJ, et al. A clinical trial comparing three antithrombotic-drug regimens after coronary-artery stenting. *N Engl J Med.* 1998;339:1665–1671.

55. Colombo A, Hall P, Nakamura S, et al. Intracoronary stenting without anticoagulation accomplished with ultrasound guidance. *Circulation.* 1995;91:1676–1688.

56. Nakamura S, Hall P, Gaglione A, et al. High pressure assisted coronary stent implantation accomplished without intravascular ultrasound guidance and subsequent anticoagulation. *J Am Coll Cardiol.* 1997;29:21–27.

57. Karrillon G, Morice MC, Benveniste E, et al. Intracoronary stent implantation without ultrasound guidance and with replacement of conventional anticoagulation by antiplatelet therapy. *Circulation.* 1996;94:1519–1527.

58. Wong P, Lau KW, Lim YL, et al. Catheterization curriculum: Stent placement for non-STRESS/BENESTENT lesions: a critical review. *Cath CV Intervent.* 2000;51:223–233.

59. Konig R, Eltchaninoff H, Commeau P, et al. for the BESMART (BeStent in Small Arteries) Trial Investigators. Stent placement compared with balloon angioplasty for small coronary arteries. *Circulation.* 2001;104:1604–1608.

60. Kastrati A, Schomig A, Dirschinger J, et al. for the ISAR-SMART Investigators. A randomized trial comparing stenting with balloon angioplasty in small vessels in patients with symptomatic coronary artery disease. *Circulation.* 2000;102:2593–2598.

61. Savage MP, Fischman DL, Rake R, et al. for the Stent Restenosis Study (STRESS) Investigators. Efficacy of coronary stenting versus balloon angioplasty in small coronary arteries. *J Am Coll Cardiol.* 1998;31:307–311.

62. Suwaidi JA, Tey W, Williams DO, et al. Comparison of immediate and one-year outcome after coronary angioplasty of narrowing <3 mm with those ≥3 mm (The National Heart, Lung, and blood Institute Dynamic registry). *Am J Cardiol.* 2001;87:680–686.

63. Kornowski R, Bhargava B, Fuchs S, et al. Procedural results and late clinical outcomes after percutaneous interventions using long (>25 mm) versus short (<20 mm) stents. *J Am Coll Cardiol.* 2000;35:612–618.

64. Briguori C, Nishida T, Adamian M, et al. Coronary stenting versus balloon angioplasty in small coronary artery with complex lesions. *Cath CV Intervent.* 2000;50:390–397.

65. Lemos PA, Martinez EE, Quintella E, et al. Stenting vs. balloon angioplasty with provisional stenting for the treatment of vessels with small reference diameter. *Cath CV Intervent.* 2002;55:309–314.

66. Moreno R, Fernandez C, Alfonso F, et al. Coronary stenting versus balloon angioplasty in small vessels: A meta-analysis from 11 randomized studies. *J Am Coll Cardiol.* 2004;43:1964–1972.

67. Di Sciasio G, Patti G, Nasso G, et al. Early and long-term results of stenting diffuse coronary artery disease. *Am J Cardiol.* 2000;86:1166–1170.

68. Tuzcu EM, Berkalp B, De Franco AC, et al. The dilemma of diagnosing coronary calcification: angiography versus intravascular ultrasound. *J Am Coll Cardiol.* 1996;27:832–838.

69. Warth DC, Leon MB, O'Neill W, et al. Rotational atherectomy multicenter registry: acute results and 6-month angiographic follow-up in 709 patients. *J Am Coll Cardiol.* 1994;24:641–648.

70. Ahmed JM, Hong MK, Mehran R, et al. Comparison of debulking followed by stenting versus stenting alone for saphenous vein graft aortoostial lesions: Immediate and one-year clinical outcomes. *J Am Coll Cardiol.* 2000;35:1560–1568.

71. Iakovou I, Ge L, michev, et al. Clinical and angiographic outcome after sirolimus-eluting stent implantation in aorto-ostial lesions. *J Am Coll Cardiol.* 2004;44:967–971.

72. Melikian N, DiMario C. Treatment of bifurcation Coronary Lesions: a review of current techniques and outcome. *J Interven Cardiol.* 2003;16:507–513.

73. Lefevre T, Louvard Y, Morice M-C, et al. Stenting of bifurcation lesions; classification, treatments, and results. *Cathet CV Intervent.* 2000;49:274–283.

74. Iakovou I, Ge L, Colombo A. Contemporary stent treatment of coronary bifurcations. *J Am Coll Cardiol.* 2005;46:1446–1455.

75. Rubartelli P, Niccoli L, Verna E, et al. Stent implantation versus balloon angioplasty in chronic coronary occlusions: results from the GISSOC trial. Gruppo Italiano di Studio sullo Stent nelle Occlusioni Coronariche. *J Am Coll Cardiol*. 1998;32:90–96.

76. Buller CE, Dzavik V, Carere RG, et al. Primary stenting versus balloon angioplasty in occluded coronary arteries: the Total Occlusion Study of Canada (TOSCA). *Circulation*. 1999;100:236–242.

77. Goldberg SL, Colombo A, Maiello L, et al. Intracoronary stent insertion after balloon angioplasty of chronic total occlusions. *J Am Coll Cardiol*. 1995;26:713–719.

78. Ozaki Y, Violaris AG, Hamburger J, et al. Short- and long-term clinical and quantitative angiographic results with the new, less shortening Wall-stent for vessel reconstruction in chronic total occlusion: a quantitative angiographic study. *J Am Coll Cardiol*. 1996;28:354–360.

79. Sirnes PA, Golf S, Myreng Y, et al. Stenting in Chronic Coronary Occlusion (SICCO): a randomized, controlled trial of adding stent implantation after successful angioplasty. *J Am Coll Cardiol*. 1996;28:1444–1451.

80. Baim DS, Wahr D, George B, et al. on behalf of the saphenous vein graft angioplasty free of emboli randomized (SAFER) trial investigators. Randomized trial of a distal embolic protection device during percutaneous intervention of saphenous vein aorto-coronary bypass grafts. *Circulation*. 2002;105:1285–1290.

81. Grube E, Gerckens U, Yeung AC, et al. Prevention of distal embolization during coronary angioplasty in saphenous vein grafts and native vessels using porous filter protection. *Circulation*. 2001;104:2436–2441.

82. Stone GW, Roger C, Ramee S, et al. Distal filter protection during saphenous vein graft stenting: technical and clinical correlates of efficacy. *J Am Coll Cardiol*. 2002;40:1882–1888.

83. Savage MP, Douglas JS, Fischman DL, et al. Stent placement compared with balloon angioplasty for obstructed coronary bypass grafts. *N Engl J Med*. 1997;337:740–747.

84. Antoniucci D, Santoro G, Bolognese L, et al. A clinical trial comparing primary stenting of the infarct-related artery with optimal primary angioplasty for acute myocardial infarction. Results from the Florence Randomized Elective Stenting in Acute Coronary Occlusions (FRESCO) Trial. *J Am Coll Cardiol*. 1998;31:1234–1239.

85. Stone GW, Brodie BR, Griffin 11, et al. Prospective, multicenter study of the safety and feasibility of primary stenting in acute myocardial infarction: in-hospital and 30-day results of the PAMI Stent Pilot Trial. *J Am Coll Cardiol*. 1998;31:23–30.

86. The EPISTENT Investigators. Randomized placebo-controlled and balloon-angioplasty controlled trial to assess safety of coronary stenting with use of platelet glycoprotein IIb/IIIa blockade. *Lancet*. 1998;352:87–92.

87. Lefkovits J, Ivanhoe RJ, Califf RM, et al. for the EPIC Investigators. Effects of platelet glycoprotein IIb/IIIa receptor blockade by a chimeric monoclonal antibody (Abciximab) on acute and six-month outcomes after percutaneous transluminal coronary angioplasty for acute myocardial infarction. *Am J Cardiol*. 1996;77:1045–1051.

88. Brener SJ, Barr LA, Burchenal JEB, et al. on behalf of the ReoPro and Primary PTCA Organization and Randomized Trial (RAPPORT) Investigators. Randomized, placebo-controlled trial of platelet glycoprotein IIb/IIIa blockade with primary angioplasty for acute myocardial infarction. *Circulation*. 1998;98:734–741.

89. Antoniucci D, Valenti R, Migliorini A, et al. Abciximab therapy improves survival in patients with acute myocardial infarction complicated by early cardiogenic shock undergoing coronary artery stent implantation. *Am J Cardiol*. 2002;90:353–357.

90. Morice M-C, Serruys PW, Sousa JE, et al. for the RAVEL Study Group. A randomized comparison of a sirolimus-eluting stent with a standard stent for coronary revascularization. *N Engl J Med*. 2002;346:1773–1780.

91. Moses JW, Leon MB, Popma JJ, et al. for the SIRIUS Investigators. Sirolimus-eluting stents versus standard stents in patients with stenosis in a native coronary artery. *N Engl J Med*. 2003;349:1315–1323.

92. Stone GW, Ellis SG, Cox DA, et al. for the TAXUS-IV investigators. A polymer-based, paclitaxel-eluting stent in patients with coronary artery disease. *N Engl J Med*. 2004;350:221–231.

93. Babapulle MN, Joseph L, Belisle P, et al. A hierarchical Bayesian meta-analysis of randomized clinical trials of drug-eluting stents. *Lancet*. 2004; 364:583–591.

94. Lemos PA, Serruys PW, an Domburg RT, et al. Unrestricted utilization of sirolimus-eluting stents compared with conventional bare stent implantation in the "real world." The rapamycin-eluting stent evaluated at Rotterdam Cardiology Hospital (RESEARCH) Registry. *Circulation*. 2004;109: 190–195.

95. Kastrati A, Mehilli J, von Beckerath N, et al. for the ISAR-DESIRE Study Investigators. Sirolimus-eluting stent or paclitaxel-eluting stent vs. balloon angioplasty for prevention of recurrences in patients with coronary restenosis. A randomized controlled trial. *JAMA*. 2005;293:165–171.

96. Lemos PA, Lee C-h, Degertekin M, et al. Early outcome after sirolimus-eluting stent implantation in patients with acute coronary syndromes. *J Am Coll Cardiol*. 2003;41:2093–2099.

97. Lemos PA, Saia F, Hofma SH, et al. Short and long-term clinical benefit of sirolimus-eluting stents compared to conventional bare stents for patients with acute myocardial infarction. *J Am Coll Cardiol*. 2004;43:704–708.

98. Saia F, Lemos PA, Lee C-h, et al. Sirolimus-eluting stent implantation in ST-elevation acute myocardial infarction: a clinical and angiographic study. *Circulation*. 2003;108:1927–1929.

CHAPTER 20

Special Subgroups: Women

Alexandra J. Lansky and Cody G. Pietras

Cardiovascular disease, primarily coronary heart disease, is the leading cause of death in both men and women: in 2003, 6 million women had CHD, and 234,000 died as a result (1). Despite the fact that more women than men die each year of CVD, only 33% of the more than 1.2 million percutaneous coronary interventions (PCIs) and 38% of the 1.4 million diagnostic cardiac catheterizations performed annually in the United States are in women, and women continue to be underrepresented in studies of CAD (1,2). There are important sex-related differences in the natural history, pathophysiology, and response to revascularization in patients with CAD, with implications for the appropriate interventional management of women.

Referral and Physician Awareness

Awareness of the severity of cardiovascular disease in women has been increasing among both physicians and patients, but gender disparities remain. Fewer than one in five physicians are aware that more women than men die each year of cardiovascular disease, and women with CVD are more likely to be assigned a lower-risk category than men with a similar calculated risk (3). In a study of physician awareness and adherence to cardiovascular disease prevention guidelines, while 80% of cardiologists and 60% of PCPs were aware of the AHA Evidence-Based Guidelines for Women, only about 40% of those who were aware incorporated the guidelines into their practice (3).

Women experience greater delays to intervention and are less often referred for diagnostic cardiac catheterization compared with men (4,5). Once referred for cardiac catheterization, it appears that interventional therapy is utilized similarly in men and women; although some studies report lower unadjusted rates of coronary revascularization in women, this sex difference disappears when data is adjusted for clinical variables (6–8).

Suggested reasons for the lower referral rates and procedural delays include women's older age and increased comorbidities at presentation predisposing toward conservative management, more frequent "atypical" chest pain presentation (9,10), and the lower predictive value of noninvasive testing in women due to a lower prevalence of obstructive CAD; however, current evidence does not exclude the possibility of a sex bias.

Pathophysiology and Risk Factors

Although contemporary interventional therapies have improved outcomes in both sexes following coronary intervention, women continue to have higher rates of short- and long-term mortality, nonfatal myocardial infarction, and emergency coronary bypass surgery. Much of this disparity is due to the worse risk profiles of women undergoing PCI: the delayed onset of cardiovascular disease in women compared with men causes women to present for treatment at an older age and with more comorbidities (11–22).

Adjustments for age and comorbid clinical conditions often (23–25), but not always (26), eliminate outcome differences following revascularization. Additional confounding risk factors are thought to include smaller vessel caliber and a greater susceptibility to vascular complications in women, more diffuse atherosclerosis and microvascular dysfunction, and humoral factors.

Gender and the Age Paradox

The risk of death after PCI has been reported to increase by 65% for each 10-year increase in age (22). Because women tend to present with CAD 10 to 15 years later than men, older age is clearly a large contributor to womens' higher rates of mortality and morbidity after PCI. However, while the prevalence of CAD is low among young premenopausal women compared with age-matched men, young women who do develop CAD have significantly worse outcomes than their male counterparts. Approximately 6% of PCIs are performed in patients 44 years of age or younger (27).

In the National Registry of Myocardial Infarction-2 (NRMI-2) (N = 384,878, 40% female), among patients aged 30 to 89 years who had sustained a myocardial infarction, the excess mortality in the female population was more pronounced in younger than older patients and was no longer significant after the age of 74 (p <0.001 for the interaction between sex and age) (28). The odds of death were an estimated 11.1% greater for women than men for every 5-year *decrease* in age (95% CI, 10.1 to 12.1), even after adjustment for differences in medical history, clinical severity of the infarction, and early management (OR = 1.07; 95% CI, 1.06–1.08) (28). Younger women were more likely than younger men to present with diabetes or a history of CHF or stroke, differences that were not apparent in older patients.

Similar patterns have been documented after coronary artery bypass graft (CABG) surgery (29) and PCI (30). It remains unclear why young women are at increased risk of death after MI and death or MI after PCI compared with age-matched men. One possibility is that premenopausal estrogen deficiency, much more prevalent in young women with CAD than those without (in one study, 69% versus 29%, p = 0.01), could predispose this population to more adverse outcomes (31). The higher frequency of plaque erosion in young women (rather than the plaque rupture seen in men and older women) may also contribute to their higher mortality (32,33).

Gender and Diabetes

Diabetes is a particularly strong risk factor for CAD incidence and mortality in women (34–36). Some studies indicate that much of the gender difference in diabetes-related risk is mediated by traditional modifiable risk factors, and adjusting for these reduces the gender disparity (37,38). Compared with men, women with diabetes are more likely to have elevation in systolic and diastolic blood pressure, worse glycemic control, greater elevations in circulating lipids, and central obesity, all of which contribute to increased CAD risk (39–43).

Among patients undergoing PCI, diabetes is more common in women than men and is particularly prevalent among younger women. In an older cohort of patients undergoing PCI in the New Approaches to Coronary Intervention (NACI) registry (N = 2855, 34% female; average age 65.6 years for women, 61.5 years for men), 28% of women and 19.6% of men had diabetes (21), compared with the 37.5% prevalence reported in an observational study of women under the age of 40 undergoing PCI (30). In addition to being more prevalent, diabetes also confers a greater risk of CAD mortality in younger women: in one report (44), diabetic women younger than 55 years with no other risk factors for CAD had a 16-fold higher risk of dying from CAD than women without diabetes, compared with the three- to fivefold risk increase seen in women overall (36,37).

Intravascular ultrasound (IVUS) studies have shown that, compared with non diabetics, the insulin-treated diabetic patient develops more extensive lumen compromise due to reductions in arterial dimensions (as measured by the external elastic membrane), rather than increases in plaque burden. This "impaired remodeling" results in a higher propensity for luminal obstruction for any given amount of plaque deposition (45). The combination of impaired arterial remodeling and smaller coronary arterial caliber (46,47) may explain the particular risk attributable to diabetes in women. Premenopausal women with diabetes have also been shown to have reduced coronary vasodilator function and impaired vascular resistance, similar to that observed in healthy postmenopausal women (48).

Diabetes can be described as a "risk equalizer" in that diabetic women seem to lose most of their inherent protection against CVD (49), particularly in the young female patient who may be dismissed as low-risk on the basis of age alone. Among 121,046 women in the Nurses' Health Study aged 30 to 55 at baseline and followed for 20 years, risk of death from CAD in women with diabetes was similar to that in women with known CAD (RR = 2.75–11.9, increasing with diabetes duration, p 0.001 for trend). Women with long-duration diabetes (>15 years) and CAD had a 30-fold increase (95% CI, 20.7–43.5) in CAD mortality compared to those with neither condition (50).

The relatively high prevalence and CAD risk associated with diabetes in young women emphasizes the need for aggressive screening and early risk factor detection and modification (49).

Increased overall use of evidence-based therapies appears to particularly benefit diabetic women in the setting of MI. Data from the National Registry of Myocardial Infarction (NRMI) 2, 3, and 4 of STEMI and NSTEMI patients (N = 1,428,956, 40% women) found that between 1994 and 2002, hospital mortality decreased more for women with diabetes than for any other group, from an OR of 1.28 to 1.10 (compared to women without diabetes, p <0.0001) (51).

Gender and Vessel Size

Women generally have smaller caliber vessels than men. It is unclear whether sex has an independent effect on vessel caliber or if the difference is solely attributable to women's smaller body size; thus far, studies have had conflicting results (46,47,52–54). In a series of 257 normal left main coronary arteries assessed by intravascular ultrasound (IVUS), mean arterial areas were smaller in women than in men (17.2 versus 20.6 mm^2, p <0.001), as were mean luminal areas (14.0 versus 16.7 mm^2, p <0.001). Both body surface area (BSA) (p < 0.001) and gender (p <0.003) were independent predictors of coronary artery size, although BSA had a greater influence than gender (55).

Regardless of its determining factors, smaller vessel caliber in women may account for some of the outcome differences following revascularization. Following PCI, women experience a higher incidence of acute complications associated with interventions in small vessels, including more frequent intimal dissections and perforations (56–59). The majority of angiographic studies find that differences in mortality after PCI are abolished after correcting for BSA or vessel caliber (23,24,56,60,61). In the Coronary Artery Surgery Study (CASS), operative mortality for both men and women decreased as vessel diameter increased and vessel diameter was found to be a predictor of operative mortality by univariate analysis, although gender was not an independent predictor of mortality after adjustment for BSA (60).

Gender and Lesion Morphology

Cardiovascular morbidity and mortality vary with the extent of CAD (62,63) and overall plaque burden (64,65). No prospective angiographic or pathologic studies have been performed to examine potential gender-related differences in lesion morphology. A published series of preinterventional IVUS in 718 patients (24% female) with chronic stable angina found that lesion characteristics were similar in men and women, including calcification frequency (71% versus 72%) and magnitude (total arc of calcium, arc of superficial calcium, arc of reference segment calcium, and length of lesion calcium), percentage of eccentric lesions (44% in women versus 48% in men, p = 0.4771), and target lesion and reference segment plaque burden (46). When normalized for the proximal reference, the lesion external elastic membrane cross-sectional area was similar in women and in men. Coupled with the lack of a sex-specific effect on plaque burden, this finding indicates that adaptive remodeling response to plaque accumulation is sex-independent, a conclusion supported by necropsy studies (66).

Beyond Morphology—The WISE Findings

Although no differences in the morphology of coronary lesions requiring intervention between men and women have been identified, there is evidence that women develop a different form of vascular disease than men, characterized by more diffuse atherosclerosis and more microvascular dysfunction (67). Results from the National Institutes of Health-National Heart, Lung, and Blood Institute-sponsored Women's Ischemic Syndrome Evaluation (WISE) study (N = 936 women referred for diagnostic coronary angiography) have added to the growing body of evidence indicating that the multifactorial nature of ischemic heart disease in women, mediated by interactions between sex hormones and traditional and conditional risk factors, may require an adjustment of current strategies for the diagnosis and treatment of CAD in women to emphasize functional rather than structural abnormalities (68).

Women who present with angina have less severe and less frequent obstructive CAD than men (69), yet the majority demonstrates test abnormalities suggestive of ischemia and continue to suffer from persistent and worsening symptoms and adverse cardiovascular events. More than half the women in WISE had endothelial dysfunction, an independent predictor of adverse outcomes regardless of CAD severity (70).

Because women's vessels are exposed to varying hormonal influences over a long period of time, they may be predisposed to more severe alterations in both endothelial and smooth muscle vascular reactivity compared with men. Risk conditions unique to women, including preeclampsia and delivering a low-birth weight baby, have been linked with endothelial dysfunction (71,72). Microvascular structural damage such as retinal microvascular abnormalities have also been linked with endothelial dysfunction, and predict ischemic heart disease outcomes in women but not men (73). Women have higher frequencies of vasculitis than men (e.g., lupus, temporal arteritis, coronary artery spasm), indicative of alterations in vascular smooth muscle function (67). In addition, many of the WISE women demonstrated coronary flow reserve attenuation with intracoronary adenosine, suggesting microvascular smooth muscle impairment (74). The WISE study showed that coronary artery flow velocity response to adenosine was associated with reduced functional capacity as measured by the Duke Activity Status Index (DASI) (75), which in turn carries an increased risk of death or MI for women (76).

Women's higher levels of inflammation together with the clustering of risk factors that occurs with menopause may cause further disruptions in endothelial and microvascular function, resulting in more frequent myocardial flow heterogeneity (77,78). In the WISE study, global measures of inflammation were shown to predict mortality in women with suspected myocardial ischemia, despite being only weakly associated with the extent of angiographic CAD (79). Levels of inflammatory markers including C-reactive protein and fibrinogen correlate with metabolic syndrome and high BMI (80,81), risk conditions with a high prevalence in women with suspected CAD: among 780 such women from the WISE study, 34% were overweight, 42% were obese, and 58% had the metabolic syndrome (81). These conditions increase oxidative stress to the endothelium in both large and small vessels (82,83). The WISE study also found that anemia was an independent predictor of adverse events (84), and anemia is associated with chronic inflammatory states, particularly in older men and women.

Some of the sex-related differences in atherosclerosis may be attributed to differences in atherogenic factors following estrogen withdrawal. The protective effects of endogenous estrogen on the cardiovascular system have been well-documented: estrogen alters serum lipid concentrations, coagulation, and fibrolytic systems; improves endothelial function; has antioxidant properties; and down-regulates expression of adhesion molecules (85). Postmenopausal women taking estrogen (without progestin) have lower fibrinogen and factor VII levels (86); increases of both are known to be associated with atherosclerosis (87). Women of any age with a family history of early CAD demonstrate hyperreactive platelet aggregation (88). Estrogen also contributes to plaque stabilization, evidenced by the higher rate of plaque erosion in premenopausal women compared with the more frequent plaque rupture in men and postmenopausal women (32). The implications of estrogen withdrawal are not limited to postmenopausal women: in premenopausal women with suspected ischemia in the WISE study, hypoestrogenemia resulting from stress-induced central disruption in ovulatory cycling was associated with a 7.4-fold increased risk of obstructive CAD (31).

In summary, the recent findings of the WISE study and others help illuminate sex differences in the pathophysiology of CAD and may begin to explain why women tolerate ACS poorly compared with men and have worse outcomes after coronary intervention despite a lesser severity of obstructive CAD.

Diagnostic and Prognostic Testing in Women

Underrecognition and underdiagnosis of CAD in women continue to contribute to their worse outcomes. Up to 40% of initial cardiac events in women are fatal (89), and women are consistently shown to experience greater delays to diagnosis and treatment and are less often referred for appropriate diagnostic testing (90–93). As the gender gap in the outcomes of current treatments continues to narrow or disappear, timely and appropriate testing and risk stratification is critical to improving the outcomes of women with CAD.

Compared with men, women have significant differences in the natural history and pathophysiology of CAD, yet clinical decision-making is hampered by the continued underrepresentation of women in studies of noninvasive testing—much of the evidence supporting current recommendations is extrapolated from studies involving middle-aged men. A high prevalence of single-vessel disease and nonobstructive CAD results in decreased diagnostic accuracy and a higher false-positive rate for noninvasive testing in women compared with men (94). Approximately half of all women referred for evaluation of suspected myocardial ischemia do not have obstructive coronary artery disease, yet these women are at risk for future CAD events and persistent symptoms.

Recommendations for Noninvasive Testing in Women with Suspected CAD

Asymptomatic Women

The risk of CHD is generally low in asymptomatic premenopausal women, with the exception of women who have diabetes or peripheral arterial disease (both are CAD risk equivalents). In low-risk asymptomatic women (10-year Framingham risk 5% or less), evidence does not support the use of diagnostic imaging. In asymptomatic women at intermediate-to-high risk (10-year Framingham risk 6%–20% or higher), screening for subclinical disease should be considered (ankle brachial index, carotid intima-media thickness, retinogram, or computed tomography calcium scan). If the results of subclinical tests suggest high risk of disease, ischemia testing should be considered (stress testing with ECG, echocardiography, single photon emission computed tomography, or cardiac magnetic resonance). Asymptomatic women with a calcium score ≥400 should be considered high risk, since this indicates an annual risk of death or MI of about 2% (95). In patients with low risk on ischemia testing, "watchful waiting" that involves symptomatic treatment and risk factor modification is appropriate. Women with high-risk results from ischemia testing should undergo cardiac catheterization, anti-ischemic therapy, and risk factor modification.

Symptomatic Women

Imaging is recommended for symptomatic women at intermediate-to-high risk (10-year Framingham risk 6%–20% or higher). Evidence does not support the use of diagnostic imaging in low-risk symptomatic women (10-year Framingham risk 5% or less or ≤1 risk factor and nonanginal/atypical symptoms).

Intermediate pretest likelihood of CAD may be crudely defined as atypical or typical angina at 50 years of age or younger or typical angina in women older than 50 (96). The exercise ECG test is generally the first-line noninvasive stress test for the assessment of symptomatic women because of its strong negative predictive value, despite having a lower diagnostic accuracy in women than in men (96). Women with a positive or nondiagnostic test should undergo further noninvasive testing rather than immediate cardiac catheterization. In patients with a positive exercise ECG and a normal noninvasive imaging test, the latter has a superior prognostic value and cardiac catheterization can be avoided (97,98).

Cardiac imaging is recommended as a follow-up to exercise treadmill testing in women with an indeterminate or intermediate-risk test, as well as those with an intermediate Duke treadmill score. Women with diabetes, an abnormal resting 12-lead ECG, or questionable exercise capacity should be evaluated with stress cardiac imaging, either exercise or pharmacological. Stress echocardiography or gated SPECT myocardial perfusion imaging provide accurate diagnostic and prognostic information in women. In patients with normal or mildly abnormal stress test results and preserved LV function, anti-ischemic therapy in addition to risk factor modification should be considered (99). Patients with moderately or severely abnormal stress test results or reduced ejection fraction should be referred for diagnostic cardiac catheterization.

Chronic Stable Coronary Artery Disease and Elective Interventions

Results after Conventional Coronary Angioplasty

Early studies of balloon angioplasty identified female gender as an independent predictor of early mortality and complications. In the 1985 NHLBI PTCA registry (N = 2136, 36% female), women had a 10-fold higher rate of in-hospital death compared with men (2.6% versus 0.3%, p = 0.02) (100). Women's worse short-term outcomes following conventional angioplasty continued into the early 1990s, despite improvements in angiographic success in both sexes (23,25,26). The early sex disparity in outcomes may partially account for the subsequent referral bias and less aggressive treatment of women with CAD (101–105).

New devices, including newer-generation balloons, have improved angiographic and clinical success rates in women. Procedural success ranged from 60% to 70% with the original balloon devices available before 1985 (100), increased to 80% to 90% after 1985 (24,25,106,107), and are above 90% with contemporary balloon devices. Although women continue to have higher mortality than men, new-device angioplasty has reduced in-hospital mortality rates for women to <1.5% (108,109), compared with as high as 4.1% previously reported with balloon angioplasty alone (107).

The changing practice of interventional cardiology has resulted in improved outcomes for both men and women, and a reduction or elimination of the gender difference in outcomes: a database of 33,666 PCIs conducted between 1994 and 1999 showed that despite a worsening case-mix, mortality rates decreased for both sexes over time, with no significant gender difference (109).

Gender Differences in Long-Term Outcome after Conventional and New-Device

Angioplasty

Compared with men, women are consistently reported to have similar or lower rates of target vessel revascularization (TVR) after angioplasty (25,56,110,111), despite having smaller vessels, smaller postprocedural lumen diameters, and more prevalent diabetes mellitus, which are factors typically associated with higher restenosis rates (112–116). Gender differences in restenosis rates have not been well-defined, and lower repeat revascularization rates in women may represent either a true reduction in need or a referral bias resulting in women being less likely to undergo appropriate repeat revascularization.

Late clinical outcomes of women with new-device angioplasty are favorable compared to those in historical balloon angioplasty series (23–25). In a registry of new-device angioplasty that included 7,372 patients, women had lower target lesion revascularization rates at 1 year (15.0% versus 18.1%, p = 0.001) and fewer major adverse clinical events (MACE) than men, though 1-year mortality remained higher for women than men (4.39% versus 3.26%, p = 0.018). Female gender was an independent predictor of in-hospital but not late mortality (108). Despite the slight increase in in-hospital cardiac mortality in women, "new-device" angioplasty is a safe and effective treatment strategy for women with symptomatic CAD.

Results after Elective Stenting in Women

Stent implantation, increasingly drug-eluting stents, has recently become the treatment modality of choice for elective PCI. Stents are used in an estimated 84% of coronary interventions with no evidence of a sex bias (117,118). The introduction of stents for the lower range of coronary vessel sizes including 2.0 mm, 2.5 mm, and 2.75 mm diameters have eliminated women's small vessel caliber as an impediment to stent use, and lesions inappropriate for stenting are seldom encountered.

Compared with conventional balloon angioplasty, stents improve acute procedural success and in-hospital outcomes and lower long-term restenosis rates (119,120). Initial studies comparing balloon-only angioplasty with stenting in women were disappointing; women in the EPISTENT trial (N = 2399, 25% female) treated with stent and abciximab had higher 30-day event rates than those treated with balloon angioplasty and abciximab (121). However, a gender-based pooled analysis of seven prospective Investigational Device Exemption (IDE) stent trials of 7,171 patients (30% female) undergoing elective stenting with a tubular slotted stent design (3.0–4.0 mm diameter) found that, despite being older and having smaller vessels and a higher prevalence of hypertension and diabetes, women had a similar unadjusted in-hospital mortality to men (0.28% versus 0.14%, p = NS) (122). There was no gender difference in other acute complications such as periprocedural MI or need for CABG surgery. Mortality at 1 year was higher in women than in men (2.25% versus 1.44%, p = 0.015), a difference that was no longer significant after adjusting for dif-

ferences in comorbid conditions (OR = 1.2, p = 0.383), and TVR was similar between women and men (12% versus 11%).

Post-approval registries comparing outcomes after stenting in a broader range of lesion and patient subsets indicate that while overall outcomes have improved in patients of both sexes who receive stents, female gender remains an independent predictor of mortality. In a study from the Nationwide Inpatient Sample, 59% of 118,548 angioplasties performed in 1997 involved stenting. Among patients who underwent elective stenting, women had higher in-hospital mortality (1.1% versus. 0.5%, p <0.0001), and a greater need for CABG (1.5% versus 1.0%, p <0.0001) compared with men, differences that were maintained even after multivariable adjustment for risk factors (123). Another registry of elective coronary stenting (N = 4,264, 23% female) reported an increased risk of the 30-day combined endpoint of death and MI in women compared with men (3.1% versus 1.8%, p = 0.02; OR = 2.02, 95% CI, 1.27–3.19) (124). One-year outcome was similar between genders. Despite the persistent gender gap in outcomes following revascularization, the benefits of elective stenting compared with balloon-only angioplasty on restenosis and the need for repeat revascularization appear to be generalizable to women.

Two recent trials evaluating drug-coated stents, the SIRIUS trial with the Cordis/Johnson & Johnson sirolimus-eluting Cypher® stent (125) and the TAXUS trial of Boston Scientific's paclitaxel-eluting Taxus® stent (126), have enabled generalization of the restenosis-reducing effects of these devices to women. In a gender substudy of the TAXUS-IV trial (N = 1,314, 28% women), women had higher absolute revascularization rates compared to men (driven by increased risk factors for restenosis in women, including diabetes and smaller reference vessel diameter and BSA); however, female gender was not an independent predictor of target lesion (OR = 1.72; 95% CI, 0.68–4.37) or target vessel (OR = 0.89; 95% CI, 0.41–1.97) revascularization (126). Taxus stent implantation significantly reduced 9-month angiographic restensosis (8.6% versus 29.2%, p = 0.001) and 1-year target lesion revascularization (7.6% versus 14.9%, p = 0.02) in women compared to the Express bare metal stent. Randomization to the Taxus stent was the only independent predictor of a lower restenosis rate in women (OR = 0.28; 95% CI, 0.11–0.74, p = 0.01) (126).

Treatment of Acute Coronary Syndromes in Women

The optimal treatment strategy for women with acute coronary syndromes (ACS, defined as unstable angina or non-ST elevation MI) remains controversial. The benefits of an early invasive strategy (consisting of GP IIa/IIIb inhibitor use, catheterization within 48 hours, and revascularization for patients at increased risk of death and MI) compared with a conservative strategy have been consistently demonstrated in men (127–129), but results in women have been conflicting.

In the TACTICS-TIMI 18 study (N = 2220 patients, 34% female), women benefited from an aggressive early invasive strategy with GP IIb/IIIa inhibitor use, early (within 48 hours) catheterization, and coronary intervention with stenting when necessary compared with a conservative medical strategy (129). Women treated with the early invasive strategy had a lower rate of death, MI, or rehospitalization for ACS (OR = 0.72, 95% CI, 0.47 –1.11) than men, with a significant benefit seen among women with elevated troponin T levels (OR = 0.47, 95% CI, 0.26–0.83). The benefit of early (within 24 hours) invasive interventional treatment was corroborated in a registry of 1,450 patients presenting with ACS: women had a lower rate of death and MI at 20 months compared with men (OR = 0.65, 95% CI, 0.42–0.99) (130).

In contrast, the Fragmin and fast Revascularization during InStability in Coronary artery disease (FRISC) II trial (N = 2,457, 30% female) found that an early invasive strategy (catheterization within 7 days) benefited men but not women compared to a conservative strategy (127). Men treated invasively experienced a lower rate of death and MI at 1 year (9.6% versus 15.8%, p <0.001), whereas there was no difference in women's outcomes between the invasive and conservative groups (12.4% versus 10.5%, p = NS), and women did worse with invasive treatment compared to men (p = 0.008). A subset analysis of the RITA-3 trial reported similar results (131).

The reasons for the incongruent findings of the TACTICS-TIMI 18, FRISC-II, and RITA-3 trials are unclear. Delayed timing of intervention is one potential explanation: in FRISC-II, patients could be enrolled if they had symptoms within 48 hours, whereas TACTICS-TIMI 18 required enrollment within 24 hours of symptom onset. FRISC-II and RITA-3 allowed a longer course of medical therapy prior to intervention (several days), whereas 60% of patients in TACTICS underwent intervention within 48 hours. Women in the conservative strategy group in FRISC-II and RITA-3 appeared to be at a lower risk of death and MI, possibly "unmasking" increased procedural risk in women. Other possible factors include increased use of glycoprotein (GP) IIb/IIIa inhibitors in the TACTICS TIMI-18 trial and more frequent use of CABG, with an accompanying increase in female mortality (9.9% versus 1.2% for men, p <0.001), in the FRISC-II trial.

Despite continued questions as to whether the benefits of an early invasive strategy apply equally well to men and women in the setting of ACS, it appears that high-risk women with UA or NSTEMI benefit from early intervention within 48 hours accompanied by adjunctive GP IIb/IIIa use (132).

Treatment of Acute Myocardial Infarction in Women

Women have higher short-term mortality rates after AMI compared with men, regardless of reperfusion modality (123,133–135). Much of this increased risk is attributable to the unfavorable risk profiles of women with AMI compared with men, but treatment delays also contribute to women's worse outcomes. Among 1,044 patients (30% women) who underwent primary angioplasty for AMI in the state of New York in 1995 (136), women had more hypertension (59% versus 44%, p <0.05), diabetes (19% versus 14%, p <0.05), peripheral vascular dis-

ease (9.5% versus 5.5%, p <0.05), cardiogenic shock, and hemodynamic instability compared to men (25% versus 17%, p <0.05). Men were more likely to be treated sooner (within 6 hours of symptom onset) than women (74% versus 63%, p < 0.05). Women had a significantly higher in-hospital mortality (7.9% versus 2.3%, p <0.05), which persisted even after adjustment for all the above differences (OR = 2.3, 95% CI, 1.2–4.6).

Recommended treatments for women with acute ST-segment elevation MI include primary PCI and thrombolytic therapy. The superiority of primary PCI has been clearly demonstrated, with a similar relative risk reduction in men and women translating to increased relative benefit for women due to their unfavorable risk profiles (137). Thrombolytic therapy should therefore be reserved for patients presenting within 3 hours of symptom onset and without access to primary PCI, or in whom access to primary PCI will be excessively delayed.

Outcome of Thrombolysis for Acute Myocardial Infarction in Women

A metaanalysis of 9 controlled, randomized thrombolytic versus placebo trials for AMI (N = 58 600) demonstrated a 12% reduction in 35-day mortality among women treated with thrombolytics (16.0% versus 14.1%, p = 0.003) (138). In the National Registry of Myocardial Infarction-2 (NRMI-2) study (N = 67 597, 36% female), tissue plasminogen activator (tPA) reduced the risk of in-hospital death or nonfatal stroke (13.3% versus 20.9%, p = 0.001). However, the absolute event rate in women remained more than twice that of men (13.3% versus 5.8%, p = 0.001), and female sex was an independent predictor of intracranial hemorrhage (OR = 1.59; 95% CI, 1.31–1.92) (139). In the GISSI 2 and GUSTO trials, women treated with thrombolytics were 2 to 3 times more likely to suffer hemorrhagic stroke than men were (OR = 2.2, p <0.001, OR = 3.3, p <0.0001, respectively) (133,140). Given the relatively high risk of hemorrhagic stroke in women receiving thrombolysis, the superiority of primary angioplasty (which virtually eliminates this risk) over fibrinolytic therapy for patients with AMI is particularly pronounced in women.

Outcome of Primary Angioplasty for Acute Myocardial Infarction in Women

The Primary Angioplasty in Acute Myocardial Infarction (PAMI) trial (N = 395, 27% women) was the first randomized trial to directly compare the outcomes of primary angioplasty and thrombolysis (with tPA) (135). Consistent with other studies, women in PAMI were older (66 versus 58 years of age, p <0.001), had more hypertension and diabetes than male patients, and on average presented to the emergency room 1 hour later (3.8 versus 2.9 hours, p = 0.0004). In-hospital mortality was significantly greater for women than for men (9.3% versus 2.8%, p = 0.005), mainly attributable to increased mortality in women receiving thrombolytic therapy (14%) compared with

PTCA (4.0%, p = 0.07). Overall women had a higher rate of hemorrhagic stroke (2.8% versus 0.3%, $P = 0.03$), but there were no strokes among women treated with PTCA. These findings, in addition to those of nonrandomized studies, strongly support primary PCI as the preferred treatment for women with AMI.

Outcomes after Primary Stenting for Acute Myocardial Infarction in Women

Although primary balloon angioplasty has improved outcomes in women (141), mortality and restenosis rates remain high (142,143). Recent studies have examined whether women's outcomes can be further improved with contemporary interventional techniques including stent implantation and glycoprotein IIb/IIIa inhibitors, although there are limited gender-specific data.

The Stent PAMI trial (N = 900, 25% female) was the first randomized trial to compare primary stenting with conventional angioplasty for AMI (144). Mortality at 6 months was higher in women than in men (7.9% versus 2.0%, p <0.0001). The highest female mortality rate occurred in patients treated with stents (10.2%), possibly attributable to the use of a relatively bulky, inflexible heparin-coated stent. Overall, stents were superior to balloons in terms of target vessel revascularization, restenosis, and vessel reocculusion.

Subsequent studies have established the superiority of stenting over balloon-only angioplasty and demonstrated that these findings are generalizable to female patients. The Controlled Abciximab and Device Investigation to Lower Late Angioplasty Complications (CADILLAC) trial (145), a trial of 2,082 (27% female) patients with AMI randomized to the MultiLink stent (Guidant, Santa Clara, CA) or PTCA, and abciximab or placebo, identified primary stenting (with or without the glycoprotein IIb/IIIa inhibitor abciximab) as the optimal reperfusion strategy for patients presenting with AMI. Compared to men, women were older, had a smaller body surface area, more diabetes, hypertension, and hyperlipidemia, experienced significant delays to treatment, and had better baseline and final TIMI grade 3 flow. Unadjusted 1-year event rates were higher for women, including death (7.6% versus 3.0%, p < 0.001), ischemic TVR (16.7% versus 12.1%, p = 0.006), and MACE (23.9% versus 15.3%, p <0.001). Female gender was an independent predictor of MACE and bleeding complications, although BSA and comorbid risk factors, but not gender, were predictive of mortality at 1 year.

Despite worse outcomes compared with men, stent implantation improved clinical and angiographic outcomes for women, independent of abciximab use. At 1 year, primary stenting resulted in a 32% reduction in MACE (19.1% versus 28.1%, p = 0.01) and a 47% reduction in target vessel revascularization (10.8% versus 20.4%, p = 0.002) compared to PTCA, without an impact on death, MI, or stroke (146).

While stenting improves outcomes compared to PTCA, women with AMI continue to have a relatively poor prognosis, with a higher risk of short-term mortality compared to men, independent of elevated baseline risk factors. Considering that 345,000 women experience a new or recurrent MI each year (1), a continued search for new adjunctive approaches is required to address the gender gap in AMI outcomes.

Adjunctive Pharmacology with Glycoprotein IIb/IIIa Inhibitors

The use of glycoprotein IIb/IIIa inhibitors as an adjunct to elective PCI or PCI for ACS reduces ischemic complications, with the greatest benefit in high-risk patients, including women, particularly those who are older, diabetic, or troponin-positive. Use of GP IIb/IIIa inhibitors in this setting does not confer an increased risk of major vascular complications (147,148), although increases in minor bleeding in women have been reported (148). The benefits of GP IIb/IIIa use occur regardless of the particular interventional device employed (149). As adjunctive therapy for primary PCI for ST-elevation MI, GP IIb/IIIa inhibition with abciximab may reduce ischemic complications in women without shock, although benefits have not been conclusively demonstrated. There have been no randomized trials examining the efficacy of adjunctive GP IIb/IIIa inhibition during rescue PCI for failed thrombolysis, but their use in this setting has been linked with an increased risk of bleeding, particularly in elderly and female patients (150,151).

Numerous studies have demonstrated the benefits of GP IIb/IIIa inhibition as an adjunct to unfractionated heparin in patients undergoing elective PCI or PCI for ACS. A pooled analysis of the EPIC, EPILOG, and EPISTENT trials (N = 6,595, 27% female) showed that abciximab treatment during PCI was beneficial in men and women, reducing the incidence of the combined endpoint of death, MI, or urgent revascularization in women from 12.7% to 6.5% (p <0.001) at 30 days and 16.0% to 9.9% (p <0.001) at 6 months, with similar reductions in men (148). At 1 year, abciximab significantly reduced mortality in women (4.0% versus 2.5%, p = 0.03), but not in men. While women experienced more major bleeding than men, this increase was independent of abciximab, though women did experience a significant increase in minor bleeding compared with placebo (6.7% versus 4.7%, p = 0.01). The ESPRIT trial (N = 2,064, 27% female) reported similar results, and female gender was not an independent predictor of bleeding complications (147).

Evidence for benefits of GP IIb/IIIa inhibition in women in the setting of ST-elevation MI have been less conclusive. The ADMIRAL study (N = 300, 18% women) demonstrated a significant early and 6-month reduction in death, MI, or urgent TVR for abciximab among AMI patients undergoing primary stenting (7.4% versus 15.9%, p <0.02) (152). This benefit was not significant in the female subgroup (9.1% versus 9.3%), possibly due to the small number of women in this study. In CADILLAC, although abciximab did not lower death, MI, or stroke at 6 months in STEMI patients, the addition of abciximab to primary stenting significantly reduced 30-day ischemic TVR in women (and men) without increasing bleeding or stroke rates (146). Despite the lack of conclusive evidence, abciximab may reduce ischemic complications in patients undergoing primary angioplasty for STEMI, particularly when used as pretreatment before revascularization; the ACC/AHA guidelines for the treatment of STEMI note that it is reasonable to initiate abciximab treatment as early as possible in patients undergoing primary PCI (153).

Vascular Complications

In studies from the 1990s, vascular complications were three to four times more frequent in women than in men. Rates of vascular complications in women have subsequently decreased with the development of less aggressive anticoagulation regimens, weight-adjusted heparin dosing, and the availability of smaller sheath sizes made possible by the smaller profile of newer third- and fourth-generation devices (132). Adjunctive use of GP IIb/IIIa inhibitors does not increase the risk of vascular complications in women, and the use of the direct thrombin inhibitor bivalirudin during elective PCI lowers the risk of periprocedural ischemic complications and major bleeding in both women and men (154).

Despite improvements, women continue to have a 1.5- to 4-fold increased risk of vascular complications compared with men in the modern era (132). In a study of 1,166 consecutive patients (31% female) undergoing "real-world" PCI for de novo CAD in the first year after the introduction of DES to the U.S. market, women had a higher risk of vascular complications than men (12.0% versus 4.2%, p <0.0001), an association that persisted even after adjustment for age, BSA, sheath size, heparin dose, and GP IIb/IIIa inhibitor use (OR = 3.38; 95% CI, 1.81–6.31, p = 0.0001) (155). In the CADILLAC trial, female gender remained an independent predictor of moderate/severe bleeding at 1 year (HR = 2.09; 95% CI, 1.19–3.68, p = 0.01) (146). Additional studies are needed to determine strategies to minimize vascular complications in women.

Conclusions

Coronary disease is the leading cause of mortality for women in the United States. Despite improved outcomes in women and reduced gender differences, the majority of studies comparing outcomes after contemporary coronary intervention in men and women continue to demonstrate worse outcomes in women, with approximately 30% of this difference attributable to delayed presentation and associated risk factors. Published studies have historically focused on comparing women's outcomes to those of men, and reports of women's worse outcomes may have led, in part, to the treatment disparities currently facing women. Clinical trials focusing on treatment alternatives in women have demonstrated improvements in outcomes, with advances in technologies and contemporary therapies such as stenting and drug-eluting stents achieving excellent results in this population. Future efforts should be focused on the proper diagnosis and treatment of women with CAD to counteract increasing mortality trends in this high-risk population.

REFERENCES

1. Thom T, Haase N, Rosamond W, et al. Heart disease and stroke statistics–2006 update: a report from the American Heart Association Statistics Committee and Stroke Statistics Subcommittee. *Circulation*. 2006;113:85–151.
2. Grady D, Chaput L, Kristof M. *Results of Systematic Review of Research on Diagnosis and Treatment of Coronary Heart Disease in Women. Evidence Report/Technology Assessment No. 80*. Rockville, MD: Agency for Healthcare Research and Quality; 2003. AHRQ Publication No. 03-0035.
3. Mosca L, Linfante AH, Benjamin EJ, et al. National study of physician awareness and adherence to cardiovascular disease prevention guidelines. *Circulation*. 2005;111:499–510.
4. Angeja BG, Gibson CM, Chin R, et al. Predictors of door-to-balloon delay in primary angioplasty. *Am J Cardiol*. 2002;89:1156–1161.
5. Schulman KA, Berlin JA, Harless W, et al. The effect of race and sex on physicians' recommendations for cardiac catheterization. *N Engl J Med*. 1999;340:618–626.
6. Ghali WA, Faris PD, Galbraith PD, et al. Sex differences in access to coronary revascularization after cardiac catheterization: importance of detailed clinical data. *Ann Intern Med*. 2002;136:723–732.
7. Roeters van Lennep JE, Zwinderman AH, Roeters van Lennep HW, et al. Gender differences in diagnosis and treatment of coronary artery disease from 1981 to 1997. No evidence for the Yentl syndrome. *Eur Heart J*. 2000;21:911–918.
8. Anand SS, Xie CC, Mehta S, et al. Differences in the management and prognosis of women and men who suffer from acute coronary syndromes. *J Am Coll Cardiol*. 2005;46:1845–1851.
9. Canto JG, Fincher C, Kiefe CI, et al. Atypical presentations among Medicare beneficiaries with unstable angina pectoris. *Am J Cardiol*. 2002;90:248–253.
10. Roger VL, Farkouh ME, Weston SA, et al. Sex differences in evaluation and outcome of unstable angina. *JAMA*. 2000;283:646–652.
11. Wingard DL, Cohn BA, Kaplan GA, et al. Sex differentials in morbidity and mortality risks examined by age and cause in the same cohort. *Am J Epidemiol*. 1989;130:601–610.
12. Lerner DJ, Kannel WB. Patterns of coronary heart disease morbidity and mortality in the sexes: a 26-year follow-up of the Framingham population. *Am Heart J*. 1986;111:383–390.
13. Wenger NK. Gender, coronary artery disease, and coronary bypass surgery. *Ann Intern Med*. 1990;112:557–558.
14. Greenland P, Reicher-Reiss H, Goldbourt U, et al. In-hospital and 1-year mortality in 1,524 women after myocardial infarction. Comparison with 4,315 men. *Circulation*. 1991;83:484–491.
15. Vaccarino V, Krumholz HM, Berkman LF, et al. Sex differences in mortality after myocardial infarction. Is there evidence for an increased risk for women? *Circulation*. 1995;91:1861–1871.
16. Goldberg RJ, Gorak EJ, Yarzebski J, et al. A communitywide perspective of sex differences and temporal trends in the incidence and survival rates after acute myocardial infarction and out-of-hospital deaths caused by coronary heart disease. *Circulation*. 1993;87:1947–1953.
17. Wong ND, Cupples LA, Ostfeld AM, et al. Risk factors for long-term coronary prognosis after initial myocardial infarction: the Framingham Study. *Am J Epidemiol*. 1989;130:469–480.
18. Pohjola S, Siltanen P, Romo M. Five-year survival of 728 patients after myocardial infarction. A community study. *Br Heart J*. 1980;43:176–183.
19. Tofler GH, Stone PH, Muller JE, et al. Effects of gender and race on prognosis after myocardial infarction: adverse prognosis for women, particularly black women. *J Am Coll Cardiol*. 1987;9:473–482.
20. Dittrich H, Gilpin E, Nicod P, et al. Acute myocardial infarction in women: influence of gender on mortality and prognostic variables. *Am J Cardiol*. 1988;62:1–7.
21. Robertson T, Kennard ED, Mehta S, et al. Influence of gender on in-hospital clinical and angiographic outcomes and on one-year follow-up in the New Approaches to Coronary Intervention (NACI) registry. *Am J Cardiol*. 1997;80:26K–39K.

22. Taddei CF, Weintraub WS, Douglas JS, Jr., et al. Influence of age on outcome after percutaneous transluminal coronary angioplasty. *Am J Cardiol.* 1999;84:245–251.

23. Weintraub WS, Wenger NK, Kosinski AS, et al. Percutaneous transluminal coronary angioplasty in women compared with men. *J Am Coll Cardiol.* 1994;24:81–90.

24. Welty FK, Mittleman MA, Healy RW, et al. Similar results of percutaneous transluminal coronary angioplasty for women and men with postmyocardial infarction ischemia. *J Am Coll Cardiol.* 1994;23:35–39.

25. Kelsey SF, James M, Holubkov AL, et al. Results of percutaneous transluminal coronary angioplasty in women. 1985–1986 National Heart, Lung, and Blood Institute's Coronary Angioplasty Registry. *Circulation.* 1993;87:720–727.

26. Bell MR, Holmes DR, Jr., Berger PB, et al. The changing in-hospital mortality of women undergoing percutaneous transluminal coronary angioplasty. *JAMA.* 1993;269:2091–2095.

27. DeFrances CJ, Hall MJ, Podgornik MN. *2003 National Hospital Discharge Survey. Advance data from vital and health statistics. No. 359.* Hyattsville, MD: National Center for Health Statistics; 2005.

28. Vaccarino V, Parsons L, Every NR, et al. Sex-based differences in early mortality after myocardial infarction. National Registry of Myocardial Infarction 2 Participants. *N Engl J Med.* 1999;341:217–225.

29. Lytle BW, Kramer JR, Golding LR, et al. Young adults with coronary atherosclerosis: 10 year results of surgical myocardial revascularization. *J Am Coll Cardiol.* 1984;4:445–453.

30. Lansky AJ, Mehran R, Dangas G, et al. Comparison of differences in outcome after percutaneous coronary intervention in men versus women <40 years of age. *Am J Cardiol.* 2004;93:916–919.

31. Bairey Merz CN, Johnson BD, Sharaf BL, et al. Hypoestrogenemia of hypothalamic origin and coronary artery disease in premenopausal women: a report from the NHLBI-sponsored WISE study. *J Am Coll Cardiol.* 2003; 41:413–419.

32. Burke AP, Farb A, Malcom G, et al. Effect of menopause on plaque morphologic characteristics in coronary atherosclerosis. *Am Heart J.* 2001;141:S58–62.

33. Arbustini E, Dal Bello B, Morbini P, et al. Plaque erosion is a major substrate for coronary thrombosis in acute myocardial infarction. *Heart.* 1999;82:269–272.

34. Kannel WB, McGee DL. Diabetes and cardiovascular disease. The Framingham Study. *JAMA.* 1979;241:2035–2038.

35. Natarajan S, Liao Y, Sinha D, et al. Sex differences in the effect of diabetes duration on coronary heart disease mortality. *Arch Intern Med.* 2005;165:430–435.

36. Natarajan S, Liao Y, Cao G, et al. Sex differences in risk for coronary heart disease mortality associated with diabetes and established coronary heart disease. *Arch Intern Med.* 2003;163:1735–1740.

37. Kanaya AM, Grady D, Barrett-Connor E. Explaining the sex difference in coronary heart disease mortality among patients with type 2 diabetes mellitus: a meta-analysis. *Arch Intern Med.* 2002;162:1737–1745.

38. Juutilainen A, Kortelainen S, Lehto S, et al. Gender difference in the impact of type 2 diabetes on coronary heart disease risk. *Diabetes Care.* 2004;27:2898–2904.

39. Hypertension in Diabetes Study (HDS). I. Prevalence of hypertension in newly presenting type 2 diabetic patients and the association with risk factors for cardiovascular and diabetic complications. *J Hypertens.* 1993;11:309–317.

40. Wei M, Gaskill SP, Haffner SM, et al. Effects of diabetes and level of glycemia on all-cause and cardiovascular mortality. The San Antonio Heart Study. *Diabetes Care.* 1998;21:1167–1172.

41. Barrett-Connor EL, Cohn BA, Wingard DL, et al. Why is diabetes mellitus a stronger risk factor for fatal ischemic heart disease in women than in men? The Rancho Bernardo Study. *JAMA.* 1991;265:627–631.

42. Haffner SM, Lehto S, Ronnemaa T, et al. Mortality from coronary heart disease in subjects with type 2 diabetes and in nondiabetic subjects with and without prior myocardial infarction. *N Engl J Med.* 1998;339:229–234.

43. Beckles GLA, Thompson-Reid PE. Socioeconomic status of women with diabetes: United States 2002. *Morb Mortal Wkly Rep.* 2002;51:147–159.

44. DeStefano F, Newman J. Comparison of coronary heart disease mortality risk between black and white people with diabetes. *Ethn Dis.* 1993;3:145–151.

45. Kornowski R, Mintz GS, Kent KM, et al. Increased restenosis in diabetes mellitus after coronary interventions is due to exaggerated intimal hyperplasia. A serial intravascular ultrasound study. *Circulation.* 1997;95:1366–1369.

46. Kornowski R, Lansky AJ, Mintz GS, et al. Comparison of men versus women in cross-sectional area luminal narrowing, quantity of plaque, presence of calcium in plaque, and lumen location in coronary arteries by intravascular ultrasound in patients with stable angina pectoris. *Am J Cardiol.* 1997;79:1601–1605.

47. Dodge JT, Brown BG, Bolson EL, et al. Lumen diameter of normal human coronary arteries. Influence of age, sex, anatomic variation, and left ventricular hypertrophy or dilation. *Circulation.* 1992;86:232–246.

48. Di Carli MF, Afonso L, Campisi R, et al. Coronary vascular dysfunction in premenopausal women with diabetes mellitus. *Am Heart J.* 2002;144:711–718.

49. Grundy SM, Benjamin IJ, Burke GL, et al. Diabetes and cardiovascular disease: a statement for healthcare professionals from the American Heart Association. *Circulation.* 1999;100:1134–1146.

50. Hu FB, Stampfer MJ, Solomon CG, et al. The impact of diabetes mellitus on mortality from all causes and coronary heart disease in women: 20 years of follow-up. *Arch Intern Med.* 2001;161:1717–1723.

51. McGuire DK, Khera A, de Lemos JA. Women with diabetes mellitus have the greatest reduction in myocardial infarction mortality over the past decade: evaluation of 1,428,596 patients enrolled in the National Registry of Myocardial Infarction 2, 3, and 4 from 1994–2002. *J Am Coll Cardiol.* 2004;43 (suppl):284A.

52. MacAlpin RN, Abbasi AS, Grollman JH, et al. Human coronary artery size during life. A cinearteriographic study. *Radiology.* 1973;108:567–576.

53. Roberts CS, Roberts WC. Cross-sectional area of the proximal portions of the three major epicardial coronary arteries in 98 necropsy patients with different coronary events. Relationship to heart weight, age, and sex. *Circulation.* 1980;62:953–959.

54. Sheifer SE, Canos MR, Weinfurt KP, et al. Sex differences in coronary artery size assessed by intravascular ultrasound. *Am Heart J.* 2000;139: 649–653.

55. Kim SG, Apple S, Mintz GS, et al. The importance of gender on coronary artery size: in vivo assessment by intravascular ultrasound. *Clin Cardiol.* 2004;27:291–294.

56. Arnold AM, Mick MJ, Piedmonte MR, et al. Gender differences for coronary angioplasty. *Am J Cardiol.* 1994;74:18–21.

57. Ellis S, Ajluni S, Arnold A, et al. Increased coronary perforation in the new device era. Incidence, classification, management, and outcome. *Circulation.* 1994;90:2725–2730.

58. Gruberg L, Pinnow E, Flood R, et al. Incidence, management, and outcome of coronary artery perforation during percutaneous coronary intervention. *Am J Cardiol.* 2000;86:680–682, A688.

59. Fasseas P, Orford JL, Panetta CJ, et al. Incidence, correlates, management, and clinical outcome of coronary perforation: analysis of 16,298 procedures. *Am Heart J.* 2004;147:140–145.

60. Fisher LD, Kennedy JW, Davis KB, et al. Association of sex, physical size, and operative mortality after coronary artery bypass in the Coronary Artery Surgery Study (CASS). *J Thorac Cardiovasc Surg.* 1982;84:334–341.

61. Cantor WJ, Miller JM, Hellkamp AS, et al. Role of target vessel size and body surface area on outcomes after percutaneous coronary interventions in women. *Am Heart J.* 2002;144:297–302.

62. Deupree RH, Fields RI, McMahan CA, et al. Atherosclerotic lesions and coronary heart disease. Key relationships in necropsied cases. *Lab Invest.* 1973;28:252–262.

63. Daoud AS, Florentin RA, Goodale F. Diffuse coronary arteriosclerosis versus isolated plaques in the etiology of myocardial infarction. *Am J Cardiol.* 1964;14:69–74.

64. Goffman JW. The quantitative nature of the relationship of coronary atherosclerosis and coronary heart disease. *Cardiol Digest.* 1969;4:28–38.

65. Kagan AR, Uemura K. Atherosclerosis of the aorta and coronary arteries in five towns. Material and methods. *Bull World Health Organ.* 1976;53:489–499.

66. Varnava AM, Davies MJ. Relation between coronary artery remodelling (compensatory dilatation) and stenosis in human native coronary arteries. *Heart.* 2001;86:207–211.

67. Pepine CJ, Kerensky RA, Lambert CR, et al. Some thoughts on the vasculopathy of women with ischemic heart disease. *J Am Coll Cardiol.* 2006;47:30–35.

68. Shaw LJ, Bairey Merz CN, Pepine CJ, et al. Insights from the NHLBI-sponsored women's ischemia syndrome evaluation (WISE) study: part I: gender differences in traditional and novel risk factors, symptom evaluation, and gender-optimized diagnostic strategies. *J Am Coll Cardiol.* 2006;47:4–20.

69. Hochman JS, McCabe CH, Stone PH, et al. Outcome and profile of women and men presenting with acute coronary syndromes: a report from TIMI IIIB. TIMI investigators. Thrombolysis in myocardial infarction. *J Am Coll Cardiol.* 1997;30:141–148.

70. von Mering GO, Arant CB, Wessel TR, et al. Abnormal coronary vasomotion as a prognostic indicator of cardiovascular events in women: results from the National Heart, Lung, and Blood Institute-Sponsored Women's Ischemia Syndrome Evaluation (WISE). *Circulation.* 2004;109:722–725.

71. Raijmakers MT, Dechend R, Poston L. Oxidative stress and preeclampsia: rationale for antioxidant clinical trials. *Hypertension.* 2004;44:374–380.

72. Norman M, Martin H. Preterm birth attenuates association between low birth weight and endothelial dysfunction. *Circulation.* 2003;108:996–1001.

73. Wong TY, Klein R, Sharrett AR, et al. Retinal arteriolar narrowing and risk of coronary heart disease in men and women. The Atherosclerosis Risk in Communities Study. *JAMA.* 2002;287:1153–1159.

74. Reis SE, Holubkov R, Lee JS, et al. Coronary flow velocity response to adenosine characterizes coronary microvascular function in women with chest pain and no obstructive coronary disease. Results from the pilot phase of the Women's Ischemia Syndrome Evaluation (WISE) study. *J Am Coll Cardiol.* 1999;33:1469–1475.

75. Handberg E, Johnson BD, Arant CB, et al. Impaired coronary vascular reactivity and functional capacity in women: results from the NHLBI Women's Ischemia Syndrome Evaluation (WISE) study. *J Am Coll Cardiol.* 2006;47:S44–49.

76. Shaw LJ, Olson MB, Kip K, et al. The value of estimated functional capacity in estimating outcome: results From the NHBLI-sponsored Women's Ischemia Syndrome Evaluation (WISE) study. *J Am Coll Cardiol.* 2006;47:S36–43.

77. Bairey Merz CN, Shaw LJ, Reis SE, et al. Insights from the NHLBI-sponsored Women's Ischemia Syndrome Evaluation (WISE) study: part II: gender differences in presentation, diagnosis, and outcome with regard to gender-based pathophysiology of atherosclerosis and macrovascular and microvascular coronary disease. *J Am Coll Cardiol.* 2006;47:S21–S29.

78. Marroquin OC, Holubkov R, Edmundowicz D, et al. Heterogeneity of microvascular dysfunction in women with chest pain not attributable to coronary artery disease: implications for clinical practice. *Am Heart J.* 2003;145:628–635.

79. Kip KE, Marroquin OC, Shaw LJ, et al. Global inflammation predicts cardiovascular risk in women: a report from the Women's Ischemia Syndrome Evaluation (WISE) study. *Am Heart J.* 2005;150:900–906.

80. Ford ES, Giles WH, Dietz WH. Prevalence of the metabolic syndrome among US adults: findings from the third National Health and Nutrition Examination Survey. *JAMA.* 2002;287:356–359.

81. Kip KE, Marroquin OC, Kelley DE, et al. Clinical importance of obesity versus the metabolic syndrome in cardiovascular risk in women: a report from the Women's Ischemia Syndrome Evaluation (WISE) study. *Circulation.* 2004;109:706–713.

82. Cankar K, Finderle Z, Strucl M. Gender differences in cutaneous laser doppler flow response to local direct and contralateral cooling. *J Vasc Res.* 2000;37:183–188.

83. Algotsson A, Nordberg A, Winblad B. Influence of age and gender on skin vessel reactivity to endothelium-dependent and endothelium-

84. Arant CB, Wessel TR, Olson MB, et al. Hemoglobin level is an independent predictor for adverse cardiovascular outcomes in women undergoing evaluation for chest pain: results from the National Heart, Lung, and Blood Institute Women's Ischemia Syndrome Evaluation Study. *J Am Coll Cardiol.* 2004;43:2009–2014.

85. Mendelsohn ME, Karas RH. The protective effects of estrogen on the cardiovascular system. *N Engl J Med.* 1999;340:1801–1811.

86. Salomaa V, Rasi V, Pekkanen J, et al. Association of hormone replacement therapy with hemostatic and other cardiovascular risk factors. The FINRISK Hemostasis Study. *Arterioscler Thromb Vasc Biol.* 1995;15:1549–1555.

87. Meade TW, Mellows S, Brozovic M, et al. Haemostatic function and ischaemic heart disease: principal results of the Northwick Park Heart Study. *Lancet.* 1986;2:533–537.

88. Roberts JW, Goldschmidt-Clermont P, Bray P. Effect of gender on thrombogenic factors in asymptomatic people at high risk for coronary artery disease. *Circulation.* 1994;90(Suppl I):I–283.

89. Mosca L, Grundy SM, Judelson D, et al. Guide to preventive cardiology for women. *Circulation.* 1999;99:2480–2484.

90. Shaw LJ, Miller DD, Romeis JC, et al. Gender differences in the noninvasive evaluation and management of patients with suspected coronary artery disease. *Ann Intern Med.* 1994;120:559–566.

91. Steingart RM, Packer M, Hamm P, et al. Sex differences in the management of coronary artery disease. Survival and ventricular enlargement investigators. *N Engl J Med.* 1991;325:226–230.

92. Bowling A, Bond M, McKee D, et al. Equity in access to exercise tolerance testing, coronary angiography, and coronary artery bypass grafting by age, sex, and clinical indications. *Heart.* 2001;85:680–686.

93. Battleman DS, Callahan M. Gender differences in utilization of exercise treadmill testing: a claims-based analysis. *J Healthc Qual.* 2001;23:38–41.

94. Shaw LJ, Peterson ED, Johnson LL. Non-invasive stress testing. In: Charney P, ed. *Coronary Artery Disease in Women: What All Physicians Need to Know.* Philadelphia, PA: American College of Physicians; 1999:327–350.

95. Mosca L, Appel LJ, Benjamin EJ, et al. Evidence-based guidelines for cardiovascular disease prevention in women. American Heart Association scientific statement. *Arterioscler Thromb Vasc Biol.* 2004;24:e29–50.

96. Gibbons RJ, Balady GJ, Timothy Bricker J, et al. ACC/AHA 2002 guideline update for exercise testing: summary article. A report of the American College of Cardiology/American Heart Association Task Force on Practice Guidelines (Committee to Update the 1997 Exercise Testing Guidelines). *J Am Coll Cardiol.* 2002;40:1531–1540.

97. Gibbons RJ, Hodge DO, Berman DS, et al. Long-term outcome of patients with intermediate-risk exercise electrocardiograms who do not have myocardial perfusion defects on radionuclide imaging. *Circulation.* 1999;100:2140–2145.

98. Sawada SG, Ryan T, Conley MJ, et al. Prognostic value of a normal exercise echocardiogram. *Am Heart J.* 1990;120:49–55.

99. Mieres JH, Shaw LJ, Arai A, et al. Role of noninvasive testing in the clinical evaluation of women with suspected coronary artery disease: consensus statement from the Cardiac Imaging Committee, Council on Clinical Cardiology, and the Cardiovascular Imaging and Intervention Committee, Council on Cardiovascular Radiology and Intervention, American Heart Association. *Circulation.* 2005;111:682–696.

100. Cowley MJ, Mullin SM, Kelsey SF, et al. Sex differences in early and long-term results of coronary angioplasty in the NHLBI PTCA Registry. *Circulation.* 1985;71:90–97.

101. Maynard C, Litwin PE, Martin JS, et al. Gender differences in the treatment and outcome of acute myocardial infarction. Results from the myocardial infarction triage and intervention registry. *Arch Intern Med.* 1992;152:972–976.

102. Behar S, Gottlieb S, Hod H, et al. Influence of gender in the therapeutic management of patients with acute myocardial infarction in Israel. The Israeli Thrombolytic Survey Group. *Am J Cardiol.* 1994;73:438–443.

103. Giacomini MK. Gender and ethnic differences in hospital-based procedure utilization in California. *Arch Intern Med.* 1996;156:1217–1224.

104. Kudenchuk PJ, Maynard C, Martin JS, et al. Comparison of presentation, treatment, and outcome of acute myocardial infarction in men versus women (the Myocardial Infarction Triage and Intervention Registry). *Am J Cardiol.* 1996;78:9–14.

105. Chiriboga DE, Yarzebski J, Goldberg RJ, et al. A community-wide perspective of gender differences and temporal trends in the use of diagnostic and revascularization procedures for acute myocardial infarction. *Am J Cardiol.* 1993;71:268–273.

106. Ruygrok PN, de Jaegere PP, van Domburg RT, et al. Women fare no worse than men 10 years after attempted coronary angioplasty. *Cathet Cardiovasc Diagn.* 1996;39:9–15.

107. Keelan ET, Nunez BD, Grill DE, et al. Comparison of immediate and long-term outcome of coronary angioplasty performed for unstable angina and rest pain in men and women. *Mayo Clin Proc.* 1997;72: 5–12.

108. Lansky AJ, Mehran R, Dangas G, et al. New-device angioplasty in women: clinical outcome and predictors in a 7,372-patient registry. *Epidemiol.* 2002;13:S46–S51.

109. Malenka DJ, Wennberg DE, Quinton HA, et al. Gender-related changes in the practice and outcomes of percutaneous coronary interventions in northern New England from 1994 to 1999. *J Am Coll Cardiol.* 2002;40: 2092–2101.

110. McEniery PT, Hollman J, Knezinek V, et al. Comparative safety and efficacy of percutaneous transluminal coronary angioplasty in men and in women. *Cathet Cardiovasc Diagn.* 1987;13:364–371.

111. Bell MR, Grill DE, Garratt KN, et al. Long-term outcome of women compared with men after successful coronary angioplasty. *Circulation.* 1995;91:2876–2881.

112. Foley DP, Melkert R, Serruys PW. Influence of coronary vessel size on renarrowing process and late angiographic outcome after successful balloon angioplasty. *Circulation.* 1994;90:1239–1251.

113. Fishman RF, Kuntz RE, Carrozza JP, Jr., et al. Long-term results of directional coronary atherectomy: predictors of restenosis. *J Am Coll Cardiol.* 1992;20:1101–1110.

114. Carrozza JP, Jr., Kuntz RE, Levine MJ, et al. Angiographic and clinical outcome of intracoronary stenting: immediate and long-term results from a large single-center experience. *J Am Coll Cardiol.* 1992;20:328–337.

115. Kuntz RE, Safian RD, Carrozza JP, et al. The importance of acute luminal diameter in determining restenosis after coronary atherectomy or stenting. *Circulation.* 1992;86:1827–1835.

116. Dussaillant GR, Mintz GS, Pichard AD, et al. Small stent size and intimal hyperplasia contribute to restenosis: a volumetric intravascular ultrasound analysis. *J Am Coll Cardiol.* 1995;26:720–724.

117. Centers for Disease Control and Prevention. QuickStats: use of stents among hospitalized patients undergoing coronary angioplasty, by race. United States, 2003. *MMWR.* 2005:54.

118. Anderson HV, Shaw RE, Brindis RG, et al. A contemporary overview of percutaneous coronary interventions. The American College of Cardiology-National Cardiovascular Data Registry (ACC-NCDR). *J Am Coll Cardiol.* 2002; 39:1096–1103.

119. Fischman DL, Leon MB, Baim DS, et al. A randomized comparison of coronary-stent placement and balloon angioplasty in the treatment of coronary artery disease. *N Engl J Med.* 1994;331:496–501.

120. Serruys PW, de Jaegere P, Kiemeneij F, et al. A comparison of balloon-expandable-stent implantation with balloon angioplasty in patients with coronary artery disease. Benestent study group. *N Engl J Med.* 1994;331:489–495.

121. Randomised placebo-controlled and balloon-angioplasty-controlled trial to assess safety of coronary stenting with use of platelet glycoprotein-IIb/IIIa blockade. The EPISTENT Investigators. Evaluation of platelet IIb/IIIa inhibitor for stenting. *Lancet.* 1998;352:87–92.

122. Lansky AJ, Popma J, Mehran R, et al. Tubular slotted stents: a breakthrough therapy for women undergoing coronary interventions. Pooled results from the STARS, ASCENT, SMART and NIRVANA randomized clinical trials. *J Am Coll Cardiol.* 1999;33 (Suppl A):58A.

123. Watanabe CT, Maynard C, Ritchie JL. Comparison of short-term outcomes following coronary artery stenting in men versus women. *Am J Cardiol.* 2001;88:848–852.

124. Mehilli J, Kastrati A, Dirschinger J, et al. Differences in prognostic factors and outcomes between women and men undergoing coronary artery stenting. *JAMA.* 2000;284:1799–1805.

125. Holmes DR, Jr, Leon MB, Moses JW, et al. Analysis of 1-year clinical outcomes in the SIRIUS trial: a randomized trial of a sirolimus-eluting stent versus a standard stent in patients at high risk for coronary restenosis. *Circulation.* 2004;109:634–640.

126. Lansky AJ, Costa RA, Mooney M, et al. Gender-based outcomes after paclitaxel-eluting stent implantation in patients with coronary artery disease. *J Am Coll Cardiol.* 2005;45:1180–1185.

127. Lagerqvist B, Safstrom K, Stahle E, et al. Is early invasive treatment of unstable coronary artery disease equally effective for both women and men? FRISC II Study Group Investigators. *J Am Coll Cardiol.* 2001;38:41–48.

128. Fox KA, Poole-Wilson P, Clayton TC, et al. 5-year outcome of an interventional strategy in non-ST-elevation acute coronary syndrome: the British Heart Foundation RITA 3 randomised trial. *Lancet.* 2005;366:914–920.

129. Glaser R, Herrmann HC, Murphy SA, et al. Benefit of an early invasive management strategy in women with acute coronary syndromes. *JAMA.* 2002;288:3124–3129.

130. Mueller C, Neumann FJ, Roskamm H, et al. Women do have an improved long-term outcome after non-ST-elevation acute coronary syndromes treated very early and predominantly with percutaneous coronary intervention: a prospective study in 1,450 consecutive patients. *J Am Coll Cardiol.* 2002;40:245–250.

131. Clayton TC, Pocock SJ, Henderson RA, et al. Do men benefit more than women from an interventional strategy in patients with unstable angina or non-ST-elevation myocardial infarction? The impact of gender in the RITA 3 trial. *Eur Heart J.* 2004;25:1641–1650.

132. Lansky AJ, Hochman JS, Ward PA, et al. Percutaneous coronary intervention and adjunctive pharmacotherapy in women: a statement for healthcare professionals from the American Heart Association. *Circulation.* 2005;111:940–953.

133. Weaver WD, White HD, Wilcox RG, et al. Comparisons of characteristics and outcomes among women and men with acute myocardial infarction treated with thrombolytic therapy. GUSTO-I Investigators. *JAMA.* 1996;275:777–782.

134. Vaccarino V, Parsons L, Every NR, et al. Impact of history of diabetes mellitus on hospital mortality in men and women with first acute myocardial infarction. The National Registry of Myocardial Infarction 2 Participants. *Am J Cardiol.* 2000;85:1486–1489; A1487.

135. Stone GW, Grines CL, Browne KF, et al. Comparison of in-hospital outcome in men versus women treated by either thrombolytic therapy or primary coronary angioplasty for acute myocardial infarction. *Am J Cardiol.* 1995;75:987–992.

136. Vakili BA, Kaplan RC, Brown DL. Sex-based differences in early mortality of patients undergoing primary angioplasty for first acute myocardial infarction. *Circulation.* 2001;104:3034–3038.

137. Tamis-Holland JE, Palazzo A, Stebbins AL, et al. Benefits of direct angioplasty for women and men with acute myocardial infarction: results of the Global Use of Strategies to Open Occluded Arteries in Acute Coronary Syndromes Angioplasty (GUSTO II-B) Angioplasty Substudy. *Am Heart J.* 2004;147:133–139.

138. Indications for fibrinolytic therapy in suspected acute myocardial infarction: collaborative overview of early mortality and major morbidity results from all randomised trials of more than 1,000 patients. Fibrinolytic Therapy Trialists' (FTT) Collaborative Group. *Lancet.* 1994;343:311–322.

139. Angeja BG, Rundle AC, Gurwitz JH, et al. Death or nonfatal stroke in patients with acute myocardial infarction treated with tissue plasminogen activator. Participants in the National Registry of Myocardial Infarction 2. *Am J Cardiol.* 2001;87:627–630, A629.

140. Maggioni AP, Franzosi MG, Santoro E, et al. The risk of stroke in patients with acute myocardial infarction after thrombolytic and antithrombotic treatment. Gruppo Italiano per lo Studio della Sopravvivenza nell'Infarto Miocardico II (GISSI-2), and the International Study Group. *N Engl J Med.* 1992;327:1–6.

141. Jacobs AK, Johnston JM, Haviland A, et al. Improved outcomes for women undergoing contemporary percutaneous coronary intervention: a report from the National Heart, Lung, and Blood Institute Dynamic registry. *J Am Coll Cardiol.* 2002;39:1608–1614.

142. Zijlstra F, Hoorntje JC, de Boer MJ, et al. Long-term benefit of primary angioplasty as compared with thrombolytic therapy for acute myocardial infarction. *N Engl J Med.* 1999;341:1413–1419.

143. Stone G, Grines C, Browne K, et al. Implications of recurrent ischemia after reperfusion therapy in acute myocardial infarction: a comparison of thrombolytic therapy and primary angioplasty. *J Am Coll Cardiol.* 1995;26:66–72.

144. Stone GW, Marcovitz P, Lansky AJ, et al. Differential effects of stenting and angioplasty in women versus men undergoing a primary mechanical reperfusion strategy in acute myocardial infarction—the PAMI Stent randomized trial. *J Am Coll Cardiol.* 1999:832A.

145. Stone GW, Grines CL, Cox DA, et al. Comparison of angioplasty with stenting, with or without abciximab, in acute myocardial infarction. *N Engl J Med.* 2002;346:957–966.

146. Lansky AJ, Pietras C, Costa RA, et al. Gender differences in outcomes after primary angioplasty versus primary stenting with and without abciximab for acute myocardial infarction: results of the Controlled Abciximab and Device Investigation to Lower Late Angioplasty Complications (CADILLAC) trial. *Circulation.* 2005;111:1611–1618.

147. Fernandes LS, Tcheng JE, O'Shea JC, et al. Is glycoprotein IIb/IIIa antagonism as effective in women as in men following percutaneous coronary intervention? Lessons from the ESPRIT study. *J Am Coll Cardiol.* 2002;40:1085–1091.

148. Cho L, Topol EJ, Balog C, et al. Clinical benefit of glycoprotein IIb/IIIa blockade with Abciximab is independent of gender: pooled analysis from EPIC, EPILOG, and EPISTENT trials. Evaluation of 7E3 for the prevention of ischemic complications. Evaluation in percutaneous transluminal coronary angioplasty to improve long-term outcome with Abciximab GP IIb/IIIa blockade. Evaluation of platelet IIb/IIIa inhibitor for stent. *J Am Coll Cardiol.* 2000;36:381–386.

149. Bhatt DL, Lincoff AM, Califf RM, et al. The benefit of abciximab in percutaneous coronary revascularization is not device-specific. *Am J Cardiol.* 2000;85:1060–1064.

150. Jong P, Cohen EA, Batchelor W, et al. Bleeding risks with abciximab after full-dose thrombolysis in rescue or urgent angioplasty for acute myocardial infarction. *Am Heart J.* 2001;141:218–225.

151. Cantor WJ, Kaplan AL, Velianou JL, et al. Effectiveness and safety of abciximab after failed thrombolytic therapy. *Am J Cardiol.* 2001;87:439–442, A434.

152. Montalescot G, Barragan P, Wittenberg O, et al. Platelet glycoprotein IIb/IIIa inhibition with coronary stenting for acute myocardial infarction. *N Engl J Med.* 2001;344:1895–1903.

153. Antman EM, Anbe DT, Armstrong PW, et al. ACC/AHA guidelines for the management of patients with ST-elevation myocardial infarction: a report of the American College of Cardiology/American Heart Association Task Force on Practice Guidelines (Committee to Revise the 1999 Guidelines for the Management of Patients with Acute Myocardial Infarction). 2004; Available at: http://www.acc.org/clinical/guidelines/stemi/index.pdf.

154. Lincoff AM, Bittl JA, Harrington RA, et al. Bivalirudin and provisional glycoprotein IIb/IIIa blockade compared with heparin and planned glycoprotein IIb/IIIa blockade during percutaneous coronary intervention: REPLACE-2 randomized trial. *JAMA.* 2003;289:853–863.

155. Thompson CA, Kaplan AV, Friedman BJ, et al. Gender-based differences of percutaneous coronary intervention in the drug-eluting stent era. *Catheter Cardiovasc Interv.* 2006;67:25–31.

CHAPTER 21

Renal Failure, Diabetics

Mark J. Ricciardi, Joel D. Robbins, James D. Flaherty, and Charles J. Davidson

Chronic kidney disease (CKD) and diabetes mellitus are frequently present in patients presenting for percutaneous coronary intervention (PCI), and both represent important markers of adverse events. At least 19 million Americans have CKD (defined as a glomerular filtration rate (GFR) of less than 60 mL/min per 1.73 m^2 for ≥ 3 months or biopsy evidence of renal damage), and the number requiring hemodialysis or transplantation is expected to exceed 650,000 by 2010 (1). Patients with CKD are more likely to die from cardiovascular causes than from renal failure, with patients on dialysis with coronary artery disease (CAD) at highest risk. The risk of worsening renal function is highest in patients with pre-existing CKD, and its development may have significant impact on post-PCI outcome. Similarly, the diabetic patient has a disproportionate burden of CAD compared to the nondiabetic and is more likely to succumb to CAD than from any other cause. CAD in the diabetic is pathologically distinct and, independent of revascularization status, prone to a more malignant course than CAD in the nondiabetic. CKD and diabetes each magnify the risk of cardiovascular disease, and compound the patient's risk when both conditions exist. (Table 21–1) (2).

Renal Failure

End-Stage Renal Disease and Revascularization Outcomes

Patients with concomitant end-stage renal disease (ESRD) and CAD are estimated to have annual mortality rates 10 to 30 times greater than the general population (1). The precise reasons for the increased mortality are not known but likely include several renal failure–related factors such as increased oxidative stress, decreased endothelial function, increased thrombogenicity and coronary calcification, and comorbid diseases like hypertension and diabetes (3). These same factors may account for the long known increases in perioperative complications and mortality after coronary artery bypass graft surgery (CABG) (4,5) and for the increased procedural complication, restenosis, and mortality rates after balloon-only PCI (6–9). Bare metal stent (BMS) PCI has significantly reduced target vessel revascularization (TVR) rates in ESRD, although not to the level of nondialysis controls. In one representative study,

BMS reduced TVR to 35%, which was still double that of patients with normal renal function (10). The relative improvement in TVR offered by drug-eluting stents (DES) in ESRD is yet to be fully elucidated. Very small published case series suggest TVR rates of 0–5% in this patient population (11,12). In a retrospective study of 2,229 consecutive patients undergoing DES, renal failure was an independent predictor of stent thrombosis and had the second highest hazard ratio (HR 6.49, CI 2.60–16.15, p <0.001) after premature antiplatelet therapy discontinuation (13). The severity of renal failure was not further defined in the study.

Retrospective analyses of early revascularization techniques offer the only basis for evidence-based discussion regarding the optimal method of coronary revascularization in patients with ESRD suitable for either CABG or PCI. Using the U.S. Renal Data System database, Herzog et al. (14) reported on 6,668 CABG, 4,836 balloon PCI, and 4,280 BMS patients with dialysis-dependent ESRD. Hospital mortality was 8.6%, 6.4%, and 4.1%, respectively. The 2-year all-cause survival (mean $\pm$ SEM) was 56.4 $\pm$ 1.4%, 48.2 $\pm$ 1.5%, and 48.4 $\pm$ 2.0%, respectively (p <0.0001). After comorbidity adjustment, the relative risk for CABG versus balloon PCI was 0.80 (95% CI 0.76 to 0.84, p <0.0001) and for BMS versus balloon PCI, 0.94 (95% CI 0.88 to 0.99, p = 0.03). It has been suggested, based on these and similar data, that CABG is preferable to PCI in dialysis patients who require revascularization, especially those with diabetes (15,16).

Mild to Moderate Renal Disease and Revascularization Outcomes

To a lesser extent, the relatively poor outcomes observed after mechanical revascularization in patients with ESRD applies to less severe forms of CKD. In the cardiovascular literature, non–end stage CKD is variably defined using different creatinine or creatinine clearance (CrCl) levels. The stages of CKD outlined by the National Kidney Foundation provide a useful reference when interpreting clinical data (Table 21–2) (15). Compared to patients with normal renal function, CABG surgery in the nondialysis CKD patient is associated with increased morbidity and mortality (17,18). In one representative study, patients with CKD (serum creatinine concentration 1.5

Table 21–1

Incidence Rates of Cardiovascular Disease in Patients with and without CKD and DM

	AMI	ASVD[b]	Death
(−) DM (−) CKD	1.6 (0.01)	14.1 (0.03)	5.5 (0.02)
(+) DM (−) CKD	3.2 (0.03)	25.3 (0.10)	8.1 (0.05)
(−) DM (+) CKD	3.9 (0.10)	35.7 (0.36)	17.7 (0.21)
(+) DM (+) CKD	6.9 (0.16)	49.1 (0.51)	19.9 (0.27)

[a]Rates are reported per 100 patient-years, with SE in parentheses.
[b]ASVD was defined as first occurrence of AMI, CVA/TIA, or PVD.
Adapted from: Foley RN, Murray AM, Li S, et al. Chronic kidney disease and the risk for cardiovascular disease, renal replacement, and death in the United States Medicare population, 1998 to 1999. *J Am Soc Nephrol.* 2005;16:489–495, with permission.

to 3.0 mg/dL) had significantly greater 30-day mortality (16% versus 6%, p = 0.001), postoperative bleeding (16% versus 8%, p = 0.023), respiratory complications (29% versus 16%, p = 0.02), and cardiac complications (18% versus 7%, p = 0.002) compared to those with serum creatinine <1.5 mg/dL (19). Similarly, a retrospective single center study of 1,427 patients undergoing CABG found baseline creatinine levels of 1.5 mg/dL or greater associated with a threefold increase in mortality and a significant increase in the need for postoperative dialysis (OR 24.43: CI, 10.37–57.52, p <0.0001) (20).

As has been demonstrated with CABG surgery, there are now data showing a relationship between lesser degrees of baseline renal dysfunction and morbidity and mortality after PCI, albeit most of the large studies are an admixture of balloon PCI and BMS and none evaluated DES. Best et al. reported on 5,327 consecutive patients who presented for either urgent or elective PCI (roughly 2/3 received BMS, 1/3 balloon PCI or atherectomy, and 1/4 glycoprotein IIb/IIIa inhibitors) and showed that the risks of death and adverse cardiac events were proportional to the degree of CKD at the time of the procedure (21). One-year mortality rates correlated with worsening CrCl: 1.5% when the CrCl was greater than 70 mL/min and 18.3% when less than ≤30 mL/min. The patients with renal dysfunction more frequently had multivessel disease, vein graft degeneration, and complex lesions. Morbidity was also linked to the degree of renal insufficiency with increasing risk of myocar-

dial infarction (MI), procedural failure, and need for bypass surgery with decreasing CrCl. Similarly, a subanalysis of the REPLACE-2 trial demonstrated that the risk of ischemic and bleeding complications after PCI were 1.4-fold and 1.7-fold higher, respectively, in patients with CrCl <60 mL/min compared to patients with normal renal function (22). More mild degrees of CKD (CrCl >60 to 70 mL/min) were not evaluated in these trials.

A similar relationship between CrCl and outcomes appears to exist in the acutely ill. A subanalysis of the CADILLAC trial evaluated 350 patients with a CrCl ≤60 mL/min presenting for PCI within 12 hours of an acute MI (23). One-year mortality was markedly increased in patients with CKD versus patients with normal baseline renal function (7.5% versus 0.8%, p <0.0001) and mortality rates increased for every 10 mL/min decrease in baseline CrCl. There was an increased risk of bleeding and need for transfusion in the CKD group as well, and restenosis and infarct artery reocclusion rates were more common in patients with CKD (restenosis: 20.6% versus 11.8%, p = 0.024; reocclusion: 14.7% versus 7.3%, p = 0.02.). Multivariate analysis showed that CKD was one of the strongest independent predictors of decreased survival after PCI for acute MI.

Whether the ubiquitous use of stents improves outcomes in the mild to moderate CKD patient is not fully addressed by the previously mentioned studies, although available data are

Table 21–2

Stages of CKD as Outlined by the National Kidney Foundation Kidney Disease Outcomes Quality Initiative

Stage	Clinical Features	GFR (mL/min/1.73 m²)
1	Renal damage with normal or increased GFR	≥90
2	Renal damage with mild decrease in GFR	60–89
3	Moderate decrease in GFR	30–59
4	Severe decrease in GFR	15–29
5	Kidney failure	<15 or dialysis

Modified from: Best PJ, Reddan DN, Berger PB, et al. Cardiovascular disease and the chronic kidney disease: insights and an update. *Am Heart J.* 2004;148:230–242, with permission.

encouraging. In one study of 1,879 patients, the composite 3-year risk of need for revascularization, MI, or death was improved with stent use compared to balloon PCI nondialysis CKD. In addition, it appears that the improvement in TVR with DES applies to the CKD population, although data is limited. In a study of 543 consecutive patients receiving BMS compared to a subsequent group of 537 receiving sirolimus DES, 92 BMS and 94 DES patients with CrCl <60 mL/min at the time of PCI were identified, and the use of sirolimus DES was associated with a significant reduction in TVR at 1 year compared to BMS (6.9% versus 13.1%, p <0.01) (25). Six hundred forty-two patients with more mild degrees of CKD enrolled in TAXUS IV (419 with CrCl 60–89 and 223 with CrCl <60 mL/min) were similarly analyzed. The paclitaxel stent reduced one-year TVR compared to BMS irrespective of renal function (6.9 vs. 19%, p <0.0001, for CrCl >90 mL/min, 8.0 vs. 15.5%, p = 0.009, for CrCl 60–89 mL/min, 6.6 vs. 15.2%, p = 0.04, for CrCl <60 mL/min.). There was no significant difference in TVR for differing degrees of CKD within the paclitaxel group (26).

Although restenosis rates in patients with mild renal dysfunction (CrCl >60 mL/min) are similar to those with normal renal function, some controversy exists regarding whether death and MI rates are elevated in patients with just mild CKD. A posthoc analysis of the large elective stent restenosis PRESTO trial, comparing tranilast to placebo in patients with creatinine less than 1.8 mg/dL, 9-month angiographic restenosis was not increased with CKD, and there were no differences in MI, PCI, CABG, or TVR between the highest and lowest CrCl groups (more than 89 mL/min and less than 60 mL/min) (27). The lowest CrCl group did have a nearly threefold increased risk of death at 9 months compared to the highest CrCl group. However, after adjusting for other variables, CrCl was no longer independently associated with mortality.

How this study squares with others showing worse PCI outcomes in the setting of just mild CKD is unclear. For example, in one study, baseline creatinine level greater than 1.3 mg/dL was associated with a twofold increase in mortality and a 10% reduction in cumulative survival over 3 years in patients undergoing PCI (28). It may be that the variability in study design, controlling for confounders, and populations studied account for the differences between studies of mild CKD. Clearly, there is more certainty about the greater risk of poor outcomes in patients with more moderate CKD, especially when coexistent with conditions associated with rapid progression of CAD, like diabetes.

Given that the heightened risks of revascularization are apparent at nearly all levels of nondialysis CKD, how do CABG and PCI compare? While there are limited data on contemporary revascularization techniques, a substudy of the ARTS trial offers some insight (29). In this study, 290 patients, or 25% of the trial population, had CKD with roughly half receiving BMS and half CABG. At 3 years, there was no difference in the frequency of the individual outcomes of stroke, MI, or death between the treatment groups, and CABG was associated with one-third the rate of repeat revascularization compared with non-DES PCI (HR 0.28, 95% CI 0.14 to 0.54, p < 0.01). Additionally, this substudy corroborates older studies

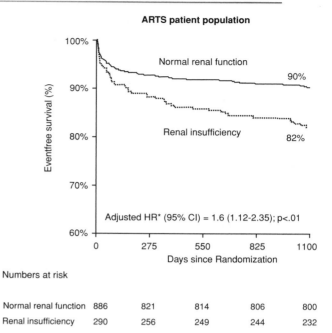

ARTS patient population

Figure 21–1.

Three-year Kaplan-Meier eventfree survival curves for death, stroke, or MI stratified according to renal function. Adjusted for diabetes mellitus, hypertension, ejection fracton, ACE inhibitor use, aspirin use, peripheral vascular disease, hemoglobin, silent ischemia, COPD, and hyperlipidemia. (Adapted from: Ix JH, Mercado N, Shlipak MG, et al. Association of chronic kidney disease with clinical outcomes after coronary revascularization: the Arterial Revascularization Therapies Study [ARTS]. *Am Heart J.* 2005;149:512–519, with permission.)

demonstrating the increased risk of adverse cardiac events in CKD patients undergoing PCI and CABG (Fig. 21–1). The acute coronary syndrome (ACS) patient with CKD undergoing revascularization may represent a special population. A non–randomized study in nondialysis–dependent patients with CrCL <60 mL/min presenting with ACS showed that patients undergoing PCI had better survival compared to CABG and medical therapy arms (30).

Adjunctive Medical Therapy

Most randomized trials demonstrating the efficacy of glycoprotein IIb/IIIa inhibitor use during PCI excluded patients with CKD, which is associated with numerous coagulation abnormalities and platelet dysfunction. Despite this, several subsequent studies have reported efficacy at a cost of at least mild bleeding. Abciximab, tirofiban, and eptifibatide all appear to improve ischemic outcomes in patients with CKD undergoing PCI to the degree it benefits patients with normal renal function, with reasonable overall safety. There is, however, a higher risk of at least minor bleeding (31–34). In an analysis of CKD patients in the TARGET trial, both ischemic and bleeding complications were highest in the lowest CrCl quartile of patients (less than 70 mL/min) treated with abciximab or tirofiban, with no significant difference between the two agents regarding ischemic or bleeding events (35).

As with the IIb/IIIa inhibitor trials, those evaluating the safety and efficacy of low molecular weight heparins excluded CKD patients. Enoxaparin is primarily renally excreted, is not approved for use in dialysis patients, but appears to be safe in patients with CrCl <30 mL/min when dose adjusted (1 mg/kg subcutaneously a day) (36). A study evaluating 174 patients presenting with non-ST MI with mean CrCl of 46 ± 27.6 mL/min showed that renally dosed enoxaparin provided adequate anti-Xa levels and no excess bleeding in the roughly 25% of patients who underwent PCI (37).

A subanalysis of patients with renal insufficiency enrolled in the REPLACE-2 trial, where bivalirudin with provisional glycoprotein IIb/IIIa inhibition was compared to heparin plus glycoprotein IIb/IIIa inhibition in elective PCI, bivalirudin resulted in ischemic event rates comparable to heparin and IIb/IIIa inhibitors (38). Fewer major bleeding events in renally impaired patients occurred in the bivalirudin group. Prospective randomized studies will be needed to determine the optimal procedural anticoagulation regimen in patients with CKD undergoing PCI.

Declining Renal Function after PCI

Acute renal dysfunction is a recognized potential complication of coronary angiography and intervention, particularly in the presence of CKD. Contrast-induced nephropathy (CIN) is the most common cause of worsening renal function after angiography and intervention and is defined as an absolute increase in the serum creatinine concentration of at least 0.5 mg/dL or relative increase of at least 25% from baseline at 48 hours. It typically presents 24 to 48 hours post contrast administration with a peak creatinine level in 3 to 5 days. In most cases, CIN is mild and self-limiting. The creatinine level usually returns to normal within a week, and dialysis is infrequently required. However, up to 30% of affected patients have residual renal impairment. Atheroembolic disease can contribute to acute renal failure after angiography and can be difficult to differentiate from CIN. An assessment for embolic phenomenon as a source of worsening renal impairment following contrast administration should be considered in selected patients (39).

Recent studies have shown that the development of CIN post-PCI portends a worse prognosis, irrespective of baseline renal function (40). The risk of CIN increases exponentially for patients with baseline creatinine of >1.2 mg/dL (Fig. 21–2) (41), although the risk of CIN is quite low in patients with normal renal function. In an analysis of 7,230 consecutive patients undergoing elective PCI, approximately with 19.2% with existing CKD (baseline Cr >1.5 mg/dL), and 13.1% without CKD, developed CIN (17). In an analysis of 7,230 consecutive patients undergoing elective PCI, major adverse cardiac events at 1 year occurred more frequently in patients with baseline CKD, especially those who developed CIN. Seventy-five percent of the small number of patients with CIN requiring in-hospital dialysis (n = 39) were dead at 1 year (42).

Risk Factors for CIN

Traditionally, baseline renal dysfunction and diabetes have been considered the strongest risk factors for CIN. Other fac-

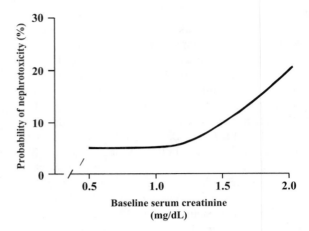

Figure 21–2.

The risk of developing CIN increases exponentially for patients with a baseline creatinine ≥1.2 mg/dL in patients presenting for cardiac catheterization. (Adapted from: Davidson CJ, Hlatky M, Morris KG, et al. Cardiovascular and renal toxicity of a nonionic radiographic contrast agent after cardiac catheterization. A prospective trial. *Ann Intern Med.* 1989;110:119–124, with permission.)

tors shown to independently predict the development of CIN after PCI include hypotension, intra-aortic balloon pump use, congestive heart failure, LVEF <40%, age >75 years, anemia, and volume of contrast used (17,43). Patients undergoing primary PCI for acute MI are at particularly high risk of developing CIN. In a study of 208 consecutive patients undergoing primary PCI for ST-segment elevation MI, fully 19% developed CIN (44). Patients who developed CIN were older and more frequently had anterior MI, higher baseline serum creatinine (40% when CrCl <60 mL/min and 13% when CrCl <60 mL/min, p <0.0001), longer time-to-reperfusion, greater cardiac enzyme peaks, and lower left ventricular ejection fractions. They also had longer hospital stays, more arrhythmias, and higher mortality rates (31% versus 6.2% in patients without CIN).

Strategies to Limit CIN

The risk of CIN can be modulated and is often preventable. Although many strategies have been tested (Table 21–3), adequate periprocedural hydration with 0.9% or 0.45% saline, typically at a rate of 1mL/kg for 12 hours before and after elective angiography, has the most proven benefit in reducing CIN. A comparison of saline, saline plus mannitol, or saline plus furosemide demonstrated no added benefit of mannitol or furosemide (45).

The specific contrast agent used impacts on the risk of developing CIN and cardiovascular events. The earliest contrast agents were hypertonic (1500 to 1800 mOsm/kg) and had frequent adverse hemodynamic and arrhythmogenic effects. Second generation agents with a 3:1 iodine to particle ratio were either nonionic or ionic low osmolar (between 600 to 850 mOsm/kg). Studies demonstrated that second generation contrast agents led to a reduction in CIN and cardiotoxicity compared to high osmolar agents (46). The newest contrast

Table 21–3

Measures to Prevent CIN

Proven
- Periprocedural hydration with normal saline
- Low or isosmolar contrast
- Contrast dose reduction (<30 mL) for diagnostic studies (<100 mL) for PCI

Possibly Beneficial
- Sodium bicarbonate infusion
- Ascorbic acid
- Theophylline
- N-acetylcysteine
- Hemofiltration
- Statin therapy

No Benefit or Deleterious
- Selective dopamine agonist fenoldopam
- High osmolar contrast media
- Furosemide
- Mannitol
- Dopamine
- Hemodialysis
- Endothelin antagonists
- Calcium channel blockers

The above table summarizes the efficacy of current treatment options to prevent CIN.

agent, iodixanol, has a 6:1 ratio, is isosmolar to human serum, and appears to further reduce the risk of CIN and major cardiovascular events (47,48).

There are conflicting data on the role of N-acetylcysteine (NAC) in preventing CIN. The most comprehensive meta-analysis reviewed 20 of the published trials involving 2,195 patients (49). There was a nonsignificant trend toward decreased CIN in patients treated with NAC. A large prospective randomized trial is needed before NAC can be routinely recommended for CIN prevention. Although the benefit of NAC is uncertain, it is safe, inexpensive, and has few reported side effects.

Paramount to the prevention of CIN is identifying patients at high risk (pre-existing CKD with CrCl <60 mL/min or creatinine >1.3 mg/dL, diabetes, periprocedural hypotension, anemia, and advanced age). All patients should be adequately hydrated pre- and postprocedure. Cardiac catheterization laboratories should ideally have biplane capabilities to minimize contrast dose in higher risk patients. Clinicians should have a low threshold to stage complex multivessel PCI procedures in high-risk patients when a high contrast load is anticipated. A nonionic isosmolar agent should be used in at-risk patients. Nephrototoxic agents and metformin should be held during the recovery period.

The Diabetic Patient

Patients with CKD and diabetes mellitus have significantly worse short- and long-term outcomes after PCI than those with either of these conditions alone (50). Mortality rates are higher during the index hospitalization and at 1 year, and the duration of hospital stay after PCI is longer. However, patients with diabetic nephropathy also have higher rates of MI, pulmonary edema, cardiogenic shock, neurologic events, and gastrointestinal bleeding after PCI than diabetic patients with preserved renal function. Diabetic patients already on dialysis have substantially worse survival after PCI than those with CKD but not on dialysis. Diabetic patients with proteinuria and normal creatinine clearance have worse long-term survival after PCI than diabetic patients without proteinuria. Even diabetic patients with normal renal function are at increased risk for CIN compared to nondiabetic patients.

Several clinical and anatomic features of CAD in diabetic patients contribute to worse outcomes after PCI compared to nondiabetics. Atherosclerotic plaques in diabetic patients are more lipid-rich, have larger necrotic cores, and contain more thrombus, fissures, inflammatory cells, and neovascularization. These features likely increase their risk of plaque rupture. The platelets of diabetic patients express more glycoprotein IIb/IIIa receptors and are more prone to aggregation, particularly in the presence of hyperglycemia. Diabetic patients undergoing PCI, on average, have lower left ventricular ejection fractions and worse angiographic profiles (51). They are more likely to have significant left main and multivessel disease. CAD in diabetic patients tends to be more diffuse, which corresponds to smaller angiographic reference segments. They also have a greater number of distal lesions. Although diabetic patients have more completely occluded segments, their ability to develop coronary collaterals is impaired. In addition, intravascular ultrasound has shown that diabetic patients are less likely to undergo favorable coronary remodeling in response to atherosclerosis. Diabetic patients also more frequently develop new coronary lesions after PCI compared to nondiabetic patients, particularly in instrumented vessels.

Revascularization Outcomes

Although the prevalence of diabetes is less than 10% in the United States, diabetic patients account for approximately 25% of all coronary revascularization procedures performed. Diabetic patients experience worse outcomes after CABG surgery or PCI compared to those without diabetes. Following CABG, they have increased perioperative morbidity and mortality as well as long-term mortality, particularly those who are insulin dependent. Diabetic patients who undergo PCI also have worse long-term survival and much higher rates of repeat revascularization, primarily due to target vessel restenosis. Diabetic patients also have more completely occlusive restenosis after PCI, a finding that independently correlates with increased long-term mortality. The interventionalist is frequently faced with the difficult choice in the diabetic patient with multivessel CAD between surgical consultation, PCI, or medical management. In making this decision, the latest outcome evidence available, ACC/AHA guidelines, and patient preferences must be taken into consideration.

There is a paucity of data from randomized controlled trials comparing CABG surgery and PCI in diabetic patients. Since its publication in 1996, the results of the Bypass Angioplasty

Revascularization Investigation (BARI) have formed the foundation for revascularization decisions in diabetic patients with multivessel CAD. In BARI, CABG and balloon-only PCI yielded similar rates of in-hospital and 5-year survival. However, in the subset of treated diabetic patients (n = 353), there was a 15% absolute survival advantage for CABG at 5 years (81.6% versus 64.5%, p = 0.003) (52). This survival advantage was limited to patients who received at least one internal mammary artery graft (81% in BARI). Diabetic patients in BARI who underwent CABG and subsequently suffered a spontaneous Q-wave MI in the first 5 years gained the most mortality benefit compared to PCI. The relative risk of death after a spontaneous Q-wave MI in CABG patients was 0.09 (95% CI 0.03 to 0.29) compared to 0.65 (95% CI 0.45 to 0.94) for those who did not suffer an MI (53). The CABG benefit was also more apparent in diabetic patients on insulin.

CABG provided more complete and durable revascularization than PCI in diabetic patients studied in the BARI trial (54). A greater percentage of significant lesions were successfully treated with CABG than PCI in BARI (87% versus 76%). Substantially more diabetic patients in the PCI arm of the BARI trial underwent at least one repeat revascularization procedure (69.9% versus 11.1% at 7 years). Angina rates at 5 years were higher after PCI than CABG (28% versus 18%, p = 0.03). Also, diabetic patients who underwent PCI had more jeopardized myocardium (territory supplied by arteries with >50% lesions) on follow-up angiography. However, after both PCI and CABG, new areas of myocardial jeopardy were more commonly due to arteries that were not initially revascularized. This illustrates the potential for rapid CAD progression following revascularization in diabetic patients.

Importantly, those patients eligible for BARI who elected not to be randomized were followed in a registry. Revascularization method was physician and patient-driven, and the majority underwent percutaneous revascularization (182 versus 117). There was no significant mortality difference between CABG and PCI at 5 years (14.4% versus 14.9%, p = 0.86) (55). Registry patients with three-vessel CAD and proximal LAD lesions more often underwent CABG, which suggested that patients with "surgical anatomy" were more likely referred for CABG.

PCI as performed in the BARI study does not resemble the current standard of care, which now includes drug-eluting stents, glycoprotein IIb/IIIa inhibitors, and improved medical therapy. The need for emergent CABG following PCI is much lower in the current era, primarily due to decreased abrupt vessel closure with stenting. In the diabetic subgroup (n = 208) of the Arterial Revascularization Therapy Study (ARTS), there was no significant mortality advantage for CABG over stent-assisted PCI at 1 or 3 years (56). This result occurred despite 89% internal mammary artery use in the CABG group. Although the use of stents decreased restenosis rates after PCI, diabetic patients in ARTS still required substantially more revascularization procedures after PCI than after CABG. The Angina with Extremely Serious Operative Mortality Evaluation (AWESOME) compared PCI (with stenting in 54%) and CABG in patients deemed to have very high operative risk. In the diabetic subgroup (n = 144), there was no statistically sig-

nificant difference in mortality throughout a 5-year follow-up period (57).

There are no specific ACC/AHA guidelines for PCI or CABG in diabetic patients. Although treated diabetes is defined as a specific cohort within the PCI guidelines, the CABG guidelines do not separately classify diabetic patients. When feasible, CABG is preferred in all patients with significant left main stenosis (>50%). CABG is also more highly recommended for patients with treated diabetes and multivessel CAD that includes a significant lesion of the proximal LAD. For diabetic patients with single-vessel CAD or two-vessel CAD not involving the proximal LAD, there is no consensus recommendation. With the most recent data in diabetic patients in mind, the algorithm depicted in Figure 21–3 (58) offers a strategy in deciding between CABG and PCI.

Adjunctive Medical Therapy

Aggressive antiplatelet therapy has further improved outcomes after PCI. The use of glycoprotein IIb/IIIa inhibitors has proved to be particularly effective in diabetic patients undergoing PCI. In a pooled analysis of diabetics in three PCI trials (n = 1462), abciximab led to a 2% mortality advantage (4.5% versus 2.5%, p = 0.03) at 1 year (59). In another meta-analysis of six studies, glycoprotein IIb/IIIa inhibitor use in diabetic patients (n = 1279) who underwent PCI while hospitalized for an acute coronary syndrome had a significant 30-day mortality reduction (4.0% versus 1.2%, p = 0.002) (60). In a subgroup of diabetic patients who underwent primary PCI with stenting (n = 53) for STEMI, treatment with abciximab was associated with a marked reduction in 6-month mortality (0% versus 16.7%, p = 0.02) (61). Based on the strength of the data in diabetic patients, glycoprotein IIb/IIIa inhibitors are strongly recommended in diabetic patients undergoing PCI, especially during an acute coronary syndrome.

Recent data support consideration for alternatives to glycoprotein IIb/IIIa inhibition in lower-risk diabetic patients undergoing PCI. In ISAR-SWEET, 701 diabetic patients received 600 mg of clopidogrel at least 2 hours before a planned PCI. Abciximab use did not reduce the composite incidence of death or MI at 1 year (8.3% versus 8.6%, p = 0.91) (62). Patients with recent acute coronary syndromes were excluded. Approximately 20% did not require medication for their diabetes. The use of abciximab was associated with a reduction in TLR at 1 year compared to the clopidogrel-only arm (23.2% versus 30.4%, p = 0.03). However, given the low use of DES, this is of questionable relevance in the DES era. It is important to emphasize the low-risk nature of the patients enrolled in ISAR-SWEET. For example, patients with recent acute coronary syndromes were excluded, and approximately 20% did not require medication for their diabetes.

In REPLACE-2, patients undergoing PCI were randomized to the direct thrombin inhibitor bivalirudin with provisional glycoprotein IIb/IIIa inhibition (7.7% of patients) versus heparin plus glycoprotein IIb/IIIa inhibition (abciximab or eptifibatide) (63). There were 1,624 diabetic patients included. Patients with acute MI, undergoing PCI as reperfusion therapy

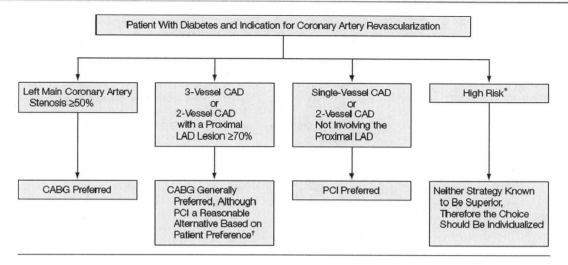

Figure 21–3.

Decision algorithm to help decide between CABG and PCI in diabetic patients. CABG indicates coronary artery bypass graft surgery; CAD, coronary artery disease; LAD, left anterior descending artery; PCI, percutaneous coronary intervention. (Reproduced from: Flaherty JD, Davidson CJ. Diabetes and coronary revascularization. *JAMA.* 2005;293:1501–1508, with permission.)

*Based on AWESOME criteria: medical refractory unstable angina plus one other high-risk feature (prior heart surgery, myocardial infarction within 7 days, left ventricular ejection fraction <35%, older than 70 years, or the use of a balloon pump).

†Based on the BARI trial and registry and ARTS.

were excluded. There was no statistically significant difference between bivalirudin and planned IIb/IIIa inhibition in the composite of death, MI, or urgent revascularization at 30 days (5.72% versus 5.88%) or in death at 1 year (2.28% versus 3.90%). There was less minor bleeding in the bivalirudin arm but no difference in major bleeding. Of note, more than 85% of patients were pretreated with clopidogrel. These studies suggest that in lower-risk diabetic patients undergoing PCI, glycoprotein IIb/IIIa use may be optional, particularly when pretreatment with clopidogrel is feasible.

Restenosis and Drug-Eluting Stents

Restenosis has long been a major limitation of PCI in diabetic patients. Insulin dependent diabetics have the highest restenosis rates, followed by those treated with oral hypoglycemic agents, and then diet-controlled individuals. When stents are used, the increased rates of restenosis observed in diabetic patients are entirely attributable to neointimal hyperplasia. The degree of hyperplasia correlates with glycemic control. Diabetic patients who achieve optimal glycemic control have rates of target vessel revascularization after PCI similar to nondiabetic patients. The use of thiazolidinediones in diabetic patients receiving bare-metal stents has been associated with reduced neointimal hyperplasia and less restenosis.

The introduction of the DES is a landmark advancement in interventional cardiology, especially for diabetic patients. Both rapamycin-eluting and paclitaxel-eluting stents have produced striking reductions in rates of angiographic restenosis and TLR in diabetic patients. In both the SIRIUS (rapamycin) and TAXUS IV (paclitaxel) trials, diabetic patients treated with DES had rates of TLR at 1 year of less than 10%, which was

roughly one third of the rate for bare-metal stents (64,65). Nevertheless, the rates of restenosis and TLR observed in diabetic patients treated with DES are still greater than those in patients without diabetes. The favorable results with DES in diabetic patients have been observed in both those treated with insulin and oral hypoglycemic agents. Small subgroup analysis suggest that insulin-dependent diabetic patients experience higher rates of restenosis and repeat revascularization after DES placement than the noninsulin-dependent or diet-controlled diabetic patients.

Data directly comparing rapamycin-eluting and paclitaxel-eluting stents suggest that the former DES may lead to less late-lumen loss and need for TLR in diabetic patients due to a smaller degree of neointimal hyperplasia (66). The impact of this on clinical outcomes is unknown, and further data are needed to demonstrate superiority of either product. No significant difference in death or MI has been observed between the two drug-eluting designs. The increased in-segment late-lumen loss observed in diabetic patients with both DES types suggest that deployment of DES from "normal-to-normal" arterial segments may have heightened importance in diabetic patients. Rather than focusing on the small differences that may exist in the two commercially available DES, it is more important to embrace the drug-eluting concept as the treatment of choice for PCI in diabetic patients. Further advances in drugs, polymers, elution platforms, and strut design hold promise to improve on the dramatic early success. The use of DES in unselected patients for difficult lesion types, such as restenosis, chronic total occlusion, left main lesions, and diffuse disease, has shown favorable early results and may eventually impact the breadth of revascularization that can be accomplished by PCI in diabetic patients.

Summary Points

- Dialysis patients have higher risk of death, MI, and restenosis after balloon or bare-metal stent PCI compared to controls.
- All-cause mortality in dialysis patients eligible for mechanical revascularization appears better with CABG than with PCI, especially in diabetics.
- In the nondialysis CKD patient, there is a strong association between death and MI and CrCl after BMS, but likely not TVR (especially true with DES).
- In the nondialysis CKD patient, CABG and BMS short/intermediate-term risk of death and MI may be equivalent, but the need for repeat revascularization is less with CABG. DES has not yet been fully studied.
- GP IIb/IIIa inhibitors improve ischemic outcomes in CKD patients undergoing PCI but at the cost of at least more minor bleeding.
- Abciximab can be used in dialysis patients and does not require renal dosing.
- Tirofiban can be used in dialysis patients, with renal dose adjustment.
- Eptifibitide is contraindicated in dialysis patients.
- The risk of CIN is highest in patients with pre-existing CKD and diabetes.
- The development of CIN portends worse outcomes.
- CIN requiring dialysis is particularly lethal.
- Effective means of preventing CIN include periprocedural hydration, limiting contrast volumes, staging interventions, and correctly identifying those at risk.
- Diabetic patients have worse angiographic profiles, including more left main, multivessel, and diffuse CAD.
- In the BARI trial, treated diabetics with multivessel CAD undergoing CABG had improved long-term survival compared to those undergoing balloon-only PCI. This benefit was limited to those receiving an internal mammary artery graft and was not observed in nondiabetics.
- According to the most recent AHA/ACC guidelines, CABG is the revascularization method of choice for diabetic patients with multivessel CAD involving the proximal LAD.
- The use of IIb/IIIa inhibitors with PCI in diabetic patients has been shown to improve survival, particularly in those with acute coronary syndromes.
- The increased rates of restenosis in diabetic patients following PCI with stenting (BMS or DES) is due to enhanced neointimal hyperplasia. Insulin use and poor glycemic control correlate with increased neointimal hyperplasia.
- Diabetic patients treated with DES have shown substantial reductions in angiographic restenosis and TLR. MACE rates are still higher than for nondiabetic patients.

REFERENCES

1. Sarnak MJ, Levy AS, Schoolwerth AC, et al. Kidney disease as a risk factor for development of cardiovascular disease. *Circulation.* 2003;108:2154–2169.
2. Foley RN, Murray AM, Li S, et al. Chronic kidney disease and the risk for cardiovascular disease, renal replacement, and death in the United States Medicare population, 1998 to 1999. *J Am Soc Nephrol.* 2005;16:489–495.
3. Luke RG. Chronic renal failure, a vasculopathic state. *N Engl J Med.* 1998;339:841–843.
4. Owen CH, Cummings RG, Sell TL, et al. Coronary artery bypass grafting in patients with dialysis-dependent renal failure. *Ann Thorac Surg.* 1994;58:1729–1733.
5. Ko W, Kreiger KH, Isom OW. Cardiopulmonary bypass procedures in dialysis patients. *Ann Thorac Surg.* 1993;55:677–684.
6. Kahn JK, Rutherford BD, McConahay DR, et al. Short and long-term outcome of percutaneous transluminal coronary angioplasty in chronic dialysis patients. *Am Heart J.* 1990;119:484–489.
7. Ahmed WH, Shubrooks SJ, Gibson M, et al. Complications and long-term outcome after percutaneous coronary angioplasty in chronic hemodialysis patients. *Am Heart J.* 1995;128:252–255.
8. Reusser LM, Osborn LA, White HJ, et al. Increased morbidity and mortality after coronary angioplasty in patients on chronic hemodialysis. *Am J Cardiol.* 1994;73:965–967.
9. Schoebel FC, Gradaus F, Ivens K, et al. Restenosis after elective coronary balloon angioplasty in patients with end stage renal disease: a case-control study using quantitative coronary angiography. *Heart.* 1997;778:337–342.
10. Azar RR, Prpic R, Ho KKL, et al. Impact of end-stage renal disease on clinical and angiographic outcomes after coronary stenting. *Am J Cardiol.* 2000;86:485–489.
11. Daemen J, Lemos P, Aoki J, et al. Treatment of coronary artery disease in dialysis patients with sirolimus-eluting stents: 1-year clinical follow-up of a consecutive series of cases. *J Invasive Cardiol.* 2004;16:685–687.
12. Hassani SE, Chu WW, Wolfram RM, et al. Clinical outcomes after percutaneous coronary intervention with drug-eluting stents in dialysis patients. *J Invasive Cardiol.* 2006;18:273–277.
13. Iakovou I, Schmidt T, Bonizzoni E, et al. Incidence, predictors, outcome of thrombosis after successful implantation of drug-eluting stents. *JAMA.* 2005;293:2126–2130.
14. Herzog CA, Ma JZ, Collins AJ. Comparative survival of dialysis dependent patients in the United States after coronary angioplasty, coronary artery stenting, and coronary artery bypass surgery and impact of diabetes. *Circulation.* 2002;106:2207–2211.
15. Best PJ, Reddan DN, Berger PB, et al. Cardiovascular disease and the chronic kidney disease: insights and an update. *Am Heart J.* 2004;148:230–242.
16. Tadros GM, Herzog CA. Percutaneous coronary intervention in chronic kidney disease patients. *J Nephrol.* 2004;17:364–368.
17. Mangano CM, Diamondstone LS, Ramsay JG, et al. Renal dysfunction after myocardial revascularization: risk factors, adverse outcomes, and hospital resource utilization. The Multicenter Study of Perioperative Ischemia Research Group. *Ann Intern Med.* 1998;128:194–203.
18. Shroyer AL, Grover FL, Edwards FH. 1995 coronary artery risk model: The Society of Thoracic Surgeons Adult Cardiac National Database. *Ann Thorac Surg.* 1998;65:879–884.
19. Anderson RJ, O'Brien M, MaWhinney S, et al. Renal failure predisposes patients to adverse outcomes after coronary bypass surgery. VA cooperative study #5. *Kidney Int.* 1999;55:1057–1062.
20. Weerasinghe A, Hornick P, Smith P, et al. Coronary artery bypass grafting in non-dialysis-dependent mild-to-moderate renal dysfunction. *J Thorac Cardiovasc Surg.* 2001;121:1083–1089.
21. Best PJM, Lennon R, Ting HH, et al. The impact of renal insufficiency on clinical outcomes in patients undergoing percutaneous coronary interventions. *J Am Coll Cardiol.* 2002;39:1113–1119.
22. Chew DP, Lincoff M, Gurm H, et al. Bivalirudin versus heparin and glycoprotein IIb/IIIa inhibition among patients with renal impairment undergoing percutaneous coronary intervention (a subanalysis of the REPLACE-2 trial). *Am J Cardiol.* 2005;95:581–585.
23. Sadeghi HM, Stone GW, Grines CL, et al. Impact of renal insufficiency in patients undergoing primary angioplasty for acute myocardial infarction. *Circulation.* 2003;108:2769–2775.
24. Stigant C, Izadnegahdar M, Levin A, et al. Outcomes after percutaneous coronary intervention in patients with CKD: improved outcome in the stenting era. *Am J Kidney Dis.* 2005;45:1002–1009.
25. Lemos PA, Arampatzis CA, Hoye A, et al. Impact of baseline renal function on mortality after percutaneous coronary intervention with

sirolimus-eluting stents or bare metal stents. *Am J Cardiol.* 2005;95:167–172.

26. Halkin A, Mehran R, Casey CW, et al. Impact of moderate renal insufficiency on restenosis and adverse clinical events after paclitaxel-eluting and bare metal stent implantation: Results from the TAXUS-IV Trial. *Am Heart J.* 2005;150:1163–1170.

27. Best PJ, Berger PB, Davis BR, et al. Impact of mild or moderate chronic kidney disease on the frequency of restenosis: results from the PRESTO trial. *J Am Coll Cardiol.* 2004;44:1786–1791.

28. Reinecke H, Trey T, Matzkies F, et al. Grade of chronic renal failure, and acute and long-term outcome after percutaneous coronary interventions. *Kidney Int.* 2003;63:696–701.

29. Ix JH, Mercado N, Shlipak MG, et al. Association of chronic kidney disease with clinical outcomes after coronary revascularization: the Arterial Revascularization Therapies Study (ARTS). *Am Heart J.* 2005;149:512–519.

30. Keeley EC, Kadakia R, Soman S, et al. Analysis of long-term survival after revascularization in patients with chronic kidney disease presenting with acute coronary syndromes. *Am J Cardiol.* 2003;92:509–514.

31. Freeman RV, Mehta RH, Al Badr W, et al. Influence of concurrent renal dysfunction on outcomes of patients with acute coronary syndromes and implications of the use of glycoprotein IIb/IIIa inhibitors. *J Am Coll Cardiol.* 2003;41:718–724.

32. Jeremias A, Bhatt DL, Chew DP, et al. Safety of abciximab during percutaneous coronary intervention in patients with chronic renal insufficiency. *Am J Cardiol.* 2002;89:1209–1211.

33. Best PJM, Lennon R, Gersh BJ, et al. Safety of abciximab in patients with chronic renal insufficiency who are undergoing percutaneous coronary interventions. *Am Heart J.* 2003;146:345–350.

34. Januzzi JL Jr, Snapinn SM, DiBattiste PM, et al. Benefits and safety of tirofiban among acute coronary syndrome patients with mild to moderate renal insufficiency: results from the Platelet Receptor Inhibition in Ischemic Syndrome Management in Patients Limited by Unstable Signs and Symptoms (PRISM-PLUS) trial. *Circulation.* 2002;105:2361–2366.

35. Berger PB, Best PJ, Topol EJ, et al. The relation of renal function to ischemic and bleeding outcomes with 2 different glycoprotein IIb/IIIa inhibitors: the do Tirofiban and ReoPro Give Similar Efficacy Outcome (TARGET) trial. *Am Heart J.* 2005;149:869–875.

36. Hulot J-S, Montalescot G, Lechat P, et al. Dosing strategy in patients with renal failure receiving enoxaparin for the treatment of non-ST segment elevation acute coronary syndrome. *Clin Pharmacol Ther.* 2005;77:542–552.

37. Collet J-P, Montalescot G, Fine E, et al. Enoxaparin in unstable angina patients who would have been excluded from randomized pivotal trials. *J Am Coll Cardiol.* 2003;41:8–14.

38. Chew DP, Lincoff M, Gurm H, et al. Bivalirudin versus heparin and glycoprotein IIb/IIIa inhibition among patients with renal impairment undergoing percutaneous coronary intervention (a subanalysis of the REPLACE-2 trial). *Am J Cardiol.* 2005;95:581–585.

39. Murphy SW, Barrett BJ, Parfrey PS. Contrast nephropathy. *J Am Soc Nephrol.* 2000;11:177–182.

40. Aspelin P, Aubry P, Fransson SG, et al. Nephrotoxic effects in high-risk patients undergoing angiography. *N Engl J Med.* 2003;348:491–499.

41. Davidson CJ, Hlatky M, Morris KG, et al. Cardiovascular and renal toxicity of a nonionic radiographic contrast agent after cardiac catheterization. A prospective trial. *Ann Intern Med.* 1989;110:119–124.

42. Dangas G, Iakovou I, Nikolsky E, et al. Contrast-induced nephropathy after percutaneous coronary interventions in relation to chronic kidney disease and hemodynamic variables. *Am J Cardiol.* 2005;95:13–19.

43. Mehran R, Aymong ED, Nikolsky E, et al. A simple risk score for prediction of contrast-induced nephropathy after percutaneous intervention. *J Am Coll Cardiol.* 2004;44:1393–1399.

44. Marenzi G, Lauri G, Assanelli E, et al. Contrast-induced nephropathy in patients undergoing primary angioplasty for acute myocardial infarction. *J Am Coll Cardiol.* 2004;44:1780–1785.

45. Solomon R, Werner C, Mann D, et al. Effects of saline, mannitol, and furosemide on acute decreases in renal function induced by radiocontrast agents. *N Engl J Med.* 1994;331:1416–1420.

46. Rudnick MR, Goldfarb S, Wexler L, et al. Nephrotoxicity of ionic and nonionic contrast media in 1196 patients: a randomized trial. The Iohexol Cooperative Study. *Kidney Int.* 1995;47:254–261.

47. Aspelin P, Aubry P, Fransson SG, et al. Nephrotoxic effects in high-risk patients undergoing angiography. *N Engl J Med.* 2003;348:491–499.

48. Davidson CJ, Laskey WK, Hermiller JB, et al. Randomized trial of contrast media utilization in high-risk PTCA: The COURT trial. *Circ.* 2000;101:2172–2177.

49. Nallamothu BK, Shojania KG, Saint S, et al. Is acetylcysteine effective in preventing contrast–related nephropathy? A meta-analysis. *Am J Med.* 2004;117:938–947.

50. Nikolsky E, Mehran R, Turcot D, et al. Impact of chronic kidney disease on prognosis of patients with diabetes mellitus treated with percutaneous coronary intervention. *Am J Cardiol.* 2004;94:300–305.

51. Ledru F, Ducimetiere P, Battaglia S, et al. New diagnostic criteria for diabetes and coronary artery disease: insights from an angiographic study. *J Am Coll Cardiol.* 2001;37:1543–1550.

52. Bypass Angioplasty Revascularization Investigation (BARI) Investigators. Comparison of coronary bypass surgery with angioplasty in patients with multivessel disease. *N Engl J Med.* 1996;335:217–225.

53. Detre KM, Lomardero MS, Brooks MM, et al. The effects of previous coronary-artery bypass surgery on the prognosis of patients with diabetes who have acute myocardial infarction. *N Engl J Med.* 2000;342:989–997.

54. Bypass Angioplasty Revascularization Investigation (BARI) Investigators. Seven-year outcome in the Bypass Angioplasty Revascularization Investigation (BARI) by treatment and diabetic status. *J Am Coll Cardiol.* 2000;35:1122–1129.

55. Detre KM, Guo P, Holubkov R, et al. Coronary revascularization in diabetic patients: a comparison of the randomized and observational components of the Bypass Angioplasty Revascularization Investigation (BARI). *Circulation.* 1999;99:633–640.

56. Legrand VM, Serruys PW, Unger R, et al. Three-year outcome after coronary stenting versus bypass surgery for the treatment of multivessel disease. *Circulation.* 2004;109:1114–1120.

57. Sedlis SP, Morrison DA, Lorin JD, et al. Percutaneous coronary intervention versus coronary bypass graft surgery for diabetic patients with unstable angina and risk factors for adverse outcomes with bypass: outcome of diabetic patients in AWESOME randomized trial and registry. *J Am Coll Cardiol.* 2002;40:1555–1566.

58. Flaherty JD, Davidson CJ. Diabetes and coronary revascularization. *JAMA.* 2005;293:1501–1508.

59. Bhatt DL, Marso SP, Lincoff M, et al. Abciximab reduces mortality in diabetics following percutaneous coronary intervention. *J Am Coll Cardiol.* 2000;35:922–928.

60. Roffi M, Chew DP, Mukherjee D, et al. Platelet glycoprotein IIb/IIIa inhibitors reduce mortality in diabetic patients with non-ST-segment-elevation acute coronary syndromes. *Circulation.* 2001;104:2767–2771.

61. Montalescot G, Barragan P, Wittenberg O, et al. ADMIRAL investigators. Platelet glycoprotein IIb/IIIa inhibition with coronary stenting for acute myocardial infarction. *N Engl J Med.* 2001;344:1895–1903.

62. Mehilli J, Kastrati A, Schuhlen H, et al. ISAR-SWEET Investigators. Randomized clinical trial of abciximab in diabetic patients undergoing elective percutaneous coronary intervention after treatment with a high loading dose of clopidogrel. *Circulation.* 2004;110:3627–3635.

63. Gurm HS, Sarembock IJ, Kereiakes DJ, et al. Use of bivalirudin during percutaneous intervention in patients with diabetes mellitus: an analysis from the Randomized Evaluation in Percutaneous Coronary Linking Angiomax to Reduced Clinical Events (REPLACE)-2 Trial. *J Am Coll Cardiol.* 2005;45:1932–1938.

64. Moussa I, Leon MB, Baim DS. Impact of sirolimus-eluting stents on outcome in diabetic patients: a SIRIUS (SIRolImUS-coated Bx Velocity balloon-expandable stent in the treatment of patients with de novo coronary artery lesions) substudy. *Circulation.* 2004;109:2273–2278.

65. Hermiller JB, Raizner A, Cannon L, et al. TAXUS-IV Investigators. Outcomes with the polymer-based paclitaxel-eluting TAXUS stent in patients with diabetes mellitus: the TAXUS-IV trial. *J Am Coll Cardiol.* 2005;45:1172–1179.

66. Dibra A, Kastrati A, Mehilli J, et al. Paclitaxel-eluting or sirolimus-eluting stents to prevent restenosis in diabetic patients. *N Engl J Med.* 2005;353:663–670.

CHAPTER 22

Acute Non-ST Segment Elevation Myocardial Infarction

Timothy A. Sanborn

Clinical Pathophysiology

As compared to previous views that a progressive narrowing of a coronary lumen by obstructive plaque led to unstable angina or myocardial infarction, it is now well established that rupture of an atherosclerotic plaque and resultant coronary thrombosis leads to the clinical presentation of acute coronary syndromes. If the thrombosis is 100% occlusive and sustained, then the clinical presentation is that of an ST segment elevation myocardial infarction (STEMI), which is discussed further in the chapter on Acute Myocardial Infarction. However, if the thrombus formation remains nonocclusive or lyses, then the clinical picture may be that of unstable angina or a non-ST segment myocardial infarction (NSTEMI). If the thrombotic occlusion is transient, then the clinical manifestation is that of unstable angina without myocardial damage. A more prolonged occlusion results in cell death and myocardial damage as NSTEMI. NSTEMI is also caused by dislodgement and embolization of platelet-rich microthrombi into the coronary microvasculature, which blocks blood flow and causes heart muscle death.

Blood platelets are now known to play a central role in the pathophysiology of NSTEMI. With disruption of an atherosclerotic plaque from internal or external triggers there is an effort to protect against blood loss. The subendothelial matrix of collagen and tissue factor is exposed to circulating blood, and a monolayer of platelets adheres to the site of injury. Platelets then become activated, degranulate, change their shape, and activate glycoprotein IIb-IIIa receptors (GP IIb-IIIa) on the platelet surface. Circulating platelets are likewise activated by the degranulation products of the platelet monolayer, and their GP IIb-IIIa receptors are also activated. Adhesive glycoproteins, such as fibrinogen, which is capable of binding two GP IIb-IIIa receptors, then cross links two platelets together. Repetitive platelet activation and fibrinogen cross linking brings about platelet aggregation, which can then lead to occlusive thrombus formation and/or microembolization downstream to the microvasculature. Thus, the platelet GP IIb-IIIa receptor is the final common pathway in platelet aggregation leading to NSTEMI.

Initial Evaluation

When evaluating a patient who may or may not have a NSTEMI, it is important to consider several factors. While chest pain from an acute myocardial infarction is classically described as being a substernal tightness or heaviness with associated shortness of breath and sweating, atypical presentations (epigastric pain, pain in jaw or neck, etc.) must also be considered, particularly in women. The physical examination may also be noncontributory. However, diaphoresis or cool skin, an unexplained sinus tachycardia, basal rales, a third or fourth heart sound, and hypotension should be an alert to consider NSTEMI.

An immediate baseline 12-lead electrocardiogram (performed within 10 minutes) and continuous ECG monitoring for at least 24 hours are ACC/AHA Guidelines Class I recommendations for the evaluation and management of patients with suspected NSTEMI (1). It should be remembered that patients presenting with ST depression have an increased risk for long term mortality compared to patients with T wave inversions, right bundle branch block, or nonspecific ST-T wave changes (2).

Cardiac-specific troponin measurement is the preferred biomarker of cardiac injury for patients who present with signs and symptoms consistent with NSTEMI, as it provides greater sensitivity and specificity than other biochemical markers of cardiac injury and is important for risk stratification (1). Elevated troponin concentrations provide prognostic information beyond that supplied by clinical characteristics and the initial ECG. Furthermore, there is a quantitative relationship between the quantity of troponin measured and the risk of death (3). If the initial 12-lead ECG and cardiac marker levels are normal, a patient suspected of having a NSTEMI should be observed in a facility for cardiac monitoring and repeat ECG and troponin levels should be obtained in 6 to 12 hours, as the sensitivity of cardiac troponins are lower in the very early phase of myocardial infarction.

Immediate Medical Management

Algorithms for the risk stratification of patients with symptoms suggestive of acute coronary syndromes including NSTEMI and acute ischemia pathways were published as ACC/AHA Guidelines in 2000 (4) and updated in 2002 (1). The reader should be thoroughly familiar with the Class I and II recommendations for anti-ischemic therapy including bed rest, nitrates, oxygen, morphine, beta blocker, and intra-aortic balloon pump counterpulsation if necessary for (a) severe ischemia that is recurring or continuing despite intensive medical therapy or (b) hemodynamic instability before or after coronary angiography. Based on the results of the CURE trial (5) and the trials of GP IIb/IIIa antagonists (6,7), the 2002 update to the guidelines (1) revised the recommendations for antiplatelet therapy (aspirin, clopidogrel, and platelet GP IIb/IIIa inhibitors) for patients with NSTEMI. Again, the reader should be very familiar with these recommendations, including the use of clopidogrel in patients intolerant of aspirin and the use of these drugs for patients in whom either an interventional (PCI or CABG) or a noninterventional approach is planned. Anticoagulation therapy (heparin or low molecular weight heparin) is also recommended. The Class III recommendations for which there is evidence and/or general agreement that the procedure/treatment is not useful/effective and in some cases may be harmful should also be remembered. For example, intravenous fibrinolytic therapy is not recommended in patients without acute ST-segment elevation, a true posterior MI, or a presumed new left bundle-branch block (Class III recommendation). The guidelines also caution against the use of nitrates within 24 hours of sildenafil (Viagra) use and the use of immediate-release dihydropyridine calcium antagonists in the absence of a beta blocker. The new ACC/AHA Guideline Class I, II, and III recommendations are listed in Table 22–1.

Rationale for an Aggressive Approach

Two different treatment strategies based on an "early conservative" or an "early invasive" approach were outlined in the 2000 ACC/AHA Guidelines. The early invasive strategy recommended that patients without clinically obvious contraindication to coronary revascularization should undergo coronary angiography and appropriate revascularization as compared to waiting for evidence of recurrent ischemia or a positive stress test despite medical therapy in the conservative strategy. Since those guidelines were published, two important randomized clinical trials (FRISC II and TACTICS-TIMI 18) comparing these two strategies were reported (8,9). Of these two trials, TACTICS-TIMI 18 is the most relevant in today's clinical practice, as routine coronary angiography was performed within 48 hours and was followed by revascularization when suitable in the early invasive strategy. In this trial, major cardiac events of death, myocardial (re)infarction, or rehospitalization within 6 months occurred significantly less in the invasive as compared to the conservative strategy. The occurrence of death or MI was also reduced at 6 months. Patients at high-risk or those with elevated troponin levels benefited the most from this early invasive strategy. These high-risk indicators are summarized in Table 22–2 and included the following: recurrence of angina/ischemia at rest, elevated troponin, ST-segment de-

---

Table 22–1

ACC/AHA Guideline Class I, II, and III Recommendations for Antiplatelet and Anticoagulant Therapy

Class I

- Administer ASA immediately and continue indefinitely. (Level of evidence A.)
- Use clopidogrel for patients unable to take ASA. (Level of evidence A.)
- For an early noninvasive approach, add clopidogrel to ASA as soon as possible and give at least 1 month (Level of evidence A) and for up to 9 months. (Level of evidence B.)
- For early PCI, clopidogrel should be started and given for at least 1 month (Level of evidence A) and up to 9 months in patients not at high risk for bleeding. (Level of evidence B.)
- In patients taking clopidogrel, for elective CABG, the drug should be withheld for 5 to 7 days. (Level of evidence B.)
- Anticoagulation with subcutaneous LMWH or IV unfractionated heparin (UFH) should be added to antiplatelet therapy with ASA and/or clopidogrel. (Level of evidence A.)
- A platelet IIb/IIIa antagonist should be administered, in addition to ASA and heparin, to patients in whom catheterization and PCI are planned. This may be done just prior to the PCI. (Level of evidence A.)

Class IIa

- Eptifibatide or tirofiban should be administered, in addition to ASA and LMWH or UFH, to patients with continuing ischemia, an elevated troponin, or with other high-risk features in whom an invasive strategy is *not* planned. (Level of evidence A.)
- Enoxaparin is preferable to UFH as an anticoagulant in patients with UA/NSTEMI unless CABG is planned within 24 hours. (Level of evidence A.)
- A IIb/IIIa antagonist should be administered to patients already receiving heparin, ASA, and clopidogrel in whom catheterization and PCI are planned. (Level of evidence B.)

Class IIb

- Eptifibatide or tirofiban should be administered, in addition to ASA and LMWH or UFH, to patients *without* continuing ischemia who have no other high-risk features and in whom PCI is *not* planned. (Level of evidence A.)

Class III

- Intravenous fibrinolytic therapy should be used in patients without acute ST-segment elevation, a true posterior MI, or a presumed new left bundle branch block (LBBB). (Level of evidence A.)
- Abciximab should be administered to patients in whom PCI is not planned. (Level of evidence A.)

---

pression, CHF, high-risk findings on noninvasive stress testing, LVEF less than 40%, hemodynamic instability, PCI within 6 months, or prior CABG. In the absence of these high-risk factors, the outcomes with these two strategies were the same. The routine use of GP IIb/IIIa inhibitors in the TACTICS-TIMI

Table 22–2

High-Risk Indicators for NSTEMI Patients

- Recurrent angina/ischemia at rest or with minimal activity on intensive anti-ischemic therapy
- Elevated troponin (I or T)
- New or presumably new ST depression
- Recurrent ischemia with CHF, S3, pulmonary edema, worsening rales, or worsening MR
- High-risk stress test findings
- Depressed LVEF (<0.40) on noninvasive testing
- Hemodynamic instability
- Sustained VT
- PCI within 6 months
- Prior CABG

Adapted from: Braunwald E, Antman EWM, Beasley JW, et al. ACC/AAHA 2002 guideline update for the management of patients with unstable angina and non-ST-segment elevation myocardial infarction-summary article. A report of the American College of Cardiology/American Heart Association task force on practice guidelines (committee on the management of patients with unstable angina). *J Am Coll Cardiol.* 2002;40:1366–1374.

18 trial may have prevented the excess risk of early acute MI in the invasive arm of the study. Thus, an invasive strategy is associated with a better clinical outcome in high-risk NSEMI patients who receive a GP IIb/IIIa inhibitor. Specific recommendations for the use of an invasive strategy were revised in the ACC/AHA 2002 guidelines update (1).

In terms of the type of coronary revascularization that is performed (PCI or CABG), the indications for revascularization versus medical therapy in patients with NSTEMI are the same as those for patients with chronic stable angina and the 1999 ACC/AHA/ACP-ASIM Guidelines for the Management of Patients With Chronic Stable Angina (10) should be reviewed. The specific Class I and II recommendations for PCI and CABG for left main, one-, two-, or three-vessel coronary artery disease as well as Class III recommendations for revascularization are summarized on pages 2161–2162 of this document.

Risk Factor Modification

While it is now established that patients with NSTEMI who are at high risk benefit from an early aggressive strategy of coronary angiography and appropriate revascularization, it is also important to follow this aggressive invasive strategy with prevention of recurrent ischemia through secondary prevention. Drugs that have been shown to provide long-term benefit include aspirin, clopidogrel, beta blockers, ACE inhibitors, and statins. The specific recommendations for the use of these drugs postdischarge are summarized in the ACC/AHA Guideline for NSTEMI (1,4).

REFERENCES

1. Braunwald E, Antman EWM, Beasley JW, et al. ACC/AAHA 2002 guideline update for the management of patients with unstable angina and non-ST-segment elevation myocardial infarction-summary article. A report of the American College of Cardiology/American Heart Association task force on practice guidelines (committee on the management of patients with unstable angina). *J Am Coll Cardiol.* 2002;40:1366–1374.
2. Savonitto S, Ardissino D, Granger CB, et al. Prognostic value of the admission electrocardiogram in acute coronary syndromes. *JAMA.* 1999;281:707–713.
3. Antman EM, Tanasijevic MJ, Thompson B, et al. Cardiac-specific troponin I levels to predict the risk of mortality in patients with acute coronary syndromes. *N Engl J Med.* 1996;335:1342–1349.
4. Braunwald E, Antman EWM, Beasley JW, et al. ACC/AAHA guidelines for the management of patients with unstable angina and non-ST-segment elevation myocardial infarction: executive summary and recommendations. A report of the American College of Cardiology/American Heart Association task force on practice guidelines (committee on the management of patients with unstable angina). *Circulation.* 2000;102:1193–1209.
5. Yusuf S, Zhao F, Mehta SR, et al. Effects of clopidogrel in addition to aspirin in patients with acute coronary syndromes without ST-segment elevation. *N Engl J Med.* 2001;345:494–502.
6. The ESPRIT Investigators. Novel dosing regimen of eptifibatide in planned coronary stent implantation (ESPRIT): a randomized, placebo-controlled trial. *Lancet.* 2000;356:2034–2037.
7. Topol EJ, Moliterno DJ, Herrmann HC, et al. Comparison of two platelet glycoprotein IIb/IIIa inhibitors, tirofiban and abciximab, for the prevention of ischemic events with percutaneous coronary revascularization. *N Engl J Med.* 2001;344:1888–1894.
8. The FRagmin and Fast Revascularisation during InStability in Coronary artery disease Investigators. Invasive compared with non-invasive treatment in unstable coronary-artery disease: FRISC II prospective randomized multicentre study. *Lancet.* 1999;354:708–715.
9. Cannon CP, Weintraub WAS, Demopoulos LA, et al. Comparison of early invasive and conservative strategies in patients with unstable coronary syndromes treated with the glycoprotein IIb/IIIa inhibitor tirofiban. *N Engl J Med.* 2001;344:1879–1887.
10. Gibbons RJ, Chatterjee K, Levy D, et al. ACC/AHA/ACP-ASIM guidelines for the management of patients with chronic stable angina. *J Am Coll Cardiol.* 1999;33:2092–2198.

CHAPTER 23

Cardiogenic Shock

Timothy A. Sanborn

Cardiogenic shock represents the most serious complication of acute myocardial infarction because it is associated with an extremely high mortality rate and is responsible for the majority of deaths associated with acute myocardial infarction (1–8). Historically, the mortality rate for cardiogenic shock was 80% to 90%. In the SHOCK Trial (8), early revascularization with percutaneous coronary intervention (PCI) or bypass surgery (CABG) was shown to significantly decrease mortality when compared to conservative medical management; however, there is still room for improvement in treatment strategies and adjunctive therapies.

Incidence

The incidence of cardiogenic shock has remained relatively constant for the last few decades (3,4). In a longitudinal single community study, from 1975 to 1997, the incidence averaged 7.1% (3), whereas in the second National Registry of Myocardial Infarction (NRMI) from 1994 to 1997, the incidence was 6.2% (9). Cardiogenic shock may occur in the setting of ST-segment elevation myocardial infarction (STEMI) as well as non–ST-segment elevation myocardial infarction (NSTEMI) (5–7), although with NSTEMI, the frequency is only approximately one half of that seen with STEMI.

The timing of shock also varies (2,6,9,10). Typically, only 10% to 15% of the patients have shock on admission. More commonly, shock develops within 48 hours of infarction. In the TRACE registry (6), 59% of the patients developed shock within 48 hours of symptom onset. In the remainder of the patients, it may develop considerably later sometimes as late as two weeks post infarction. Patients with early shock development in days 1 to 2 had significantly lower 30-day mortality than those with later shock development.

Etiology

The pathophysiology of shock also varies. Most commonly, in approximately three quarters of patients, cardiogenic shock is the result of left ventricular failure (11). However, other etiologies should always be considered. In the SHOCK Trial Registry (11), the incidence of other etiologies of cardiogenic shock were as follows: severe mitral regurgitation (8.3%), ventricular septal rupture (4.6%), right ventricular infarction (3.4%),

and cardiac tamponade (1.7%). It is extremely important to recognize these other causes of cardiogenic shock because of the different therapeutic options such as emergency surgery, which must be considered for optimal management. Emergent echocardiography or right and left heart catheterization is crucial for the early diagnosis of these mechanical complications of cardiogenic shock. Hypotension due to aggressive diuresis is sometimes confused with cardiogenic shock. Patients with right ventricular infarction may also present with cardiogenic shock. Mortality is unexpectedly high in patients with predominant right ventricular shock and is similar to patients with shock due to left ventricular dysfunction (12). As with patients with left ventricular dysfunction, these patients had a similar benefit from revascularization. For patients in cardiogenic shock, left ventricular function and the culprit vessel were independent correlates of 1-year survival (13).

Treatment Strategies

Given the high mortality rate associated with cardiogenic shock, there has been intense interest in developing treatment strategies. Emergent management should include oxygen, pressors (dobutamine, dopamine, or norepinephrine), intra-aortic balloon counterpulsation, and a temporary pacemaker for symptomatic bradycardia. Although thrombolytic therapy, one of the mainstays of reperfusion therapy for infarction has been studied in this group, the results have been variable. It appears that in patients with acute myocardial infarction who have been treated with fibrinolytic therapy, the chances of subsequently developing shock are decreased (14,15). Once shock develops, however, fibrinolytic therapy has not been shown to have a significant survival benefit. This may be due to poor delivery of IV fibrinolytic agents to the site of coronary occlusion in shock patients.

Circulatory support devices have also been used empirically (16–18). Intra-aortic balloon pump counterpulsation (IABP) has been used in the setting of cardiogenic shock for 30 years, and placement of this device is an ACC/AHA Guideline Class 1 recommendation (19). It is almost always used in combination with either fibrinolytic therapy or revascularization. Combined with fibrinolysis in the NRMI-2 Database, intra-aortic balloon counter pulsation was associated with a significant reduction in mortality from 67% to 49% (16). Similarly, in the Shock

Registry, this combination was also associated with a significant reduction of mortality from 63% to 47% (17). This synergy, which has also been noted in GUSTO I and GUSTO III, may relate to several factors including improved delivery of drugs to the site of occlusion or improved penetration into the thrombus (20). The independent role of IABP when used in combination with PCI is harder to define, although it appears to facilitate PCI and may improve its safety.

Other circulatory devices have also been used (21–23), including peripheral cardiopulmonary bypass and a variety of ventricular assist devices. Partial left heart bypass has also been evaluated. Recently, trans-septal placed bypass systems have also been released for percutaneous cardiac support. Although these devices can improve and stabilize hemodynamics, they are not readily available and require specialized skill, in part because of the large-sized catheters required for system operation.

Early Revascularization

Given the severity of the underlying coronary anatomy (7), and the limited success rates with medical therapy for cardiogenic shock, revascularization has received considerable interest and attention. Beginning in the 1980s, PCI was applied, initially in single center observational series. In a recent review, Lane identified 22 reports and made several important observations (24). Lane stated that the procedural success rate was associated with improved outcome compared to historical controls. Even with a successful procedure, however, mortality was still high at 35%. Lane also stated that if PTCA failed, the mortality was substantially higher, averaging 79.9%.

In parallel with these single institutional experiences, in large-scale randomized fibrinolytic trials, patients who either had shock or developed it were included, and some of these patients underwent PTCA. In one of the largest experiences of shock published to date, the GUSTO-I investigators evaluated the outcome of shock in 2,972 patients (2). In this trial, PCI was associated with a 30-day mortality of 30% to 40% compared to 60% 30-day mortality in those patients treated with fibrinolytic therapy. Several other studies have also documented the association between aggressive treatment strategies with revascularization and improved survival, including the Worcester Heart Attack Study (3), NRMI-2 Registry (9), California State Database (25), and GUSTO-III (4). In these studies, using multivariate logistic regression analyses, an invasive strategy was independently associated with a reduction in mortality. It must be remembered that selection bias may play a major role in affecting outcome. Patients in randomized fibrinolytic trials who underwent intervention have been typically younger with fewer other adverse baseline characteristics. For this reason, the SHOCK trial (8) was conducted, which randomly assigned patients with shock due to predominately impaired left ventricular function in the setting of ST-segment elevation myocardial infarction or new left bundle branch block to either an early revascularization strategy (angioplasty 55%,

bypass surgery 38%) within 6 hours of randomization or intensive medical stabilization and delayed (≥54 hours) revascularization if clinically and angiographically appropriate. IABP support was used in both limbs in 86% of patients. The primary endpoint in this trial was 30-day survival. While there was a difference with 53% survival at 30 days in the emergency revascularization group compared to 44% in the initial medical stabilization group, it did not reach statistical significance (95% CI 0.96, 1.53; p = 0.109). However, at 6 and 12 months, the survival differences had increased and were statistically significant (26). The survival benefit was, however, limited to those patients less than 75 years of age. This trial, in part, led to the ACC/AHA Guidelines that cardiogenic shock is a Class 1 indication for PCI at least for younger patients (27).

Early Revascularization in Elderly Patients

Although the randomized SHOCK Trial initially identified that patients aged ≥75 years did not appear to derive a mortality benefit from early revascularization versus initial medical stabilization, further analysis of the SHOCK Trial suggested that the elderly patients randomized to initial medical stabilization were a lower risk group with more favorable baseline characteristics. Specifically, those assigned to early revascularization had a lower ejection fraction at baseline compared to the initial medical stabilization group (28). Other studies have also reported different results. For example, in the SHOCK Registry, which enrolled patients during the same time frame as the randomized SHOCK Trial, there was a lower mortality in elderly patients with an early invasive strategy (29). Support for the advantage of an invasive strategy also comes from a report by Prasad et al. (30), who evaluated a consecutive series of 61 cardiogenic shock patients with a mean age of 79.5 ± 3 years. In this group, percutaneous coronary intervention was performed 8.0 ± 7.2 hours after the onset of the myocardial infarction. Angiographic success was high at 91%. In this population, 56% survived to discharge, and of the hospital survivors, 75% remained alive in 1 year. Finally, in a multicenter, decade-long report from the Northern New England Cardiovascular Disease Study Group, the hospital mortality rate for 310 patients (>75 years of age) undergoing PCI was 46%, which is significantly less than previously reported for elderly patients in the SHOCK Trial (31). These later studies support an aggressive approach to the elderly patient with cardiogenic shock.

It must be remembered that in selected patients with cardiogenic shock, surgical revascularization is also effective in improving outcome. In fact, in series reported to date, including GUSTO-I (2), the SHOCK Registry (11), the California Experience (25), and a community-based experience, shock patients undergoing surgical revascularization have somewhat better outcome than PCI. Obviously, selection bias also plays a significant role and must be kept in mind in interpreting the results. Other factors involved with surgery must be considered, including hypothermia, venting the ventricle, cardioplegia techniques, and complete revascularization, any of which may also improve outcome.

Advances in PCI

Earlier series of patients with shock undergoing PCI mainly included patients treated with conventional PTCA. Since then, stents have become the dominant approach. In randomized trials of PCI for acute myocardial infarction not restricted to shock, stents have been found to improve initial success rates with less severe residual stenosis and improved TIMI flow as well as decreased reocclusion (32–34). This has particular relevance for shock patients. In the SHOCK registry, achievement of PCI success had a major impact on in-hospital mortality. In patients in whom the final residual stenosis was <50%, the mortality was 38% compared to patients with a residual stenosis ≥50 % in whom it was 81% (34). Achievement of PCI success as assessed by TIMI flow was also an important predictor of in-hospital mortality; in those patients with TIMI-3 flow, mortality was 33% compared to those patients in whom only TIMI 0/1 flow was achieved in whom it was 86% (35). TIMI flow rates may be improved in patients treated with stent implantation versus conventional PTCA (36).

During performance of the SHOCK Trial, stent utilization patterns changed significantly, increasing from 0% in 1993 to 1994, to 74% in 1997 to 1998. This change was associated with an improvement in success rates. In those patients in whom a stent was used, PCI success was achieved in 93% versus 67% in patients in whom no stent was used (37). In patients treated with the combination of stenting and IIB/IIIA-inhibitors, 1-year survival was lower, although the number of patients was small. This finding may be spurious and be the result of the fact that IIB/IIIA-inhibition may have only been used in salvage situations when a complication was seen to be developing. The use of IIB/IIIA agents in combination with PCI remains somewhat controversial. In the CADILLAC trial (36), patients with acute myocardial infarction were randomly assigned to one of four groups (PTCA versus stent and abciximab versus placebo). The primary endpoint was a composite of death, reinfarction, disabling stroke, and ischemia-driven revascularization of the target vessel at 6 months. This trial indicated that when stent implementation was performed, the addition of an IIB/IIIA agent offered relatively little with the exception of significantly reducing the incidence of late subacute stent closure. The CADILLAC trial did not enroll patients with shock. A more recent prospective study suggests that the combination of stent implantation and abciximab resulted in higher TIMI 3 flow and a long-term mortality benefit in patients with cardiogenic shock complicating acute myocardial infarction (38).

Other mechanical devices, including thrombectomy catheters and embolic protection devices, have also been tested in the setting of cardiogenic shock and acute myocardial infarction. Whether these devices, which are more complicated, will offer a significant improvement compared to conventional stent-based PCI remains to be determined in the setting of shock. In patients with a large thrombus burden (e.g., in a large RCA vein graft), thrombectomy may offer an advantage and might be useful in preventing no reflow. To date, results with embolic protection for acute myocardial infarction have not shown a benefit.

Adjunctive Therapies

Even though survival is improved in patients to cardiogenic shock who undergo urgent revascularization compared to traditional medical therapy, mortality rates remain high and alternative approaches are being tested. Nitric oxide has a biphasic effect on myocardial function. At low levels, it is beneficial in promoting coronary and myocardial relaxation. However, at high levels, nitric oxide results in adverse effects by decreasing contractility and inhibiting the positive inotropic effect of beta-adrenergic stimulation. Blocking the effect of high levels of nitric oxide during shock by the competitive antagonist LNMMA has been postulated to improve outcome. Cotter et al. (39) performed a small, single center trial of LNMMA infusion in 11 patients with persistent cardiogenic shock and found an improvement in mean arterial pressure and a reduction in wedge pressure. Of the 11 patients, ten were able to be weaned off the ventilator and the intra-aortic balloon pump; and in 1 month, seven (64%) were alive. Subsequent to this another nitric oxide antagonist LNAME was studied by the same authors in a small randomized trial of 30 patients with cardiogenic shock and successful percutaneous coronary intervention. In this group, the 4-month survival in patients treated with LNAME was 73% compared to 33% in those patients treated with placebo. These data formed the basis for the upcoming Shock II Randomized Clinical Trial.

Conclusion

Early revascularization with PCI is now an ACC/AHA Guideline Class 1 indication for patients in cardiogenic shock. Cardiac surgery is also of benefit for acute mitral regurgitation, ventricular rupture, and extensive left main or three-vessel coronary artery disease. We await the results of emerging technologies such as nitrous oxide antagonists, catheter-based cooling systems, and cardiac myocyte cell implantation to further improve the prognosis of patients in cardiogenic shock.

REFERENCES

1. Leor J, Goldbourt U, Reicher-Reiss H, et al. Cardiogenic shock complicating acute myocardial infarction in patients without heart failure on admission: incidence, risk factors, and outcome. SPRINT Study Group. *Am J Med.* 1993;94:265–273.
2. Holmes DR, Jr., Bates ER, Kleiman NS, et al. Contemporary reperfusion therapy for cardiogenic shock: the GUSTO-I trial experience. The GUSTO-I Investigators. Global Utilization of Streptokinase and Tissue Plasminogen Activator for Occluded Coronary Arteries. *J Am Col Cardiol.* 1995;26:668–674.

3. Goldberg RJ, Samad NA, Yarzebski J, et al. Temporal trends in cardiogenic shock complicating acute myocardial infarction. *N Engl J Med*. 1999; 340:1162–1168.

4. Hasdai D, Holmes DR. Jr., Topol EJ, et al. Frequency and clinical outcome of cardiogenic shock during acute myocardial infarction among patients receiving reteplase and alteplase: requests from Gusto III. *Eur Heart J*. 1999;20:128–135.

5. Holmes DR, Jr., Berger PB, Hochman JS, et al. Cardiogenic shock in patients with acute ischemic syndromes with and without ST-segment elevation. *Circulation*. 1999;100:2067–2073.

6. Lindholm MG, Kober L, Boesgaard S, et al. Cardiogenic shock complicating acute myocardial infarction. *Eur Heart J*. 2003;24:258–265.

7. Jacobs AK, French JK, Col J, et al. Cardiogenic shock with non-ST-segment elevation myocardial infarction: a report from the SHOCK Trial Registry. Should we emergently revascularize occluded coronaries for cardiogenic shock? *J Am Coll Cardiol*. 2000;36:1091–1096.

8. Hochman JS, Sleeper LA, Webb JG, et al. Early revascularization in acute myocardial infarction complicated by cardiogenic shock. SHOCK Investigators. Should we emergently revascularize occluded coronaries for cardiogenic shock. *N Engl J Med*. 1999;341:625–634.

9. Goldberg RJ, Gore JM, Thompson CA, et al. Recent magnitude of and temporal trends (1997–1997) in the incidence and hospital death rates of cardiogenic shock complicating acute myocardial infarction: the second national registry of myocardial infarction. *Am Heart J*. 2001;141:65–72.

10. Webb JG, Sleeper LA, Buller CE, et al. Implications of the timing of onset of cardiogenic shock after acute myocardial infarction: a report from the SHOCK Trial Registry. Should we emergently revascularize occluded coronaries for cardiogenic shock? *J Am Coll Cardiol*. 2000;36:1084–1090.

11. Hochman JS, Buller CE, Sleeper LA, et al. Cardiogenic shock complicating acute myocardial infarction—etiologies, management and outcome: a report from the SHOCK Trial Registry. Should we emergently revascularize occluded coronaries for cardiogenic shock? *J Am Col Cardiol*. 2000;36:1063–1070.

12. Jacobs AK, Leopold JA, Bates E, et al. Cardiogenic shock caused by right ventricular infarction. A report from the SHOCK registry. *J Am Coll Cardiol*. 2003;42:1273–1279.

13. Sanborn TA, Sleeper LA, Webb JG, et al. Correlates of one-year survival in patients with cardiogenic shock complicating acute myocardial infarction. angiographic findings from the SHOCK trial. *J Am Coll Cardiol*. 2003;42:1373–1379.

14. AIMS Trial Study Group. Effect of intravenous APSAC on mortality after acute myocardial infarction: preliminary report of a placebo controlled clinical trial. *Lancet*. 1988;1:545–549.

15. Wilcox RG, van der Lippe G, Olsson CG, et al. Trial of tissue plasminogen activator for mortality reduction in acute myocardial infarction: Anglo-Scandanavian Study of Early Thrombolysis (ASSET). *Lancet*. 1988;1:525–530.

16. Barron HV, Every NR, Parsons LS, et al. The use of intra-aortic balloon counterpulsation in patients with cardiogenic shock complicating acute myocardial infarction: data from the National Registry of Myocardial Infarction 2. *Am Heart J*. 2001;141:933–939.

17. Sanborn TA, Sleeper LA, Bates ER, et al. Impact of thrombolysis, intra-aortic balloon pump counterpulsation, and their combination in cardiogenic shock complicating acute myocardial infarction: a report from the SHOCK Trial Registry. Should we emergently revascularize occluded coronaries for cardiogenic shock? *J Am Coll Cardiol*. 2000;36:1123–1129.

18. Anderson RD, Ohman EM, Holmes DR, Jr., et al. Use of intraaortic balloon counterpulsation in patients presenting with cardiogenic shock: observations from the GUSTO-I Study. Global utilization of streptokinase and TPA for occluded coronary arteries. *J Am Coll Cardiol*. 1997;30:708–715.

19. Ryan TJ, Antman EM, Brooks NH, et al. 1999 update: ACC/AHA guidelines for the management of patients with acute myocardial infarction: executive summary and recommendations: A report of the American College of Cardiology/American Heart Association Task Force on Practice Guidelines (Committee on Management of Acute Myocardial Infarction) *Circulation*. 1999;100:1016–1030.

20. Hudson MP, Granger CB, Stebbins A, et al. Cardiogenic shock survival and use of intra anti balloon counterpulsation: results from the GUSTO I and III trials. *Circulation*. 1999;100:I–370.

21. Thiele H, Lauer B, Boudroit E, et al. Reversal of cardiogenic shock by left atrial-to-femoral arterial bypass assistance. *Circulation*. 2001;104:2917–2922.

22. Smalling RW, Sweeney M, Lachterman B, et al. Transvalvular left ventricular assistance in cardiogenic shock secondary to acute myocardial infarction. Evidence for recovery from near fatal myocardial stunning. *J Am Col Cardiol*. 1994;23:637–644.

23. Kurose M, Okamoto K, Sato T, et al. Emergency and long term extracorporsal life support following acute myocardial infarction: rescue from severe cardiogenic shock related to stunned myocardium. *Clin Cardiol*. 1994;17:552–557.

24. Lane GE, Holmes DR. The modern strategy for cardiogenic shock. In: Cannon CP, ed. *Management of Acute Coronary Syndromes*. Totowa, NJ: Humana Press; 2003:603–651.

25. Edep ME, Brown DL. Effect of early revascularization in mortality from cardiogenic shock complicating acute myocardial infarction in California. *Am J Cardiol*. 2000;85:1185–1188.

26. Hochman JS, Sleeper LA, White HD, et al. One-year survival following early revascularization for cardiogenic shock. *JAMA*. 2001;285:190–192.

27. Ryan TJ, Antman EM, Brooks, NH, et al. 1999 update: ACC/AHA guidelines for the management of patients with acute myocardial infarction. A report of the American College of Cardiology/American Heart Association Task Force on Practice Guidelines (Committee on Management of Acute Myocardial Infarction). *J Am Col Cardiol*. 1999;34:890–911.

28. Dzavik V, Sleeper LA, Picard MH, et al. Outcome of patients aged >75 years in the Should we emergently revascularize Occluded Coronaries in cardiogenic shocK (SHOCK) trial: Do elderly patients with acute myocardial infarction complicated by cardiogenic shock respond differently to emergent revascularization? *Am Heart J*. 2005;149:1128–1134.

29. Dzavik V, Sleeper LA, Cocke TP, et al. Early revascularization is associated with improved survival in elderly patients with acute myocardial infarction complicated by cardiogenic shock: a report from the Shock Trial Registry. *Eur Heart J*. 2003;24:828–837.

30. Prasad A, Lennon RJ, Rihal CS, et al. Outcomes of elderly patients with cardiogenic shock treated with early percutaneous revascularization. *Am Heart J*. 2004;147:1066–1077.

31. Dauerman HL, Ryan TJ, Winthrop WD, et al. Outcomes of percutaneous coronary intervention among elderly patients in cardiogenic shock: a multicenter, decade-long experience. *J Invas Cardiol*. 2003;15:380–384.

32. Al Suwaidi J, Berger PB, Holmes DR. Coronary artery stents. *JAMA*. 2000;284:1828–1836.

33. Wilson SH, Bell MR, Rihal CS, et al. Infarct reocclusion after primary angioplasty, stent placement and thrombolytic therapy for acute myocardial infarction. *Am Heart J*. 2001;141:704–710.

34. Hasdai D, Topol EJ, Califf RM, et al. Cardiogenic shock complicating acute coronary syndromes. *Lancet*. 2000;356:749–756.

35. Webb JG, Sanborn TA, Sleeper LA, et al. Percutaneous coronary intervention for cardiogenic shock in the SHOCK Trial Registry. *Am Heart J*. 2001;141:964–970.

36. Stone GW, Grines CL, Cox DA. The controlled abciximab and device investigation to lower late angioplasty complications (CADILLAC) investigators. Comparison of angioplasty with stenting with or without abciximab in acute myocardial infarction. *New Eng J Med*. 2002;346:957–966.

37. Webb JG, Lowe AM, Sanborn TA, et al. Percutaneous coronary intervention for cardiogenic shock in the shock trial. *J Am Coll Cardiol*. 2003;42:1380–1386.

38. Chan AW, Chen DP, Bhatt DL, et al. Long-term mortality benefit with the combination of stents and abciximab for cardiogenic shock complicating acute myocardial infarction. *Am J Cardiol*. 2002;89:132–136.

39. Cotter G, Kaluski E, Blatt A, et al. L-NMMA (a nitric oxide synthase inhibitor) is effective in the treatment of cardiogenic shock. *Circulation*. 2000;101:1358–1361.

Adult Congenital Heart Disease and Valvuloplasty

Peter C. Block

CHAPTER 24

Percutaneous Balloon Valvuloplasty

Thomas M. Bashore

Percutaneous balloon procedures began in 1964 when Dotter and Judkins (1) reported 11 patients who had large vessel angioplasty, and the concept of catheter expansion of stenotic lesions was born. In 1971, Rashkind described the use of a balloon catheter to create an atrial septal defect in congenital heart disease patients (2). By 1979, "rupturing of the fused pulmonic valve" in a desperately ill neonate with valvular pulmonary stenosis triggered the concept for balloon therapy of stenotic valves (3). Reports of balloon valvuloplasty during surgery for congenital aortic stenosis emerged in the early 1980s, and percutaneous methods quickly followed in neonates and then adults (4). By the mid-1980s, encouraging results from percutaneous valvuloplasty of mitral stenosis led the National Heart Lung and Blood Institute (NHLBI) to initiate a registry to better understand the emerging technology. Reports from this registry (5), the Mansfield balloon catheter registry, and large institutional experiences (6) have all helped shape the current knowledge base regarding the utility of percutaneous balloon procedures for stenotic valvular lesions.

Early on, the procedure was variously called valvuloplasty, valvotomy, or commissurotomy. The term *commissurotomy* stemmed from the surgical procedure, and some thought valvuloplasty should be reserved for procedures that more directly altered the valvular structure. As a compromise, the NHLBI working group suggested the terms *valvotomy* for aortic and pulmonic procedures and *commissurotomy* for mitral procedures. However, the term *valvuloplasty* had been fixed in the minds of most of the cardiology community, and the majority of physicians still use that descriptor for all the percutaneous valvular procedures.

Table 24–1 outlines the indications, definition of a successful procedure, the major complications, and the long-term results to be expected from the use of percutaneous balloon valvuloplasty procedures. For the purposes of board review, this is the summary statement.

Pulmonary Valve Stenosis

Pathophysiology

The most common form of isolated right ventricular (RV) outflow obstruction, pulmonary valve stenosis (PS), occurs in about 7% of the population with congenital heart disease. It may be associated with significant RV hypertrophy and infundibular narrowing. Although multiple morphologic types have been described, two forms dominate isolated PS: the doming variety and the dysplastic. Fusion of the valvular cusps produces a classic systolic "doming" appearance angiographically (Fig. 24–1). Tissue pads within the valve sinuses may be present at times and result in a thickened, rigid valve considered dysplastic. This excessive thickening renders the dysplastic valve generally unsuitable for percutaneous valvuloplasty in most instances, although there have been occasional reports of some success. The dysplastic form is especially common in Noonan's syndrome. The greater the severity of congenital valvular pulmonic stenosis, the more likely the RV outflow tract will be narrowed and the lesion will resemble pulmonary valve atresia. The presence of annular hypoplasia is a contraindication for the use of balloon valvuloplasty. Fortunately, in adults the most common form of PS is due to commissural fusion, making this lesion one of the most amenable lesions to approach with percutaneous balloon methods.

At times, the RV outflow tract has considerable muscular subpulmonic hypertrophy, and multiple levels of outflow tract stenosis may be present. In some patients, branch PS and peripheral PS may also be present. The sudden reduction in the valvular gradient following valvuloplasty has been reported to result in acute RV decompensation due to marked infundibular obstruction, sometimes referred to as the "suicide RV." Fluid loading, calcium channel blockers, and beta blockers have all been used to treat the condition acutely following the procedure. This subpulmonic hypertrophy usually regresses over the next several months.

Indications for Pulmonary Balloon Valvuloplasty

In a patient with less than 2+ pulmonic insufficiency and a doming pulmonic valve, it has been generally accepted that a peak pulmonary valve gradient of 50 mm Hg at the time of cardiac catheterization is sufficient to warrant balloon valvuloplasty even in the absence of symptoms. Recent guidelines from the AHA/ACC Task Force on valvular heart disease (7) have suggested a lowering of the peak pulmonary gradient indication to 40 mm Hg in the asymptomatic and 30 mm Hg in the symptomatic patient, considering these as Class II indications for the procedure. Any evidence for RV dysfunction or associated RV failure and tricuspid regurgitation should clearly prompt intervention. Procedural success is much less likely in patients with pulmonary valve dysplasia, and these are

Table 24–1

Balloon Valvuloplasty Summary

Valvular Anatomy	Indications	Successful Result	Major Complications	Comments
Pulmonary Stenosis Good results: Classical doming valve. (Poor results in patients with dysplastic valves.)	1. Symptomatic patients with peak gradient >40 mm Hg. Class II indication: Peak gradient >30 mm Hg. 2. Asymptomatic patients with peak gradient >40 mm Hg.	About 90% success rate. <20 mm Hg pulmonary gradient.	Complications rare (1%–2%). Mild pulmonic insufficiency. "Suicide" RV.	Dilate to 1.2–1.4 annulus size. One or two balloons used. Inoue balloon can be used. Excellent short-and long-term results.
Aortic Stenosis Acceptable results: Bicuspid valves in adolescents. (Poor results in calcific AS in elderly.)	1. Neonates with symptoms. 2. Symptomatic adolescents with peak gradient >50 mm Hg. 3. Asymptomatic adolescents with peak gradient >60 mm Hg or peak gradient >50 mm Hg plus LVH with strain.	About 80% initial success rate. AVA >1.0 cm^2 **or** 50% reduction in gradient **or** 50% increase in AVA.	Complications frequent (3%–15%) acutely. Transfusion Vascular injury CVA Systemic emboli Myocardial infarction Aortic insufficiency Complete heart block	Dilate only to annulus size. In elderly, only value is as a temporizing measure in patients with a preserved LV systolic function.
Mitral Stenosis Good results: Rheumatic etiology. (Poor results in congenital or calcific MS.)	1. Severe MS and symptoms. 2. Severe MS and pulmonary systolic pressure >50 mm Hg at rest or >60 mm Hg with stress. 3. Class IIb indication: Severe MS and atrial fibrillation.	MVA ≥1.5 cm^2 **or** 50% reduction in gradient **or** 50% increase in MVA.	Complications infrequent (3%–4%) acutely ASD (from trans-septal) MR Tamponade	Echo score helps determine suitability 0–4 points for mobility, calcium, valvular thickening, submitral scar. Long-term results similar to surgical commissurotomy, especially if echo score ≤8. Worse if score >12. Pulmonary pressures regress over time (weeks to months).
Tricuspid Stenosis (Rheumatic or Carcinoid)	Mean gradient >5 mm Hg.	Zero gradient and no TR.	TR frequent.	Not recommended.
Bioprosthetic Valve Stenosis (Degenerative)	None.	None.	Regurgitation frequent.	Not recommended.

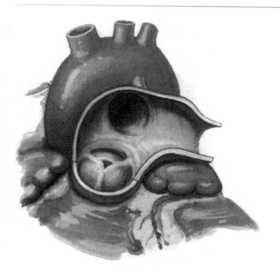

Figure 24–1.

Pulmonary valve stenosis. The classic doming pulmonary valve is shown. (From: Bashore T. Percutaneous balloon valvuloplasty. In: Runge M, Ohman M, eds. *Netter's Cardiology*. Teterboro, NJ: Icon Learning Systems; 2004:308–323, with permission.)

generally not amenable to valvuloplasty. The procedure also has had limited success in patients with carcinoid valvular involvement of the pulmonic valve, usually because pulmonic insufficiency dominates.

The Technique of Pulmonary Balloon Valvuloplasty

Prior to the procedure, an RV angiogram, using the cranial RAO and straight lateral views, is performed. Pulmonary angiography is also used to assess preprocedural pulmonic insufficiency and the presence of branch or peripheral PS. The annular size can be determined prior to the procedure by echocardiography, MRI, or in the cath lab by contrast angiography. A marker catheter (with radio-opaque markers a known distance apart) may be used for angiography at the level of the valve in order to determine the appropriate balloon size. Quantitative angiographic methods may also be applied for this purpose. The dilating balloon or balloons are percutaneously inserted into the femoral vein without a sheath. The maximal balloon diameter at inflation should be equal to or up to 1.2 to 1.4 times the annular size. The pulmonary arterial wall is elastic, often requiring oversizing to achieve an adequate valvotomy result. The goal of the procedure is to achieve a final peak valvular gradient of <20 mm Hg, because the recurrence rates are much lower if that threshold is reached. A single balloon, often 23 mm in diameter in adults, may be used, although two balloons side-by-side may be necessary in patients with a large annulus. In some laboratories, trefoil or bifoil balloon catheters are available and preferred. When two balloons are used (Fig. 24–2A), the effective balloon diameters can be calculated by using the formula

Combined diameters (D_1 and D_2)

$$= \frac{D_1 + D_2 + \pi(D_1/2 + D_2/2)}{\pi} \quad (24.1)$$

where D_1 and D_2 are the maximal diameters of each respective balloon. More recently, the single Inoue mitral balloon has increasing been used for pulmonary valvuloplasty given its stability during the balloon inflation (Fig. 24–2B).

Acute Results and Complications

Multiple studies have reported excellent acute results in children, adolescents, and adults. Representative results are exemplified by a report of 66 infants and children by Rao (8). In this series, the peak gradient across the pulmonic valve fell from 92+/−43 mm Hg to 29+/−20 mm Hg with no change in the cardiac output. The NHLBI adult registry included 37 adult patients. The procedure was completed in 97%, and the peak gradients fell from an average of 46 to 18 mm Hg. Larger balloon sizes, up to 30% to 50% larger than the annulus, have resulted in improved gradient reductions without increasing complications.

Complications from the procedure have been minimal. In the acute setting, vagal symptoms predominate. Catheter-induced ventricular ectopy often occurs as well. Pulmonary edema, presumably from increasing pulmonary flow to previously underperfused lungs, perforation of a cardiac chamber, high-grade AV nodal block, and the transient RV outflow obstruction noted previously have all been reported. Pulmonary valve insufficiency occurs in up to two thirds of the patients after the procedure, but it is rarely clinically significant.

Long-Term Results

Long-term follow-up data for up to 10 years are now available. In one representative study (9), 62 children had an average balloon-to-pulmonary annulus ratio of 1.4 employed. A mean follow-up of 6.4+/−3.4 years was available. Persistent pulmonary valve insufficiency was found in 39%. There was evidence for a progressive resolution of infundibular hypertrophy, and the restenosis (>35 mm Hg gradient at follow-up) rate was only 4.8%. Restenosis in this study was much more common in patients with dysplastic valves. Should restenosis occur, a repeat valvuloplasty procedure appears to be effective in patients without a dysplastic pulmonary valve. Rao compared percutaneous results to surgical valvotomy in children (8) and noted a surgical mortality estimated at 3% with a poor surgical result (residual gradient >50 mm Hg) in 4%. Restenosis rates after surgery ranged from 14% to 33% at up to 34 months after the procedure. Based on data such as this, percutaneous valvuloplasty for classic domed valvular PS is the treatment of choice and can be performed at low risk.

Aortic Valve Stenosis
Pathophysiology

The normal aortic valve has thin, flexible cusps composed of three tissue layers sandwiched between layers of endothelium on both the aortic and ventricular sides of the valve. Congenital deformities of the aortic valve are generally of two types:

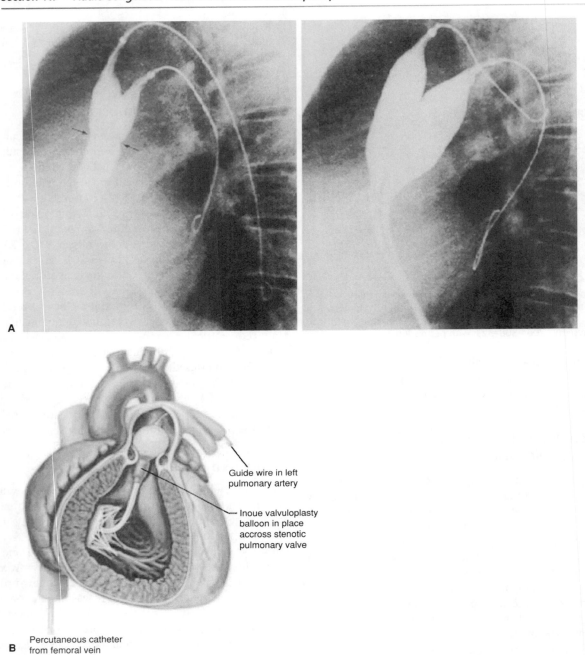

Guide wire in left
pulmonary artery

Inoue valvuloplasty
balloon in place
accross stenotic
pulmonary valve

Percutaneous catheter
B   from femoral vein

Figure 24–2.

Percutaneous balloon pulmonary valvuloplasty techniques. **A:** Double balloon. Arrows indicate valvular waist in balloons at initiation of dilatation. **B:** Inoue mitral balloon being used for pulmonary valvuloplasty. The distal balloon inflates initially, and then the entire balloon inflates to dilate the valve. (From: Bashore TM, Davidson CJ. Acute hemodynamic effects of percutaneous balloon aortic valvuloplasty. In: Bashore TM, Davidson CJ, eds. *Percutaneous Balloon Valvuloplasty and Related Techniques.* Baltimore: Williams and Wilkins; 1991:99–111, with permission.

Unicuspid and bicuspid. Unicuspid valves are inherently stenotic at birth and result in symptoms early in life, although up to 10% of isolated aortic stenosis (AS) in adulthood will be due to a unicuspid valve. Of patients with isolated AS aged 15 to 65, about 60% have bicuspid valves. The bicuspid valve generally has two nearly equal-sized cusps with variable commissural fusion. There is usually a residual false commissure (raphe) present in one cusp. Over time, there is progressive fibrosis and calcium deposition within the valve.

The AS seen in the elderly generally involves a trileaflet valve and may be pathophysiologically similar to the atherosclerotic process with calcium deposition predominating. It initially presents as an aortic sclerosis process and is progressive in nature. In recent natural history studies, the prevalence of aortic sclerosis has been reported to be around 25% in those over 65, with frank AS being evident in 1% to 2% of the elderly population. In this type of valvular pathology, there is little commissural fusion, but rather there are literally mounds of calcium

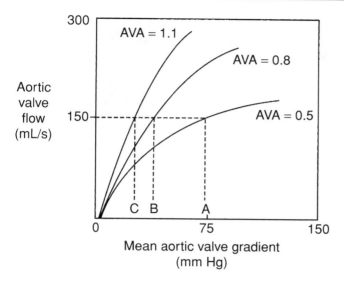

Figure 24–3.

The effect of valvuloplasty on the aortic valve area. Note that the gradient change for 0.3 cm^2 reduction in the valve area differs depending on the initial severity of the lesion. At any one level of cardiac output (aortic valve flow), the gradient change from 0.5 cm^2 to 0.8 cm^2 (A to B) is much greater than the change from 0.8 cm^2 to 1.1 cm^2 (B to C). This makes the use of only an incremental change in aortic valve area a difficult measure by which to grade the success of the procedure. (From: Bashore TM, Davidson CJ. Acute hemodynamic effects of percutaneous balloon aortic valvuloplasty. In: Bashore TM, Davidson CJ, eds. *Percutaneous Balloon Valvuloplasty and Related Techniques:* Baltimore: Williams and Wilkins; 1991:99–111, with permission.)

deposits within the cusps that restrict the valve opening. As there is little commissural fusion, any reduction in the aortic valve gradient afforded by balloon procedures has been attributed to cracks in the calcific nodules, cuspal tears, and aortic wall expansion. As one might expect from the pathology, results from balloon valvuloplasty are poor in the calcific form of AS.

Hemodynamically, the gradient change in the valve area after aortic valvuloplasty is a complex one dependent upon the cardiac output (aortic flow) and the valve area. As noted in Figure 24–3, a change in the AVA of 0.3 cm^2 will have a dramatic effect on the peak LV systolic pressure if the baseline AVA is severe (i.e., going from 0.5 to 0.8 cm^2), but the same incremental change may have much less consequence on the gradient if the baseline AVA is less severe (i.e., going from 0.8 to 1.1 cm^2). Interpreting a successful procedure is therefore complex, and for these reasons, improvement in both the gradient and in the final valve area are used to define a successful result (i.e., a final valve gradient of <50 mm Hg or a 50% improvement in the AVA).

Indications for Percutaneous Aortic Valvuloplasty

The decision to intervene in aortic stenosis is usually dependent upon symptoms of exertional dyspnea, angina, or presyncope. The latest guidelines from the ACC/AHA (7) define *mild AS* as a valve area of 1.5 cm^2, a mean gradient of <25 mm Hg,

or maximal aortic Doppler jet of 3.0 m/sec. *Moderate AS* is defined as a valve area of 1.0 to 1.5 cm^2, a mean gradient of between 25 to 40 mm Hg, or a maximal Doppler jet of 3.0 to 4.0 m/sec. *Severe AS* is considered present when the valve area is <1.0 cm^2, the mean gradient is >40 mm Hg, or the Doppler jet is >4.0 m/sec. Echo-Doppler gradients are particularly useful for following individuals, and when the maximal velocity exceeds 4 m/sec (estimated gradient of 64 mm Hg), symptoms emerge relatively quickly. A change in the Doppler gradient of >0.3 m/sec in a 1-year period also portends early symptoms. Although guidelines are changing to take into account echocardiographic indices and to consider surgery or intervention in asymptomatic patients, most cardiologists still use symptoms as a basis for the decision to proceed with intervention.

In symptomatic patients with reduced LV systolic function and poor forward cardiac output, the use of an inotropic agent or nitroprusside to augment aortic flow has become popular in order to determine whether the low output (and the subsequently low gradient) is a consequence of the valvular stenosis or attributable to the poor ventricular function. If one can show that the valve area increases with improved C.O., then the presumption is that the associated cardiomyopathy is predominant over the narrowed valve orifice.

Whether to use a percutaneous intervention in AS is dependent on the clinical situation and on the type of valvular disease that has resulted in the AS. In the rare case of rheumatic AS without significant AI, commissural fusion is present. The procedure would be expected to be beneficial in that setting, but the number of patients with isolated AS due to rheumatic disease is quite small. In neonates and young children, the initial success rates have not been great, although older children clearly may benefit and should be considered for the procedure prior to valve replacement. Current guidelines (7) recommend valvuloplasty in symptomatic adolescents with a peak gradient >50 mm Hg. Asymptomatic patients with a peak gradient >60 mm Hg or a peak gradient >50 mm Hg plus LVH with strain on ECG should also be considered candidates for the procedure. In adults, surgical intervention has consistently proven superior to valvuloplasty (10). The use of valvuloplasty in adults is restricted to those in high-risk situations (i.e., during pregnancy or in cardiogenic shock) where it may be useful as a bridge to eventual aortic valve replacement. In addition, there is the rare adult with preserved LV systolic function and severe AS, for whom a surgical AVR is prohibitive due to comorbid conditions. In this latter situation, the procedure can be utilized for short-term symptomatic benefit (11).

Technique of Balloon Aortic Valvuloplasty

Following crossing of the aortic valve retrograde from the femoral artery, the balloon catheters are generally inserted with or without a sheath over a 0.038-inch guide wire with its tip coiled in the LV (Fig. 24–4). A backup pacemaker is usually placed at the RV apex. The maximum dilated size of the balloon chosen is usually slightly less than the size of the aortic root at the valve plane. Longer balloons, (i.e., 5.5 cm versus 3 cm in length) are advantageous to help prevent movement in

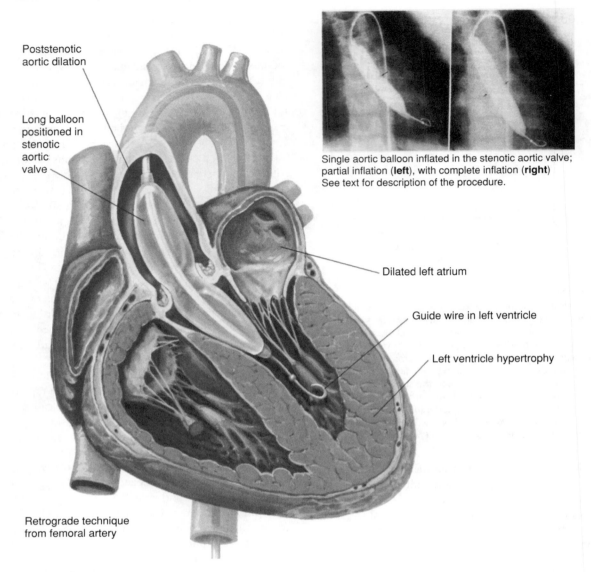

Poststenotic aortic dilation

Long balloon positioned in stenotic aortic valve

Single aortic balloon inflated in the stenotic aortic valve; partial inflation (**left**), with complete inflation (**right**) See text for description of the procedure.

Dilated left atrium

Guide wire in left ventricle

Left ventricle hypertrophy

Retrograde technique from femoral artery

Figure 24–4.
Balloon aortic valvuloplasty. The balloon catheter is placed in retrograde manner across the aortic valve and is inflated momentarily to its maximum dimension. (From: Bashore T. Percutaneous balloon valvuloplasty. In: Runge M, Ohman M, eds. *Netter's Cardiology.* Teterboro, NJ: Icon Learning Systems; 2004:308–323, with permission.)

the stenotic valve orifice during balloon inflation. Many operators use transient rapid right ventricular pacing (usually 180 to 200/min) during balloon inflation to further minimize to and fro balloon motion. For most adults, a 20-mm diameter balloon is used, although a 23-mm balloon may be required in larger patients. In children, the balloon size is estimated from the echo or angiogram in much the same manner as with pulmonic valvuloplasty. After baseline hemodynamics are obtained, the balloon catheter is placed in the middle of the valve plane and inflated using dilute (25%) contrast in saline. Inflation pressures are usually not measured, because they appear to have little effect on the outcome.

A brachial artery approach has also been employed by some groups, as well as a trans-septal antegrade approach to the aortic valve via the right femoral vein. Results appear to be similar regardless of the access site utilized.

Acute Results and Complications

In general, the mean aortic gradient can be expected to fall from a baseline of about 55 mm Hg to 29 mm Hg acutely, with the AVA increasing from 0.5 to 0.8 cm^2. Results in children and neonates vary widely depending on the clinical status of the patient and the associated cardiac anomalies. Many neonates with critical AS have severe LV hypoplasia or endocardial fibroelastosis and do poorly with either percutaneous valvuloplasty or surgery. Once out of the neonatal period, the results of percutaneous aortic valvuloplasty are much better. Rao (8) reviewed the data from 232 children and adolescents with a mean age of about 9 years and found the aortic gradients fell about 60% from around 75 mm Hg to 30 mm Hg. The procedure thus appears to work reasonably well in the adolescent age group, although restenosis will eventually occur at a later date.

In the elderly, serious life-threatening complications from the aortic valvuloplasty procedure are fairly common. Because of that, almost all of the reported studies require elderly patients to be noncandidates for surgical intervention. In-hospital mortality from all the initial series of patients is around 5% with a 0% to 1.5% risk of CVA, cardiac perforation, myocardial infarction, or serious aortic insufficiency. Not surprisingly, vascular complications are a dominant complicating feature with about a 10% incidence reported.

In the NHLBI registry of 671 patients (5), at least one complication was reported in 25% of the patients within 24 hours, and 31% had some complication before hospital discharge. The most common complication was the need for transfusion (23%). This was followed by vascular surgery (7%), CVA (3%), systemic embolization (2%), and myocardial infarction (2%). All cause mortality was 3% with death usually related to multiorgan failure and poor LV function before the procedure. In patients who survived to 30 days, 75% had improved at least one NYHA functional class.

Long-Term Results

Short-term studies after aortic valvuloplasty in the elderly revealed evidence for an increase in the aortic gradient (restenosis) as early as 2 days following the procedure. Some of this is undoubtedly due to aortic recoil, and there is also some progressive early improvement in cardiac output over this initial time period that may contribute to the increased gradient. By 6 months, almost all patients have evidence for hemodynamic restenosis. Of note is that the re-emergence of symptoms at follow-up appears more related to diastolic dysfunction than to either the measured aortic valve area or gradient.

At a follow-up of 1 year, Davidson (11) noted that the probability of recurrent symptoms could be predicted by simply

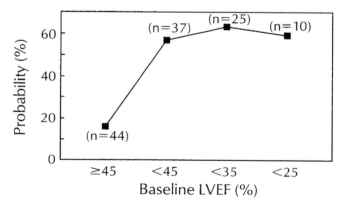

Figure 24–5.

Probability of recurrent symptoms based on initial LV ejection fraction (EF) following balloon aortic valvuloplasty. (From: Davidson CJ, Harrison JK, Pieper KS, et al. Determinants of one-year outcome from balloon aortic valvuloplasty. *Am J Cardiol.* 1991;68:75–80, with permission.)

observing the baseline ejection fraction. In that study, the majority of patients with a reduced baseline EF of <45% was symptomatic by the 1-year anniversary (Fig. 24–5). The implication from this study was that patients with poor LV systolic function should not be considered for aortic valvuloplasty. Because most patients with preserved LV systolic function and AS would likely be candidates for aortic valve replacement surgery, there is only a small fraction of the population of adult patients with AS that benefits from the short-term symptomatic improvement from the procedure. Currently, this is most prevalent in the severely symptomatic group of AS patients who are at an extreme age (over 90 years) and where the risk of surgery is prohibitive due to comorbid disease.

Mitral Valvuloplasty
Pathophysiology

In the adult, obstruction to LV inflow through the mitral valve is usually attributed to the effects of rheumatic heart disease. In children, congenital mitral stenosis may occur and generally reflects fusion of the mitral chordae, often to each other, or abnormal positioning of the papillary muscles. The papillary muscles may be so close together that a single papillary muscle is evident (parachute mitral valve). On rare occasions, a mitral web is present on the atrial side of the mitral leaflet and can obstruct flow. In the elderly, mitral annular calcification may result in stiffening of the leaflets and clinical mitral stenosis. In this latter situation, calcium virtually invades from the annulus toward the center of the valve, and mitral regurgitation is frequently associated. Other causes of mitral stenosis are extremely rare including carcinoid (usually associated with a patent foramen ovale or atrial septal defect), systemic lupus erythematosus, rheumatoid arthritis, Fabry disease, and amyloidosis.

The interval between an episode of acute rheumatic fever and symptomatic mitral stenosis averages about 16 years, and most patients in this country do not recall having the acute event by the time the valvular lesion manifests itself. The most characteristic feature of rheumatic mitral stenosis is the fusion of the commissures between the anterior and posterior leaflets. Fusion, thickening, and retraction of the chordae, thickening of the valvular leaflets themselves, and calcium deposition all contribute in various degrees to the obstruction. The severity of these features has led to an echocardiographic semiquantitative scoring system wherein numbers from 0 to 4 are assigned to each characteristic (12) (Table 24–2). Thus, mobility of the anterior leaflet, valvular thickening, submitral scarring, and evidence for calcification are all weighted into an echo score to help define the suitability of the valve for percutaneous valvuloplasty. Echo scores >8 have been shown to result in poorer results from the valvuloplasty procedure.

Because the balloon valvuloplasty procedure works by tearing the commissural fibrosis that causes the leaflet fusion, it is important to document that commissural fusion is present. Echocardiography readily provides these data. In addition, if there is eccentric commissural fusion on only one side of the

Table 24–2

The Massachusetts General Hospital Mitral Valve Morphology Scoring System

Leaflet Mobility

1. Highly mobile valve with restriction only of the leaflet tips.
2. Midportion and base of leaflets have reduced mobility.
3. Valve leaflets move forward in diastole mainly at the base.
4. No or minimal forward movement of the leaflets in diastole.

Valvular Thickening

1. Leaflets near normal (4 to 5 mm).
2. Midleaflet thickening, pronounced thickening of the margins.
3. Thickening extends through the entire leaflets (5 to 8 mm).
4. Pronounced thickening of all leaflet tissue (>8 mm).

Subvalvular Thickening

1. Minimal thickening of chordal structures just below the valve.
2. Thickening of the chordae extending up to one third of chordal length.
3. Thickening extending to the distal third of the chordae.
4. Extensive thickening and shortening of all chordae extending down to the papillary muscle.

Valvular Calcification

1. A single area of bright echo density.
2. Scattered areas of brightness confined to the leaflet margins.
3. Brightness extending into the midportion of the leaflets.
4. Extensive brightness through most of the leaflet tissue.

Each is graded for 0 to 4 with 0 being normal. The range in scoring is, therefore, 0 to 16. It weights each characteristic equally, however.
Modified from: Wilkins GT, Weyman AE, Abascal VM, et al. Percutaneous balloon dilatation of the mitral valve: an analysis of echocardiographic variables related to outcome and the mechanism of dilatation. *Br Heart J*. 1988;60:299–308, with permission.

leaflet, the inflated balloon(s) might be forced to the nonfused side of the leaflet, increasing the risk of valvular or ventricular tearing.

Indications for Percutaneous Balloon Mitral Valvuloplasty

Mitral stenosis (MS) results in obstruction to LV inflow and an elevation in left atrial pressure. Any activity that increases flow (i.e., exercise) or shortens diastolic filling time (i.e., the onset of a rapid tachycardia, such as atrial flutter or fibrillation) increases the mitral gradient. When left atrial pressure is elevated, symptoms of dyspnea and pulmonary congestion emerge. For the most part, the decision to intervene in MS is based on exertional symptoms or evidence for pulmonary hypertension. The pulmonary hypertension present in MS is, at times, greater than would be expected from the magnitude of left atrial pressure el-

evation alone. Although the trigger for this excessive elevation of the pulmonary artery pressure is unknown, endothelin and adrenomedullin, both pulmonary vasoconstrictors, may play a role. Because there is evidence that the pulmonary hypertension in this situation regresses following balloon valvuloplasty, the presence of pulmonary hypertension or right heart failure even without congestive symptoms should be considered an indication for intervention in MS.

Before the procedure, each patient should undergo a transesophageal echocardiogram (TEE) both to insure no atrial thrombus is present and to provide a further assessment of valvular morphology. If an atrial thrombus is present, then the patients are generally placed on warfarin for 4 to 6 weeks, and the TEE repeated. The procedure can be done in the presence of atrial thrombus deep inside the appendage, but the better part of valor is to try to resolve any atrial clot before proceeding.

The age of the patient or a history of prior surgical commissurotomy does not seem to play a major factor in the acute results from the procedure, as long as the valvular morphology is favorable.

In general, a symptomatic patient (or one with a resting pulmonary systolic pressure >50 mm Hg or an exercise pulmonary systolic pressure >60 mm Hg) with a low echocardiographic morphology score should be considered for percutaneous mitral valvuloplasty if there is less than 2+ mitral regurgitation (MR). Essentially all of the patients with symptoms due to MS will have a calculated mitral valve area of <1.5 cm^2.

The Technique of Percutaneous Mitral Valvuloplasty

Antegrade and retrograde approaches are possible, although most laboratories use an antegrade method that requires trans-septal catheterization. Ventriculography to help quantitate the degree of MR and a right heart catheterization are done prior to the valvuloplasty to determine the cardiac output, the pulmonary pressure, the valve gradient, and MVA. Some interventionalists utilize a right atrial angiogram with levophase filling of the LA to help guide trans-septal needle placement.

There are several available balloons systems that have been used for mitral valvuloplasty. When using balloons similar to that with aortic or pulmonic valvuloplasty, double balloons have been favored over the single balloon due to the shape of the mitral orifice in mitral stenosis (often being compared to the mouth of a catfish). The balloons are thus positioned side-by-side and inflated (Fig. 24–6). With either single or double balloon methods, the intra-atrial septum is first dilated with an 8-mm balloon catheter to allow for the advancement of the larger balloon catheter or catheters. The most common approach using double balloons places them side-by-side using two guide wires. Other systems are available that use two balloons on a single catheter (the bifoil system) (13) or two balloons on a single guide wire (the Multi-Track system) (14). A reusable metallic valvuloplasty catheter has also been developed wherein the business end resembles the Tubbs dilator formerly used for closed surgical commissurotomy (15). In addition,

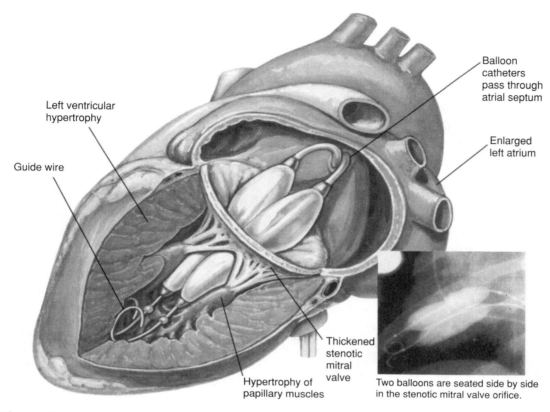

Figure 24–6.

Double balloon technique for mitral valvuloplasty. See text for description. (From: Bashore T. Percutaneous balloon valvuloplasty. In: Runge M, Ohman M, eds. *Netter's Cardiology*. Teterboro, NJ: Icon Learning Systems; 2004:308–323, with permission.)

a retrograde transarterial approach has been advocated by some laboratories (18). In this latter method, the catheter is placed over a wire that has been advanced from the femoral artery across the aortic valve then retrograde into the LA.

Most mitral valvuloplasty procedures, though, are now performed using the Inoue balloon. The maximal size of

the balloon used can be determined from echocardiographic measurements of the mitral annulus or can be estimated simply by using the patient's height. The most commonly used sizes are 26- and 28-mm maximal diameters.

The 12F Inoue balloon catheter is designed so the distal end of the balloon inflates before the proximal end, allowing

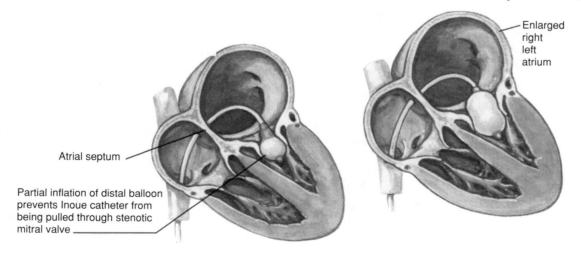

Figure 24–7.

Inoue balloon technique for mitral valvuloplasty. See text for description. (From: Bashore T. Percutaneous balloon valvuloplasty. In: Runge M, Ohman M, eds. *Netter's Cardiology*. Teterboro, NJ: Icon Learning Systems; 2004:308–323, with permission.)

positioning of the balloon across the mitral valve, inflation of the distal end, and the retraction of the remainder of the balloon before inflating the entire balloon within the mitral orifice (Fig. 24–7). With double balloons, the maximal diameter is predetermined and dependent on the inflated maximal balloon diameter (using the formula described earlier). With the Inoue system, the diameter is dependent upon the amount of diluted contrast used to inflate the balloon. This feature allows for graded increases in the diameter of the balloon during the procedure without having to replace the entire balloon catheter to achieve a larger dilating orifice.

Before insertion into the patient, the Inoue balloon is also prestretched. Following the trans-septal, a stainless steel guide wire with a spring coil end is placed through the Mullins sheath into the LA. The atrial septum and the femoral vein insertion site are then dilated with a long 14F dilator. The stretched balloon is then placed into the LA through the septal puncture site. The stretching tube is subsequently removed, and a specially designed control wire is then inserted into the catheter to guide the balloon across the mitral valve into the LV.

Once in the LV, the balloon is sequentially inflated in the mitral valve orifice. The diameter of the balloon at maximal inflation is progressively increased in increments of 1 to 2 mm. The LA pressure and mitral gradient are re-evaluated following each balloon inflation. In most laboratories, a chest wall echocardiogram is performed between each inflation to observe any change in the mitral valve and any Doppler evidence for MR. If MR (17) is present or if the valvular gradient has been satisfactorily reduced, the procedure is completed. The balloon is then restretched before removal from the LA.

Acute Results and Complications

Immediate improvement in both the hemodynamic and the clinical state is universal in successful procedures. Dixon and Safian recently reviewed 19 studies, and as a generality, one should expect a 50% to 70% decrease in the transmitral gradient with an accompanying 50% to 100% increase in the mitral valve area (18). A representative example would be a valve area of 0.9 cm^2 at baseline improving to a MVA of 1.9 cm^2 following the procedure. Similarly, a representative preprocedural mitral gradient would be around 14 mm Hg before and 6 mm Hg following valvuloplasty. Acutely cardiac output tends to remain unchanged. The postprocedural valve areas achieved are similar between the double balloon method and the Inoue system (19). About 8% to 10% of the patients will not improve their valve area over 1.0 cm^2, however.

Pulmonary pressure falls immediately consistent with the change in LA pressure. In patients with severe pulmonary hypertension, by 24 hours the pulmonary pressure drops further (20) and continues to decline over the ensuing months.

The issues surrounding the relationship between the valve area and valve flow discussed above in the interpretation of the results of aortic valvuloplasty also pertain to the results of mitral valvuloplasty. Because of these basic hemodynamic issues, a successful procedure is generally defined as either an improvement in the MVA by 50% or a final MVA of >1.5 cm^2 plus no more than 2+ mitral regurgitation. Contemporary studies suggest an acute success rate of around 90% can be expected depending on the valvular morpholophy (21–25). The major factors that have been identified as predictive of a successful procedure are a low valvular score by whatever method (24,26,27) and the absence of significant baseline mitral regurgitation (24).

Complications from percutaneous mitral valvuloplasty have declined over the years as the learning curve for the procedure has been completed (28) and as programs with a particular interest in the procedure have done the highest volumes. Since the advent of the routine use of TEE prior to the procedure, the risk of embolic events has virtually disappeared, and the major complications are related to the trans-septal puncture and to the development of significant mitral regurgitation due to injury to the mitral valve apparatus.

Long-Term Results: Survival and Event-Free Survival Data

Ten-year data regarding overall survival and event-free survival are available. Ten-year survival rates range from 85% to 97% in the more contemporary studies (29) with event-free survival rates between 61% and 72%. Event-free survival appears dependent upon favorable valve morphology, the presence of sinus rhythm, lower initial left atrial pressures, and ≤2+ mitral regurgitation following the procedure. Recently, Palacios et al. reviewed the MGH experience (24) and found that although adverse events (death, mitral valve surgery, and redo-valvuloplasty) were low within the first 5 years of follow-up, a progressive number of events occurred beyond this period. Survival (82% versus 57%) and event-free survival (38% versus 22%) at 12-year follow-up was greater in patients with an echo score of ≤8 than in those with an echo score >8. Cox regression analysis identified postvalvuloplasty mitral regurgitation ≥3+, an echo score of >8, older age, prior surgical commissurotomy, NYHA functional class IV, prevalvuloplasty mitral regurgitation ≥2+, and higher postvalvuloplasty pulmonary artery pressure as independent predictors of combined events at long-term follow-up. Others have found that the presence of atrial fibrillation imparts a negative effect on event-free survival, and some reports have focused on the negative impact of valvular calcium. As one might expect, those with suboptimal initial results do less well clinically. In some reports, the presence of baseline mitral regurgitation has been the greatest predictor of a poor late outcome.

Symptomatic Improvement and Restenosis

Essentially all studies emphasize the impressive improvement in clinical symptoms in those patients who have undergone balloon mitral valvuloplasty. Symptoms more likely recur in patients with suboptimal results and in those with unfavorable valve morphology. Anatomic valvular restenosis after the procedure is not simple to define due to the same issues noted previously regarding valve area, gradient, and cardiac output.

Initial studies defined restenosis as $\geq 50\%$ loss of the initial MVA gain, whereas others have advocated including an MVA of <1.5 cm^2 as part of the definition.

Clinical restenosis may not correlate well with anatomic restenosis. Wang et al. (26) recently reported anatomic data using serial echocardiographic examinations in 310 patients with generally high baseline echo scores. Restenosis, defined as mitral valve area <1.5 cm^2 and $\geq 50\%$ loss of initial MVA increase, was assessed by serial 2-D and Doppler echocardiography over a 6-year period. Acute procedural success (defined as a final valve area >1.5 cm^2) occurred in 206 patients (66%). The cumulative restenosis rate was approximately 40% at 6 years after successful PMC (44% by 2D and 40% by Doppler MVA). The only independent predictor of restenosis was the echocardiographic score (restenosis at 5 years was 20% for score <8 versus 61% for score ≥ 8). The decline in MVA and the occurrence of restenosis was gradual and progressive during the follow-up period.

Clinical restenosis data are more impressive than anatomic, although mitral valve anatomy always appears to predict the symptomatic outcome. A recent study by Ben-Farhat et al. (30) from Tunisia suggests a 10-year clinical restenosis rate of 23% for those with an echo score ≤ 8, 55% for those with an echo score of 9 to 11, and 50% for those with a score ≥ 12.

Comparative Data with Surgical Commissurotomy

Because both surgical and balloon procedures work similarly to improve the mitral valve orifice in mitral stenosis (commissurotomy), the results are similar. In a study of 60 patients with favorable anatomy randomized to valvuloplasty (using the double balloon technique) versus open surgical commissurotomy, at 3 years, the mitral valve areas of the balloon valvuloplasty patients were actually better than the surgical group (2.4 cm^2 versus 1.8 cm^2), and 72% of the valvuloplasty patients were in NYHA functional class 1 versus 57% of the surgical group (31).

In another study, 90 patients randomized to valvuloplasty versus open commissurotomy or closed commissurotomy were followed for 7 years. There appeared to be little difference between the valvuloplasty patients and the open commissurotomy patients at the study's conclusion (32). Both the valvuloplasty and the open surgical procedure groups had less clinical restenosis than the closed commissurotomy group (0% for the valvuloplasty and open commissurotomy group and 27% for the closed surgical group). At 7 years, 87% of the valvuloplasty patients and 90% of the open commissurotomy patients were in NYHA functional class 1 compared to only 33% of the closed surgical commissurotomy patients.

Given the available data, it would appear that balloon valvuloplasty is either equivalent or even superior to surgical commissurotomy for symptomatic mitral stenosis, at least through the first 7 years after the procedure. This has generally led most to advocate for the percutaneous approach in those with appropriate valve morphology.

Tricuspid Valve Stenosis

Pathophysiology

Tricuspid valve anatomy is more variable than mitral anatomy. The three leaflets are of unequal size, with the septal leaflet the smallest, the anterior leaflet the largest and the posterior leaflet in-between. While some chordae attach to distinct papillary muscles in the RV, chordae also attach directly to the RV endocardium. Tricuspid regurgitation is therefore a frequent occurrence when the RV dilates from any cause. The orifice of the tricuspid valve is considerable larger than the mitral orifice, the normal tricuspid valve area being about 10 cm^2. Considerable stenosis of the valve must be present to obstruct the RV inflow. Although a mean gradient of 2 mm Hg is enough to establish the diagnosis, most feel a mean gradient of ≥ 5 mm Hg or a calculated valve area <2.0 cm^2 is considered significant tricuspid stenosis.

Tricuspid valve stenosis (TS) is decidedly uncommon, with rheumatic disease accounting for 90% of all cases. It is never an isolated lesion. About 3% to 5% of all patients with rheumatic mitral valve disease will have associated TS. Commissural fusion is present, and the fibrosis and/or fusion of the chordae are seen less often than in rheumatic MS. Leaflet calcium is also quite uncommon.

In this country, the second most common cause of TS is in the carcinoid syndrome, where tricuspid regurgitation is usually present as well. Carcinoid plaque thickens the leaflets and chordae, but commissural fusion is not the rule. Congenital forms of tricuspid stenosis exist and are generally due to abnormalities in the leaflets (absent or decreased number), chordae (absent, reduced, or shortened), and the papillary muscles (reduced number). Congenital tricuspid stenosis has been approached by percutaneous balloon techniques, although it has a very limited role.

Open surgical commissurotomy on the tricuspid valve is also rarely performed because of the high risk of tricuspid regurgitation. It is particularly inadvisable to open the commissure between the anterior and posterior leaflets, although surgical commissurotomy may be successful if fusion is relieved between the anterior and septal or posterior and septal leaflets. It is obviously impossible to restrict the commissural tear that any percutaneous balloon might make to a specific commissure. Based purely on the surgical experience, the use of balloon valvuloplasty has a limited role.

Indications for Tricuspid Valvuloplasty

Patients with TS usually present with low output, fatigue, abdominal swelling due to hepatomegaly and ascites, and anasarca. A wave may be visible in the JVP and may even be felt by the patient. Symptomatic TS would be an acceptable reason to consider valvuloplasty. Clinically, the limiting issue is almost always the presence of associated tricuspid regurgitation. If there is a situation where the patient is not a surgical candidate, and there is either limited tricuspid regurgitation or there is a sense that the risk of converting the patient from tricuspid stenosis to tricuspid regurgitation would not create a hemodynamic disadvantage, then the procedure could be considered. This is a distinctly unusual circumstance.

The Tricuspid Valvuloplasty Procedure and Results

There are few data on the use of percutaneous balloon tricuspid valvuloplasty. The technical aspects are much the same as with percutaneous mitral valvuloplasty with the obvious exception that no trans-septal is required. In the NHLBI Balloon Valvuloplasty Registry, there were only three patients who underwent the procedure on a native valve. Double balloons were used in all. Other reports have reported the use of either double balloons or the Inoue balloon system.

Most of the tricuspid valvuloplasty procedures have been in patients who have undergone both mitral and tricuspid valvuloplasty at the same setting. Mixed results have been note in the treatment of tricuspid stenosis due to the carcinoid syndrome. There are no long-term reports regarding the efficacy of tricuspid valvuloplasty in any setting.

Bioprosthetic Valve Stenosis

Pathophysiology

Porcine or bovine pericardial prosthetic valves may be implanted in any valvular position. They all suffer from a limited lifespan due to a process of mineralization and collagen degeneration over time. Cuspal tears, fibrin deposition, disruption of the fibrocollagenous structure, perforation, fibrosis, and calcium infiltration begin to appear after a few years, and by 10 years, tissue valve failure occurs in about 30%. The process then accelerates, and by 15 years, over half of the valves will have failed. There are some data that pericardial valves may degenerate slower than porcine. The degenerative structural changes occur earlier in valves in the mitral position compared to the aortic position due to the greater hemodynamic stress on the mitral valve. Patients on dialysis appear to be particularly susceptible to early failure. Other factors that have been identified include younger age, pregnancy, and hypercalcemia.

Commissural fusion is uncommon in these valves, the major problem being leaflet immobility. At times, these valves become relatively stenotic due to undersizing (patient-prosthetic mismatch). From an anatomic standpoint, the use of percutaneous balloon valvuloplasty procedures would appear to be problematic given the lack of commissural fusion present.

The Use of Prosthetic Valvuloplasty

There are limited data regarding the use of balloon procedures in prosthetic valve stenosis. It has been reported successfully in two patients with porcine tricuspid valve stenosis, although limited follow-up was available and "restenosis" had quickly occurred in one (33). The NHLBI Balloon Valvuloplasty reported four successful procedures but with no follow-up. There are no prospective studies that have addressed the safety and efficacy of this procedure, and it is not recommended based on the anecdotal evidence for poor results.

REFERENCES

1. Dotter CT, Judkins MP. Transluminal treatment of arteriosclerotic obstruction. Description of a new technic and a preliminary report of its application. *Circulation.* 1964;30:654–670.
2. Rashkind WJ. Atrioseptostomy by balloon catheter in congenital heart disease. *Radiol Clin North Am.* 1971;9(2):193–202.
3. Semb BK, Tjonneland S, Stake G, et al. "Balloon valvulotomy" of congenital pulmonary valve stenosis with tricuspid valve insufficiency. *Cardiovasc Radiol.* 1979;2:239–241.
4. Buchanan JW, Anderson JH, White RI. The 1st balloon valvuloplasty: an historical note. *J Vet Intern Med.* 2002;16:116–117.
5. NHLBI Balloon Valvuloplasty Registry Participants. Percutaneous balloon aortic valvuloplasty: acute and 30-day follow-up results in 671 patients from the NHLBI Balloon Valvuloplasty Registry. *Circulation.* 1991;84:2383–2394.
6. Palacios IF, Lock JE, Keane JF, et al. Percutaneous transvenous balloon valvotomy in a patient with severe calcific mitral stenosis. *J Am Coll Cardiol.* 1986;7:1416–1419.
7. Bonow RO, Carabello BA, Chatterjee K, et al. ACC/AHA 2006. Guidelines for the management of patients with valvular heart disease. *J Am Coll Cardiol.* 2006;48:598–675.
8. Rao PS. Percutaneous balloon valvotomy/angioplasty in congenital heart disease. In: Bashore TM, Davidson CJ, ed. *Percutaneous Balloon Valvuloplasty and Related Techniques.* Lippincott Williams and Wilkins Baltimore, 1991:251–277.
9. Jarrar M, Betbout F, Farhat MB, et al. Long-term invasive and noninvasive results of percutaneous balloon pulmonary valvuloplasty in children, adolescents, and adults. *Am Heart J.* 1999;138:950–954.
10. Lieberman EB, Bashore TM, Hermiller JB, et al. Balloon aortic valvuloplasty in adults: failure of procedure to improve long-term survival. *J Am Coll Cardiol.* 1995;26:1522–1528.
11. Davidson CJ, Harrison JK, Pieper KS, et al. Determinants of one-year outcome from balloon aortic valvuloplasty. *Am J Cardiol.* 1991;68:75–80.
12. Wilkins GT, Weyman AE, Abascal VM, et al. Percutaneous balloon dilatation of the mitral valve: an analysis of echocardiographic variables related to outcome and the mechanism of dilatation. *Br Heart J.* 1988;60:299–308.
13. Rath PC, Tripathy MP, Das NK, et al. Balloon mitral valvuloplasty with bifoil catheter: immediate and long-term follow-up results. *Cathet Cardiovasc Diagn.* 1998;43:43–47.
14. Bonhoeffer P, Piechaud JF, Sidi D, et al. Mitral dilatation with the Multi-track system: an alternative approach. *Cathet Cardiovasc Diagn.* 1995;36:189–193.
15. Cribier A, Rath PC, Letac B. Percutaneous mitral valvotomy with a metal dilatator. *Lancet.* 1997;349:1667.
16. Stefanadis CI, Stratos CG, Lambrou SG, et al. Retrograde nontransseptal balloon mitral valvuloplasty: immediate results and intermediate long-term outcome in 441 cases—a multicenter experience. *J Am Coll Cardiol.* 1998;32:1009–1016.
17. Wang A, Harrison JK, Pieper KS, et al. What does the left atrial v wave signify during balloon commissurotomy of mitral stenosis? *Am J Cardiol.* 1998;82:1388–1393.
18. Dixon S, Safian RD. Balloon Valvuloplasty. In Manual of Interventional Cardiology, Safian RD, Freed MS eds. *Physicians Press.* Royal Oak, Michigan, 2002;903–927.
19. Leon MN, Harrell LC, Simosa HF, et al. Comparison of immediate and long-term results of mitral balloon valvotomy with the double-balloon versus Inoue techniques. *Am J Cardiol.* 1999;83:1356–1363.
20. Fawzy ME, Mimish L, Sivanandam V, et al. Immediate and long-term effect of mitral balloon valvotomy on severe pulmonary hypertension in patients with mitral stenosis. *Am Heart J.* 1996;131:89–93.
21. Tuzcu EM, Block PC, Griffin B, et al. Percutaneous mitral balloon valvotomy in patients with calcific mitral stenosis: immediate and long-term outcome. *J Am Coll Cardiol.* 1994;23:1604–1609.

22. Reid CL, Otto CM, Davis KB, et al. Influence of mitral valve morphology on mitral balloon commissurotomy: immediate and six-month results from the NHLBI Balloon Valvuloplasty Registry. *Am Heart J.* 1992;124:657–665.

23. Multicenter experience with balloon mitral commissurotomy. NHLBI Balloon Valvuloplasty Registry Report on immediate and 30-day follow-up results. *Circulation.* 1992;85:448–461.

24. Palacios IF, Sanchez PL, Harrell LC, et al. Which patients benefit from percutaneous mitral balloon valvuloplasty? Prevalvuloplasty and post-valvuloplasty variables that predict long-term outcome. *Circulation.* 2002; 105:1465–1471.

25. Krasuski RA, Warner JJ, Peterson G, et al. Comparison of results of percutaneous balloon mitral commissurotomy in patients aged ≥65 years with those in patients aged <65 years. *Am J Cardiol.* 2001;88:994–1000.

26. Wang A, Krasuski RA, Warner JJ, et al. Serial echocardiographic evaluation of restenosis after successful percutaneous mitral commissurotomy. *J Am Coll Cardiol.* 2002;39:328–334.

27. Padial LR, Abascal VM, Moreno PR, et al. Echocardiography can predict the development of severe mitral regurgitation after percutaneous mitral valvuloplasty by the Inoue technique. *Am J Cardiol.* 1999;83:1210–1213.

28. Sanchez PL, Harrell LC, Salas RE, et al. Learning curve of the Inoue technique of percutaneous mitral balloon valvuloplasty. *Am J Cardiol.* 2001;88:662–667.

29. Iung B, Garbarz E, Michaud P, et al. Late results of percutaneous mitral commissurotomy in a series of 1024 patients. Analysis of late clinical deterioration: frequency, anatomic findings, and predictive factors. *Circulation.* 1999;99:3272–3278.

30. Ben Farhat M, Ayari M, Maatouk F, et al. Percutaneous balloon versus surgical closed and open mitral commissurotomy: seven-year follow-up results of a randomized trial. *Circulation.* 1998;97:245–250.

31. Reyes VP, Raju BS, Wynne J, et al. Percutaneous balloon valvuloplasty compared with open surgical commissurotomy for mitral stenosis. *N Engl J Med.* 1994;331:961–967.

32. Ben Farhat M, Ayari M, Maatouk F, et al. Percutaneous balloon versus surgical closed and open mitral commissurotomy: seven-year follow-up results of a randomized trial. *Circulation.* 1998;97:245–250.

33. Block PC, Smalling R, Owings RM. Percutaneous double balloon valvotomy for bioprosthetic tricuspid stenosis. *Cathet Cardiovasc Diagn.* 1994; 33:342–344.

CHAPTER 25

Percutaneous Interventions in Adults with Congenital Heart Disease

Thomas M. Bashore

Percutaneous catheter intervention is now feasible in a variety of disorders affecting adults with congenital heart disease (1–7). This chapter will focus on the congenital diseases most likely to be seen in the adult patient. Other chapters review the valvuloplasty procedure for pulmonary valve stenosis and the use of occluder devices for closure of atrial septal defects and the patent foramen ovale.

For most of these less common noncoronary procedures, there are no randomized trials of clinical results, few comparative studies, and many series are quite small, often reflecting the bias of single institutions. For these reasons, most of these interventions should be done in a facility with a particular interest in the adult with congenital heart disease. This allows for an adequate volume of cases so that the operators can achieve an appropriate skill level. In the majority of situations, procedures of this nature are best done by adult cardiologists in concert with their pediatric colleagues or by pediatric cardiologists with experience in this area (3,8).

Because the indications and interpretation of the results in many of these situations require an understanding of the measurement of shunts and the calculations of vascular resistance, a brief review of how one should approach the cardiac catheterization of the adult with congenital heart disease will be presented as a review prior to the discussion of the various interventional procedures.

The Measurement of Cardiac Output, Intracardiac Shunts, and Vascular Resistances

Although shunt locations and sizes can be measured in a variety of ways using indicator dilution techniques, most laboratories now use simple oximetric methods. These methods are based on the Fick equations and an understanding of how the cardiac output is determined by Fick allows for an explanation of how the shunt equations are derived. Figure 25–1 graphically represents flow through the lungs. If one knows how much hemoglobin is in the pulmonary artery (PA) and how much of it is saturated with oxygen, then one can determine the oxygen content in the PA. When the hemoglobin passes through

the lungs, it picks up more oxygen. If one knows the oxygen content in the PA, the oxygen consumption rate, and the subsequent oxygen content in the pulmonary veins (PV), then one can determine how fast the blood flowed through the lungs. This is demonstrated by the Fick equation. The number 10 is used in the denominator to make the units come out correctly:

$$\text{Cardiac output (L/min)} = \frac{\text{oxygen consumption (mL/min)}}{(\text{PV} - \text{PA oxygen content}) \times 10} \quad (25.1)$$

To determine oxygen content, one needs the hemoglobin, a constant, and the oxygen saturation of the blood:

$$\text{Oxygen content} = \text{Hb} \times 1.36 \times O_2 \text{ saturation} \quad (25.2)$$

For the sake of simplicity, the pulmonary blood flow can thus be represented by the abbreviated equation:

$$\text{PBF} = \frac{O_2 \text{ consumption}}{\text{PV} - \text{PA}} \quad (25.3)$$

In the absence of any shunt, the pulmonary blood flow and the systemic blood flow should be the same. The systemic blood flow represents the flow from the aorta (AO) through the body to the right atrium (RA). Unfortunately, there is a normal variation in the saturation of blood arriving to the RA; the inferior vena caval (IVC) blood has higher oxygen content than the superior vena caval (SVC) blood because the kidneys remove far less oxygen relative to their degree of perfusion. The coronary sinus (CS) has very desaturated blood due to the high oxygen extraction rate of the heart, but the amount of CS blood is minor, and its contribution is ignored in the equations. The IVC saturation is high enough normally that one needs at least an 11% step up in the sat from the SVC to the RA to be sure there is an atrial level shunt. As the blood mixes further downstream in the RV, a 7% step up in the RV versus the SVC should be used to confirm a ventricular level shunt, and a 5% step up is recommended in the PA to be confident of a pulmonary arterial left-to-right shunt. To normalize for the higher IVC oxygen content, a mixed venous (MV) saturation is derived from the formula:

$$\text{MV} = \frac{3\,\text{SVC} + \text{IVC}}{4} \quad (25.4)$$

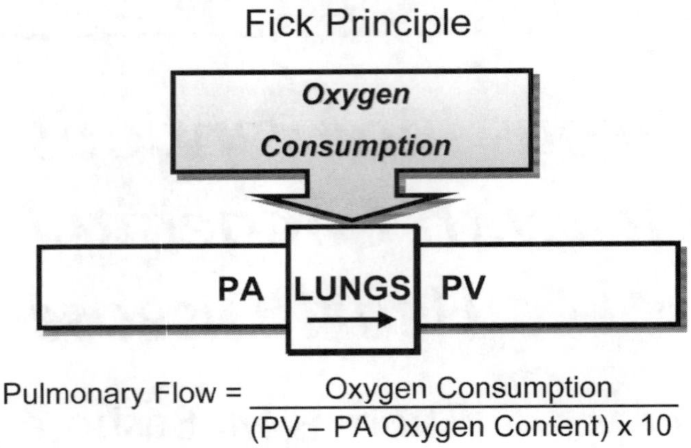

Fick Principle

Oxygen Consumption

PA LUNGS PV →

$$\text{Pulmonary Flow} = \frac{\text{Oxygen Consumption}}{(\text{PV} - \text{PA Oxygen Content}) \times 10}$$

Figure 25–1.

The Fick equation concept. Knowing the oxygen content of the blood entering the lungs, the oxygen content of the blood leaving the lungs, and the rate at which the oxygen has been consumed, the flow rate across the lungs can be determined.

The systemic blood flow (SBF) is, therefore, determined by:

$$\text{SBF} = \frac{O_2 \text{ consumption}}{\text{AO} - \text{MV}} \qquad (25.5)$$

If there is no shunt present,

$$\text{SBF} = \text{PBF} = \frac{O_2 \text{ consumption}}{\text{AO} - \text{MV}} = \frac{O_2 \text{ consumption}}{\text{PV} - \text{PA}} \qquad (25.6)$$

In other words, if there is no shunt, the AO oxygen content should be the same as the PV oxygen content. Similarly, the MV oxygen content should be the same as the PA oxygen content. This is shown in Figure 25–2.

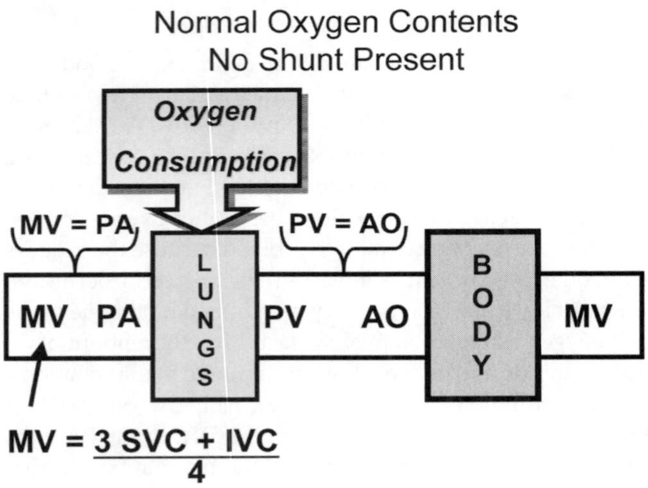

Normal Oxygen Contents
No Shunt Present

Oxygen Consumption

MV = PA   PV = AO

MV PA LUNGS PV AO BODY MV

$$\text{MV} = \frac{3 \text{ SVC} + \text{IVC}}{4}$$

Figure 25–2.

The normal oxygen contents. Because the inferior vena cava (IVC) oxygen saturation is greater than the superior vena cava (SVC), normalization to achieve a mixed venous (MV) saturation is necessary. In the normal situation, the oxygen saturations of the MV and the pulmonary artery (PA) are the same. Similarly, the oxygen saturations of the pulmonary vein (PV) and the aorta (Ao) are identical. Pulmonary blood flow and systemic blood flow are thus equal.

Left-to-Right Shunt Present

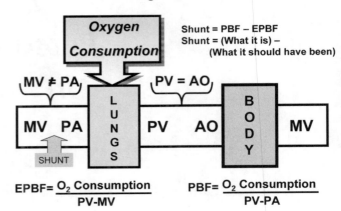

Shunt = PBF − EPBF
Shunt = (What it is) −
(What it should have been)

MV ≠ PA   PV = AO

MV PA LUNGS PV AO BODY MV

SHUNT

$$\text{EPBF} = \frac{O_2 \text{ Consumption}}{\text{PV} - \text{MV}} \qquad \text{PBF} = \frac{O_2 \text{ Consumption}}{\text{PV} - \text{PA}}$$

Figure 25–3.

The effect of a left-to-right shunt. When there is a left-to-right shunt present, the oxygen content of the mixed venous (MV) is no longer the same as the pulmonary artery (PA). The size of the shunt is therefore the difference between the pulmonary blood flow (PBF) and the anticipated pulmonary blood flow (EPBF).

Another way to express the same thing is to use a term known as the *effective blood flow*. Because the PA saturations and the MV saturations are the same, the PBF and the effective pulmonary blood flow (EPBF) should be the same:

$$\text{EPBF} = \frac{O_2 \text{ consumption}}{\text{PV} - \text{MV}} = \text{PBF} = \frac{O_2 \text{ consumption}}{\text{PV} - \text{PA}} \qquad (25.7)$$

By the same token, because the PV saturation and the AO saturation are the same, the SBF and the effective systemic blood flow should be the same:

$$\text{ESBF} = \frac{O_2 \text{ consumption}}{\text{PV} - \text{MV}} = \text{SBF} = \frac{O_2 \text{ consumption}}{\text{AO} - \text{MV}} \qquad (25.8)$$

Note that the equation for the effective pulmonary blood flow (EPBF) is the same as the equation for the effective systemic blood flow (ESBF).

Figure 25–3 now shows how the equations change when there is a left-to-right shunt. Now, the effective pulmonary blood flow does not equal the systemic blood flow because of the shunt. The amount of shunt present is simply:

$$\text{Shunt} = \text{PBF} - \text{EPBF} \qquad (25.9)$$

In effect, the EPBF equation represents what the pulmonary blood flow should have been, and the pulmonary blood flow represents what it actually was. The difference is the size of the shunt.

Figure 25–4 shows the same thing when there is a right-to-left shunt. The effective systemic blood flow no longer is the same as the systemic blood flow because of the shunt. The amount of the shunt is simply:

$$\text{Shunt} = \text{SBF} - \text{ESBF} \qquad (25.10)$$

Just like for a left-to-right shunt, the ESBF equation represents what the systemic blood flow should have been, and the SBF

Right-to-Left Shunt Present

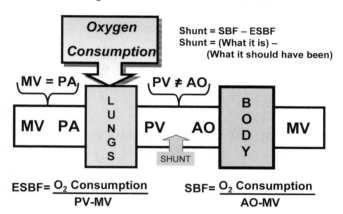

Shunt = SBF − ESBF
Shunt = (What it is) −
(What it should have been)

$$ESBF = \frac{O_2\ Consumption}{PV - MV}$$

$$SBF = \frac{O_2\ Consumption}{AO - MV}$$

Figure 25–4.

The effect of a right-to-left shunt. When there is a right to left shunt, the oxygen content of the PV and the AO are no longer the same. The blood flow across the body (SBF) is thus greater than the anticipated blood flow (ESBF). The difference is the size of the shunt.

equation represents what it actually is. The difference is the size of the shunt.

Besides determining the actual size of a shunt, the ratio of the PBF (or Qp) over the SBF (or Qs) is often used to quantitate the shunt. Using the previous equations, this ratio can be determined by use of only the saturations of blood. This is because when the ratio is derived, the O_2 consumption, the hemoglobin, and constants all drop out. Note using our abbreviated nomenclature:

$$\frac{PBF}{SBF} = \frac{O_2\ consumption/(PV - PA)}{O_2\ consumption/(AO - MV)}$$

$$= \frac{AO - MV\ sats}{PV - PA\ sats} \quad (25.11)$$

Use this simplified equation if only the Qp/Qs is required to answer any board question.

Besides determining the size and locations of shunts, a further important parameter derived from the cardiac catheterization information is the estimate of vascular resistance. This equation is derived from Ohm's law, and although not hemodynamically accurate (it assumes constant flow in systole and diastole), it has been found to be useful clinically. Figure 25–5 reveals the basic concept. If one visualizes a tube with flow through the tube, one can appreciate that the flow would be inversely proportional to the resistance and directly proportional to the pressure pushing the flow past the resistance. The pressure used is the mean pressure.

$$Flow = \frac{pressure_1 - pressure_2}{resistance} \quad (25.12)$$

Or, solving the concept equation:

$$Resistance = \frac{pressure_1 - pressure_2}{flow} \quad (25.13)$$

The pulmonary vascular resistance (PVR) is thus derived from the mean PA pressure entering the lungs, the pressure on the

Pulmonary Vascular Resistance

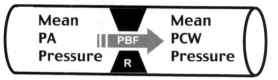

$$PBF = \frac{PA\ Pressure - PCW\ Pressure}{PVR}$$

$$PVR = \frac{PA\ Pressure - PCW\ Pressure}{PBF}$$

Figure 25–5.

Concept of resistance measurements. An analog of Ohm's law is used. Assume a tube with a resistance within it. The flow through the tube (in this case the pulmonary blood flow [PBF]) is directly related to the pressure driving the flow through the tube and inversely related to the magnitude of the resistance. In the case of pulmonary resistance, this means the flow is related to the pressure drop across the lungs and inversely related to the pulmonary vascular resistance (PVR). Solving the equation for PVR allows one to calculate the pulmonary resistance measurement.

other side of the lungs (usually the pulmonary capillary wedge pressure is used), and the flow through the lungs (PBF).

$$PVR = \frac{PA\ mean - PCW\ mean\ (mm\ Hg)}{PBF\ (L/min)} \quad (25.14)$$

Similarly, the systemic vascular resistance (SVR) is derived from the mean aortic pressure, the mean RA pressure, and the SBF.

$$SVR = \frac{AO\ mean - RA\ mean\ (mm\ Hg)}{SBF\ (L/min)} \quad (25.15)$$

When the PBF or SBF are expressed in terms of liters per minute, the units derived are referred to as Absolute or Wood Units. If there is no shunt present, the PBF and the SBF are equal. The Woods Unit number can be multiplied by 80 to derive dynes cm/second^{-5}. Table 25–1 outlines normal values and the various situations where the use of the shunt, the shunt ratio, and the pulmonary resistance has clinical relevance.

By determining the pulmonary vascular resistance, one can decipher whether the cause of pulmonary hypertension is related to a high pulmonary venous pressure (usually from left heart disease) or whether there is a pulmonary cause. An elevated PVR suggests at least some component of pulmonary vascular disease. In some situations this is reversible, whereas in others it is permanent (9). In an attempt to sort out a potential vasoactive component to an elevated PVR, a variety of drugs have been given and the resistance reassessed. These efforts include studying the acute effect of 100% oxygen and pulmonary vasoactive drugs such as adenosine, calcium channel blockers, prostacyclin, and inhaled nitric oxide. A "positive" response is generally one in which there has been both a reduction of the PVR by >20% and the final mean PA pressure is less than 45 mm Hg (10). Both primary pulmonary hypertension and secondary pulmonary hypertension patients may

Table 25–1

Clinical Generalities Regarding Pulmonary Hypertension, Pulmonary Vascular Resistance, and Shunt Values

Pulmonary Hypertension Definitions:

Mild:	Mean PA >20 mm Hg
Moderate:	Mean PA >30 mm Hg
Severe:	Mean PA >45 mm Hg

Normal Pulmonary Vascular Resistance = 0.9+/−0.3 Wood Unit

High-Risk Levels of PVR, PVR/SVR, and PA/Ao Systolic Ratio:

PVR >7.0 Wood Units. (Generally inoperable.)

PVR/SVR >5.0 (High risk for surgery)

PVR/SVR >7.0 (Generally considered inoperable)

If PVR/SVR or PA systolic/AO systolic >2/3, (then only operable if demonstrate persistent left-to-right shunt of >1.5:1.)

Positive Vasoactivity Response to Pulmonary Vasodilators:

>20% drop in PVR and mean PA pressure <45 mm Hg

Shunt Magnitude:

Intervene generally when Qp/Qs >1.5:1

Inoperable when there is shunt reversal and less than 1.5:1 left-to-right shunt

respond to these agents (11). A positive response has been associated with an improved long-term outcome, though the response may not predict clinical improvement with the various pulmonary hypertensive agents now available, such as IV prostacyclin (Flolan) (12), oral endothelin-receptor blockers (Bosentan) (13), prostacyclin agonists (14), vasodilators such as sildenafil (Viagara) (15), inhaled prostacyclin (Iloprost) (16), or subcutaneous trepostinol (Remodulin) (17). *Eisenmenger's physiology* is defined by the presence of pulmonary hypertension and evidence for shunt reversal (cyanosis). If any of these therapies decrease the systemic resistance more than the pulmonary resistance, then an increase in cyanosis may result.

■ Adult Congenital Cardiac Percutaneous Interventions

There are a variety of lesions in patients with adult congenital heart disease that are amenable to percutaneous intervention. The devices used include vascular occluders or coil occlusion for patent ductus arteriosus (PDA), aortopulmonary collaterals, coronary fistulae, pulmonary AV fistulae, and other unwanted vascular structures, such as residual Blalock-Taussig shunts. Septal occluder devices similar to that used for ASD and PFO closure are making their way as therapeutic options for certain ventricular septal defects (VSD). These devices are also being used off-label to occlude other unwanted shunts, leaks, and perforations. In addition, angioplasty and/stent pro-

cedures are being applied to the treatment of coarctation of the aorta, branch or peripheral pulmonary arterial stenosis, and stenosis of the systemic or pulmonary veins. Covered stents can also be used to repair leaks in Mustard baffles. Finally, some devices are being used to actually create a shunt to hopefully reduce right heart pressures in situations such as in Fontan patients with a protein-losing enteropathy.

■ Vascular Occluder Devices

Table 25–2 outlines the current use of vascular occluder devices, their basic indication, method, general success rate, and any additional comments. The most common application of these methods in the adult is for closure of the PDA or coronary fistulae.

A patent ductus arteriosus is the second most common congenital heart defect seen in adults (~10% to 15% of all CHD in adults). It is present in isolation in about 75% of adults, unlike in children where it is frequently associated with more complex heart defects. A substantial left-to-right shunt through the patent ductus can result in the development of pulmonary hypertension. Some feel that any residual PDA should be occluded to prevent endarteritis and to remove any excess flow to the pulmonary circuit and left heart that may result in volume overload over time. In most laboratories, the indication for closure of the PDA is the demonstration of any persistent left-to-right shunt even if there is some evidence for pulmonary hypertension. If the shunt has reversed (giving one blue toes and pink hands due to the cyanosis in the lower extremity), then the pulmonary hypertension is considered irreversible, and closure is not considered an option.

There are currently two popular options available for percutaneous closure (18): an occluder device (such as the Amplatzer PDA Occluder) or spring occlusion coils (Fig. 25–6). Either strategy appears favorable with relatively little morbidity, although coils are generally not recommended for defects in excess of 4 mm in diameter because of the higher risk for arterial embolization (19). Multiple coils, though, have been occasionally used to close defects as large as 7 mm in diameter (20).

In a representative coil occlusion technique (21), the defect is first sized angiographically to optimize coil size selection. A catheter (often a right coronary catheter) is then used to cross the defect in retrograde fashion from the aorta. A snare is then advanced from the pulmonary side. A detachable coil is pushed out the end of the aortic catheter and the tip of the coil snared in the pulmonary artery after at least one major coil loop is evident in the PA. The aortic catheter is then withdrawn, and the proximal coil loops are allowed to coil in the ductus itself. Several coils may be used, or coils may be placed from both the aortic or pulmonary directions. Detachable (22) coils are now available that allow positioning and observation of the results before detaching the coil from the delivery system. An alternative coil method uses a nylon sack attached to an end-hole catheter; wire coils are advanced into the sack, expanding it and occluding the ductus (23). More recently, PDA closure

Table 25–2

Coils and Occluder Devices and Their Use in Adult Congenital Heart Disease

	Indication	Methods	Acute Success	Comments
Patent ductus arteriosus (PDA)	Volume overload to left heart. Prevention of endocarditis. Left-to-right shunt only (no reversal of shunt).	PDA vascular occluder. Coil occlusion.	For coils, 90% success if PDA minimal diameter is <4 mm. Success >75% if minimal diameter <7 mm. Larger ductus occlusion possible with occluder devices.	High long-term success rate. Complications include residual leak, hemolysis, and embolization.
Coronary fistulae	Evidence for coronary steal.	Coil occlusion.	Technically high.	Complications include unwanted branch occlusion or embolization.
Aortopulmonary bronchial collaterals	Hemoptysis in patients with pulmonary hypertension. Prelung transplant.	Coil occlusion.	Technically high.	Regrowth of other collaterals common.
Pulmonary AV fistulae	Cyanosis. Evidence for paradoxical emboli.	Coil occlusion. Occasionally, Amplatzer or other occluder if fistula large.	Technically high in selected lesions.	Often multiple small fistulae present that are not amenable to coil occlusion. Regrowth of collaterals high.
Ventricular septal defect	Qp/Qs >1.5. Evidence for LA and LV enlargement. If pulmonary hypertension (pulmonary systolic pressure or PVR >2/3 systemic systolic pressure or SVR), then need Qp/Qs >1.5.	Ventricular septal occluder devices.	Almost 90% success rate. High rate of complications, however, with 10% major complications.	CardioSEAL approved for muscular VSDs and postinfarction VSDs. Other devices undergoing investigation for membranous and muscular VSDs.

has been popularized by delivery of a PDA occluder device from the PA side of the ductus (24) (Fig. 25–6). There are data that suggest the occluder method and the coil methods are equally effective (25).

Incomplete occlusion can be associated with hemolysis due to the injury to RBCs within the residual shunt jet lesion (26). Rare cases of endocarditis have also been reported. Coil occlusion is successful in 75% to 90% of patients; the smaller the ductus, the better the results. Occasionally, recanalization of the defect can occur during follow-up and may require further intervention. A strategy of coil occlusion has been compared head to head to surgical therapy and found to be cost beneficial.

Coronary fistulae generally arise from the proximal portion of the native coronary artery and enter either the pulmonary artery or atria. In the most extreme example, the left main may arise from the pulmonary artery (Bland-Garland-White syndrome) with the right coronary supplying the entire myo-cardium and emptying into the PA. The resultant coronary steal into the PA often results in massively dilating the RCA and portions of the left coronary system and can result in myocardial infarction or an ischemic cardiomyopathy. The right coronary may similarly arise from the PA. Coronaries arising from the PA should be surgically corrected.

Most coronary fistulae, however, are discovered during routine coronary angiography and require no therapy (27). On rare occasions, the steal from the coronary bed will be of significance and result in anginal symptoms. The resultant coronary underperfusion can usually be demonstrated by exercise imaging methods. Rarely are coronary fistulae large enough that a substantial left-to-right shunt is present, and often no oximetric step-up can be demonstrated at catheterization even in angiographically appearing large fistulae (28). Intervention is indicated only when the there is evidence for coronary steal and symptoms. Percutaneous coil implantation for coronary fistulae requires a favorable vessel size and shape in order to

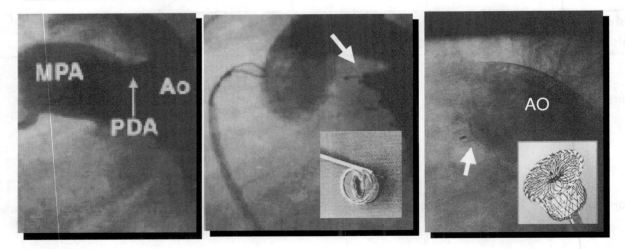

Figure 25–6.

Patent ductus occlusion. The patent ductus arteriosus is angiographically shown in the *right panel*. The *middle panel* represents coils occlusion after withdrawal of the snare in the PA. The *left panel* represents device occlusion with the Amplatzer PDA occluder.

position coils without embolization (29). Figure 25–7 demonstrates coil occlusion of a coronary fistula from the left anterior descending coronary artery to the PA.

In patients who have pulmonary arterial hypertension or pulmonary arterial underperfusion due to an RV outflow tract obstructive lesion, aorto-pulmonary or bronchial collaterals may form. These commonly arise from the aorta or the internal mammary arteries. These can rupture and produce gross and even life-threatening hemoptysis. When lung transplantation is being considered as definitive therapy, these collaterals also may be the source of excessive bleeding in the early postoperative period. For those reasons, coil occlusion of these bronchial collaterals may be clinically indicated (30,31). Fig-

ure 25–8 demonstrates the results of coil occlusion of a typical bronchial collateral.

Pulmonary AV fistulae may result in hypoxemia, or the patient may present with paradoxical embolization. These are particularly common in patients with Osler-Weber-Rendu syndrome (hereditary hemorrhagic telangiectasia) and in the right lung of patients who have undergone a classic Glenn procedure (SVC attachment to the right pulmonary artery). Multiple small fistulae may also be seen in patients with hepatopulmonary syndrome. When the fistulae are large enough to create either cyanosis or evidence for systemic embolization, then coil occlusion (32) or ductal occlusion devices (33) may be used. Figure 25–9 demonstrates coil occlusion of a

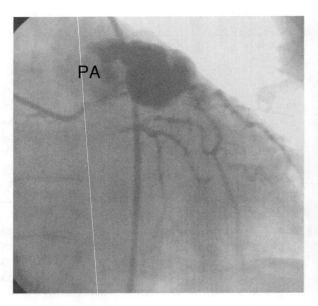
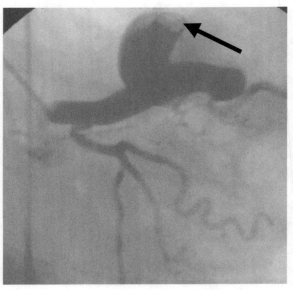

Figure 25–7.

Coil occlusion of a coronary fistula. The *right panel* reveals a proximal left anterior descending fistula to the pulmonary artery. The *left panel* reveals persistence of the proximal aneurysmal portion of the fistula, but coil occlusion of the midportion with loss of contrast flow into the PA. The *arrow* points to the coils.

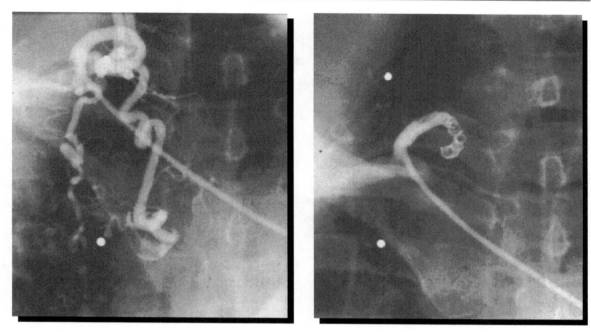

Figure 25–8.

Coil occlusion of bronchial collaterals. A large collateral from the aorta to the left pulmonary artery is shown in the *right panel*. Occlusion is achieved with coils as noted in the *left panel*.

pulmonary AV fistula in a patient with a prior classic Glenn anastomosis.

Anomalous venovenous collaterals may also occur in patients with elevated systemic venous pressure, such as those who have had the Glenn/Fontan procedure or those with occlusion of the SVC. Often, these collaterals connect the innominate vein or other systemic venous structures to the pulmonary veins or left atrium, resulting in cyanosis from the right-to-left shunt. Transcatheter coil occlusion of these anomalous channels has been used successfully (34) to reduce the right-to-left shunt.

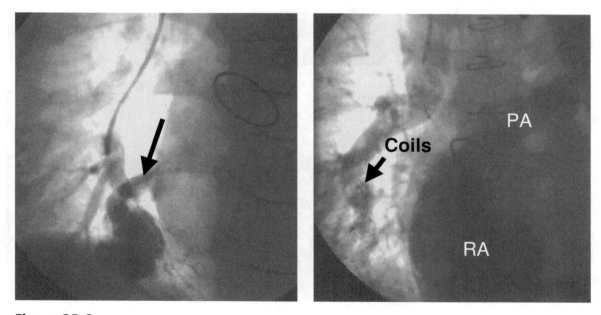

Figure 25–9.

Coil occlusion of a pulmonary AV fistula. The patient has undergone a Glenn procedure (SVC to right PA) and a Fontan procedure (in this case an RA conduit with a bioprosthetic valve to the main PA). A large AV fistula has formed in the right lung as shown by the *right panel*. In the *left panel*, the right PA is injected simultaneously with the RA. The coils have occluded the AV fistula.

Ventricular Septal Defect Occlusion

Patients with certain ventricular septal defects may also be treated with percutaneous occluder devices. As early as 1988, Lock et al. reported six patients deemed not to be operative (either congenital or postmyocardial infarction) in whom the Rashkind umbrella was successfully deployed (35). Since then, there has been increasing interest in the use of ventricular septal occluder devices for repair of congenital membranous ventricular septal defects (36), congenital muscular septal defects (37), and following acute myocardial infarction (38). As of this writing, the CardioSEAL device is approved for muscular VSD and postinfarction VSD occlusion (39), and the Amplatzer device is under investigation for muscular VSD occlusion with 75 patients reported from that registry (37). Figure 25–10 demonstrates the procedure (40).

The indication for VSD closure generally includes a Qp/Qs >1.5 and an increased LV and LA size due to the volume overload. If pulmonary hypertension is present (pulmonary systolic pressure >2/3 systemic systolic pressure or PVR >2/3

SVR), then demonstration of at least a net shunt ratio of 1.5:1 must be present or there must be evidence that the pulmonary artery pressure is responsive to pulmonary vasodilators (41).

The procedure is not without potential complications, however. In the largest series reported to date, Knauth et al. (42) examined the 13-year experience at Children's Hospital Boston involving 170 patients with congenital or postop residual VSDs that had undergone percutaneous occluder device implantation, generally with the clam-shell (STARflex-type) device. Up to seven devices were implanted per patient with multiple devices in 40%. Complications were frequent (a total of 332): 261 were related to the catheterization procedure itself and 39 related to the device. At a 2-year follow-up, 14 patients had died, and 18 devices had been surgically explanted.

Holzer et al. reported on the registry using the Amplatzer device (43), and while there was an 87% success rate, the major complication rate was 10.7% including death, embolization of the device, and cardiac perforation. Closure appeared to occur more often over time with only 47% closed at 24 hours, but 70% at 6 months and 92% at 1 year.

VSD Occlusion Procedure

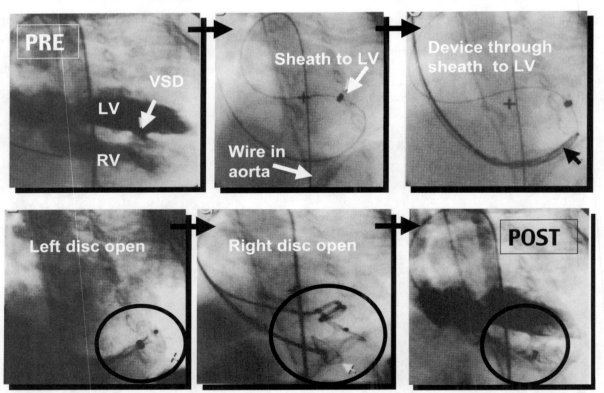

Figure 25–10.

Device occlusion of a muscular ventricular septal defect. The *first panel* reveals the preprocedural ventriculogram with the muscular VSD evident. A balloon catheter is placed in the LV and passed to the RV through the defect. A wire through this catheter is snared in the RV from a jugular venous approach. A sheath is then placed along this wire to the LV as shown in the *second panel*. The device is then placed in the sheath from the right side to the LV. Progressively, the sheath is removed and the device expanded on the left then right side of the ventricular septum. The final panel reveals the postprocedural ventriculogram. (Modified from: Chessa M, Carminati M, Cao QL, et al. Transcatheter closure of congenital and acquired muscular ventricular septal defects using the Amplatzer device. *J Invasive Cardiol.* 2002;14:322–327, with permission.)

Percutaneous closure of VSDs are made complicated by the heavily trabeculated RV restricting the opening of the RV side of the occluder in some cases. Residual shunting is frequent. The use of these devices in the postmyocardial infarction patient, where surgical mortality is extraordinarily high (around 70% in many series), is particularly of interest. The difficulty in using these devices after an acute MI, though, is that many VSDs due to septal rupture are multiple in nature, follow a serpentine course through the ventricular septum, and do not have firm enough tissue in the area of the infarction to hold a device in place.

Other Lesions Potentially Amenable to Percutaneous Occluder Devices

Other lesions that have been approached by transcatheter techniques include the coil occlusion of patent Blalock-Taussig shunts (44), device occlusion of fenestrations purposely left in the conduit of the lateral tunnel Fontan procedure (45,46),

and device or covered stent occlusion of baffle leaks in patients who have undergone the Mustard procedure (46,47). Devices have also been used off label to occlude the conduit from the LV to descending aorta (48), to close a ruptured sinus of Valsalva fistula (49) or a window-type patent ductus arteriosus (50), or to alleviate perivalvular prosthetic valve insufficiency (51,52).

Angioplasty and Stent Devices

Table 25–3 outlines the major use of angioplasty and stenting devices for adults with congenital heart disease. The devices may be used in coarctation of the aorta, branch and peripheral pulmonary artery stenosis, and to relieve obstruction of systemic venous channels (obstructed baffles in patients with a Mustard procedure, SVC occlusion) or pulmonary venous stenosis.

Coarctation of the aorta (53) is a relatively common congenital heart defect, accounting for about 8% of all congenital

Table 25–3
Use of Angioplasty and Stenting in Adult Congenital Heart Disease

	Indications	Methods	Acute Success	Comments
Coarctation of the aorta	>20 mm Hg peak gradient. Angiographically amenable to stent placement. Proximal systemic hypertension.	Balloon angioplasty. Stent placement (now preferred).	>60% acute success rate. Success variably defined but recommended as final gradient <10 mm Hg. Higher success rate with stenting than angioplasty.	Originally, balloon angioplasty for postop coarctation due to aneurysmal formation in native coarctation angioplasty. Now stent placement acceptable for both native and postop. Complications include aortic rupture, aneurysm formation. Hypertension may not always resolve after procedure.
Branch pulmonary artery stenosis	>50% diameter lesion with gradient across stenosis.	Balloon angioplasty. Stent placement.	Technically high early success rate.	Restenosis common.
Peripheral pulmonary artery stenosis	>50% diameter lesion with gradient across stenosis. Pulmonary hypertension.	Balloon angioplasty. Stent placement.	Angiographic success high.	Restenosis very common.
Systemic and pulmonary venous stenoses	>50% diameter lesion with gradient across stenosis.	Balloon angioplasty. Stent placement.	Variable success rates. Angiographically high success rate initially.	In Mustard baffle, if associated baffle leak, a covered stent can also be deployed to cover leak. Restenosis rates are high, particularly if only balloon angioplasty used.

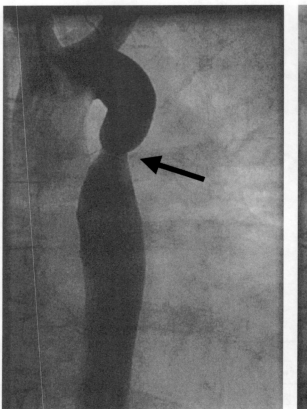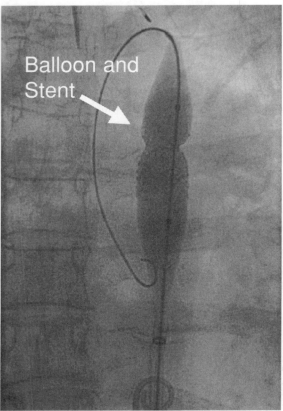

Figure 25–11.

Stenting of coarctation of the aorta. The *left panel* reveals the native coarctation prior to stenting and the *right panel* reveals the positioning of the stent during balloon inflation.

defects. Anatomically, it can occur proximal, at, or distal to the takeoff of the ductus arteriosus. It likely results from extraneous ductal tissue in the aorta that contracts following birth. Adults with previously undiagnosed coarctation generally present with postductal lesions. The most common presentation in adults is the fortuitous discovery during secondary work-up for systemic hypertension. Renal hypoperfusion leads to a resetting of the renin-angiotensin system and a hyper-renin state that, unfortunately, may not abate even after repair of the coarctation (54). In most patients, there is upper extremity hypertension with the development of collateral vessels around the coarctation to the lower body. These collateral channels often create a continuous murmur heard in the back, and involvement of the intercostals arteries leads to the familiar "rib notching" noted on the chest x-ray. An associated bicuspid aortic valve is present 50% to 85% of patients with aortic coarctation, and a significant aortic gradient is particularly important to exclude when deciding on definitive therapy. An association with berry aneurysms in the circle of Willis can lead to CNS hemorrhage in up to 10% of patients (55).

Echocardiography can be used to interrogate the descending aorta, with a resting peak systolic velocity ≥3.2 m per second or a diastolic velocity of ≥1.0 m per second suggestive of significant coarctation. Echo also allows interrogation of the aortic valve and assessment of the ascending aortic root. Magnetic resonance imaging has now become the favorite imaging

modality both pre- and postoperatively to size the aorta and evaluate the coarctation region. It also provides anatomic data regarding the aortic valve. In the event of a contraindication to MRI (pacemaker or severe claustrophobia) or the lack of availability, computer tomography with contrast provides an acceptable alternative. In particular, multi-detector CT allows for three-dimensional reconstruction similar to magnetic resonance angiographic methods.

Symptomatic patients with a peak gradient over 20 mm Hg across the coarctation when invasive measurement is performed or a similar gradient in asymptomatic patients with upper extremity hypertension, and left ventricular hypertrophy should be considered for intervention therapy. A successful procedure is usually defined as a reduction in the peak gradient to less than 20 mm Hg (56), though some data suggests that a final residual gradient of less than 10 mm Hg is preferred (57). Other evolving indications for treatment include the presence of aortic aneurysms and symptomatic aneurysms of the circle of Willis. Young women who wish to bear children are also at risk, as there may be inadequate placental flow should they become pregnant.

Percutaneous angioplasty for coarctation has been performed since 1982, and the availability of stents has recently led to improved outcomes, to the extent that percutaneous intervention is now considered the procedure of choice in patients with recoarctation following surgery (56,58). More

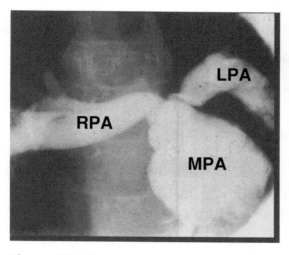
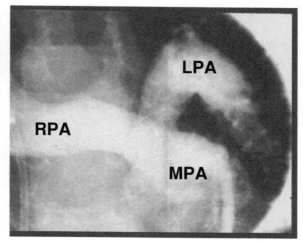

Figure 25–12.

Pulmonary branch stenosis. The *left panel* reveals the lesions at the origins of both the left and right pulmonary arteries. The *right panel* demonstrates an excellent result from stenting.

recently, aortic stents of adequate size have been available, and these are particularly effective in preventing complications from recoil of the aorta following angioplasty (Fig. 25–11). The size of the stent is never larger than the native aorta. Intravascular ultrasound has been useful in insuring that there is adequate apposition of the stent against the aortic wall.

Several large series of angioplasty/stent reports suggest that success rates of 65% to 100% with a complication rate of ∼13% are to be expected (58,59). Problems to watch for include recoarctation and aneurysm formation at the site of intervention

and persistent blood pressure elevation. Older patients and those with an associated bicuspid aortic valve are at greatest risk for long-term complications (60). Endocarditis prophylaxis remains indicated.

Postcoarctation aneurysm formation was particularly a concern early in the experience of using angioplasty for native coarctation, resulting in the recommendation that native coarctation is better treated with surgical intervention (61,62). This concern has lessened more recently with the greater use of stenting, and many advocate a percutaneous approach in both

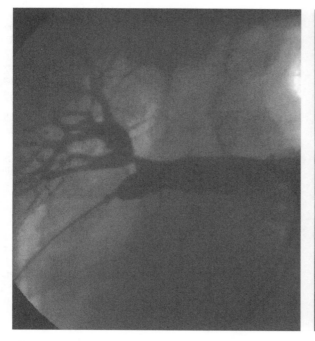
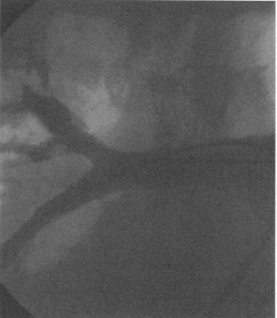

Figure 25–13.

Peripheral pulmonary artery stenosis. The *left panel* reveals two areas of peripheral PS. The *right panel* demonstrates the results of stenting in both of these lesions.

native and postop coarctation if the anatomy is suitable for stent placement (58,63).

Branch pulmonary artery stenosis is sometimes associated with tetralogy of Fallot or may be an isolated lesion. When it occurs, the main pulmonary arterial pressure may be elevated, and symptoms consistent with any RV outflow tract lesion may become manifest. When a "significant" angiographic lesion is noted (usually defined as one >50% diameter narrowing) and a demonstrable gradient across the lesion can be found, then it may be appropriate to intervene. Balloon angioplasty studies have revealed excellent early results, but the highly elastic pulmonary vessels result in early restenosis. Stenting has fared a little better and is currently the recommended approach to these lesions (64) (Fig. 25–12). When restenosis occurs, surgical patch intervention is possible in some cases.

Peripheral pulmonary artery stenosis may present with a similar clinical scenario as primary pulmonary hypertension. The presence of peripheral lung murmurs may be a clue to their presence. These lesions are associated with a variety of congenital lesions and may be the sequelae of the maternal rubella syndrome. Similar to other right-sided vascular lesions, the balloon angioplasty has not been proven effective, though much better results have been obtained using stent procedures (3,64). These lesions are not generally considered amenable to surgical approaches. Figure 25–13 demonstrates the effect of stenting in peripheral pulmonary arterial stenosis.

Other Uncommon Applications of Angioplasty/Stenting in Adults with Congenital Heart Disease

There are also case reports or very small series where stents have been used to relieve stenosis in patients with an obstructed Glenn shunt or at the SVC site following sinus venosus repair (2). Stents have also been used to relieve obstruction in pulmonary venous stenoses and narrowed Fontan conduits (64), to increase the outflow tract size in patients with subpulmonic stenosis (65) and hypertrophic cardiomyopathy (66), and to relieve right heart conduit stenoses (67) when present.

REFERENCES

1. Holzer R, Hijazi ZM. Interventional approach to congenital heart disease. *Curr Opin Cardiol.* 2004;19:84–90.
2. O'Laughlin MP, Perry SB, Lock JE, et al. Use of endovascular stents in congenital heart disease. *Circulation.* 1991;83:1923–1939.
3. Allen HD, Beekman RH III, Garson A Jr, et al. Pediatric therapeutic cardiac catheterization: a statement for healthcare professionals from the Council on Cardiovascular Disease in the Young, American Heart Association. *Circulation.* 1998;97:609–625.
4. Andrews RE, Tulloh RM. Interventional cardiac catheterisation in congenital heart disease. *Arch Dis Child.* 2004;89:1168–1173.
5. Faella HJ. Congenital heart defects in the adult: towards nonsurgical interventionism. *Rev Esp Cardiol.* 2004;57:33–38.
6. Krasuski RA, Bashore TM. The emerging role of percutaneous intervention in adults with congenital heart disease. *Rev Cardiovasc Med.* 2005;6:11–22.
7. Verma R, Keane JF. Percutaneous therapy of structural heart disease: pediatric disease. *Prog Cardiovasc Dis.* 1997;40:37–54.
8. Grown-up congenital heart (GUCH) disease: current needs and provision of service for adolescents and adults with congenital heart disease in the UK. *Heart.* 2002;88 (suppl):1–14.
9. Bush A, Busst CM, Haworth SG, et al. Correlations of lung morphology, pulmonary vascular resistance, and outcome in children with congenital heart disease. *Br Heart J.* 1988;59:480–485.
10. Krasuski RA, Wang A, Harrison JK, et al. The response to inhaled nitric oxide in patients with pulmonary artery hypertension is not masked by baseline vasodilator use. *Am Heart J.* 2005;150:725–728.
11. Krasuski RA, Warner JJ, Wang A, et al. Inhaled nitric oxide selectively dilates pulmonary vasculature in adult patients with pulmonary hypertension, irrespective of etiology. *J Am Coll Cardiol.* 2000;36:2204–2211.
12. Rosenzweig EB, Kerstein D, Barst RJ. Long-term prostacyclin for pulmonary hypertension with associated congenital heart defects. *Circulation.* 1999;99:1858–1865.
13. Apostolopoulou SC, Manginas A, Cokkinos DV, et al. Effect of the oral endothelin antagonist bosentan on the clinical, exercise, and haemodynamic status of patients with pulmonary arterial hypertension related to congenital heart disease. *Heart.* 2005;91:1447–1452.
14. Suzuki H, Sato S, Tanabe S, et al. Beraprost sodium for pulmonary hypertension with congenital heart disease. *Pediatr Int.* 2002;44:528–529.
15. Preston IR, Klinger JR, Houtches J, et al. Acute and chronic effects of sildenafil in patients with pulmonary arterial hypertension. *Respir Med.* 2005;99:1501–1510.
16. Carroll CL, Backer CL, Mavroudis C, et al. Inhaled prostacyclin following surgical repair of congenital heart disease—a pilot study. *J Card Surg.* 2005;20:436–439.
17. Simonneau G, Barst RJ, Galie N, et al. Continuous subcutaneous infusion of treprostinil, a prostacyclin analogue, in patients with pulmonary arterial hypertension: a double-blind, randomized, placebo-controlled trial. *Am J Respir Crit Care Med.* 2002;165:800–804.
18. O'Donnell C, Neutze JM, Skinner JR, et al. Transcatheter patent ductus arteriosus occlusion: evolution of techniques and results from the 1990s. *J Paediatr Child Health.* 2001;37:451–455.
19. Sommer RJ, Gutierrez A, Lai WW, et al. Use of preformed nitinol snare to improve transcatheter coil delivery in occlusion of patent ductus arteriosus. *Am J Cardiol.* 1994;74:836–839.
20. Hijazi ZM, Geggel RL. Results of anterograde transcatheter closure of patent ductus arteriosus using single or multiple Gianturco coils. *Am J Cardiol.* 1994;74:925–929.
21. Sommer RJ, Gutierrez A, Lai WW, et al. Use of preformed nitinol snare to improve transcatheter coil delivery in occlusion of patent ductus arteriosus. *Am J Cardiol.* 1994;74:836–839.
22. Galal MO, Bulbul Z, Kakadekar A, et al. Comparison between the safety profile and clinical results of the Cook detachable and Gianturco coils for transcatheter closure of patent ductus arteriosus in 272 patients. *J Interv Cardiol.* 2001;14:169–177.
23. Grifka RG, Vincent JA, Nihill MR, et al. Transcatheter patent ductus arteriosus closure in an infant using the Gianturco-Grifka Vascular Occlusion Device. *Am J Cardiol.* 1996;78:721–723.
24. Lee CH, Leung YL, Chow WH. Transcatheter closure of the patent ductus arteriosus using an Amplatzer duct occluder in adults. *Jpn Heart J.* 2001;42:533–537.
25. Santoro G, Bigazzi MC, Palladino MT, et al. Comparison of percutaneous closure of large patent ductus arteriosus by multiple coils versus the Amplatzer duct occluder device. *Am J Cardiol.* 2004;94:252–255.
26. Shim D, Fedderly RT, Beekman RH III, et al. Follow-up of coil occlusion of patent ductus arteriosus. *J Am Coll Cardiol.* 1996;28:207–211.
27. Harikrishnan S, Jacob SP, Tharakan J, et al. Congenital coronary anomalies of origin and distribution in adults: a coronary arteriographic study. *Indian Heart J.* 2002;54:271–275.
28. Lacombe P, Rocha P, Marchand X, et al. High flow coronary fistula closure by percutaneous coil packing. *Cathet Cardiovasc Diagn.* 1993;28:342–346.
29. Dorros G, Thota V, Ramireddy K, et al. Catheter-based techniques for closure of coronary fistulae. *Catheter Cardiovasc Interv.* 1999;46:143–150.
30. Rothman A, Tong AD. Percutaneous coil embolization of superfluous vascular connections in patients with congenital heart disease. *Am Heart J.* 1993;126:206–213.

31. Lois JF, Gomes AS, Smith DC, et al. Systemic-to-pulmonary collateral vessels and shunts: treatment with embolization. *Radiology*. 1988;169:671–676.

32. Rath PC, Tripathy MP, Panigrahi NK, et al. Successful coil embolization and follow-up result of a complex pulmonary arterio-venous fistula. *J Invasive Cardiol*. 1999;11:83–86.

33. Bialkowski J, Zabal C, Szkutnik M, et al. Percutaneous interventional closure of large pulmonary arteriovenous fistulas with the amplatzer duct occluder. *Am J Cardiol*. 2005;96:127–129.

34. Beekman RH III, Shim D, Lloyd TR. Embolization therapy in pediatric cardiology. *J Interv Cardiol*. 1995;8:543–556.

35. Lock JE, Block PC, McKay RG, et al. Transcatheter closure of ventricular septal defects. *Circulation*. 1988;78:361–368.

36. Kalra GS, Verma PK, Dhall A, et al. Transcatheter device closure of ventricular septal defects: immediate results and intermediate-term follow-up. *Am Heart J*. 1999;138:339–344.

37. Holzer R, Balzer D, Cao QL, et al. Device closure of muscular ventricular septal defects using the Amplatzer muscular ventricular septal defect occluder: immediate and mid-term results of a U.S. registry. *J Am Coll Cardiol*. 2004;43:1257–1263.

38. Anantharaman R, Walsh KP, Roberts DH. Combined catheter ventricular septal defect closure and multivessel coronary stenting to treat post-myocardial infarction ventricular septal defect and triple-vessel coronary artery disease: a case report. *Catheter Cardiovasc Interv*. 2004;63:311–313.

39. Ruiz CE, Austin EH, Cheatham JP, et. al. First Food and Drug Administration approval under humanitarian device exemption of a septal occluder for fenestrated Fontan and muscular ventricular septal defects. *Circulation*. 2000;101:E9042.

40. Chessa M, Carminati M, Cao QL, et al. Transcatheter closure of congenital and acquired muscular ventricular septal defects using the Amplatzer device. *J Invasive Cardiol*. 2002;14:322–327.

41. Therrien J, Dore A, Gersony W, et al. CCS Consensus Conference 2001 update: recommendations for the management of adults with congenital heart disease. Part I. *Can J Cardiol*. 2001;17:940–959.

42. Knauth AL, Lock JE, Perry SB, et al. Transcatheter device closure of congenital and postoperative residual ventricular septal defects. *Circulation*. 2004;110:501–507.

43. Holzer R, Latson L, Hijazi ZM. Device closure of iatrogenic membranous ventricular septal defects after prosthetic aortic valve replacement using the Amplatzer membranous ventricular septal defect occluder. *Catheter Cardiovasc Interv*. 2004;62:276–280.

44. Perry SB, Radtke W, Fellows KE, et al. Coil embolization to occlude aortopulmonary collateral vessels and shunts in patients with congenital heart disease. *J Am Coll Cardiol*. 1989;13:100–108.

45. Kay JD, O'Laughlin MP, Ito K, et al. Five-year clinical and echocardiographic evaluation of the Das AngelWings atrial septal occluder. *Am Heart J*. 2004;147:361–368.

46. Apostolopoulou SC, Laskari CV, Kiaffas M, et al. Diverse experience with the CardioSEAL and STARFlex septal occluders. *Cardiol Young*. 2004;14:367–372.

47. Daehnert I, Hennig B, Wiener M, et al. Interventions in leaks and obstructions of the interatrial baffle late after Mustard and Senning correction for transposition of the great arteries. *Catheter Cardiovasc Interv*. 2005;66:400–407.

48. Amin Z, Leatherbury L, Moore HV, et al. A novel use of Amplatzer duct occluder. *Pediatr Cardiol*. 2000;21:180–182.

49. Arora R, Trehan V, Rangasetty UM, et al. Transcatheter closure of ruptured sinus of valsalva aneurysm. *J Interv Cardiol*. 2004;17:53–58.

50. Bialkowski J, Szkutnik M, Kusa J, et al. Percutaneous closure of window-type patent ductus arteriosus: using the CardioSEAL and STARFlex devices. *Tex Heart Inst J*. 2003;30:236–239.

51. Webb JG, Pate GE, Munt BI. Percutaneous closure of an aortic prosthetic paravalvular leak with an Amplatzer duct occluder. *Catheter Cardiovasc Interv*. 2005;65:69–72.

52. Cabalka AK, Hagler DJ, Mookadam F, et al. Percutaneous closure of left ventricular-to-right atrial fistula after prosthetic mitral valve rereplacement using the Amplatzer duct occluder. *Catheter Cardiovasc Interv*. 2005;64:522–527.

53. Bashore TM, Lieberman EB. Aortic/mitral obstruction and coarctation of the aorta. *Cardiol Clin*. 1993;11:617–641.

54. de Divitiis DM, Pilla C, Kattenhorn M, et al. Ambulatory blood pressure, left ventricular mass, and conduit artery function late after successful repair of coarctation of the aorta. *J Am Coll Cardiol*. 2003;41:2259–2265.

55. Connolly HM, Huston J III, Brown RD Jr, et al. Intracranial aneurysms in patients with coarctation of the aorta: a prospective magnetic resonance angiographic study of 100 patients. *Mayo Clin Proc*. 2003;78:1491–1499.

56. Hamdan MA, Maheshwari S, Fahey JT, et al. Endovascular stents for coarctation of the aorta: initial results and intermediate-term follow-up. *J Am Coll Cardiol*. 2001;38:1518–1523.

57. Zabal C, Attie F, Rosas M, et al. The adult patient with native coarctation of the aorta: balloon angioplasty or primary stenting? *Heart*. 2003;89:77–83.

58. Fawzy ME, Awad M, Hassan W, et al. Long-term outcome (up to 15 years) of balloon angioplasty of discrete native coarctation of the aorta in adolescents and adults. *J Am Coll Cardiol*. 2004;43:1062–1067.

59. Ebeid MR, Prieto LR, Latson LA. Use of balloon-expandable stents for coarctation of the aorta: initial results and intermediate-term follow-up. *J Am Coll Cardiol*. 1997;30:1847–1852.

60. Oliver JM, Gallego P, Gonzalez A, et al. Risk factors for aortic complications in adults with coarctation of the aorta. *J Am Coll Cardiol*. 2004;44:1641–1647.

61. Cooper RS, Ritter SB, Rothe WB, et al. Angioplasty for coarctation of the aorta: long-term results. *Circulation*. 1987;75:600–604.

62. Cowley CG, Orsmond GS, Feola P, et al. Long-term, randomized comparison of balloon angioplasty and surgery for native coarctation of the aorta in childhood. *Circulation*. 2005;111:3453–3456.

63. Piechaud JF. Stent implantation for coarctation in adults. *J Interv Cardiol*. 2003;16:413–418.

64. O'Laughlin MP, Slack MC, Grifka RG, et al. Implantation and intermediate-term follow-up of stents in congenital heart disease. *Circulation*. 1993;88:605–614.

65. Gibbs JL, Uzun O, Blackburn ME, et al. Right ventricular outflow stent implantation: an alternative to palliative surgical relief of infundibular pulmonary stenosis. *Heart*. 1997;77:176–179.

66. Anzuini A, Uretsky BF. Covered stent septal ablation for hypertrophic obstruction cardiomyopathy. *Circulation*. 2004;109:e6.

67. Sugiyama H, Williams W, Benson LN. Implantation of endovascular stents for the obstructive right ventricular outflow tract. *Heart*. 2005;91:1058–1063.

Transcatheter Closure of Atrial Septal Defects & Patent Foramen Ovale

Ralf J. Holzer, Qi-Ling Cao, and Ziyad M. Hijazi

Atrial septal defects (ASD) represent approximately 6% to 10% of all congenital cardiac anomalies, with females being affected more commonly (2:1) than males (1). Percutaneous or surgical closure of ASDs is indicated in patients with large defects to prevent long-term complications, such as reduced exercise tolerance, atrial arrhythmias, or pulmonary vascular disease that may develop in up to 5% to 10% of affected individuals (2). Transcatheter device closure has established itself as the first line of treatment in suitable patients with hemodynamically significant ASD's, thereby replacing the surgical approach (3,4).

King and colleagues in 1976 (5) reported the first successful transcatheter closure of a secundum ASD in a human. Since that time, procedural technique and available devices have significantly improved. At present, only two devices are currently in use: the Amplatzer Septal Occluder and the Helex device (6).

In 1997, the Amplatzer Septal Occluder [ASO] (AGA Medical Corporation, Golden Valley, MN) was introduced and results of its use have been excellent (7). Closure rates with the ASO have been superior to those with other devices (8), and complications associated with this device have been very low (7,9–11). Additionally, the device has been successfully used even in cases with large ASDs or ASDs with deficient rims (12).

Many of the devices that are used to close secundum ASD's have also been successfully used to close patent foramen ovale (PFO). However, the morphological characteristics of a PFO when compared to secundum defects within the oval fossa, have lead to the development of several devices that are specifically designed for transcatheter PFO closure, such as the PFO-Star or the Amplatzer PFO Occluder (13,14).

Anatomy of The Atrial Septum

The true atrial septum is considerably smaller than the size of the atrial tissue that separates left atrium from right atrium. This is mainly due to the fact that a large extent of the superior rim is made up through an infolded groove between the right pulmonary veins and superior vena cava, rather than a true atrial septum (15). In contrast, the inferior rim is predominantly made up of septum primum, which is in direct continuation with the atrioventricular valves. The anterior rim of the atrial septum is mainly defined through its close relationship to the aortic root, whereas the posterior rim is in continuation with the inferior caval vein and only partly a true septum (15).

ASDs have been classified to be of secundum type, superior or inferior sinus venosus type, coronary sinus type or ostium-primum type (partial atrioventricular septal defect). The most common of these defects and the only one amenable for transcatheter device closure is the secundum type ASD. Embryologically, this defect results from a deficiency of the septum primum, thereby producing incomplete overlap between septum primum and septum secundum. Most defects are solitary (90%) and the margins are formed through septum primum as well as the limbus of the fossa ovalis (septum secundum). In contrast to abnormal intra-atrial communications, a PFO represents a normal, physiological communication of fetal life. In up to 30% of healthy people, the septum primum fails to form a permanent cohesion with the limbus of the fossa ovalis, thereby producing a persist opening, a PFO (1).

Patient Selection—Clinical Background

ASD Device Closure

ASDs are associated with left-to-right shunts of variable degree, depending on the size of the defects and ventricular compliance. This shunt may lead to right-atrial and right ventricular volume overload. If the shunt is large, patients may develop symptoms related the ASD, such as reduced exercise tolerance, shortness of breath or palpitations, in the second or third decade of life.

Even though the risk of procedure or device related complications are low, this does not eliminate the need to carefully evaluate in each individual patient the indications for ASD closure. Small intra-atrial communications with a diameter of <5 mm and absence of evidence of right atrial or ventricular volume overload do not impact upon the natural history of the individual and therefore do not require closure, unless associated with paradoxical embolism.

The situation is different in patients with large ASDs and evidence of right ventricular volume overload on echocardiography. In this instance potential long-term complications such as reduced exercise tolerance, atrial arrhythmias, or pulmonary vascular disease, which may develop in up to 5% to 10% of affected individuals (2), clearly present valid indications to proceed with closure of the ASD.

Percutaneous closure has replaced the surgical approach as the standard treatment to close intra-atrial communications, with surgical closure being reserved for those defects that are unsuitable for the transcatheter approach. However, through increasing operator experience and the availability of specialized devices, the range of defects that can be closed safely using percutaneous closure has increased significantly, and includes large ASDs up to 35 mm in diameter as well as defects with one or more deficient rims (12).

Contraindications for ASD (or PFO) device closure include the presence of associated cardiac anomalies requiring cardiac surgery, pulmonary vascular disease with a pulmonary vascular resistance index in excess of 7 Woods units, acute or recent septic events, as well as the presence of bleeding disorders or other contraindications to anti-platelet therapy. Reports have documented that Nickel is being released from the device into the systemic circulation for a limited period after implantation, and therefore caution is necessary in patients with a known Nickel allergy (16). However, from our own experience we have implanted ASO in two patients with known Nickel allergy without any adverse events.

PFO Device Closure

Stroke is the third leading cause of death in the United States after heart disease and cancer, accounting for more than 160,000 deaths in the United States in 2002 (17). Up to 40% of cerebral ischemic events have no identifiable etiology and are therefore classified as cryptogenic (18). The incidence of PFO ranges between 10% to 35% (19), and several studies have identified an association between the presence of a PFO and ischemic cerebrovascular events, particularly in young patients (20,21). Paradoxical embolism through a PFO may account for these cryptogenic events with a recurrence risk of 3.4% to 3.8% per year (22,23). If a PFO is associated with an atrial septal aneurysm, the recurrence risk has been reported to be as high as 15% after 4 years (24). Not surprisingly therefore, percutaneous closure of a PFO in patients with a cryptogenic cerebrovascular event has emerged as an alternative to medical treatment. Results of the procedure have generally been favourable with a low incidence of procedure or device related complications (21,25).

However, at present there is no evidence based data available, comparing percutaneous PFO device closure with standard medical treatment in their efficacy to reduce the incidence of recurrent cerebrovascular events. This is currently being investigated in two trials: the RESPECT trial ("**R**andomized **E**valuation **of** Recurrent **S**troke, TIA, **or** **P**eripheral **e**mbolism **c**omparing **P**FO Closure to **E**stablished **C**urrent Standard of **C**are **T**reatment") using the Amplatzer PFO device and the CLOSURE 1 trial using the CardioSeal device, with the primary endpoint being "recurrent symptomatic cryptogenic stroke or cardiovascular death."

There is some suggestion that other potential indications for PFO closure may include patients with orthodeoxia/platypnea and patients who suffer from migraine with aura (26), even though prospective data to support this treatment option is not yet available.

Pre-Procedure Evaluation

In addition to basic clinical assessment, all patients with secundum ASDs should undergo full transthoracic echocardiographic evaluation. The atrial septum is best assessed using subcostal views, as well as apical four-chamber and parasternal short axis views. Of particular importance is to confirm normal pulmonary venous drainage, as well as evaluating the size of the ASD and surrounding septal rims. Right atrial dimensions should be obtained (standard apical four-chamber view) as well as measurement of the right ventricular diastolic diameter obtained from standard long-axis m-mode recordings. The right ventricular pressure should be estimated using the peak tricuspid regurgitant jet velocity. Associated anomalies, such as pulmonary valve stenosis, should be identified.

A standard 12-lead ECG may demonstrate right axis deviation and intraventricular conduction delay with RSR' configuration in V1 and V3R. A chest radiograph as well as 24-hour ambulatory ECG recordings (optional) will complete the pre-procedure evaluation. Often, due to poor transthoracic echo windows in adults, transesophageal echocardiography (TEE) should be performed for a full assessment of the ASD anatomy and determination for suitability for device closure.

Patients, who are considered for PFO device closure, should additionally undergo full specialist neurological evaluation, to identify potential causes of the cerebral ischemic event. Among others, this work-up usually includes Doppler examination of the carotid arteries as well as a thrombophilia screen. PCB Note—what tests are recommended for the latter? Transthoracic echocardiography (TTE) may be insufficient to demonstrate a PFO in larger-sized adult patients, and therefore, evaluation using TEE should be considered. It is essential to prove an existing right-to-left shunt, using either contrast bubble-echocardiography and/or transcranial Doppler (TCD), which has been identified as a sensitive non-invasive tool to detect and semi-quantify right-to-left shunting (27,28). Patients with a previous history of deep vein thrombosis may benefit from Doppler ultrasound examination of the femoral vessels to document patency and absence of any thrombus in these vessels. Furthermore, the right and left atrium, especially the left atrial appendage require careful assessment for the presence of thrombus.

The Amplatzer Devices

General Description

The Amplatzer devices (AGA Medical Corporation, Golden Valley, MN) are made of Nitinol wire, which is an alloy of Nickel and Titanium. All devices are self-expandable and can be recaptured into the delivery sheath to allow re-positioning of the device if required. Most devices have polyester fabric incorporated into the disks and connecting waist to enhance thrombosis and fibrous ingrowth.

Several different Amplatzer devices have been produced for a variety of lesions, such as the Amplatzer septal occluder (ASO) for ASDs and the Amplatzer PFO occluder for occlusion of PFOs, both of which consist of two flat disks that are linked via a central connecting waist. A variation of these devices is the Amplatzer multi-fenestrated septal occluder or "Cribriform" device, which is useful for occlusion of multiple intra-atrial communications or multifenestrated ASDs (29).

The Amplatzer Septal Occluder (ASO)

The ASO consists of two flat disks, the left atrial disk exceeding the right atrial disk by about 4 mm in diameter. The right atrial disk itself exceeds the diameter of the connecting waist by about 8 to 10 mm. The waist diameter determines the size of the device, which is available from 4 to 40 mm, and can be delivered through a 6 to 12 Fr delivery sheath.

The Amplatzer PFO Occluder

In contrast to the ASO, the PFO occluder has a thin connecting waist of 3 mm length, with the right atrial disk exceed or equal to the size of the left atrial disk. This design is specifically useful for the tunnel-like PFO that may otherwise distort the configuration of a standard ASO through its much wider waist. The device is available in three sizes, with dimensions of right/left atrial disk measuring 18/18 mm (18 mm device), 25/18 mm (25 mm device), or 35/25 mm (35 mm device). All devices can be passed through an 8 to 9 Fr delivery sheaths.

The Amplatzer Multi-Fenestrated Septal Occluder

The Amplatzer Multi-Fenestrated Septal Occluder (Cribriform device) is very similar to the PFO occluder. The device has a thin 3 mm connecting waist and both disks are equally sized, either 15 mm, 25 mm, or 35 mm in diameter. All devices can be passed through an 8 to 9 Fr delivery system. Its design makes the device specifically helpful to close multifenestrated atrial communications (29).

The Delivery System

The delivery system is supplied separately from the device and contains a 45 degree angle, 60–80 cm length, delivery sheath with a dilator, a 0.081″ delivery cable, a loader that facilitates collapsing of the device and introduction into the delivery sheath, as well as a plastic pin vise that facilitates unscrewing of the device. In addition a hemostatic valve with a side arm is included that can be passed onto the end of the delivery sheath to avoid blood loss during device delivery. An alternative to this hemostatic valve is the use of a standard Touhy-Borst adapter, which more securely connects to the delivery sheath. Should an angiogram be needed prior to device release, the Touhy-Borst can be used for this purpose and it accepts higher pressure of injection than the side arm provided by the manufacturer.

Procedure—Protocol and Technique

General Technique

Preparation

With the exception of very uncooperative young children, all procedures are usually performed under local anaesthesia, using conscious sedation. This is specifically important in patients who undergo closure of a PFO, as their cooperation using appropriate valsalva techniques to detect any residual right-to-left shunting is required throughout the procedure. All relevant pre-procedure investigations (TTE, CXR, ECG, ambulatory 24-hour ECG) should be available for review and antiplatelet doses of Aspirin should be stated about 48 hours prior to the procedure.

Closure of large defects in the elderly requires careful evaluation for complicating factors such as left ventricular diastolic dysfunction that may result in increased left atrial pressures after closing an intra-atrial communication (30). Therefore, these patients may benefit from pre-treatment using diuretic therapy prior to ASD device closure (31). The procedure is performed using anticoagulation with intravenous Heparin to achieve and maintain an activated clotting time (ACT) in excess of 200 seconds (once vascular access has been obtained). The ACT should be evaluated every 30 minutes throughout the procedure. Antibiotic coverage using a first generation cephalosporin is required before as well as after the procedure (three doses in total).

Vascular Access and Hemodynamic Evaluation

After sterile draping, vascular access is obtained placing a 7 Fr or 8 Fr short introducer sheath in the right femoral vein. Arterial monitoring is optional. Where intracardiac echocardiography (ICE) is used to guide ASD closure, an additional 8 or 11 Fr sheath is placed in the same femoral venous vessel via a separate puncture. Device closure using transhepatic access is an alternative in patients, where the femoral venous route is occluded. However, an in situ vena-cava filter does not pose a contraindication to using the transfemoral approach, as reports have documented that percutaneous device closure of an intra-atrial communication can be safely performed through an in-situ vena cava filter (32). Standard

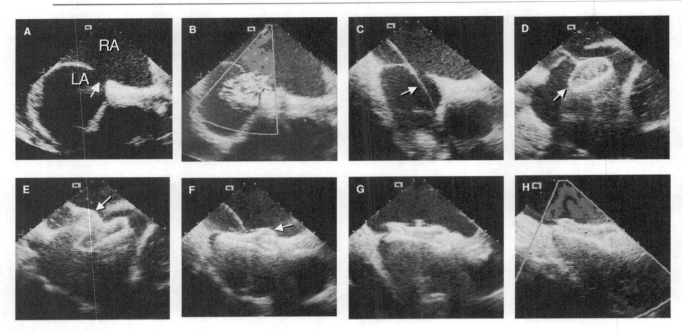

Figure 26–1.

Intracardiac echocardiographic (ICE) images in a 79-year-old female patient with a 18 x 25-mm secundum atrial septal defect demonstrating the various steps during assessment and device closure of the defect. **A, B:** Septal views (without and with color Doppler) demonstrating the right atrium (RA), left atrium (LA) and the defect (arrow). **C:** Septal view during passage of the guide wire into the left atrium (arrow). **D:** Modified septal view during deployment of the left atrial disk of a 26-mm Amplatzer Septal Occluder (arrow). **E:** Deployment of the connecting waist (arrow) in the defect. **F:** Deployment of the right atrial disk (arrow) in the right atrium. **G, H:** Images without and with color Doppler after the device has been released demonstrating good device position and no residual shunt.

right and anterograde left heart catheterization is performed, specifically evaluating the distal pulmonary artery pressures as well as calculating the Qp:Qs ratio and the pulmonary vascular resistance index. The mean gradient across the intra-atrial communication has to be documented. Elderly patients may not tolerate sudden complete occlusion of their intra-atrial communication and therefore test occlusion of the ASD should be performed, while evaluating any rise in left atrial pressure. From our own experience, we have documented that patients with a moderate rise in left atrial pressure during test occlusion, may benefit from the use of a fenestrated ASO (33).

Echocardiography

ASD and PFO device closure can be performed using either TEE or ICE. Recently, an 8 Fr ICE catheter has become available; therefore, placement of an additional 8 Fr sheath instead of the 11 Fr is an obvious advantage. A full echocardiographic evaluation should be performed, assessing the dimensions of the intra-atrial communication in different echocardiographic planes (short/long axis view, four-chamber view, SVC view). It is important to document normal pulmonary venous drainage as well as the size of the anterior, posterior, superior or inferior rim. Du and colleagues evaluated twenty-three patients with deficient septal margins and they were able to demonstrate that closure of ASDs with deficient anterior, inferior or posterior rim is feasible using the ASO (12). However, this should only be performed by experienced operators that have per-

formed many ASD closures (>50 cases), especially if multiple rims are deficient (<5 mm).

The atrial chambers have to be carefully evaluated for the presence of any intracardiac thrombus. In patients with a PFO, assessment of the right to left shunt using contrast bubbles with TCD with and without valsalva should be performed prior to device deployment (27). Figures 26–1 and 26–2 demonstrate the echocardiographic steps of closure in two patients, one with secundum ASD and one with a PFO.

Angiography

An angiogram in the right upper pulmonary vein in 35 degree left anterior oblique/35 degree cranial angulation should be performed in patients with secundum ASD. This profiles the septum and the angiogram can be used as a control image when the device is deployed, but not released.

Crossing the ASD, Balloon Sizing and Choice of Device-Size

The intra-atrial communication is usually crossed using a multipurpose catheter, which is advanced into the left upper pulmonary vein. On occasions it can be difficult to cross a tight, tunnel-like PFO, in which case the defect can be approached from a position within the IVC, using a 0.035″ glide wire, which frequently directly advances through the PFO.

A 0.035″ exchange length stiff wire, such as the Amplatz extra or super stiff wire with 1 cm floppy tip, is positioned in the left upper pulmonary vein. Depending on the size of

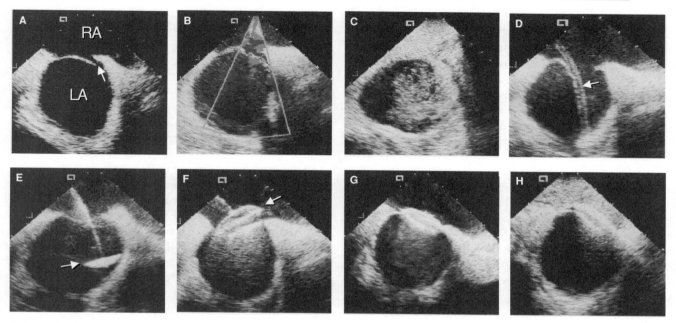

Figure 26–2.

Intracardiac echocardiographic (ICE) images in a 43-year-old female patient who sustained a cryptogenic stroke with a large PFO demonstrating the various steps during assessment and device closure of the defect. **A, B:** Septal view (without and with color Doppler) demonstrating the right atrium (RA), left atrium (LA) and the defect (*arrow*) and bidirectional shunt by color. **C:** Septal view during contrast bubble study at rest demonstrating passage of the bubbles from the right to the left atrium. **D:** Passage of an 8 Fr delivery sheath (*arrow*) through the PFO to the left atrium. **E:** Deployment of the left atrial disk (*arrow*) of a 25-mm Amplatzer PFO device in the left atrium. **F:** Deployment of the right atrial disk (*arrow*) on the right side of the PFO. **G, H:** After the device has been released and with contrast bubbles (**H**) demonstrating good device position and no residual shunt.

the defect determined by echocardiographic evaluation, either a 24 or 34 mm AGA sizing balloon is used to balloon size the defect—the balloon is passed directly through the skin without the use of a hemostatic sheath. It is important that the balloon is inflated under echocardiographic guidance, until the shunt through the ASD is just abolished (using 25% contrast). This is what is called stop-flow technique. A cine recording is obtained at this stage and the diameter of the balloon is measured. Similarly, one should also measure the diameter of the balloon by echocardiography.

The device size is chosen, using a diameter that exceeds the stop-flow diameter by about 0 to 2 mm. It is important to avoid oversizing, as this may lead to suboptimal configuration of the device and possibly increases the risk of device erosion into the aortic root (34). For patients with PFO, balloon sizing using the Amplatzer devices is not needed. TEE or ICE is used to measure the distances from the superior vena cava to the defect and from the aortic root to the defect. If both exceed 17.5 mm, then the 35 mm device should be used. If one measurement is between 12.5 to 17.5 mm, then the 25-mm device is used and if both are <12.5 mm and >9.5 mm, the 18-mm device is used.

Positioning of the Delivery Sheath

The delivery sheath is advanced over the Amplatz super/extra stiff wire into the left upper pulmonary vein, with the dilator being advanced up to mid-atrial level, followed by the sheath

itself being advanced over the dilator and wire until the tip is positioned in the left upper pulmonary vein. At this stage the dilator and wire are slowly withdrawn to avoid any negative pressure within the sheath. The sheath is allowed to back bleed freely. One should avoid aspirating and flushing the sheath due to the risk of air embolism.

Loading and Advancement of the Device

The delivery cable is passed through the Touhy-Borst adapter as well as the attached loader, and the device is then screwed onto the delivery cable. Of importance is to check and confirm integrity of the device, but also to avoid any use of force when screwing on the device: If the device does not screw on easily it is not lined up correctly. The device is pulled into the loader under water seal and the whole system is flushed using normal saline solution. The loader is then screwed onto the delivery sheath and the cable/device assembly is advanced under fluoroscopic guidance until the tip of the delivery sheath is reached.

Device Deployment

It is important that appropriate echocardiographic views are obtained that allow real-time visualization of the device deployment. Views that may be suitable include the 4-chamber view by TEE or the septal or short axis view by ICE. The delivery sheath is pulled back until it exits the pulmonary vein to the mid left atrial level, and then the delivery cable is fixed firmly while retracting the sheath over the cable, this will deploy the left atrial disk. Once the left atrial disk is deployed echocardiographic guidance is used to assess the alignment of the left atrial disk to the septum, fine adjustments can be made to achieve parallel alignment. Then, under echocardiographic guidance the entire assembly (sheath/cable) is pulled back as one unit towards the septum. At that stage, the connecting waist can be deployed partly in the left atrium and the defect itself, in essence to stent the defect. Further retraction of the sheath over the cable and continuous pulling of the entire assembly towards the inferior vena cava will deploy the right atrial disk. It is important to point out that the deployment of waist and right atrial disk may have to be performed in quick succession, especially in larger ASDs, as only the deployment of both disks achieves the best possible stability of the device. All stages of the deployment process should be documented and monitored by echocardiography as well as cine fluoroscopy recordings.

Device Release and Evaluation

After device deployment, the position of the device is assessed using echocardiography (TEE/ICE) in different views. This should specifically focus on device position in relation to the septal rims, device position in relation to SVC and coronary sinus, as well as presence of any residual shunt other than through the device itself. In patients who undergo PFO device closure, shunt assessment should be performed using contrast bubble with and without valsalva, under echocardiographic and TCD monitoring.

Different techniques to evaluate stable device position include: the "Minnesota Wiggle" which is done by gently pushing the cable forward towards the left atrium and pulling the cable backward towards the inferior vena cava. This done while the delivery sheath itself is fixed in position. A stable device position is manifested by the lack of movement of the device in either direction. Also, this can be monitored using echocardiography. During pulling the cable towards the inferior vena cava, one should be able to see the atrial septum between the two disks of the device. Another technique used to determine stable device position is by performing an angiogram in the right atrium using the same view as the initial angiogram in the right upper pulmonary vein. Good device position is manifested by opacifying the right atrial disk only when the contrast is in the right atrium and by opacifying the left atrial disk when the contrast goes through the pulmonary levophase. If all these techniques indicate stable and correct device position, it is safe then to release the device. This can be done by rotating the pin vise in a counter clock-wise direction. Often, due to the self-centering mechanism of the device and also due to the shape of the atrial septum, once the device is released, the device changes its orientation to follow the shape of the atrial septum.

"The Difficult ASD"—Technical Challenges

Large ASDs pose a great challenge, especially when associated with deficient septal rims. Our own unpublished experience

of ASD device closure documented a size of the ASD in excess of 30 mm to be significantly related to reduced procedural success, with two out of four procedural failures occurring in patients with an ASD measuring 39 and 41 mm, respectively.

The challenge in these patients is frequently in aligning the left atrial disk to be parallel to the atrial septum, as one has to avoid any tension on the device when pulled against the septum. In a small ASD tension on the device may lead to better alignment with the septum, but in a large ASD it may lead to prolapse of the left atrial disk through the superior anterior margin of the defect (35).

There are different techniques used to align the left atrial disk parallel to the atrial septum. One is to use a specially designed delivery sheath (the Hausdorf sheath) [Cook Inc., Bloomington, IN] that possesses two posterior curves at the tip (35). This allows the left atrial disk when deployed to be more parallel to the septum. Similarly, one can use a Judkins right coronary guiding catheter. However, this will limit the size of the device that can be loaded inside it to 16 to 18 mm. Another successful technique is to deploy the left atrial disk entirely in the left upper pulmonary vein (35). Once the left atrial disk is constrained inside the left upper pulmonary vein, continuous pulling of the delivery sheath towards the inferior vena cava will result in a sudden jump of the disk to align with the atrial septum. The remainder of the device is deployed as previously mentioned. Alternatively, one can deploy the left atrial disk in the right upper pulmonary vein (36). This will achieve the same result as deploying in the left upper pulmonary vein. Another technique used is to place the dilator of the long sheath from the contralateral femoral vein or from the introducer of the ICE catheter until the dilator reaches the right atrium (37). Then the stiff end of the extra stiff wire is shaped to have a curve and is advanced inside the dilator until it reaches the tip. Then the dilator is maneuvered through the ASD to the left atrium. The left atrial disk is deployed in the mid left atrium. Then with the help of an assistant, the dilator is used to hold the left atrial disk in the left atrium while the neck and right atrial disk are deployed. Once the device is in correct position, the dilator is removed. Finally, Dalvi et al reported on using a Meditech sizing balloon (Boston Scientific, Watertown, MA) over a wire positioned in the left upper pulmonary vein to hold the left atrial disk in the left atrium while deploying the remainder of the device in the defect and right atrium (38).

The frequency of device embolization has been low at about 0.5%, predominantly secondary either to the presence of deficient septal margins, or the use of undersized devices (39). It is therefore important that all operators who implant septal occluders are sufficiently technically skilled in retrieval techniques. A delivery sheath 2 Fr sizes in excess of the sheath size used to deploy the device is used for the retrieval. A gooseneck snare (ev3) is advanced inside this sheath and the microscrew of the embolized device is snared. Devices most commonly embolize to the right atrium and the ability to recapture the device inside the sheath can be enhanced by gently pulling on the device from the opposite end of the microscrew. Obviously, puncture of the right internal jugular vein is needed and one may use a bioptome or another gooseneck snare to stretch the device and enhance the chances of it being forced inside the delivery sheath (39).

Occasionally after multiple attempts in deploying and re-capturing the device inside the sheath, it may become defective and one cannot recapture the device inside the sheath and the sheath wrinkles (Accordion effect). In such example, the manufacturer provides a rescue system (9 and 12 Fr). This rescue system is similar to the delivery system with the exception of the dilator having a larger inner diameter to allow an extension cable (0.081″) to be introduced inside it. The cable of the rescue system is screwed to the proximal end of the cable inside the patient, making it similar to an exchange wire. Then, over this long cable, one advances either the 9 or 12 Fr rescue sheath with its dilator. Once the dilator reaches the microscrew of the device, one brings the dilator inside the sheath for about 10 cm, the sheath is advanced near the microscrew and then one can recapture the device inside the sheath. Laboratories that do closure of ASD or PFO should have this rescue system available.

Multiple atrial communications pose another technical challenge. They are frequently associated with aneurysmal atrial septum (present in 4% of ASDs), and are best treated using the "Cribriform" device. Ideally the device should be positioned in the central defect. The device size is chosen so that the disks of the device cover the entire distance between the defects.

Multiple ASDs that are separated by more than 7 mm of septal tissue may require more than one device to achieve complete closure of each defect. Balloon sizing may be needed for each defect. When using more than one device, it is important to cross the two defects individually and a delivery sheath is positioned in each defect. Then the smaller device is deployed but not released first, followed by the larger device being deployed. Once stable devices position have been confirmed, the smaller device is released first, followed by the large device (40).

Follow-Up

All patients should undergo echocardiographic evaluation to assess device position and residual shunts within 24 hours of device implantation. In patients with PFO, a contrast bubble study (with and without valsalva) is used to assess the presence of residual right-to-left shunt, using ideally the same imaging tool as during device implantation (echocardiography and/or TCD).

CXR and a 12-lead ECG should be performed. A 24-hour ambulatory ECG recording starting immediately after the procedure is optional. Hill and colleagues documented an increased incidence of atrial arrhythmias and conduction abnormalities early after ASD device closure (41). From our own unpublished experience, we found the incidence of non-sustained atrial tachycardias as well as the average number of premature atrial ectopic beats to steadily decline toward pre-procedure values at the 6-month and 12-month follow-up.

All patients should be seen within 6 months from implantation and after 1 year. If there is no residual shunt documented at 1-year follow-up, we recommend following patients once

every 1 to 2 years. In each visit, physical examination, chest radiograph, TTE and ECG are done. Prophylaxis against bacterial endocarditis as well as aspirin is discontinued if complete closure is documented at the 6-month visit. It has been well documented that right ventricular size undergoes rapid improvement within 1 month of percutaneous device closure. Only 29% of patients have persistent right ventricle enlargement at 1-year follow-up (42). This suggests that some degree of remodelling of the right ventricle takes place when the exposure to volume loading is eliminated. However, it is important to recognize that long-standing right ventricular dilatation may normalize more slowly or may not regress to completely normal values at all. This emphasizes the need for early percutaneous intervention in patients with hemodynamically significant ASDs.

Complications

Procedure and device-related complications after percutaneous closure of ASD are rare. The most common complications include temporary rhythm and conduction abnormalities, which usually resolve over the follow-up period. We have encountered one patient who developed complete heart block detected at the 6-month visit (41). This patient had an abnormal rhythm prior to the procedure. One of the most serious complications observed after ASD or PFO device closure is erosion of the device into the aortic root. This has been a rare complication with an approximate incidence of 0.1% in the United States (34). It has been suggested that the risk of erosion is increased in patients with deficient aortic and/or superior rims, as well as in patients who had an oversized device implanted. Therefore, the use of oversized devices should be avoided whenever possible (34).

Residual Shunts

The incidence of residual shunts after ASD device closure is low (7,9–11). Our own experience documented an incidence of residual shunts of 11.7% immediately after device closure, most of which were of small or trivial degree when assessed with echocardiography (43). The incidence of residual shunts decreased further to 9% at day 1 postprocedure and 5.9% at 6-months follow-up. At 24 months only 2% of patients had a residual shunt, with none of our patients requiring any additional surgical or percutaneous intervention for a residual shunt.

Summary

In summary, percutaneous closure of intra-atrial communications using the Amplatzer devices offers excellent mid-term results and a low rate of procedure or device related complications. Although most procedures are technically straightforward, the situation is very different when dealing with a complex ASD or PFO, which may demand a much higher degree of procedural knowledge and technical skill.

REFERENCES

1. Porter CJ, Feldt RH, Edwards WD, et al. Atrial septal defects. In: Allen HD, Gutgesell HP,Clark EB, et al., eds. *Heart Disease in Infants, Children, and Adolescents.* Lippincott Williams & Williams; 2001:603–617.

2. Steele PM, Fuster V, Cohen M, et al. Isolated atrial septal defect with pulmonary vascular obstructive disease—long-term follow-up and prediction of outcome after surgical correction. *Circulation.* 1987;76:1037–1042.

3. Kim JJ, Hijazi ZM. Clinical outcomes and costs of Amplatzer transcatheter closure as compared with surgical closure of ostium secundum atrial septal defects. *Med Sci Monitor.* 2002;8:787–791.

4. Bialkowski J, Karwot B, Szkutnik M, et al. Closure of atrial septal defects in children: surgery versus Amplatzer device implantation. *Texas Heart Inst J.* 2004;31:220–223.

5. King TD, Thompson SL, Steiner C, et al. Secundum atrial septal defect. Nonoperative closure during cardiac catheterization. *JAMA.* 1976;235:2506–2509.

6. Vincent RN, Raviele AA, Diehl HJ. Single-center experience with the HELEX septal occluder for closure of atrial septal defects in children. *J Interv Cardiol.* 2003;16:79–82.

7. Masura J, Gavora P, Formanek A, et al. Transcatheter closure of secundum atrial septal defects using the new self-centering amplatzer septal occluder: initial human experience. *Cathet Cardiovasc Diagn.* 1997;42:388–393.

8. Butera G, Carminati M, Chessa M, et al. CardioSEAL/STARflex versus Amplatzer devices for percutaneous closure of small to moderate (up to 18 mm) atrial septal defects. *Am Heart J.* 2004;148:507–510.

9. Fischer G, Stieh J, Uebing A, et al. Experience with transcatheter closure of secundum atrial septal defects using the Amplatzer septal occluder: a single centre study in 236 consecutive patients. *Heart.* 2003;89:199–204.

10. Du ZD, Hijazi ZM, Kleinman CS, et al. Comparison between transcatheter and surgical closure of secundum atrial septal defect in children and adults: results of a multicenter nonrandomized trial. *J Amer Coll Cardiol.* 2002;39:1836–1844.

11. Chessa M, Carminati M, Butera G, et al. Early and late complications associated with transcatheter occlusion of secundum atrial septal defect. *J Am Coll Cardiol.* 2002;39:1061–1065.

12. Du ZD, Koenig P, Cao QL, et al. Comparison of transcatheter closure of secundum atrial septal defect using the Amplatzer septal occluder associated with deficient versus sufficient rims. *Am J Cardiol.* 2002;90:865–869.

13. Braun M, Gliech V, Boscheri A, et al. Transcatheter closure of patent foramen ovale (PFO) in patients with paradoxical embolism. Periprocedural safety and mid-term follow-up results of three different device occluder systems. *Eur Heart J.* 2004;25:424–430.

14. Braun MU, Fassbender D, Schoen SP, et al. Transcatheter closure of patent foramen ovale in patients with cerebral ischemia. *J Am Coll Cardiol.* 2002;39:2019–2025.

15. Anderson RH, Becker AE. *The Heart: Structure in Health and Disease.* 1st ed. Gower Medical Publishing; 1992.

16. Ries MW, Kampmann C, Rupprecht HJ, et al. Nickel release after implantation of the Amplatzer occluder. *Am Heart J.* 2003;145:737–741.

17. Kochanek KD, Murphy BS, Anderson RN, et al. Deaths: final data for 2002. *Natl Vital Stat Rep.* 2004;53:1–116.

18. Sacco RL, Ellenberg JH, Mohr JP, et al. Infarcts of undetermined cause: the NINCDS Stroke Data Bank. *Ann Neurol.* 1989;25:382–390, 1989.

19. Fisher DC, Fisher EA, Budd JH, et al. The incidence of patent foramen ovale in 1,000 consecutive patients. A contrast transesophageal echocardiography study. *Chest.* 1995;107:1504–1509.

20. Di Tullio M, Sacco RL, Gopal A, et al. Patent foramen ovale as a risk factor for cryptogenic stroke. *Ann Intern Med.* 1992;117:461–465.

21. Du ZD, Cao QL, Joseph A, et al. Transcatheter closure of patent foramen ovale in patients with paradoxical embolism: intermediate-term risk of recurrent neurological events. *Cathet Cardiovasc Interv.* 2002;55:189–194.

22. Bogousslavsky J, Garazi S, Jeanrenaud X, et al. Stroke recurrence in patients with patent foramen ovale: the Lausanne Study. Lausanne Stroke with Paradoxal Embolism Study Group. *Neurology.* 1996;46:1301–1305.

23. Mas JL, Zuber M. Recurrent cerebrovascular events in patients with patent foramen ovale, atrial septal aneurysm, or both and cryptogenic stroke or transient ischemic attack. French Study Group on patent foramen ovale and atrial septal aneurysm. *Am Heart J.* 1995;130:1083–1088.

24. Mas JL, Arquizan C, Lamy C, et al. Recurrent cerebrovascular events associated with patent foramen ovale, atrial septal aneurysm, or both. *N Engl J Med.* 2001;345:1740–1746.

25. Onorato E, Melzi G, Casilli F, et al. Patent foramen ovale with paradoxical embolism: mid-term results of transcatheter closure in 256 patients. *J Interv Cardiol.* 2003;16:43–50.

26. Morandi E, Anzola GP, Angeli S, et al. Transcatheter closure of patent foramen ovale: a new migraine treatment? *J Interv Cardiol.* 2003;16:39–42.

27. Zanchetta M, Rigatelli G, Onorato E. Intracardiac echocardiography and transcranial Doppler ultrasound to guide closure of patent foramen ovale. *J Invasive Cardiol.* 2003;15:93–96.

28. Blersch WK, Draganski BM, Holmer SR, et al. Transcranial duplex sonography in the detection of patent foramen ovale. *Radiol.* 2002;225:693–699.

29. Hijazi ZM, Cao QL. Transcatheter closure of multifenestrated atrial septal defects using the new Amplatzer cribriform device. *Pediatr Cardiol Today.* 2003;1:1.

30. Ewert P, Berger F, Nagdyman N, et al. Masked left ventricular restriction in elderly patients with atrial septal defects: a contraindication for closure? *Cathet Cardiovasc Interv.* 2001;52:177–80.

31. Schubert S, Peters B, Abdul-Khaliq H, et al. Left ventricular conditioning in the elderly patient to prevent congestive heart failure after transcatheter closure of atrial septal defect. *Cathet Cardiovasc Interv.* 2005;64:333–337.

32. Awadalla H, Boccalandro F, Majano RA, et al. Percutaneous closure of patent foramen ovale guided by intracardiac echocardiography and performed through the transfemoral approach in the presence of previously placed inferior vena cava filters: a case series. *Cathet Cardiovasc Interv.* 2004;63:242–246.

33. Holzer R, Cao QL, Hijazi ZM. Closure of a large atrial septal defect with a self-fabricated fenestrated Amplatzer Septal Occluder in an 85-year-old gentleman with reduced diastolic elasticity of the left ventricle. *J Invasive Cardiol.*(In Press).

34. Amin Z, Hijazi ZM, Bass JL, et al. Erosion of Amplatzer septal occluder device after closure of secundum atrial septal defects: review of registry of complications and recommendations to minimize future risk. *Cathet Cardiovasc Interv.* 2004;63:496–502.

35. Varma C, Benson LN, Silversides C, et al. Outcomes and alternative techniques for device closure of the large secundum atrial septal defect. *Cathet Cardiovasc Interv.* 2004;61:131–139.

36. Berger F, Ewert P, Abdul-Khaliq H, et al. Percutaneous closure of large atrial septal defects with the Amplatzer Septal Occluder: technical overkill or recommendable alternative treatment? *J Interv Cardiol.* 2001;14:63–67.

37. Wahab HA, Bairam AR, Cao QL, et al. Novel technique to prevent prolapse of the Amplatzer septal occluder through large atrial septal defect. *Cathet Cardiovasc Interv.* 2003;60:543–545.

38. Dalvi BV, Pinto RJ, Gupta A. New technique for device closure of large atrial septal defects. *Cathet Cardiovasc Interv.* 2005;64:102–107.

39. Levi DS, Moore JW. Embolization and retrieval of the Amplatzer septal occluder. *Cathet Cardiovasc Interv.* 2004;61:543–547.

40. Roman KS, Jones A, Keeton BR, et al. Different techniques for closure of multiple interatrial communications with the Amplatzer septal occluder. *J Interv Cardiol.* 2002;15:393–397.

41. Hill SL, Berul CI, Patel HT, et al. Early ECG abnormalities associated with transcatheter closure of atrial septal defects using the Amplatzer septal occluder. *J Interv Card Electrophysiol.* 2000;4:469–474.

42. Veldtman GR, Razack V, Siu S, et al. Right ventricular form and function after percutaneous atrial septal defect device closure. *J Am Coll Cardiol.* 2001;37:2108–2113.

43. Boutin C, Musewe NN, Smallhorn JF, et al. Echocardiographic follow-up of atrial septal defect after catheter closure by double-umbrella device. *Circulation.* 1993;88:621–627.

Statistics and Guidelines

Warren K. Laskey

Introduction to Statistics in Clinical Research Interventional Cardiology Board Review Course

Robert A. Harrington and Karen S. Pieper

Clinical cardiologists, including interventional specialists, need to understand the quantitative issues in clinical research so that they are capable of choosing therapies and technologies that have proven benefit for their patients and avoiding therapies and technologies that are either harmful or unlikely to provide benefit to their patients. In this chapter we discuss the basic concepts of evidence-based medicine, address basic issues of designing clinical studies, and discuss common analytical techniques. All of these topics should be familiar to clinicians, whether or not they are actively engaged in clinical investigation. Interventional cardiology is a continuous learning process; an ability to read and interpret the medical literature with facility is an important part of one's professional life.

Clinical research provides the evidence upon which the practice of medicine is best and most reliably based. The results of clinical studies are typically subjected to peer review before being published in leading medical journals. However, when making decisions about care to offer to his or her patients, the individual clinician needs to have a level of comfort and understanding of basic quantitative methods so that he or she can arrive at the most appropriate medical decisions.

Evidence-Based Medicine

Evidence-based medicine has been defined as combining quantitative evidence about medical practice with expert judgment in an effort to ensure the provision of medical care with reproducible high quality (1). In addition to understanding the concept of evidence-based medicine, those preparing for the International Cardiology Board examinations must be familiar with the various American College of Cardiology/American Heart Association (ACC/AHA) guidelines for clinical practice. The ACC/AHA Guidelines Committees have issued a series of evidence-based practice recommendations that cover a variety of diseases and cardiac procedures, including percutaneous coronary intervention and coronary bypass surgery (2,3). These Guidelines are constructed using a defined, ob-

jective methodology that begins with the accumulation and weighing of evidence. All recommendations are accompanied by an assigned evidence grade (A, B, or C) (Table 27–1). Weight of evidence A means the data have been derived from many trials or at least a single large, randomized clinical trial. Weight of evidence B indicates that the data have been derived from smaller randomized trials or nonrandomized observational studies. The lowest weight of evidence is a grade C, denoting expert consensus.

After weighing the evidence, guideline writers including clinical experts, statisticians and policy makers then assign classes of recommendations I, II, or III (Table 27–1). Class II recommendations are further subdivided into IIa or IIb. For the purposes of board preparation, the candidate must be particularly familiar with Class I and III recommendations. Class I recommendations are those in which the intervention is felt to be useful and effective; Class III denotes interventions that are not deemed useful or effective and may in fact be harmful. The Class II recommendations indicate situations where the evidence has been more controversial. A Class IIa recommendation is given when the evidence conflicts or opinions differ, but overall the evidence leans towards benefit; a Class IIb recommendation indicates that the evidence conflicts or opinions differ, but the weight of the evidence leans against benefit. Despite a wealth of clinical trials information supporting many of the major decisions in cardiovascular medicine, including interventional cardiology, the majority of recommendations in the ACC/AHA guidelines are Class II recommendations, suggesting that a limited amount of evidence exists even for interventions considered routine in clinical practice.

Types of Study Designs

There are two main types of study design: observational studies and experimental studies (4). Observational studies are when patients or groups of patients are observed over a period of time while characteristics of that patient population are recorded. In an experimental design, an intervention such as a drug,

Table 27–1
Levels of Evidence for Clinical Practice Recommendations

Measure	Description
Class of Recommendation	
I	Intervention is useful and effective
IIa	Evidence conflicts/opinions differ but lean toward efficacy
IIb	Evidence conflicts/opinions differ but lean against efficacy
III	Intervention is not useful/effective and may be harmful
Level of Evidence	
A	Data from many randomized clinical trials
B	Data from single randomized trial or nonrandomized studies
C	Expert consensus

Adapted from: Gibbons RJ, Smith SC Jr, Antman E. American College of Cardiology/American Heart Association clinical practice guidelines. Part I: where do they come from? *Circulation.* 2003;107:2979–2986, with permission.

procedure, or technology is introduced into the population and the effect on the study subjects is observed.

Types of observational studies vary. We will consider a few with which the reader should be familiar. These include case control studies and cohort studies. Regarding experimental studies, we will mainly consider randomized controlled trials.

Case Control Studies

A case control study is typically performed on previously collected, retrospective data. In these studies, there are five steps to consider. First, one begins with either the presence of absence of an outcome of interest. Second, one defines a group of cases that have the measure of interest—typically this is a disease or an outcome event. Third, a control group is identified that does not have the disease or the measure of interest but may be matched on a common characteristic such as age or gender. Fourth, the investigator looks backward in time to detect possible causes or risk factors in the history of the cases, but not in the history of the controls. Step five is an attempt to answer the question of what happened or what is the difference between the cases and the controls that might explain the outcome of interest. A case control study might be useful, for example, to consider whether the use of a medication is related to the development of a disease. When considering a treatment, the cases and controls should be carefully matched on other important risk factors to be as certain as possible that only the treatment effect varies between the two groups. Figure 27–1 and Table 27–2 show examples.

Case control studies have certain advantages and disadvantages. The methodology may be the best design for studying diseases or conditions that develop over long periods of time. Additionally, case control studies may be very useful for investigating a preliminary hypothesis, because they are typically a very rapid way of performing a study provided the data on the population have already been collected. The major disadvantage is that the case control study depends upon existing records, which may have been collected for other reasons. This particular study design is subject to a fair degree of bias or er-

ror, because the data are typically collected in advance of the question being asked, so one is limited by the existing data. Specifically, factors associated with the outcome may not be equally distributed between the two treatments. If these factors are not available to be examined, one cannot test whether the differences in the factors, rather than the treatment being studied, are responsible for any statistically significant treatment results. In addition, patient care may have changed since the data were collected, making the results no longer applicable. Choosing an appropriate control group (including one that is matched for certain characteristics) is critical, but may prove to be quite difficult.

Cohort Studies

In a cohort study, information is collected on a group of subjects who have something in common and who remain part of that group for an extended period of observation or follow-up. Typically in this type of design, one begins with the identification of an exposure to some event that is felt to be relevant

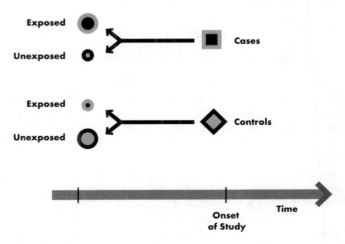

Figure 27–1.

Example of a case control study design.

Table 27–2
Example of a Case-Control Study: Is There an Association Between Use of Aspirin and the Development of Reye's Syndrome?
We have 30 patients with Reye's syndrome, of whom 28 used aspirin. There were 60 patients drawn from a large population of patients with minor viral illnesses, but not Reye's Syndrome. Of these, 35 used aspirin.
Odds of exposure in cases: 28/2 = 14
Odds of exposure in controls: 35/25 = 1.4
Odds ratio: 14/1.4 = 10
Interpretation: Odds of being on aspirin is 10 times greater with Reye's syndrome than without.

to the development of some outcome in the future. One then identifies two groups of subjects, the exposed group and the nonexposed group. In this particular type of study, one looks forward in time from the exposure to determine the effect of the defining characteristics or exposure on the outcome of interest. This design attempts to answer the prospective question: what will happen?

An example of a cohort study design is seen in Figure 27–2 and Table 27–3. A cohort study is a good design when one is interested in studying the particular causes of a condition, the course of a particular disease, or the impact of risk factors over time. The Framingham Study, which has provided so much critical information on the understanding of the association between cardiac risk factors and cardiac outcome, is an example of a cohort study (5). One of the major disadvantages of a cohort design is that studies such as the Framingham study may take a long time to conduct. Because of this they tend to be resource-intensive. It is also a difficult methodology when one is interested in causation: one may define association, but because there is no intervention being introduced into the population, it is difficult to prove causation. It may also be a difficult design when a disease is rare in the population, because the requisite large sample size may be prohibitive.

Experimental Studies

There are two types of experimental studies, the controlled and the uncontrolled study. In a controlled study an experimental drug, procedure, or technology is typically compared with another drug, procedure, or technology. This might include a comparison with placebo. In an uncontrolled study, an investigator will describe the experience with the experimental drug or procedure, but not compare it directly with another treatment. This type of experiment has less validity and is less likely to allow one to conclude that there are differences between the treatments.

Controlled clinical trials may be further grouped into two types—randomized and nonrandomized experiments. In each of these, the trial is being conducted with concurrent controls. There are typically two groups: the experimental group, who receive the experimental drug or procedure, and the control group, who receive placebo or the standard drug or procedure. Randomized clinical trials provide the strongest evidence for reaching a conclusion of causation, whereas in the nonrandomized trial, when the assignment to a treatment group is not random, there may be biases introduced that render conclusions questionable.

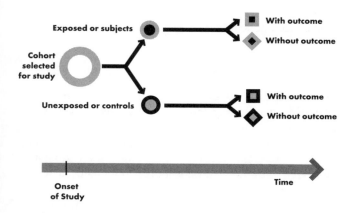

Figure 27–2.
Example of a cohort study design.

Table 27–3
Example of a Cohort Study Design
The association of smoking with coronary heart disease (CHD) is investigated by selecting a group of 3,000 smokers (exposed) and a group of 5,000 nonsmokers (unexposed) who are free of heart disease at the beginning of the study. Both groups are followed for the development of CHD and the incidence in the group is compared. Suppose CHD develops in 84 smokers and 87 nonsmokers.
Risk of CHD in smokers: 84/3,000 = 2.8%
Risk of CHD in nonsmokers: 87/5,000 = 1.74%
Relative Risk: 2.8/1.7 = 1.61
Incidence: Smokers
Incidence: Nonsmokers

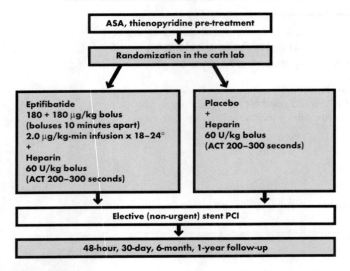

Figure 27–3.

Example of a randomized clinical trial, in this case the ESPRIT study. ESPRIT was a randomized, double-blind, placebo-controlled, parallel-group study in 2,064 patients scheduled to undergo percutaneous coronary intervention with stent implantation.

The randomized clinical trial is distinguished from other types of research by the process of randomization and the introduction of an intervention. The question being asked is, does the intervention make a difference? Because the treatments are randomly allocated, the other risk factors should fall fairly equally between the two groups. Thus only the intervention is left to be different. Figure 27–3 shows an example of a randomized clinical trial. Table 27–4 shows some of the differences between randomized trials and observational studies. Both types of research have complementary value, and the methodology employed will largely depend upon the question of interest. For example, when measuring a treatment effect, the randomized trial methodology is far superior to the observational study.

In the next section, we will discuss a variety of issues relevant to randomized clinical trials, including study endpoints, the calculation of sample size, superiority, equivalence, and noninferiority trials, and the concept of intention-to-treat.

Table 27–4
Randomized Clinical Trials Versus Observational Studies
Efficacy (RCTs)
Experimental setting (causality reduces bias)
"Ideal" circumstances
Limited population
Optimal care
Effectiveness (Observational)
Clinical practice setting
Broad range of patients/providers
Community standard of care

Study Endpoints

In any clinical study the investigator is typically interested in the outcome events, or endpoints. In very broad terms, endpoints may be thought of as consisting of two types: "hard" or "soft" endpoints. Soft endpoints are those that may be affected by individual views or interpretations, and, thus, may be difficult to define or measure. Examples of this include: quality-of-life, symptom scales, and clinical impression. Conversely, hard endpoints are those that are well-defined, measurable, and objective, including death, myocardial infarction, stroke, revascularization, or re-hospitalization. Smaller clinical trials, particularly hypothesis-generating or early-phase development trials, often employ softer endpoints that may require a smaller patient population. Harder clinical endpoints are typically required to make more definitive statements about the value of a therapy or technology in the clinical setting.

Composite Endpoints

Because some outcome events may occur infrequently, investigators commonly combine the endpoints into a composite that will increase the number of anticipated outcome events and therefore decrease the potential sample size. Examples of this would include the composites of death or myocardial infarction; death, myocardial infarction or revascularization; and death or heart failure hospitalization. Typically in a composite endpoint, one measures the occurrence of any one of the events versus none of the events occurring. In such an analysis, one must be vigilant and careful that endpoints of differing severity do not cancel each other out and potentially obscure any potential treatment effect. There should always be a secondary analysis planned that reports the individual rates of the component events by treatment groups.

A different way to view the composite endpoint is to have a ranked composite endpoint. In such an analysis, the different components are assigned a severity score. For example, death would be assigned the higher score and a nonfatal event like re-hospitalization a lower score. Although such an approach has intuitive appeal by assigning an increased amount of weight to the more severe event, the ranking scale must be properly defined. The ranking scale is typically constructed using statistical modeling that helps to quantify the severity of each particular component of the composite.

Sample Size

A proper calculation of sample size is a critical part of clinical research. Understanding this process is essential for understanding the validity of clinical research findings. The calculation of sample size depends on multiple factors, including the Type I error rate, the Type II error rate, the endpoint to be analyzed, the estimated value for the endpoint occurring in the control arm, the estimated improvement in the treatment arm, the amount of variation in the endpoint measured, and the statistical method to be used in analyzing the endpoint. In particular clinicians should feel comfortable in understanding

Table 27–5

Sample Size Estimation: Type I and II Errors

		Test Results	
		No treatment effect	Treatment has an effect
Truth	No treatment effect		Type I error (α)
	Treatment has an effect	Type II error (β)	Power ($1 - \beta$)

both Type I and Type II errors (Table 27–5). The Type I error (α) is when one observes an effect when in truth no effect exists. The Type II error (β) is when one observes no treatment effect when in fact a treatment effect does exist. One minus the Type II error ($1-\beta$) is also the trial's power. By understanding the risk of a Type II error, or, conversely, the importance of power in examining clinical trials results, one can appreciate whether or not a trial actually had adequate power to answer the desired question. Yusuf first pointed this out in the cardiovascular clinical literature nearly 20 years ago (6). Table 27–6 summarizes those results and the importance of sample size in allowing clinicians to determine whether the population was adequate to answer the question the study sought to answer.

Sample size is also dependent upon what type of trial is planned. We will briefly discuss three types of trials: superiority, noninferiority, and equivalence (7). In a superiority trial, the experiment is designed to test for a statistically significant and clinically meaningful improvement (or harm) from the use of the experimental treatment over that of the standard of care. In an equivalence trial, the experiment is designed to evaluate whether the difference in outcome for the experimental treatment compared with standard care falls within the boundary of a clinically defined minimally important difference (MID). The minimally important difference is the largest difference that one would accept between the outcome of the two groups while still considering them clinically similar or comparable. In a noninferiority trial, the results are evaluated assuming that the experimental treatment is not worse than the standard of care by a clinically meaningful amount. Although one still uses the MID to determine the boundary of noninferiority, unlike equivalence studies, a noninferiority study does not look for small improvements over the experimental therapy. Essentially

one might view this as a one-sided test as opposed to the two-sided evaluation that is the hallmark of equivalence. One can see graphically in Figure 27–4 the results of a variety of studies and the potential results in superiority, equivalence, and noninferiority studies.

Several recent examples from the cardiology literature demonstrate the concept of noninferiority. Both the Global Use of Strategies to Open Occluded Arteries in Acute Myocardial Infarction (GUSTO V) (8) and Superior Yield of the New strategy of Enoxaparin, Revascularization and GlYcoprotein IIb/IIIa inhibitors (SYNERGY) (9) Trials were designed to demonstrate the superiority of an experimental therapy over the standard of care. But in both cases it was pre-specifed that if superiority was not met, then the treatments would be compared for noninferiority. In GUSTO V, the hypothesis was that the combination of abciximab plus reteplase was superior to reteplase alone in the treatment of patients with acute ST-segment–elevation myocardial infarction. While the trial did not show the superiority of the abciximab plus reteplase combination, it did demonstrate noninferiority, with the upper boundary of the 95% confidence interval being less than the prespecified noninferiority boundary of 1.1. Similarly, SYNERGY did not demonstrate that enoxaparin was superior to unfractionated heparin among patients presenting with non-ST–elevation acute coronary syndromes. However, the protocol defined inferiority criteria that were met when the upper boundary of the confidence interval did not exceed the pre-specified ratio of 1.1.

In an era when multiple active therapies are available for patients with acute cardiovascular disease, equivalence and noninferiority trials are becoming increasingly important in the evaluation of new therapies. Noninferiority and equivalence trials have most of their value when the experimental

Table 27–6

Sample Size Calculations

Deaths	Pts Randomized (Risk = 10%)	Chance of Type II Error*	Comments on Sample Size
0–50	<500	>0.9	Utterly inadequate
50–150	1,000	0.7–0.9	Probably inadequate
150–350	3,000	0.3–0.7	Possibly inadequate
350–650	6,000	0.1–0.3	Probably adequate
>650	10,000	<0.1	Adequate

*Probability of failing to achieve P <0.01 if risk reduction = 25%. Reprinted from: Yusuf S, Peto R, Lewis J, et al. Beta blockade during and after myocardial infarction: an overview of the randomized trials. *Prog Cardiovasc Dis.* 1985;27:335–71, with permission.

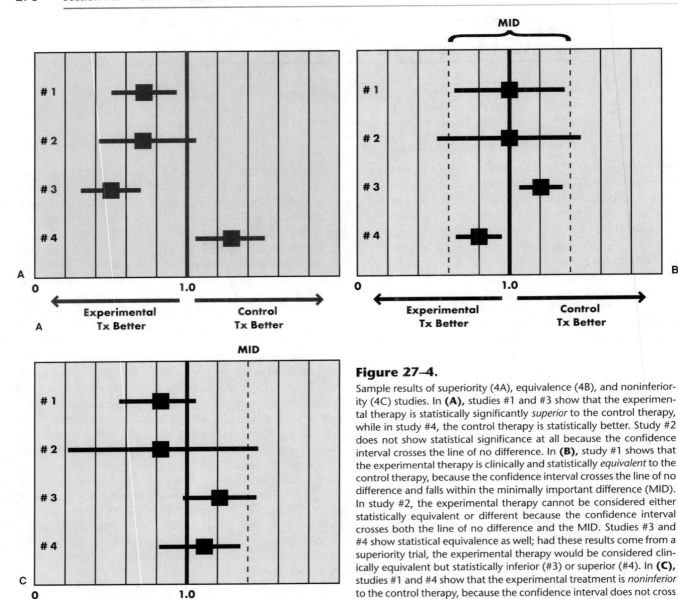

Figure 27–4.

Sample results of superiority (4A), equivalence (4B), and noninferiority (4C) studies. In **(A)**, studies #1 and #3 show that the experimental therapy is statistically significantly *superior* to the control therapy, while in study #4, the control therapy is statistically better. Study #2 does not show statistical significance at all because the confidence interval crosses the line of no difference. In **(B)**, study #1 shows that the experimental therapy is clinically and statistically *equivalent* to the control therapy, because the confidence interval crosses the line of no difference and falls within the minimally important difference (MID). In study #2, the experimental therapy cannot be considered either statistically equivalent or different because the confidence interval crosses both the line of no difference and the MID. Studies #3 and #4 show statistical equivalence as well; had these results come from a superiority trial, the experimental therapy would be considered clinically equivalent but statistically inferior (#3) or superior (#4). In **(C)**, studies #1 and #4 show that the experimental treatment is *noninferior* to the control therapy, because the confidence interval does not cross the MID. Study #2's confidence interval is too wide to draw a conclusion. Study #3 crosses the MID, indicating that the experimental treatment is inferior to the control.

therapy is felt to be unlikely to be better than the established therapy, but could offer incremental benefit with regard to, for example, improved safety, greater ease of administration, or reduced cost. The challenge for noninferiority and equivalence studies is the establishment of the minimally important difference boundary.

While a number of recent large-scale trials have used the equivalence or noninferiority methodology, there is not a firmly accepted definition of the minimally important difference. Consequently, in interpreting the medical literature one must pay particular attention to how that boundary was constructed. If the MID is quite large, the validity of a noninferiority or equivalence claim can be questioned. On the other hand, if the boundary is overly narrow, very little is gained by choosing a noninferiority or equivalence design over a more traditional

superiority design. The boundary of the MID is a clinically determined one, frequently based on a fair bit of subjectivity as to what constitutes an acceptable clinical deviation.

Intention-to-Treat Analysis

An important concept in the evaluation of clinical studies is the notion of performing an analysis based on the intention-to-treat principle (ITT). Broadly, ITT is the notion that patients are randomly assigned to a treatment group and then analyzed as if they received that treatment, regardless of whether they actually did. The purest form of ITT means that any patient who signs an informed consent and who is assigned a randomized treatment remains in that treatment arm for the purposes of analysis, even if they drop out before any treatment was received or if they received a treatment different than the allocated one.

A commonly performed analysis, particularly in blinded studies, is the ITT-treated analysis. In this adaptation of the intention-to-treat principle, the patients remain in the group that they were randomized into for the purposes of analysis, but only those patients who actually received the treatment are considered in the primary analysis. In order for this analytical method to be as valid as possible, the investigator must be blinded to the treatment that the patient is to receive when the decision is made not to give them the treatment. This helps to assure that factors other than the allocation assignment itself are responsible for the patient not receiving the assigned therapy. An example of this in percutaneous coronary intervention (PCI) trials is when a patient has been randomized prior to the final decision to perform percutaneous intervention. A recent example of this was the Integrilin to Minimise Platelet Aggregation and Coronary Thrombosis-II (IMPACT-II) Trial (10). In this study, testing the use of the glycoprotein IIb/IIIa inhibitor eptifibatide in the setting of PCI, a small group of patients were randomized prior to the final decision regarding their suitability for PCI. Approximately 3% to 4% of the patients did not actually receive their assigned therapy when it was decided not to perform PCI. The potential therapeutic effect of the glycoprotein IIb/IIIa inhibitor might best be considered when one evaluates the patients who actually received any amount of study drug. When this is done, there is little change in the absolute treatment effect, but the subtle changes in the relative treatment effect translate into a significant p-value when the treated patient analysis is considered relative to one considering the all-patient ITT analysis (10).

The decision to use an intention-to-treat analysis versus using a treated-patient analysis has particular importance in the interpretation of noninferiority trials. In a noninferiority trial, the most essential and appropriately robust analysis considers only those patients who have actually received therapy as. This is because, paradoxically, noncompliance actually improves the chances of declaring a noninferior result. An extreme example would be if in a randomized trial none of the patients received the assigned therapy, then the two groups would likely not appear different from one another, thus fulfilling the criteria of noninferiority.

◼ Considerations in Analysis Method

In order to understand what analysis method one might choose when considering clinical data one should be familiar with the scales of measurement of data. Data can be described as nominal, ordinal, or continuous. Nominal data are made up of discrete categories that have no particular order (e.g., gender). Ordinal data are data that are categorical, but with an inherent order; for example, as when describing the number of diseased vessels in patients with coronary artery disease (1, 2, or 3-vessel). Finally, continuous data are that in which the differences between numbers have actual meaning. Examples of continuous data include age and weight. When dealing with continuous measures, in addition to considering the scales of measurement one should also consider the shape of the distri-

bution. For example, are the data points normally distributed, like a bell-shaped or symmetric curve? Or are the data skewed or do they have a bimodal distribution? This is also referred to as a non-normal distribution of continuous data.

In describing continuous data, one might refer to measures of the center of the distribution. For example, one refers to the mean, which is the average of the measures, or to the median, which is the middle value of the distribution. Also important are measures of the variability around the center. This can be described as the range of the data (maximum value–minimum value), the standard deviation or variance, or percentile (e.g., the 25th to 75th range).

There are a number of ways to perform statistical tests that compare two groups. When the data are nominally distributed, these include the Chi-Square Test, Fisher's Exact Test, or logistic regression. The results are often presented as rates, odds ratios, or risk ratios. Odds ratios and risk ratios are frequently confused for one another. Although these are among the most common ways to compare two groups, it is worth understanding how they are calculated. We have included examples of calculating an odds ratio and a risk ratio in Table 27–7. Finally, a clinically important number to understand that is frequently reported in the medical literature is the so-called number needed to treat (NNT). The NNT refers to the number of patients who need to be treated with a therapy to prevent one adverse outcome. This is calculated by dividing one by the absolute risk reduction. For example, if the absolute difference between two therapies is 1.5%, the number needed to treat is 1 divided by .015, which equals 67 patients.

P-Values

A p-value is the probability of obtaining the results you have observed (or even more extreme results) if the effect is really due to random chance alone (11). For example, a p-value of ≤ 0.05 indicates that a difference of at least the amount observed in the experiment would occur in fewer than 50 out of 1,000 similar experiments if the treatment studies had absolutely no effect on the measured outcome. In designing a clinical study, particularly a randomized clinical trial, the investigators must state the hypothesis that is being tested, the statistical test that will be used on this hypothesis (to reject the null hypothesis, meaning the rejection of the statement that there is no difference between the treatment groups), and the critical (or nominal) value for declaring significance (the Type I error rate).

In most clinical research, the critical value to declare significance is set at 0.05. As this is mostly by convention, it is appropriate for certain types of studies to set a different level of nominal significance, for example at 0.025 or 0.001. When one sets a nominal level of significance, then the prestated declaration must be followed. For example, if the nominal level of significance has been set at 0.05, then for a final study p-value of 0.053, one cannot declare statistical significance, whereas if the results provide a p-value of 0.048 under the same conditions, then one could declare a statistically significant difference between the treatment groups. Understanding clinical trial results requires careful reading of the clinical study

Table 27–7

Examples of Calculating Odds Ratios and Risk Ratios in the PURSUIT Trial

Odds Ratios

The primary endpoint of CEC-adjudicated MI or death at 30 days was compared for patients receiving eptifibatide versus placebo. In the eptifibatide group, 672 out of 4,722 patients experienced an event. In the placebo group, 745 out of 4,739 experienced an event.

Odds in the eptifibatide group: 672/4050 = 0.166
Odds in the placebo group: 745/3994 = 0.187
Odds ratio: 0.166/0.187 = 0.889

Risk Ratios

The primary endpoint of CEC-adjudicated MI or death at 30 days was compared for patients receiving eptifibatide versus placebo. In the eptifibatide group, 672 out of 4,722 patients experienced an event. In the placebo group, 745 out of 4,739 experienced an event.

Risk in the eptifibatide group: 672/4722 = 14.2%
Risk in the placebo group: 745/4739 = 15.7%
Risk ratio: 14.2/15.7 = 0.905

From: The PURSUIT Investigators. Inhibition of platelet glycoprotein IIb/IIIa with eptifibatide in patients with acute coronary syndromes without persistent ST-segment elevation: a randomized, placebo-controlled, clinical trial. *N Engl J Med.* 1998,339:436–443, with permission.

methods and understanding of the Type I error that has been prospectively set for a clinical experiment. Violation of this conservation approach through activities such as data mining until one obtains a desired p-value is particularly troublesome and has been termed "random research" (12).

Confidence Intervals

As with p-values, a reader of the clinical research literature must be facile in an understanding of confidence intervals (CI). CIs are frequently misinterpreted as being the same thing as the p-value, and although these two figures might provide complementary information, they are most assuredly not the same. For example, consider the 95% CI. This suggests that if one were to perform the same study an infinite number of times, then 95% of the estimates of the effect would fall within the bounds of the interval. A ratio of two rates that are the same gives a value of 1. Thus a confidence interval that overlaps 1 implies that the treatment difference is not statistically significant. An interval that does not include 1 implies statistical significance. Data are frequently presented in ratio plots displaying the point estimate and the associated 95% confidence intervals. Figure 27-5 demonstrates study results using ratio plots that include superiority and uncertainty results.

▨ Further Interpretation

When interpreting clinical study results, it is insufficient to consider only the conclusion that the results are statistically significant. The reader should ask a series of questions to better understand the meaning of that claim. Is the effect size clinically meaningful and important? Is the study sample very homogeneous; can these results be generalized to broader

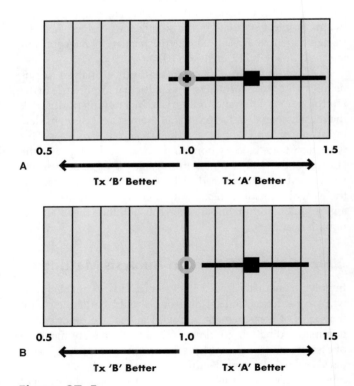

Figure 27–5.

Interpreting ratio plots. If the confidence interval crosses the value of no difference (1.0 for a ratio), as in **(A)**, then the P-value is >0.05. If it does not, as in **(B)**, the P-value is <0.05 and the comparison is statistically significant, in this case showing that Treatment A is better.

Table 27–8

Questions to Ask When Reading and Interpreting the Results of a Clinical Trial

Are the Results of the Study Valid?
Primary Guides
  Was the assignment of patients to treatment randomized?
  Were all patients who entered the study properly accounted for at its conclusion?
  Was follow-up complete?
  Were patients analyzed in the groups to which they were randomized?
Secondary Guides
  Were patients, their clinicians, and study personnel blinded to treatment?
  Were the groups similar at the start of the trial?
  Aside from the experimental intervention, were the groups treated equally?

What Were the Results
  How large was the treatment effect?
  How precise was the treatment effect (confidence intervals)?

Will the Results Help Me in Caring for My Patients?
  Does my patient fulfill the enrollment criteria for the trial? If not, how close is the patient to the enrollment criteria?
  Does my patient fit the features of a subgroup in the trial report? If so, are the results of the subgroup analysis in the trial valid?
  Were all the clinically important outcomes considered?
  Are the likely treatment benefits worth the potential harm and costs?

Reprinted from: Califf RM, Topol EJ. Considerations in the design and conduct of clinical studies and the interpretation of quantitative evidence. In: Topol EJ, ed. *Textbook of Cardiovascular Medicine.* 2nd ed. Philadelphia: Lippincott Williams & Wilkins; 2002: with permission.

---

populations? How statistically robust are the results? For example, how close is the actual p-value to the nominal level of significance? When the results are displayed as a ratio plot, do the confidence intervals include the estimate of no difference (1 for an odds ratio, 0 for absolute differences, or % change)? How wide are the CI? Other questions to ask in interpreting the results of a clinical trial are delineated in Table 27–8.

Summary

Clinicians need familiarity with common quantitative issues in order to fairly and appropriately interpret the medical literature. The essence of evidence-based medicine is thoughtful clinical care guided by the best available data on the topic. Interventional cardiologists preparing for their Board exams should understand basic statistical topics as well as how the commonly used ACC/AHA Practice Guidelines are constructed and employed.

Acknowledgment

The authors wish to thank John M. Daniel for his editorial expertise in preparing this manuscript.

REFERENCES

 1. Sackett DL, Rosenberg WMC, Gray JAM, et al. Evidence-based medicine: what it is and what it is not. *Br Med J.* 1996;312:71–72.
 2. Gibbons RJ, Smith SC Jr, Antman E. American College of Cardiology/American Heart Association Clinical Practice Guidelines: part I: where do they come from?. *Circulation.* 2003;107:2979–2986.
 3. Gibbons RJ, Smith SC Jr, Antman E. American College of Cardiology/American Heart Association Clinical Practice Guidelines: part II: evolutionary changes in a continuous quality improvement project. *Circulation.* 2003;107:3101–3107.
 4. Bailer JC, Mosteller F. *Medical uses of statistics.* 2nd ed. Boston: New England Journal of Medicine Books; 1992:149–151.
 5. Fox CS, Evans JC, Larson MG, et al. Temporal trends in coronary heart disease mortality and sudden cardiac death from 1950 to 1999: the Framingham Heart Study. *Circulation.* 2004;110:522–527.
 6. Yusuf S, Peto R, Lewis J, et al. Beta blockade during and after myocardial infarction: an overview of the randomized trials. *Prog Cardiovasc Dis.* 1985;27:335–371.
 7. Friedman LM, Furberg CD, DeMets DL. Fundamentals of clinical trials. 3rd ed. St. Louis: Mosby-Year Book, Inc.; 1996:5556.
 8. Topol EJ. Reperfusion therapy for acute myocardial infarction with fibrinolytic therapy or combination reduced fibrinolytic therapy and platelet glycoprotein IIb/IIIa inhibition: the GUSTO V randomised trial. *Lancet.* 2001;357:1905–1914.
 9. Mahaffey KW, Ferguson JJ. Exploring the role of enoxaparin in the management of high-risk patients with non–ST-elevation acute coronary syndromes: the SYNERGY trial. *Am Heart J.* 2005;149:S81–S90.
10. The IMPACT-II Investigators. Randomised placebo-controlled trial of effect of eptifibatide on complications of percutaneous coronary intervention: IMPACT-II. Integrilin to Minimise Platelet Aggregation and Coronary Thrombosis-II. *Lancet.* 1997;349:1422–1428.
11. Moyé LA. P-value interpretation, and alpha allocation in clinical trials. *Ann Epidemiol.* 1998;8:351–357.
12. Moyé LA. Random research. *Circulation.* 2001;103:3150–3153.

CHAPTER 28

Economics of Percutaneous Coronary Intervention

Larry S. Dean

Health care expenditures are increasing at a rapid rate and are estimated to consume 17% of the gross domestic product by 2011 (Fig. 28–1) and 20% by 2015 (1). The economics of coronary intervention have always been important, but did not become more central to the procedure until the advent of stenting, and in particular with the availability of drug eluting stents (DES). Over the years since the first description of percutaneous coronary angioplasty by Gruentzig in 1977 (2), balloon angioplasty catheter prices have steadily declined as more product from an increasing number of companies entered the marketplace driving cost down. With the development of bare metal stents in the mid-1990s (3,4), once again the cost of the devices, and hence the procedure, increased. However, beginning in 2004 with FDA approval of the Cypher DES and with subsequent data showing clear clinical superiority in many subsets of patients, the cost of the device central to the procedure markedly increased by approximately threefold. This caused great concern within the administration of most hospitals, because reimbursement lagged availability of the devices (5). In addition, hospital reimbursement by the Centers for Medicare and Medicaid and many private payers in the United States did not cover the complete cost of the new devices. Many institutions felt the need, in order to maintain adequate margins for the procedure, to restrict access to the devices by implementing clinical criteria for their use (6). However, the subsequent overwhelmingly positive clinical data supporting their use led to rapid adoption by physicians, particularly in the United States.

Because the economics of much of the practice of interventional cardiology has become more important in the last several years, this chapter serves as an introduction to key economic and financial concepts ultimately using DES as a model.

Basic Economic Principles

In order to understand the economics of coronary intervention several basic concepts and or terms must be understood:

- Reimbursement

Gone are the days of payment for services rendered. In today's health care environment, much of hospital reimbursement is discounted fee for service or, as in the case of Medicare, it is prospective and DRG based. This has led to essentially fixed reimbursement for services. This is true even without penetration by HMOs with their unique form of fixed payment for services delivered.

- Cost

Cost is borne by several groups including the individual patient, society, and the individual hospital. The ability to bear this cost varies widely, but impacts decisions made by all involved. Individuals in the United States have been isolated from health care cost, because typically they see only their premiums and copays as the cost of their care. However, this represents only a fraction of the true cost of the care delivered.

Society bears the brunt of health care cost, because it is passed on to all of us through a higher cost for everything we buy. For example, it is estimated that $1,000 of every new car that is built by Ford Motor Company is attributable to the cost of health care for their workers (7). Starbucks spends more on health care than it spends on coffee beans per year (8). The uninsured, estimated to make up 40 million people in the United States and many of them children, also impacts the cost borne by all of us. Ultimately, each society, decides how much it is willing to spend on health care.

Frequently hospital and procedure cost are estimated based on charges, typically by using a cost to charge ratio that is unique to the individual hospital. Therefore, much of the cost of providing services is frequently an estimate which should be kept in mind during our subsequent review of the SIRIUS trial.

Cost can be of several types, some of which physicians, by their practice patterns, can have great impact. Types of cost can be divided into:

- Direct or that which is related to the procedure (e.g., DES stent cost). This can be impacted by physician practice (e.g., the number of stents used per case). These costs can be attributed to a specific area or service.
- Indirect or that which is attributable to delivering the service (e.g., electricity to run the x-ray equipment). They are typically difficult to allocate to an individual unit or area and borne by all by some form of allocation.

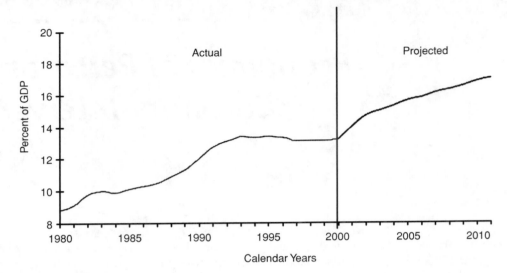

Figure 28–1.

United States health care expenditures as a percent of gross domestic product (GDP). After 2000, they are estimated. Source: http://cms.hhs.gov/charts/default.asp.

- Fixed or that which does not vary due to volume (e.g., cost allocation for the space occupied by the cath lab).
- Variable or that which varies based on volume (e.g., cath lab staff).
- Opportunity costs are those that can be realized if the available dollars are used for something else. They are related to the time value of money and net present value, concepts that are beyond the scope of this chapter. (For those interested in additional detail, an excellent general text is *Healthcare Finance. An Introduction to Accounting and Financial Management,* 2nd ed. by Louis C. Gapenski.)
- Profit

Profit is the bottom line, so to speak. Net profit is what allows equity to be returned to shareholders in for profit companies and for both profit and nonprofit institutions to maintain their physical plant, purchase capital, and plan for the future.

Related to profit is contribution margin. Contribution margin is that margin that "contributes" to offset fixed cost with any additional income going to profit. One common misconception is the idea that if a particular service has a positive margin that they can use those dollars to support that particular service. Unfortunately, many hospital services have negative margins which must be supported by those that have a margin that is positive. As an aside, specialty hospitals (e.g., the "heart hospital") is an incredible business model for those involved since positive net profit should be fairly easy to produce since they do not have to "cover" losses elsewhere. This is true because cardiovascular services, by in large, are profitable for hospitals.

Outcome Measures

Before one can discuss the value of a procedure to the patient or society, an understanding of various outcomes is necessary. Understanding outcome measures is important when consid-

ering cost effectiveness and when counseling patients on the most appropriate treatment. Common terms used to describe outcomes are:

1. *Absolute risk reduction*, which is defined as the difference in outcome between the control versus the treated arm of a study. For example, if the mortality rate in the control arm was 15% versus 10% in the treated arm, the absolute risk reduction would be 5%. See Figure 28–2.
2. *Relative risk reduction* is the difference in the treated arm divided by the control arm. Considering the previous example, the relative risk reduction is 33%. Relative risk reduction should always be interpreted with caution, because it tends to overstate the benefit of a treatment.
3. The number needed to treat or harm is a very helpful way to look at the benefit to the patient, because it gives one the ability to determine, based on the absolute risk reduction, the number of patients who must receive a treatment in order to benefit one patient. It is determined by dividing the absolute risk reduction into 100%. Using the previous example with a 5% absolute risk reduction, one would have to treat 20 patients to yield a benefit in one. Importantly, it also gives balance to relative risk. To obtain the 33% relative risk reduction noted earlier, one would need to treat 20 patients. A more extreme example would be a study that had a reduction of relative risk by let's say 50% in a population of 2 million. This would require the treatment of 1 million people! The number needed to harm is similar in concept, but would be used when harm occurred to the treatment group.

Decision Analysis

Now that we have a basic understanding of cost and outcomes, in deciding which treatment is most appropriate for society or others to pay for, it becomes necessary to look at several modifying factors over and above outcomes in and of themselves.

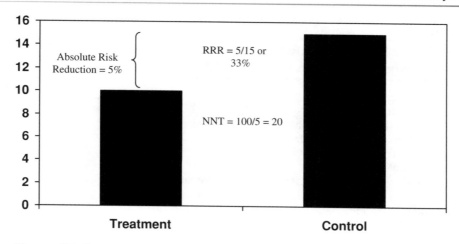

Figure 28–2.

Hypothetical outcomes of a randomized trial comparing treatment to control. RRR, relative risk reduction; NNT, number needed to treat.

This is necessary since neither the patient, payer, or society can afford all therapies. This is true even in a wealthy country such as the United States.

- Cost Effectiveness

  - *Cost effectiveness analysis* is a technique that uses outcomes and cost to determine the cost for the expected benefit. Another way to look at this is that it is a way of determining the economic efficiency with which an intervention or therapy generates benefit (9). As will be seen it balances the cost and benefit of a particular intervention allowing one to examine the impact of each on decisions of therapy (10).

    Cost effectiveness ratio is a ratio defined by the following simple formula: Cost of the therapy/benefit of the therapy. As an example lets assume that a single-vessel stenting procedure costs $50,000 and the benefit is 5 years of life. The CE ratio is, therefore, $10,000/year of life. Note that this is purely a ratio and as such is not particularly helpful in making health care decisions. A more helpful ratio is known as the incremental cost effectiveness ratio.

  - *Incremental cost effectiveness ratio* (ICER) is more helpful, because it allows evaluation of the incremental benefit of a particular therapy and is defined as: Incremental cost of a therapy (IC)/incremental benefit of a therapy (IB). Using the previous example and assuming that the comparison is with another therapy, let's consider medical therapy, which costs $25,000 and yields 2 years of life. Then the incremental cost of single-vessel stenting is $25,000 and that the incremental benefit is 2 years of life: ICER = IC/IB or $25,000/2 year or $12,500/year of additional life. Other benefits can be used for the calculation such as incremental cost avoided by a particular therapy or procedure compared to another.

  - *The cost effectiveness plane* (11) is a technique of determining, based on ICER, which therapy among several is most or least cost effective. A therapy is dominant if it is lower in cost and superior in benefit, but dominated if it is higher in cost and of less benefit (Fig. 28–3).

- *Bootstrapping* is a nonparametric statistical technique commonly used in studies of health care cost to determine the range of potential outcomes when there is concern that the data set in not normally distributed, which is frequently the case in health care cost analyses (12).

- *Quality adjusted benefit* is our last method of determining the cost benefit of a particular therapy. If one thinks about an outcome, is it worth it to a patient to give them 4 additional years of life if the benefit can only be realized with the patient likely to remain bed ridden in order to gain the benefit? Quality adjusted benefit takes into account not only the incremental cost and incremental benefit of a therapy but also the quality of the outcome. This technique uses a quality-of-life measure to "adjust" the benefit. Examples of measures that are frequently used include years free of angina or additional life. In order to add the quality adjustment, a quality-of-life measure must be used. Frequently it is what is termed utility and if one uses increased life as the benefit of the therapy, then the resultant metric

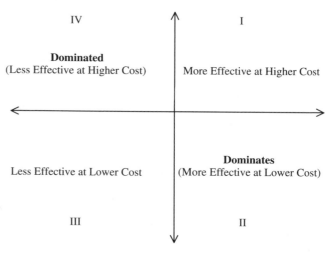

Figure 28–3.

The cost effectiveness plane.

Table 28–1

QALYs for Some Common Therapies and Procedures. This Is Commonly Known as a League Table

	$/QALY
US screening for AAA, males 60-years old	950
Hypertension screening and treatment, males 60-years-old	12,000
ICD in high-risk patients for SCD	39,000
PTCA for single-vessel disease	27,000
CABG for single-vessel disease	54,000
Hypertension screening and treatment in asymptomatic 20-year-old females	61,000
Screening for carotid disease with operation in asymptomatic 65-year-old men	130,000

Modified from: Winkelmayer WC, Cohen DJ, Berger ML, et al. Comparing cost utility analyses in cardiovascular medicine. In: WS Weintraub, ed. *Contemporary Cardiology: Cardiovascular Healthcare Economics.* Humana Press, Inc. 2003:337–353.
US, ultrasound; AAA, abdominal aortic aneurysm; ICD, implantable cardioverter defibrillator; SCD, sudden cardiac death.

is termed quality adjusted life years or QALYs. But before we discuss QALYs, we need to better understand utility, an important concept in the determination of benefit.

- Utility is a value that varies from 0 to 1 where 0 represents death and 1 is perfect heath. Typically it is determined by posing to patients multiple risks for a particular benefit; let's say longer life. It is based on some intervention, for example coronary intervention, commonly using a technique known as the gamble, until a point of indecision is reached that becomes the utility of the therapy.

Using utility and ICER (known as cost utility analysis) one can determine the quality adjusted benefit; let's use life (called QALY), of a particular therapy by the following formula: QALY = ICER × utility. Using the previous example for ICER and a utility of 0.5, the QALY = $12,500/year of additional life × 0.5 = $6,250/adjusted life year. This hypothetical represents a real bargain based on QALYs for other therapies (Table 28–1). Typically a QALY of <$50,000 is considered acceptable in the United States, but will vary from country to country based on that society's willingness to pay for the added benefit. The problem is, however, that even in the United States we have multiple therapies competing for the same resources and those resources are constrained. This technique can also be used to allocate resources, as was done several years ago in the State of Oregon with its decisions on Medicaid coverage of various therapies (13). Care must be taken in the interpretation of this type of information since estimates of benefit can vary significantly depending on the treatment used and the patient populated treated. For example, using statins as primary prevention in women with low risk cost up to $1.4 million/QALY whereas secondary prevention in men aged 45 to 55 cost $3,900/QALY (14).

QALYs can also be used to compare two or more therapies since at first glance the most effective one may not be obvious. For example, if two therapies have equal life years, how is it

possible to know which is best? If the result is adjusted based on the utility of each therapy the question is simplified such that if therapy A has a utility of 0.8 (better quality-of-life) and B is 0.3 (worse quality-of-life), therapy A would be, in general, the best choice. What happens if utility is high, but additional life years are less? Then patient choice enters the deliberation. In other words, does the patient desire a better short-term quality-of-life or a longer life, but at lower quality? Using QALYs makes this type of decision somewhat more straightforward.

There are obvious limitations of this technique. For example:

1. Many studies do not design quality-of-life measures into the study and therefore, they must be inferred.
2. If they are included in the study any benefit found is based on that unique study population. Few individual patients perfectly match study patients, which affects ones ability to generalize and therefore impacts the strength of an individual recommendation.
3. The calculated utility can have great impact on the result; therefore, its accuracy is paramount. It is really a hypothetical since no patient can truly know what they are willing to do in order to have more life for a given quality. This uncertainty is balanced by the number of people used to determine the results of the gamble.

Now we are ready to turn our attention to the economic analysis of the SIRIUS trial, a comparison of the sirolimus drug eluting Cypher stent with the bare metal Bx Velocity stent (Cordis Corporation) (15).

Case Study: The SIRIUS Trial

The economic study of SIRIUS (16) was a prospective trial designed to determine if the more costly Cypher stent was cost effective compared to the less costly bare metal Bx Velocity. The hypothesis was that there would be less repeat procedures and hospitalizations because of the lower restenosis rate in the Cypher stent and, therefore, lower cost in follow-up that would balance the higher initial cost of the DES.

The SIRIUS trial randomized 1,058 patients undergoing single vessel, nonostial, elective percutaneous coronary intervention to either the sirolimus eluting stent, n = 533 or a bare metal stent, n = 525. The stented vessels were between 2.5 and 3.5 mm in diameter and the lesions were 15 to 30 mm in length. The average number of stents used per case was 1.4 in both groups. Aggregate costs were followed for 1 year and the primary endpoint for analysis was the incremental cost of revascularization avoided by using the sirolimus stent. Pre-specified subgroup analysis was also performed based on diabetes status, reference vessel diameter, and lesion length. The secondary endpoint was quality adjusted life years. Because the data required to assess this outcome was not prospectively collected, and was not powered to assess mortality, a surrogate data set and utility was used.

Initial hospital cost were $2,881 higher in the DES group which was due to the higher cost of the stent in the Cypher arm of the study. However, because repeat hospitalizations and revascularization procedures were lower in the sirolimus arm, at 1 year follow-up, aggregate cost were only $309 higher than the control arm. The primary endpoint, incremental cost of revascularization avoided, was $1,650 favoring the Cypher stent. Subgroup analysis revealed that the Cypher stent was dominant with reference vessel size <2.5 mm and with lesion length >20 mm.

Secondary endpoint analysis showed that the Cypher stent cost $27,540 per QALY gained with acceptable ranges with bootstrap analysis. This is well within the accepted cost per life year gained in this country. However, the secondary endpoint is based on inference since the data was not collected prospectively and another study's utility was used. It should therefore be interpreted with some caution and in light of the patients studied.

Summary

Health care costs continue to increase which at some point will not be sustainable even for the United States. There are tools that can be used to determine the effectiveness of the many therapies currently available and that can be applied to those of the future. These tools can help us make decisions about which therapies are not only beneficial but can also be had at a cost that we can all bare. Having an understanding of these techniques and their strengths and limitations will allow physicians to more actively participate in the economic aspects of health care and allow us to better guide the decisions that will ultimately impact the patients who have entrusted their care and wellbeing to us.

REFERENCES

1. Gruentzig AR, Senning A, Siegenthaler WE. Nonoperative dilatation of coronary-artery stenosis. *N Engl J Med.* 1979;301:61–68.
2. Borger C, Smith S, Truffer C, et al. Health Spending Projections through 2015: Changes on the Horizon, Health Affairs. 2006;25(2);W61–73.
3. Roubin GS, King SB, Douglas JS Jr, et al. Intracoronary stenting during percutaneous transluminal coronary angioplasty. *Circulation.* 1990;81:IV92–100.
4. Schatz RA, Baim DS, Leon M, et al. Clinical experience with the Palmaz-Schatz coronary stent. Initial results of a multicenter study. *Circulation.* 1991;83:148–161.
5. Becker C. Stuck in the middle. The highly anticipated drug-eluting stents are good for heart patients, but are they bad for hospital balance sheets? *Mod Healthc.* 2002;32:4–5.
6. O'Neill WW, Leon MB. Drug-eluting stents. Cost versus clinical benefit. *Circulation.* 2003;107:3008–3011.
7. Available at: http://www.ford.com/en/company/about/publicPolicy/health Care.htm.
8. A full bodied talk with Mr. Starbucks. Edited by Patricia O'Connell. Business Week Online. November 22, 2004. Available at: http://www.businessweek.com/magazine/content/04_47/b3909098.htm.
9. Nease RF. Introduction to cost-effectiveness analysis. In: Weintraub WS, ed. *Contemporary Cardiology: Cardiovascular Healthcare Economics.* Humana Press, Inc. 2003.
10. Eisenberg JM. Clinical economics. A guide to the economics of clinical practices. *JAMA.* 1989;262:2789–2886.
11. Black WC. The CE plane. A graphic representation of cost effectiveness. *Med Decis Making.* 1990;10:212–224.
12. Barber JA, Thompson SG. Analysis of cost data in randomized trials: an application of the non parametric bootstrap. *Stat Med.* 2000;19:3219–3236.
13. Tengs TO. An evaluation of Oregon's Medicaid rationing algorithms. *Health Econ.* 1996;5:171–181.
14. Prosser LA, Stinnett AA, Goldman PA, et al. Cost-effectiveness of cholesterol-lowering therapies according to selected patient characteristics. *Ann Intern Med.* 2000;132:769–779.
15. Moses JW, Leon MB, Popma JJ, et al. Sirolimus-eluting stents versus standard stents in patients with stenosis in a native coronary artery. *N Engl J Med.* 2003;349:1315–1323.
16. Cohen, DJ, Bakhai A, Shi C, et al. Cost-effectiveness of sirolimus-eluting stents for treatment of complex coronary stenoses. Results from the sirolimus-eluting balloon expandable stent in the treatment of patients with de novo native coronary artery lesions (SIRIUS) trial. *Circulation.* 2004;110:508–514.

CHAPTER 29

PCI Guidelines for Interventional Cardiology Boards

Michael J. Lim

In November 2005, the ACC/AHA/SCAI released the 2005 update of the guidelines for percutaneous coronary intervention (1). This guideline statement offers the first update involving all types of percutaneous coronary intervention since 2001 and, thus will reflect most of the material relevant to the interventional cardiology board exam.

We must keep in mind that guideline documents are created in an attempt to define practices that meet the needs of most patients encountered in clinical practice. In creating these recommendations a writing group reviews the available scientific evidence and used it to gather a consensus around specific statements. As a rule, Class I recommendations are made when there is clear evidence that the benefit greatly outweighs the risk and thus, the procedure/treatment should be performed. Class IIa reflects a recommendation where the evidence is not as strong but it is viewed that treatments/procedures are reasonable. Class IIb recommendations are made when there is equivocal data available and the benefit to risk ration is less certain. Class III reflects those treatments/procedures where the risks outweigh the benefits and these therapies should not be provided.

This chapter summarizes many of the recommendations contained within the guideline document. Most of the basis for specific recommendations is covered in many of the other chapters in this book and therefore not duplicated here. In preparation for the interventional cardiology boards, one should always keep these guideline recommendations in mind when reviewing case descriptions, as several questions on the exam will ask for a specific treatment and the correct answer will always be the one most supported by the guidelines. Specific answers will generally reflect those recommendations that are either Class I or III, and therefore will be the focus of this chapter.

Procedural Success

Outcomes from percutaneous coronary interventions (PCI) can be divided into multiple categories: Angiographic success, procedural success, and clinical success. Clinical success remains the standard to which we are all held, but all three are measurable quantities. The definition of angiographic success in the era of intracoronary stents includes a minimum angiographic stenosis diameter reduction to <20%. A successful PCI from a procedural success standpoint involves the achievement of angiographic success without major complications (death, myocardial infarction and/or emergency coronary artery bypass surgery). Clinical success includes all criteria needed for the achievement of procedural success in addition to the relief or sings of symptoms for which the patient presented to the cardiac catheterization lab.

Complications

Percutaneous coronary interventions are not free of complications; however, the absolute rate remains very well. Complications are categorized as major or minor. Major complications include occurrence of death, myocardial infarction, or stroke. Minor complications include occurrence of transient ischemic attack, access site complications, renal insufficiency, or reactions to radiographic contrast. The rate of these complications is listed in Table 29–1.

With respect to guidelines associated with acute procedural complications, there are two:

1. Class I: All patients who have signs or symptoms of myocardial infarction during or after percutaneous coronary intervention and those with complicated procedures should all have a CK-MB and troponin measured after the procedure (Level of Evidence B).
2. Class IIa: Routine measurement of cardiac biomarkers including CK-MB and/or troponin in all patients undergoing percutaneous coronary intervention 8 to 12 hours after the procedure (Level of Evidence C).

These recommendations specifically address the complication of peri-procedure myocardial infarction. There has been a great deal of controversy surrounding the exact level of elevation of cardiac biomarkers that reflect an important level of myocardial necrosis. General consensus has settled on either a 3 times upper limit of normal or 5 times upper limit of normal elevation in troponin or CK-MB isomer.

Table 29–1
Complication Rates and PTCA

Series	Death	MI	Vascular	CVA	Total
Noto[a]	0.32%	0.61%	3.4%	0.05%	5.6%
Chandrasekar[b]	1.1%	3.4%	4%	0.10%	15.1%

[a]Noto TJ, Johnson LW, Krone RJ, et al. *Cardiac Catherization.* 1990: A report of the registry of the society for cardiac angiography and interventions (SCAI). *Cathet Cardiovasc Diag.* 1991;24:75–83.
[b]Chandrasekar B, Doucet S, Bilodeau L, et al. Complications of cardiac catherization in the current era: A single-center experience. *Cathet Cardiovasc Intervent.* 2001;52:289–295.

Predictors of Complications

The best complication remains the one that was prevented. In this light, many studies have addressed the ability to predict complications based on individual patient characteristics. Lesion morphology has been shown in multiple studies to predict complications of percutaneous coronary interventions and the currently accepted lesion classification system is listed in Table 29–2. Clinical factors have also been correlated to an increased risk of procedural complications and poor outcomes from PCI. These factors include advanced age, female gender, a procedure performed in the patient with unstable angina and/or acute coronary syndrome, congestive heart failure, diabetes, and patients with multivessel coronary artery disease.

With respect to specific lesions known to carry a higher risk of procedural complications the guideline committee specifi-

Table 29–2
Lesion Classification

SCAI Lesion Classification System

Type I Lesions (highest success expected with lowest risk)
  Does not meet criteria for C lesion
  Patent artery

Type II Lesions
  Meets any criteria for ACC/AHA C lesion: Diffuse (>2 cm in length), excessive tortuosity of the proximal segment, extremely angulated segments (>90 degrees), inability to protect major side branches, degenerated vein grafts with friable lesions
  Patent artery

Type III Lesions
  Does not meet criteria for C lesion
  Occluded vessel

Type IV Lesions (Highest risk, lowest success)
  Meets any criteria for ACC/AHA C lesion
  Occluded vessel

Krone RJ, Shaw RE, Klein LW, et al. Evaluation of the ACC/AHA/SCAI lesion classification system in the current "stent era" of coronary interventions (From the ACC-National Cardiovascular Data Registry). *Am J Cardiol.* 2003;92:394.

Table 29–3
Procedural Success and Complication Rates for PCI in Patients with Previous CABG

Conduit/Site	Success Rate	Mortality	MI
Saphenous Vein Graft	>92%	<2%	15%
Internal Mammary Artery	97%	<1%	12.5%
Left Main	95%	<2%	10%

cally addressed a patient with left main coronary artery disease. It was very clearly stated that coronary artery bypass surgery continues to be the gold standard for revascularization in patients who had unprotected left main coronary artery lesion. Currently, many small studies were evaluated by the committee that have proven the feasibility of performing unprotected left main coronary stenting with bare metal stents and/or drug-eluting stents and have also demonstrated reasonable short-term procedural outcomes. However, because of the overall number of the patients study to this point remains small, percutaneous coronary intervention for the patient with an unprotected left main should be restricted for patients who are not suitable candidates for coronary artery bypass grafting surgery.

Patients presenting to the catheterization laboratory after having already undergone a previous coronary artery bypass operation have always been thought to represent a patient at higher risk for complications when undergoing PCI. However, recent data have shown that the success and complication rate in most of these patients is equivalent to those having not undergone previous bypass grafting (Table 29–3). Specific considerations involving PCI in vein grafts will be discussed later.

Institutional and Operator Competency

A contentious issue remains the minimal procedure volume needed to be performed on a yearly basis to maintain a minimum skill level. Studies supporting these recommendations have shown a clear association with higher operator volume, as well as institutional volume, correlating with improved procedure success and reduced complications. The recommendations are as follows:

Class I

1. Elective PCI should be performed by operators with acceptable annual volume (at least 75 procedures) at high-volume centers (more than 400 procedures) with onsite cardiac surgery.
2. Primary PCI for STEMI should be performed by experienced operators who perform more than 75 elective PCI procedures per year and, ideally, at least 11 PCI procedures for STEMI per year. Ideally, these procedures should be

> ## Table 29–4
>
> ## Patient Selection for Primary PCI at Hospitals Without On-Site Cardiac Surgery
>
> **Avoid Intervention in Hemodynamically Stable Patients with:**
> - Significant ($\geq$60%) stenosis of an unprotected left main coronary artery
> - Extremely long or angulated infarct-related lesions with TIMI grade 3 flow
> - Infarct-related lesions with TIMI grade 3 flow in stable patients with three vessel disease
> - Infarct-related lesion of small or secondary vessels
> - Hemodynamically significant lesions in other than the infarct artery
>
> **Transfer for Emergency CABG with:**
> - High-grade residual left main or multivessel disease and clinical or hemodynamically instability after primary PCI of occluded vessels, preferably with IABP support

performed in institutions that perform more than 400 elective PCIs per year and more than 36 primary PCI procedures for STEMI per year.

Class III

It is not recommended that elective PCI be performed by low-volume operators (fewer than 75 procedures per year) at low-volume centers (200 to 400) with or without onsite cardiac surgery.

This update of the PCI guidelines incorporated the recommendations that were made in the ACC/AHA guidelines for unstable angina/NSTEMI as well as those for STEMI. Primary PCI for STEMI patients, thus, was recognized as a unique procedure requiring a skill set that could not be achieved by performing PCI only on elective cases.

Role of Onsite Cardiac Surgical Backup

Despite many small studies suggesting that need for emergent coronary artery bypass grafting operations is markedly low, the guideline group continued to recommend as a class I guideline that all elective PCIs should be performed by operators with acceptable annual volumes at centers that provide immediately available onsite cardiac surgical services. PCI for the patients with ST segment elevation MI should be performed at sites with onsite surgical back up as well. As a class III recommendation, elective PCI should not be performed in institutions without the ability to perform onsite cardiac surgery. Addressing the performance of primary PCI for STEMI, the following was recommended:

Class IIb

Primary PCI for patients with STEMI might be considered in hospitals without onsite cardiac surgery, provided that appropriate planning for program development has been accomplished, including appropriately experienced operators, an experienced catheterization team on a 24 hours per day, 7

days per week call schedule, and a well-equipped catheterization lab. The procedure should be limited to patients with STEMI or MI with new or presumably new left bundle-branch block on ECG and should be performed in a timely fashion (foal of balloon inflation within 90 minutes of presentation).

Several specific considerations were also addressed with respect to patient selection in labs without on-site cardiac surgery and these are shown in Table 29–4.

Indications of PCI Given the Patient Presentation

Patients present to the cardiac catheterization lab with a wide array of clinical presentations ranging from stable angina to unstable angina with hemodynamic instability. The guideline committee recommended separate recommendations for each one of these clinical presentations as follows:

1. Patients with Asymptomatic Ischemia or CCS Class I or II Angina
   Class III: PCI is not recommended who have one or more of the following:

   - Only a small area of viable myocardium
   - No objective evidence of ischemia
   - Lesions that have a low likelihood of success
   - Mild symptoms that are unlikely to be due to ischemia
   - Factors associated with increased morbidity/mortality
   - Left main disease and eligibility for CABG
   - Insignificant disease

2. Patients with CCS Class III Angina
   Class III: PCI not recommended for patients with single or multivessel disease who have no evidence for ischemia or myocardial injury, no trial of medical therapy, or who have any one of the following:

   - Only a small area of myocardium at risk
   - Lesions with a low likelihood of success
   - A high risk or procedural complications
   - Insignificant disease (<50% stenosis)
   - Significant left main disease and CABG eligibility

3. Patients with UA/NSTEMI

Class I: An early invasive PCI strategy in patients without serious comorbidities and lesions amenable to PCI and any of the following high-risk features:

- Recurrent ischemia despite intensive medical therapy
- Elevated troponin level
- New ST-segment depression
- Symptoms of CHF, new or worsening MR
- Depressed ejection fraction
- Hemodynamic instability
- PCI within previous 6 months
- Prior CABG

Class III: In the absence of high-risk features and any one of the following:

- Only a small area of myocardium at risk
- Low likelihood of success
- High risk of procedure related morbidity/mortality
- Insignificant disease (<50% stenosis)

Recommendations for Patients Presenting with ST Segment Elevation Myocardial Infarction

A class I recommendation for the performance of primary PCI in patients presenting with criteria meeting the definition of ST segment elevation myocardial infarction whose symptoms have been present for less than 12 hours if it can be performed in a timely fashion (balloon inflation within 90 minutes of presentation to a medical facility). Furthermore PCI should be performed in patients <75-years-old presenting with ST elevation myocardial infarction or a left bundle branch block developing shock within 36 hours of their symptoms of myocardial infarction, if it can be performed within 18 hours of the onset of shock. It is a class IIA recommendation to perform primary PCI in patients 75 years or older with STEMI or left bundle branch block, who develop shock within 36 hours of the myocardial infarction and can be revascularized within 18 hours of the onset of shock. Further more it is reasonable to perform primary angioplasty in patients with the onset of symptoms 12 to 24 hours induration if one or more of the following exists:

a. Severe congestive heart failure.
b. Hemodynamic or electrical instability.
c. Evidence of persistent ischemia.

There are two class III recommendations:

1. Elective percutaneous coronary intervention should not be performed in a non-infarct related artery at the time of primary percutaneous coronary intervention without evidence of hemodynamic compromise.
2. Primary percutaneous coronary intervention should not be performed in asymptomatic patients more than 12 hours after the onset of symptoms who are hemodynamically and electrically stable.

Facilitated PCI, that is a strategy incorporating pretreatment with a pharmacologic strategy followed immediately by PCI, has many unrealized potential advantages. Mainly, the hope is that the 90 minute reperfusion window will be able to be prolonged with similarly good outcomes. However, small preliminary studies have not demonstrated its ability to achieve these results and it is recommended as a Class IIb strategy.

PCI following failed fibrinolysis (rescue PCI) should be performed in all patients <75 years of age who develop cardiogenic shock within 36 hours of their index myocardial infarction. Furthermore, rescue PCI should be performed in all patients with Killip Class 3 failure within 12 hours. It is a Class IIa recommendation to perform rescue PCI for those patients failing a lytic as initial reperfusion and with persistent ischemia, hemodynamic, or electrical instability.

PCI in Patients with Prior Coronary Bypass Surgery

Recurrent ischemia after coronary bypass surgery within 30 days of the procedure often indicates a technical failure from the operation and/or incomplete revascularization achieved during the operation. Ischemia occurring more than one year postoperatively usually reflects development of new stenosis in graft conduits and/or native vessels that which may have not been previously grafted. It is clearly stated that use of glycoprotein IIB/IIIA blockers have not been shown to improve results of PCI. However, the use of distal protection devices has been recommended (see the subsequent text). As a general rule, the guidelines advise treatment of the native vessel, when feasible, instead of a failing graft conduit.

Class I

1. When technically feasible, PCI should be performed in patients with early ischemia (within 30 days) after CABG.
2. It is recommended that distal embolic protection devices be used when technically feasible in patients undergoing PCI to saphenous vein grafts.

Class III

1. PCI is not recommended in patients with prior CABG for chronic total vein graft occlusions.
2. PCI is not recommended in patients with multivessel disease, failure of multiple grafts, and impaired LV function unless repeat CABG caries excessive risk

Use of Adjunctive Technology (Intracoronary Ultrasound Imaging, Full Velocity, and Pressure)

Many operators performing enough coronary angiographic procedures have been well initiated into the limitations of the coronary angiogram in elucidating the true pathology, which may or may not be seen. Multiple modalities are now available to assist the operator and interpreting the angiogram and/or guiding the operator to treat the patients despite the lack of severe angiographic findings.

One of these modalities includes a use of intravascular ultrasound. The recommendations for use are all Class IIa and generally reflect two categories: when the operator deems that angiography is suboptimal or the result of the angioplasty and/or a coronary stent cannot be fully assessed. It is a Class III recommendation to perform IVUS when the angiographic diagnosis is clear cut and no interventional treatment is planned.

Utilizing a coronary flow or pressure is another currently accepted modality to assist the operator in understanding the physiologic significance of a coronary artery lesion. Again, its use is a Class IIa recommendation to assess intermediate stenosis (30% to 70% angiographic luminal narrowing) in patients with anginal symptoms. It also is a class IIB recommendation to utilize intracoronary physiologic measurements in patients with anginal symptoms without apparent angiographic coronary artery lesions. Routine use of intracoronary physiologic measurements in patients with an unequivocal noninvasive study demonstrating ischemia is not recommended.

Adjunctive Medical Therapy/Oral Anti-Platelet Therapy

Aspirin has long been utilized to assist the operator in inhibiting platelet activation during the performance of percutaneous coronary intervention and more recently agent such as ticlopidine and clopidogrel have also been utilized. There are multiple recommendations concerning the uses of these medications in these patients and these are important and although important to understand. They must be interpreted in context of a highly changing world with new studies suggesting the advantages and disadvantages of specific medications or combination of medications any more frequent rates and guidelines can be produced and/or changed. Table 29–5 summarizes the Class I guidelines for the use of oral anti-platelet therapy.

Glycoprotein IIB/IIIA Inhibitors

The use of glycoprotein IIB/IIIA inhibitor has been well studied within the past 10 years and the writing committee recommended:

Class I

All patients presenting with unstable angina or non-ST elevation myocardial infarction undergoing angioplasty without clopidogrel administration, should receive a glycoprotein IIB/IIIA inhibitor.

Class IIA

1. In patients with unstable angina/non-ST elevation myocardial infarction undergoing PCI with clopidogrel administration. It is reasonable to administer IIB/IIIA inhibitor.
2. In patients with ST elevation myocardial infarction undergoing PCI is reasonable to administer abciximab as early as possible.
3. In patients undergoing elective percutaneous coronary intervention with stent placement, it is reasonable to administer a glycoprotein IIB/IIIA inhibitor.

Antithrombotic Therapy

There has been a long experience with the use of unfractionated heparin within the cardiac catheterization lab; however, other agents such as low molecular weight heparin and bivalirudin have also gained prominence. As a Class I recommendation unfractionated heparin should be administered to all patients undergoing percutaneous coronary intervention and those patients who have had a history of heparin-induced thrombocytopenia should be treated bivalirudin or argatroban instead of heparin. As a Class IIA recommendation is reasonable to use bivalirudin as an alternative to unfractionated heparin in combination with glycoprotein IIB/IIIA inhibitors in patients who are deemed *low* risk for elective percutaneous coronary

---

Table 29–5

Oral Antiplatelet Therapy

Class I

Patients already taking daily chronic aspirin should take 75 to 325 mg of aspirin prior to PCI

Patients not already taking daily aspirin should be give 300 to 325 mg of aspirin prior to PCI

After PCI, 325 mg of aspirin per day should be given for at least 1 month (bare metal stents), 3 months (sirolimus-eluting stents), or 6 months (paclitaxel-eluting stents) unless the patient is allergic or at high bleeding risk. After this, aspirin should be continued indefinitely at a dose of 75 to 162 mg per day.

A loading dose of clopidogrel (300 mg) should be given at least 6 hours prior to PCI

After PCI, clopidogrel 75 mg per day should be given for at least 1 month (bare metal stents), 3 months (sirolimus-eluting stents), or 6 months (paclitaxel-eluting stents), and ideally for 12 months in patients who are not at high-risk of bleeding

intervention. Second, the use of low molecular weight heparin is a reasonable alternative to unfractionated heparin in patients with unstable angina and non-ST elevation myocardial infarction undergoing angioplasty. There is one class IIB recommendation: low molecular weight heparin may be considered alternative to unfractionated heparin in patients undergoing angioplasty with ST-segment elevation myocardial infarction.

As with the recommendations of four antiplatelet drugs, these recommendations should be considered to reflect the information that was available at the time of writing and it is understood that new information will be forthcoming which may change the overall recommendations.

Postangioplasty Management

The guidelines stressed that operator should pay careful attention to patients following preforms of percutaneous coronary intervention which involve monitoring patients for recurrent ischemia assuring adequate hemostasis and proper care of access site, detecting and preventing possible contrast induced renal failure, and assuring lack of complications from a percutaneously placed vascular closure devices.

Following this immediate post procedural care attention to assuring the implementation of secondary preventive measures to reduce the risk from coronary arthrosclerosis. As many as 50% of patients develop chest pain after PCI. Prior to the advent of drug-eluting stents, the major cause of recurrent chest pain in patients was the development of restenosis. More importantly approximately one quarter of the patients with restenosis remained asymptomatic and thereby raising the question of whether exercise testing should be routinely performed following this procedure. The writing committee favored a selective approach to evaluate patients after angioplasty including those patients at highest risk (those with decreased LV systolic function, multivessel coronary disease, proximal LAD disease, previous sudden death diabetes, left main disease, and suboptimal PCI results). Furthermore an exercise ECG in isolation was recommended as a test that was an insensitive predictor of restenosis, and therefore stress testing with adjunctive imaging was recommended in the evaluation of symptomatic patients after angioplasty. The guideline committee specifically stated that neither exercise testing nor radionucleotide imaging is indicated for *routine* periodic monitoring of asymptomatic patients after percutaneous coronary intervention without the above stated indications.

Summary

This chapter has focused on the major recommendations from the 2005 update of the guidelines for performance of percutaneous coronary interventions. It is strongly suggested that the interventional cardiologist become very familiar with these guidelines prior to taking the interventional cardiology board examination. Questions will be asked that describe a patient care scenario involving a specific recommendation and the examinee will need to identify when the performance of a procedure is appropriate (i.e., supported by a Class I recommendation). Coupled with a complete understanding of the material in the other chapters in this book, these guidelines represent the foundation for answering the majority of board examination questions properly.

REFERENCES

1. ACC/AHA/SCAI 2005 Guideline update for percutaneous coronary intervention. *J Am Coll Cardiol.* 2006;47:216–235.

Index